Human Fungal Pathogens

Human Fungal Pathogens

Editor: Perry Jacobs

AMERICAN
MEDICAL PUBLISHERS
www.americanmedicalpublishers.com

Cataloging-in-Publication Data

Human fungal pathogens / edited by Perry Jacobs.
p. cm.
Includes bibliographical references and index.
ISBN 979-8-88740-188-1
1. Mycoses. 2. Mycoses--Pathogenesis. 3. Mycoses--Treatment.
4. Pathogenic fungi. 5. Medical mycology. I. Jacobs, Perry.
RC117 .H86 2023
616.969--dc23

American Medical Publishers,
41 Flatbush Avenue,
1st Floor, New York,
NY 11217, USA

ISBN 979-8-88740-188-1 (Hardback)

Contents

Preface

Fungi are the main elements in global biogeochemical cycles. They play a significant role in biomedical research and manufacturing industries, and impact humans through their influence on biodiversity, global health and agriculture. Pathogenic fungi cause disease in human beings or other organisms. Majority of the fungi do not have pathogenic traits, but certain species result in infections which range from posturing to life threating. The fungi that are pathogenic to humans, are studied within the discipline of medical mycology. Several pathogenic fungi are microorganisms despite the fact that they are eukaryotic. There are various types of pathogenic fungi including Cryptococcus, Stachybotrys, Candida, Histoplasma, Aspergillus and Pneumocystis. Cryptococcus neoformans can result in a severe form of meningitis and meningo-encephalitis in AIDS infected patients. Stachybotrys can cause severe headaches and respiratory issues. Fungal infection usually occurs in the gastrointestinal tract, skin, genital-urinary tract and respiratory tract. This book provides comprehensive insights on human fungal pathogens. Its extensive content provides the readers with a thorough understanding of the subject. This book will prove to be immensely beneficial to students and researchers in this field.

The information contained in this book is the result of intensive hard work done by researchers in this field. All due efforts have been made to make this book serve as a complete guiding source for students and researchers. The topics in this book have been comprehensively explained to help readers understand the growing trends in the field.

I would like to thank the entire group of writers who made sincere efforts in this book and my family who supported me in my efforts of working on this book. I take this opportunity to thank all those who have been a guiding force throughout my life.

Editor

1

The Major Chromoblastomycosis Etiologic Agent *Fonsecaea pedrosoi* Activates the NLRP3 Inflammasome

Raffael Júnio Araújo de Castro[1], Isaque Medeiros Siqueira[1], Márcio Sousa Jerônimo[1], Angelina Maria Moreschi Basso[1], Paulo Henrique de Holanda Veloso Junior[1], Kelly Grace Magalhães[2], Luiza Chaves Leonhardt[1], Stephan Alberto Machado de Oliveira[1], Pedro Henrique Bürgel[1], Aldo Henrique Tavares[1†] and Anamélia Lorenzetti Bocca[1†]*

[1] Laboratory of Applied Immunology, Department of Cellular Biology, Institute of Biological Sciences, University of Brasília, Brasília, Brazil, [2] Laboratory of Immunology and Inflammation, Department of Cellular Biology, Institute of Biological Sciences, University of Brasília, Brasília, Brazil

***Correspondence:**
Anamélia Lorenzetti Bocca
albocca@unb.br

[†]These authors have contributed equally and share senior authorship.

Fonsecaea pedrosoi is the main etiologic agent of chromoblastomycosis (CBM), one of the most prevalent subcutaneous mycosis in tropical and subtropical countries. CBM is a poorly characterized chronic infection that commonly starts after transcutaneous inoculation of conidia and saprophytic hyphae of *F. pedrosoi*. Recently, we have shown that unlike conidia, hyphae and muriform cells (the parasitic morphotype) of *F. pedrosoi* promotes an intense inflammatory response pattern *in vivo*, which comprises the production of an inflammasome-derived cytokine, IL-1β. Nonetheless, the mechanisms underlying IL-1β production and maturation upon *F. pedrosoi* infection and its functional output in the course of CBM remains unknown. We show here that *F. pedrosoi* hyphae, differently from conidia, induce IL-1β secretion in both bone marrow-derived dendritic cells and macrophages. Using inhibitors and knockout cells, we demonstrated that the mechanisms underlying IL-1β production by hyphae-infected macrophages were dependent on dectin-1, -2, and -3 receptors and the Syk-NF-kB signaling pathway. Furthermore, *F. pedrosoi* promoted a NLRP3-dependent inflammasome activation, which required potassium efflux, reactive oxygen species production, phagolysosomal acidification, and cathepsin B release as triggers. IL-1β processing and release was mediated primarily by caspase-1 and, to a lesser extent, by caspase-8-dependent cleavage. Finally, we showed using a murine CBM model that *F. pedrosoi* elicits a NLRP3-regulated IL-1β and interleukin-18 release *in vivo*, but without NLRP3 inflammasome activation interfering in the course of the experimental infection.

Keywords: NLRP3 inflammasome, *Fonsecaea pedrosoi*, chromoblastomycosis, hyphae, macrophages, dendritic cells

INTRODUCTION

Chromoblastomycosis (CBM) is a chronic, granulomatous, suppurative, and often debilitating cutaneous and subcutaneous mycosis, caused by dimorphic filamentous fungi belonging to the *Dematiaceous* family (1–3). Multiple dematiaceous fungi are related to the disease etiology; of these, *Fonsecaea pedrosoi* and *Cladophialophora carrionii* are the most frequently identified fungal species in human CBM skin lesions. This disease occurs worldwide; however, it is mostly prevalent in tropical and subtropical areas (4, 5). Clinically, CBM is characterized by the slow development of polymorphic skin lesions, such as nodules, warts, tumors, plaques, and scars, after inoculation of fungal propagules consisting of conidia and hyphal fragments into host skin, more frequently into lower limbs (6–8). During infection of mammalian host, these primarily saprophyte fungal forms undergo transformation into the intensely melanized and thick-walled muriform (sclerotic) cells, the parasitic morphotype of *F. pedrosoi* (4).

Although little is known about the immune response of the host to infection by *F. pedrosoi*, it has been credited that an adaptive response mediated by T helper (Th) cell types 1 and 17 might be protective against *F. pedrosoi* infection (9–11). In this scenario, the abrogation of IL-12p35 transcription in human dendritic cells, leading to Th1-deficient development by several *Fonsecaea* species, and the Th17-mediated response suppression in experimentally infected mice, suggest that this fungal pathogen evade host immune response by complex mechanisms. These mechanisms usually encompass the evasion or subversion of the function of innate pattern recognition receptors (PRRs) in the detection of conserved fungal components or pathogen-associated molecular patterns (PAMPs) by phagocytes (10–12). A number of PRRs families have been associated with *F. pedrosoi* sensing, including the C-type lectin receptors (CLRs) mincle, dectin-1 and dectin-2, as well as toll-like receptors (TLRs). Besides these cytoplasmic membrane-bound receptors, fungal sensing by cytosolic PRRs, such as NOD-like receptors (NLRs) and AIM2-like receptors, is becoming increasingly apparent.

The members of the NLR protein family typically share three functional domains: a C-terminal leucine-rich-repeat putative ligand-binding domain, a central NACHT nucleotide-binding and oligomerization domain and an N-terminal signaling domain (13). The latter consists of different domains, most notably a pyrin domain (PYD) or a caspase recruitment domain (CARD). Certain NLRP (NLR subfamily with an N-terminal PYD), such as NLRP1 and NLRP3, and the NLR family CARD domain-containing protein 4 (NLRC4) associate with inflammatory caspase-1 (in the form of pro-caspase-1) to assemble the inflammasome, a large cytosolic multiprotein complex. Notably, NLRP3-containing inflammasome formation is dependent on the adaptor protein ASC (apoptosis-associated speck-like protein containing a CARD), which promotes the recruitment of pro-caspase-1 through CARD–CARD interactions (13). The assembly of the inflammasome complex leads to the cleavage of pro-caspase-1 into an active cysteine protease, which cleaves the proinflammatory cytokines interleukin-1β (IL-1β) and interleukin-18 (IL-18) into their mature forms. NLRP3 inflammasome, the most studied and the main inflammasome associated with fungal infection, is activated by a typical two-step mechanism: priming and activation (14, 15). The priming signal is generated by the recognition of PAMPs by PRRs, usually leading to NF-kB activation and, as a result, production of pro-IL-1β, pro-IL-18, and NLRP3. The activation step is associated with the assembly of the multiprotein complex induced by a broad variety of endogenous danger-associated molecules (DAMPs), such as potassium efflux, production of reactive oxygen species (ROS), phagolysosome acidification, and cathepsin B release. Several conditions may lead to DAMPs production, including metabolic disorders, inflammatory diseases, and infections.

The inflammasome-dependent release of IL-1β and IL-18 cytokines has a striking importance in the regulation of innate and adaptive response against many different fungal pathogens, including significant protective roles against *Candida albicans*, *Aspergillus fumigatus*, *Cryptococcus neoformans*, *Paracoccidioides brasiliensis*, and *Histoplasma capsulatum* (16–22). One aspect associated with inflammasome activation is fungal morphotype diversity and complexity. *C. albicans* hyphae are better inducers and the only fungal form of *A. fumigatus* that activates the NLRP3 inflammasome (16, 17, 23). Indeed, we have recently showed that unlike conidia, the hyphae and muriform (sclerotic) cells of *F. pedrosoi* promote intense production of proinflammatory cytokines *in vitro* and *in vivo* (24). Among these cytokines, we observed IL-1β production, suggesting that *F. pedrosoi* could activate the inflammasome. In this context, we aimed to evaluate the inflammasome activation by *F. pedrosoi* infective propagules and the role of the inflammasome in CBM experimental disease.

We show here that *F. pedrosoi* hyphae, differently from conidia, induce IL-1β secretion in both bone marrow-derived dendritic cells and macrophages. The mechanisms underlying IL-1β production by macrophage-infected hyphae were dependent on dectin-1, -2, and -3 receptors and the Syk-NF-kB signaling pathway. *F. pedrosoi* promoted a NLRP3-dependent inflammasome activation, which required K^+ efflux, ROS production, phagolysosomal acidification, and cathepsin B release. IL-1β processing and release were mediated by caspase-1 and, to a lesser extent, caspase-8-dependent cleavage. Furthermore, we demonstrated using an experimental CBM model that *F. pedrosoi* elicits a NLRP3-regulated IL-1β and IL-18 release *in vivo*. However, we did not observe an influence of the NLRP3 inflammasome on the control of the fungal infection.

MATERIALS AND METHODS

Fungal Culture and Preparation

Fonsecaea pedrosoi ATCC 46428 were maintained in Sabouraud dextrose agar medium (SDA) at 37°C after serial animal passages to enhance fungal virulence. In order to obtain purified conidia and hyphae for experiments, virulent *F. pedrosoi* propagules were grown in potato dextrose medium in a rotary shaker (120 rpm) at 30°C. A 15-day-old suspension containing conidia and hyphal fragments was submitted to successive filtrations on 70 and 40 μm cell strainers (BD), respectively. The 40 μm filter-retained cells (ranging between 40 and 70 μm) were re-suspended in phosphate-buffered saline (PBS) and consisted of more than 98% of purified hyphae. The suspension of cells smaller than 40 μm was further filtered using a 14 μm filter paper (J. Prolab) to remove small hyphal fragments and achieve a minimum of 98% purified conidia. A mix of purified hyphae and conidia at a 3:1 rate was used as *F. pedrosoi* fungal propagules for *in vivo* assays. For assays with inactivated fungi, conidia, and hyphae were heat-killed by boiling for 40 min, or fixed with 3% paraformaldehyde (PFA) for 6 h. *F. pedrosoi* cells were washed twice, counted using a hemocytometer, and used for experiments.

Cell Culture

Bone marrow-derived macrophages (BMDMs) and dendritic cells (BMDCs) were generated by a previously described method (25). Briefly, bone marrow cells were flushed out of murine femurs and tibias and submitted to erythrocyte lysis using tris-buffered ammonium chloride. Cells (2×10^6) were plated onto non-tissue culture-treated Petri dishes in 10 mL of RPMI-1640 medium (Sigma-Aldrich) supplemented with 10% heat-inactivated FBS (Gibco), 50 μM 2-mercaptoethanol, 50 μg/mL of gentamicin, and 20 ng/mL GM-CSF (Peprotech), and cultured for 8 days in a humidified 5% CO_2 atmosphere at 37°C. On day 3, another 10 mL of fresh complete medium was added to the culture. On day 6, half of the medium was exchanged. On day 8, loosely adherent/suspended BMDCs and firmly adherent BMDMs stripped with TrypLE™ Express (Gibco) were separately collected and plated at a density of 10^6 cells/mL in RPMI medium containing 10% FBS and 50 μg/mL of gentamicin, for experimental use. THP-1 cells were maintained and used under the same experimental use conditions.

In Vitro F. pedrosoi Challenge and Cell Treatments

Bone marrow-derived macrophages derived from wild-type (WT) or knockout mice were infected with *F. pedrosoi* for 6 (RT-qPCR analysis) and 24 h (other assays) at a multiplicity of infection (MOI) of 3 for conidial infection (except for fungicidal assays, performed with a MOI of 1) and of 1 for hyphal. For inhibition assays, BMDMs received 2 h prior to the infection a Myd88 inhibitor peptide (50 μM) (InvivoGen), Syk inhibitor R406 (5 μM) (InvivoGen), NF-kB inhibitor celastrol (5 μM) (InvivoGen), caspase-1 inhibitor AC-YVAD-CHO (50 μM) (Santa Cruz Biotechnology), caspase-8 inhibitor Z-IETD-FMK (50 μM) (Santa Cruz Biotechnology), intracellular potassium efflux inhibitors glyburide (150 μM) (InvivoGen) and KCl (50 mM) (Sigma-Aldrich), ROS inhibitor DPI (diphenyleneiodonium chloride) (20 μM) (Sigma-Aldrich), endosomal acidification inhibitor bafilomycin A (250 nM) (InvivoGen) or cathepsin B inhibitor CA-074 Me (50 μM) (Sigma-Aldrich). In some experiments, BMDMs and BMDCs were treated 2 h previously to the fungal infection with 500 ng/mL of LPS (Sigma-Aldrich) and/or 20 μM of nigericin (InvivoGen) during the last 40 min of incubation (1 h for fungicidal assays). Cells stimulated with both LPS and nigericin served as a positive control for NLRP3-mediated inflammasome activation.

Analysis of Fungal Cell Morphology by Flow Cytometry

In order to induce and evaluate conidial swelling, *F. pedrosoi* conidia (5×10^6 cells/mL) were incubated for 6 h with PBS or RPMI supplemented with 20% of heat-inactivated FBS at 37°C, under 120 rpm. In addition, conidia were incubated with BMDMs at a MOI of 3, for 6 and 24 h. Infected BMDMs were washed to discard nonphagocyted fungus and lysed with 0.05% SDS to release intracellular fungi. Then, fungal were fixed with PFA treatment, washed twice, and evaluated by flow cytometry analysis. Micron-size beads of 2 and 3 μm (CS&T Research Beads, BD) were used as control. Cell acquisition was performed using a FACSVerse (BD) flow cytometry, and data were analyzed with FlowJo v.10 software.

In Vitro Fungicidal Assay

Bone marrow-derived macrophages derived from WT, *Nlrp3*$^{-/-}$, and *Caspase-1/11*$^{-/-}$ mice were infected for 24 h with *F. pedrosoi* conidia or hyphae. In addition, WT macrophages were also treated, or not, with nigericin as described above, or stimulated 3 h before the infection with LPS and IFN-γ (both from Sigma-Aldrich) (500 and 20 ng/mL, respectively) to activate the mechanisms of macrophage killing [e.g., nitric oxide (NO) production]. After infection, the cell culture supernatant was harvested for NO determination. The remaining cell monolayers were carefully washed to remove non-adherent cells, lysed as described above, and re-suspended in PBS. After serial dilutions, cell suspension was plated on SDA and incubated at 30°C for 5–7 days for colony-forming unit (CFU) evaluation.

Detection of Activated Caspase-1 by Fluorochrome-Labeled Inhibitor of Caspases (FLICA)

After 24 h of infection with *F. pedrosoi* conidia or hyphae, BMDMs were detached (as mentioned above) and incubated for 1 h with a caspase-1 fluorochrome-labeled inhibitor of caspases (FLICA), FAM-YVAD-FMK (Immunochemistry Technologies), according to the manufacturer's instructions. Next, cells were washed and stained with APC-conjugated anti-CD11b antibody (eBioscience) in PBS with 2% heat-inactivated FBS (Gibco) to distinguish macrophages from non-internalized fungus. Then, cells were washed and samples were analyzed by flow cytometry as described above.

Quantitative Real-time PCR (qRT-PCR)

Total RNA from BMDMs was extracted using the TRIzol reagent (Invitrogen) and cDNA was synthesized using the high capacity RNA-to-cDNA kit (Applied Biosystems), according to manufacturer's protocols. qRT-PCR was performed using SYBR green incorporation (Applied Biosystems) and real-time PCR equipment (StepOne system) (Applied Biosystems). Expression of the genes of interest was normalized to the expression of the housekeeping gene *Rps9* and expressed as "Fold change," which was calculated by the $2^{-\Delta\Delta CT}$ method (26). The primers used were validated according Livak and Schmittgen (26) and listed in Table S1 in Supplementary Material.

Animals and *In Vivo F. pedrosoi* Infection

Clec7a$^{-/-}$ (*Dectin-1*$^{-/-}$) mice were supplied by Dr. Gordon Brown (University of Aberdeen, Scotland). *Clec4n*$^{-/-}$ (*Dectin-2*$^{-/-}$), *Clec4d*$^{+/+}$ (*Dectin-3*$^{+/+}$), *Clec4d*$^{-/-}$ (*Dectin-3*$^{-/-}$) mice were kindly provided by Dr. Bruce Klein (University of Wisconsin-Madison,

USA). All animals (C57BL/6 background), including *Nlrp3*$^{-/-}$, *Caspase-1/11*$^{-/-}$, and C57BL/6 WT mice, were maintained under pathogen-free conditions and used at 8 to 12 weeks old for experiments. For *in vivo* infection, WT, *Nlrp3*$^{-/-}$ and *Caspase-1/11*$^{-/-}$ mice were inoculated subcutaneously into the hind footpad with 50 μl (per foot) of a suspension containing 1×10^6 (2×10^7/mL) *F. pedrosoi* hyphae and conidia in the proportion of 3:1, respectively (fungal propagules). Mice were euthanized at 14, 21, and 28 days postinfection and the footpad was collected, weighed, and homogenized for ELISA assay and plated for CFU analysis.

Measurement of NO and Cytokine Production

Nitrite (NO_2^-) concentration in culture supernatants was applied as an indicator of NO generation and measured with the Griess reagent (1% sulfanilamide, 0.1% naphthylethylene diamine dihydrochloride, 2.5% H_3PO_4). For that, 50 μl of the culture supernatant was added to an equal volume (v/v) of Griess reagent and allowed to incubate at room temperature for 10 min. Absorbance was measured at 540 nm using a microplate reader. The NO_2^- concentration was determined using a standard curve of 1.56–100 μM of $NaNO_2$. Cytokine levels from the homogenized animal tissue and cell culture lysate and supernatants were determined by ELISA, according to the manufacturer's guidelines, for the following cytokines: human interleukin-1β (IL-1β) and murine IL-1β (both uncleaved and cleaved forms), IL-18 and tumor necrosis factor-α (TNF-α), all purchased from eBioscience. Results were expressed as cytokines pictogram per milliliters or per 100 mg of tissue, for samples obtained from *in vivo* assays.

Statistical Analysis

Statistical analysis was conducted using GraphPad Prism v.5.0 software. Data were analyzed by one-way ANOVA followed by Tukey's *post hoc* test. Two-way ANOVA and Bonferroni's *post hoc* test were used to compare different groups with more than one variable. *p*-Values of less than 0.05 were considered significant.

RESULTS

F. pedrosoi Hyphae, but Not Conidia, Induce IL-1β Secretion in BMDMs and THP-1 Cells

To determine whether *F. pedrosoi* could induce IL-1β secretion, we infected murine BMDMs with *F. pedrosoi* conidia or hyphae for 24 h. Hyphae cell infection resulted in IL-1β secretion, while conidia failed to induce significant levels of this cytokine (**Figure 1A**). In addition, THP-1, a human monocyte cell line, secreted IL-1β upon infection by *F. pedrosoi* hyphae, but not conidia (**Figure 1B**). To test if the size of conidia could affect the BMDM activation, we induced swollen-conidia (Figure S1 in Supplementary Material), an intermediate stage of conidia-into-hyphae transformation, and used it to stimulate BMDMs. Swollen conidia were equally unable to promote IL-1β secretion (**Figure 1A**).

Then, we evaluated if the lack of secreted IL-1β in BMDM-conidia coculture supernatant results primarily from the inability of BMDMs to trigger *Il1b* gene transcription after conidial infection. RT-qPCR analysis revealed that at 6 h of infection, hyphae and, to a lesser extent, conidia induce *Il1b* and *Tnfa*, but not *il18* transcripts in BMDMs (**Figure 1C**). ELISA assay performed with 24 h culture supernatant showed that, contrary to conidial, hyphal infection results in IL-18 and TNF-α secretion (**Figures 1D,E**), despite the observation that the *Il18* transcript is not upregulated. Further, we stimulated BMDMs with inactivated hyphae to determine whether the viability of this fungal form influences IL-1β secretion. Both PFA and heat-killed (HK) hyphae stimulus resulted in severe reduction of IL-1β in comparison to live fungus (**Figure 1F**), whereas the viability of the fungus did not significantly affect the levels of TNF-α production and only slighted affected the levels of pro-IL-1β only in the HK hyphae (**Figures 1G,H**). These finding suggest that that the viability of *F. pedrosoi* affects activation, but not priming of NLRP3 inflammasome.

Differential Inflammasome Activation Requirements in BMDMs and BMDCs Are Morphotype-Dependent in *F. pedrosoi* Infection

Since we previously showed that BMDCs differ from BMDMs regarding inflammasome activation requirements upon *P. brasiliensis* infection (27), we investigated whether this is also the case with *F. pedrosoi*. Differently from BMDM infection, conidia alone induced IL-1β secretion in BMDCs, suggesting that it acts as both the first and the second signal for inflammasome activation in this cell type (**Figures 2A,B**). When nigericin was added to BMDMs or BMDCs, these cells secreted a large amount of mature IL-1β, confirming that conidia elicit pro-IL-1β production (as indicated in **Figure 1C**), but fail to provide further inflammasome activating signals in BMDMs (**Figures 2A,B**). Regarding hyphae, this morphotype alone was able to induce IL-1β secretion not only in BMDMs (as shown in **Figure 1**) but also in BMDCs (**Figure 2B**).

The Syk-NF-kB Signaling Pathway, Coupled to Dectin-1, Dectin-2, and Dectin-3 Receptors, Enables Inflammasome Activation by BMDMs Challenged with *F. pedrosoi* Hyphae

Macrophages play central roles in host immune response against fungal infections (28). Likewise, these phagocytes are not only ubiquitous in CBM lesions but are also actively involved in the recognition of fungal cells and in the modulation of inflammatory responses against *F. pedrosoi* (4, 29, 30). In this context, we performed subsequent assays focused on macrophage-hyphae interaction, since we show here that hyphae are the *F. pedrosoi* infective morphotype most likely to be responsible for initiating the inflammatory response observed in CBM. In order to determine the mechanisms underlying BMDMs inflammasome priming in *F. pedrosoi* infection, we treated BMDMs with celastrol, an inhibitor of IKK activity, which results in the inactivation of NF-kB, the main transcriptional factor associated with pro-IL-1β

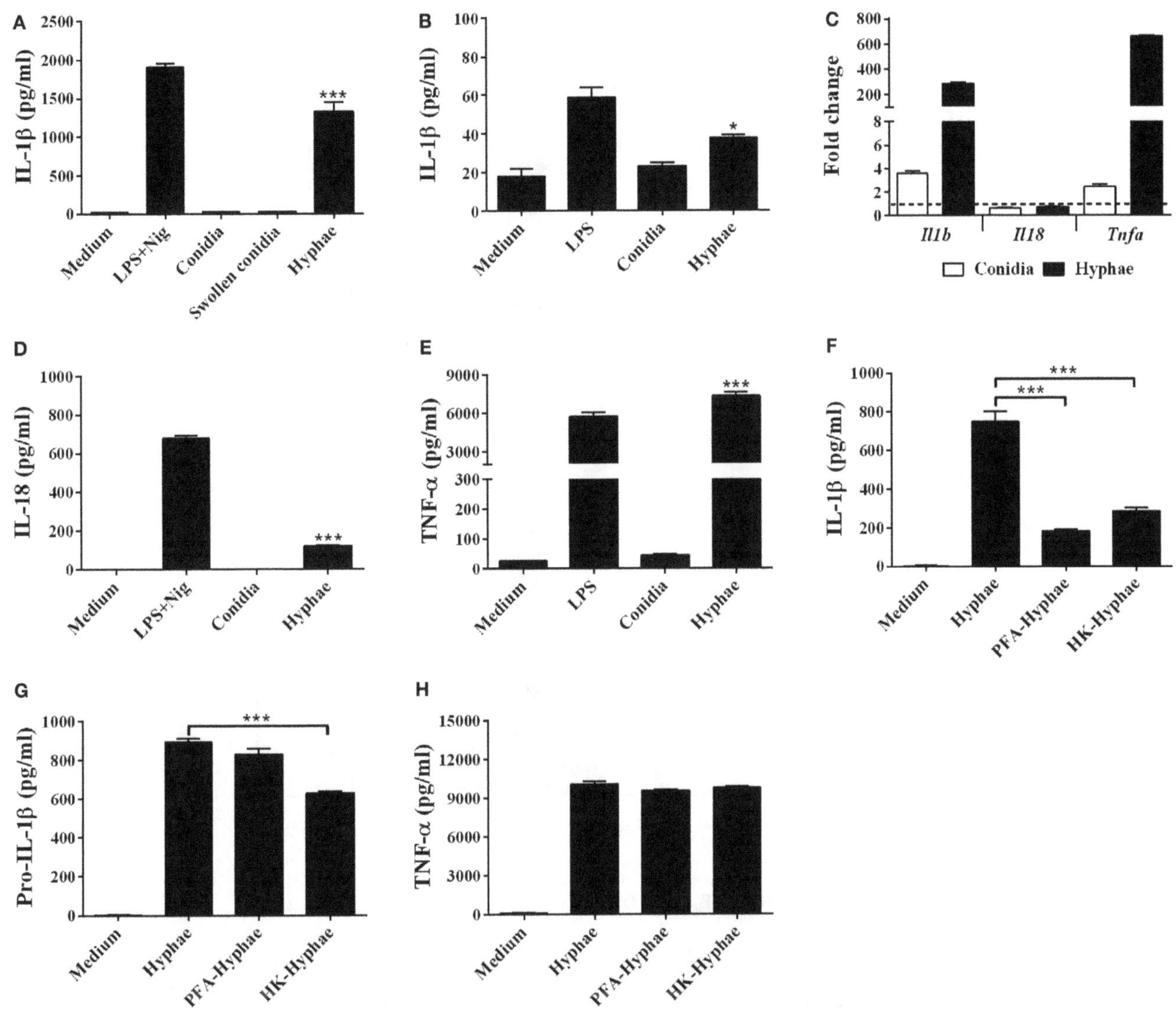

FIGURE 1 | *Fonsecaea pedrosoi* hyphae, but not conidia, induce IL-1β secretion in bone marrow-derived macrophages (BMDMs) and THP-1 cells. IL-1β levels after 24 h of BMDMs incubation with medium, *F. pedrosoi* conidia, swollen conidia, or hyphae **(A)**. IL-1β secretion after 24 h of THP-1 cell incubation with medium, *F. pedrosoi* conidia, or hyphae **(B)**. Intracellular *Il1b*, *Il18*, and *Tnfa* gene transcription of BMDMs after 6 h stimulation with hyphae or conidia were analyzed by RT-qPCR **(C)**. Interleukin-18 (IL-18) **(D)** and tumor necrosis factor-α (TNF-α) **(E)** secretion of BMDMs co-cultivated with medium, conidia, or hyphae. BMDMs were stimulated also with live, paraformaldehyde-killed, or heat-killed (HK) hyphae for IL-β **(F)**, pro-IL-β **(G)**, and TNF-α measurement **(H)**. Pro-IL-1β was evaluated in the cell lysate after 12 h of infection, while the others cytokines were assayed in the cell supernatant after 24 h. IL-1β, pro-IL-1β, IL-18, and TNF-α levels were evaluated by ELISA. Data shown are mean ± SEM and are representative of two to three independent experiments. *$p < 0.05$; ***$p < 0.001$, compared to cells with only medium or between groups indicated by brackets.

transcription. As expected, NF-kB inhibition led to a complete abolition of IL-1β, as well as a strong reduction of TNF-α secretion in cell supernatant (**Figures 3A,B**, respectively). Furthermore, it is known that NF-kB-activating PRRs license inflammasome activation by providing both pro-IL-1β and inflammasome receptors expression (31). To clarify the nature of the PRRs that are involved in the *F. pedrosoi* recognition that led to NF-kB-dependent BMDMs priming, we evaluated the transcription of *Myd88* and *Syk*, which are pivotal signal transducers of TLRs and CLRs, respectively. We observed that hyphae not only induced *Syk* and *Nfkb1* upregulation (**Figure 3C**), but also depend on Syk activity to induce IL-1β secretion, as shown in BMDMs treated with Syk inhibitor R406 (**Figure 3A**). *Myd88*, however, was poorly transcribed in BMDMs upon hyphal infection (**Figure 3C**), and its activity was indifferent to IL-1β secretion in cells treated with a Myd88 inhibitory peptide (**Figure 3A**).

It is known that CLRs, such as dectin-1, dectin-2, and dectin-3, signaling *via* Syk kinase promote NF-kB activation (32). To test whether these CLRs were responsible for recruiting Syk to signal inflammasome priming in BMDMs challenged with hyphae, we used cells from mice deficient in these receptors, and observed that *Dectin-1*$^{-/-}$, *Dectin-2*$^{-/-}$, and *Dectin-3*$^{-/-}$ BMDMs

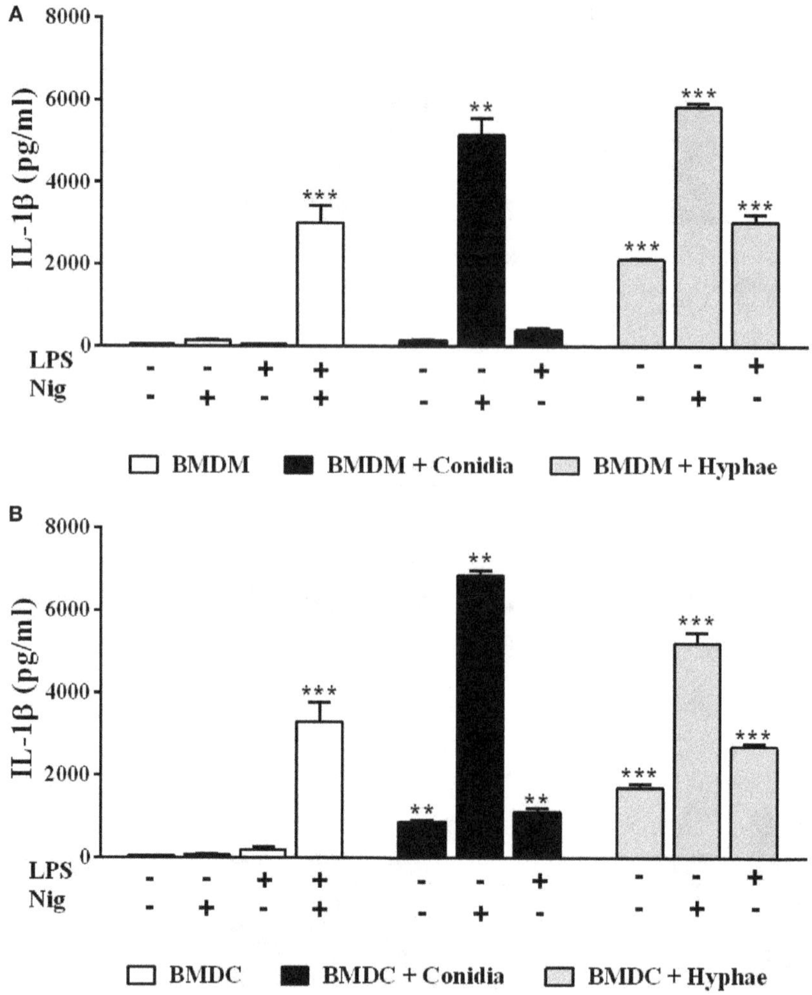

FIGURE 2 | Differential inflammasome activation requirements in bone marrow-derived macrophages (BMDMs) and dendritic cells (BMDCs) are morphotype-dependent in *Fonsecaea pedrosoi* infection. IL-1β detection by ELISA in supernatants of BMDMs **(A)** and BMDCs **(B)** incubated for 24 h with medium, *F. pedrosoi* conidia or hyphae, and co-stimulated (or not) with LPS (500 ng/mL added 2 h before fungal infection), nigericin (20 μM during the last 40 min of incubation), or both (as a positive control). Data shown are mean ± SEM and are representative of three independent experiments. $^{**}p < 0.01$; $^{***}p < 0.001$, compared to cells with only medium.

show reduced IL-1β secretion when compared to their respective controls (**Figure 3D**). Except for *Dectin-3*$^{-/-}$ cells, all tested knockout cells also exhibited a slight reduction in TNF-α levels (**Figure 3E**). Dectin-1 KO cells had the strongest depletion of IL-1β (**Figure 3D**), although WT BMDMs did not present differential regulation of *Dectin-1* transcription—only *Dectin-2* and *Dectin-3* genes were upregulated (**Figure 3F**). Further, since the inhibition of Syk signaling did not completely abrogate the IL-1B secretion (**Figure 3A**), we reasoned that an alternative Syk-independent dectin-1-NF-kB signaling pathway would be in use. To evaluate this hypothesis, we inhibited Raf-1 kinase signaling, an adaptor protein that dectin-1 engages to signal NF-kB activation independently of Syk (33); however, IL-1β levels were unaffected (data not shown). The results indicate that the Syk-NF-kB signaling pathway, coupled to dectin-1, dectin-2, and dectin-3 receptors, enables inflammasome activation by BMDMs challenged with *F. pedrosoi* hyphae.

Inflammasome Activation by *F. pedrosoi* Hyphae Is Dependent on Caspase-1 and Caspase-8

IL-1β secretion requires proteolytic cleavage of its inactive pro-form, canonically performed by caspase-1 enzyme. To assess whether *F. pedrosoi* infective morphotypes were able to activate caspase-1, we used a fluorescent probe, FAM-YVAD-FMK, which specifically binds the active protease, and analyzed stained BMDMs using flow cytometry. As expected, only hyphae, but not conidia, were able to induce caspase-1 activation (**Figure 4A**), which corroborates our ELISA data showing that only hyphae infection led to IL-1β processing and secretion in BMDMs (**Figure 2A**). Then, to confirm that IL-1β secretion was caspase-1 dependent, we challenged BMDMs from WT and *Caspase-1/11* knockout mice with hyphae. In addition, we also treated WT BMDMs with AC-YVAD-CHO, a specific caspase-1 inhibitor. Both *Caspase-1/11*$^{-/-}$ BMDMs and WT BMDMs treated with

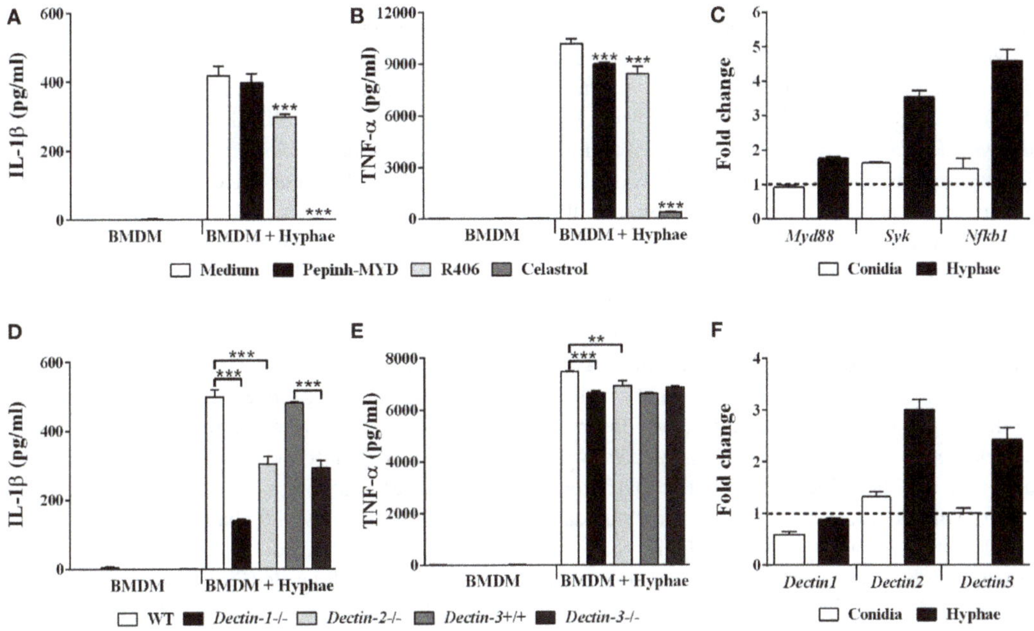

FIGURE 3 | The Syk-NF-kB signaling pathway, coupled to dectin-1, dectin-2, and dectin-3 receptors, enables inflammasome activation by bone marrow-derived macrophages (BMDMs) challenged with *Fonsecaea pedrosoi* hyphae. BMDMs were pretreated for 2 h with Myd88 inhibitor peptide (50 μM), R406 (5 μM), and celastrol (5 μM) and thereafter infected with *F. pedrosoi* hyphae for 24 h **(A,B)**. BMDMs were infected with conidia or hyphae for 6 h, and then were lysed for RT-qPCR analysis to quantify gene expression of indicated genes **(C,F)**. BMDMs obtained from wild-type (WT), *Dectin-1*$^{-/-}$, *Dectin-2*$^{-/-}$, *Dectin-3*$^{+/+}$, and *Dectin-3*$^{-/-}$ mice were infected with *F. pedrosoi* hyphae for 24 h **(D,E)**. The supernatant of 24 h cell culture assays were evaluated for IL-1β and TNF-α by ELISA. Data shown are mean ± SEM and are representative of two to three independent experiments. $^{**}p < 0.01$; $^{***}p < 0.001$, compared to infected untreated cells or between groups indicated by brackets.

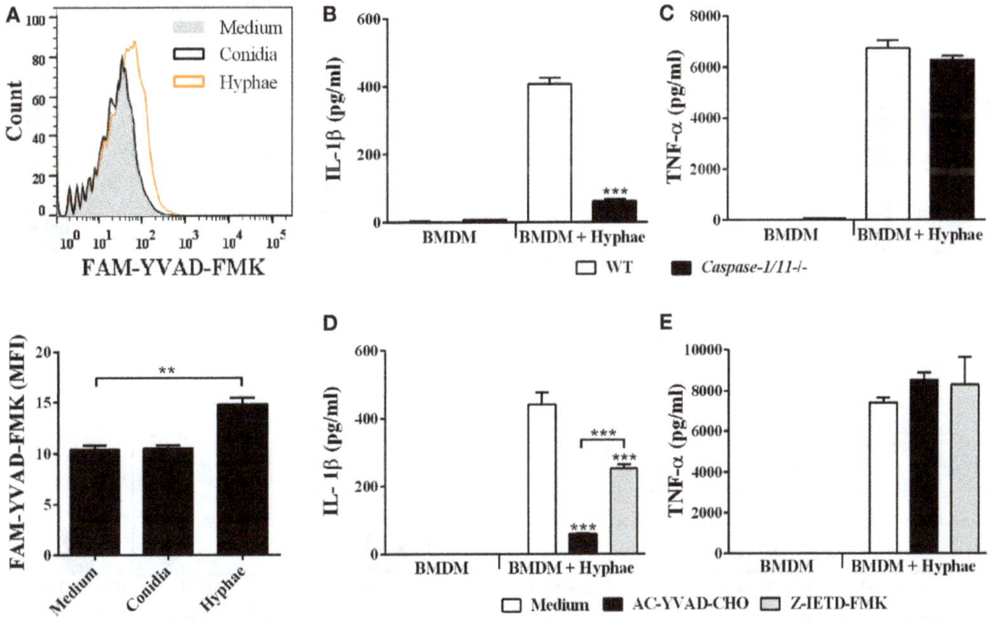

FIGURE 4 | Inflammasome activation by *Fonsecaea pedrosoi* hyphae is dependent on caspase-1 and caspase-8. Bone marrow-derived macrophages (BMDMs) were incubated with medium, *F. pedrosoi* conidia or hyphae for 24 h, and thereafter stained with anti-CD11b-APC antibody and FAM-YVAD-FMK-FITC probe to perform flow cytometry analysis. Caspase-1 activity (indicated by intensity of FAM-YVAD-FMK-FITC binding) of CD11b^{+} cells is represented in histogram and by cell mean fluorescence intensity (MFI) **(A)**. BMDMs obtained from wild-type (WT) or *Caspase-1/11*$^{-/-}$ mice were infected with *F. pedrosoi* hyphae for 24 h **(B,C)**. WT BMDMs were pretreated for 2 h with 50 μM of AC-YVAD-CHO (caspase-1 inhibitor) or Z-IETD-FMK (caspase-8 inhibitor) and then infected with *F. pedrosoi* hyphae for 24 h **(D,E)**. The supernatant of cell culture assays **(B–E)** was evaluated for IL-1β and tumor necrosis factor-α by ELISA. Data shown are mean ± SEM and are representative of two to three independent experiments. $^{**}p < 0.01$; $^{***}p < 0.001$, compared to WT-infected untreated cells or between groups indicated by brackets.

caspase-1 inhibitor showed a severe reduction in IL-1β secretion (**Figures 4B,D**, respectively). Moreover, as caspase-8 has been associated with the non-canonical processing of IL-1β in response to *C. albicans*, *A. fumigatus*, and *C. neoformans* infection, we further tested caspase-8 inhibitor Z-IETD-FMK with WT BMDMs infected with *F. pedrosoi* hyphae (34, 35). Interestingly, cells treated with caspase-8 inhibitor decreased IL-1β production, although not as dramatically as cells undergoing caspase-1 inhibition (**Figure 4D**). TNF-α secretion was not affected in the inhibition/absence of the aforementioned caspases (**Figures 4C,E**). In addition to its role in maturing inflammasome-derived cytokines, caspase-1 mediate an inflammasome-dependent cell death mechanism termed pyroptosis, which leads to plasma membrane lysis and release of cytoplasmic content, including lactate dehydrogenase (LDH). Interestingly, we observed no extracellular release of LDH from BMDMs infected with *F. pedrosoi* hyphae nor conidia, which suggests that pyroptosis does not occur in our model (data not shown). Thus, our data demonstrate that IL-1β secretion by BMDMs in response to *F. pedrosoi* hyphae infection depends on caspase-1 and, to a lesser extent, on caspase-8 activity.

F. pedrosoi Hyphae Activate the NLRP3 Inflammasome, Which Depends on K^+ Efflux, ROS Production, Phagolysosomal Acidification/Disruption, and Cathepsin B Release

With respect to inflammasome activation upon fungal infections, only the inflammasome receptors AIM2, NLRC4 and, mainly, NLRP3, are related to engaging and triggering IL-1β caspase-dependent cleavage (36). Thus, we first evaluated the gene transcription of these receptors in BMDMs upon hyphal infection, and only *Nlrp3* was upregulated (**Figure 5A**). To evaluate whether NLRP3 participates in IL-1β secretion in BMDMs stimulated with hyphae, we used BMDMs obtained from NLRP3-deficient mice. In NLRP3 absence, IL-1β secretion was almost completely abolished (**Figure 5B**), whereas inflammasome-independent TNF-α production remained unchanged (**Figure 5C**).

NLRP3 is activated in response to a myriad of microbial infections through the sensing of their common-induced cellular disturbances, principally potassium efflux, ROS production, phagolysosomal acidification, and cathepsin B release (37). In order to assess whether the aforementioned mechanisms of NLRP3-inflammasome activation are required for our model, we impaired cell potassium efflux by cell treatment with glyburide, an ATP-sensitive K^+ channel inhibitor, and also by addition of exogenous KCl. Under both conditions, we observed a drastic decrease in IL-1β levels (**Figure 5D**). To verify the role of ROS production, we used DPI, a blocker of ROS derived from the phagosome and mitochondria. In response, IL-1β secretion was impaired (**Figure 5E**). However, reduction in TNF-α secretion was also observed (data not shown). Furthermore, we measured IL-1β levels in cultures of BMDMs treated with bafilomycin A and CA-074Me, inhibitors of phagolysosomal acidification and cathepsin B cytosolic activity, respectively, which succeeds phagolysosomal damage and subsequent disruption. This inhibitory assay indicated that IL-1β secretion is strongly dependent on cathepsin B release and influenced by phagolysosomal

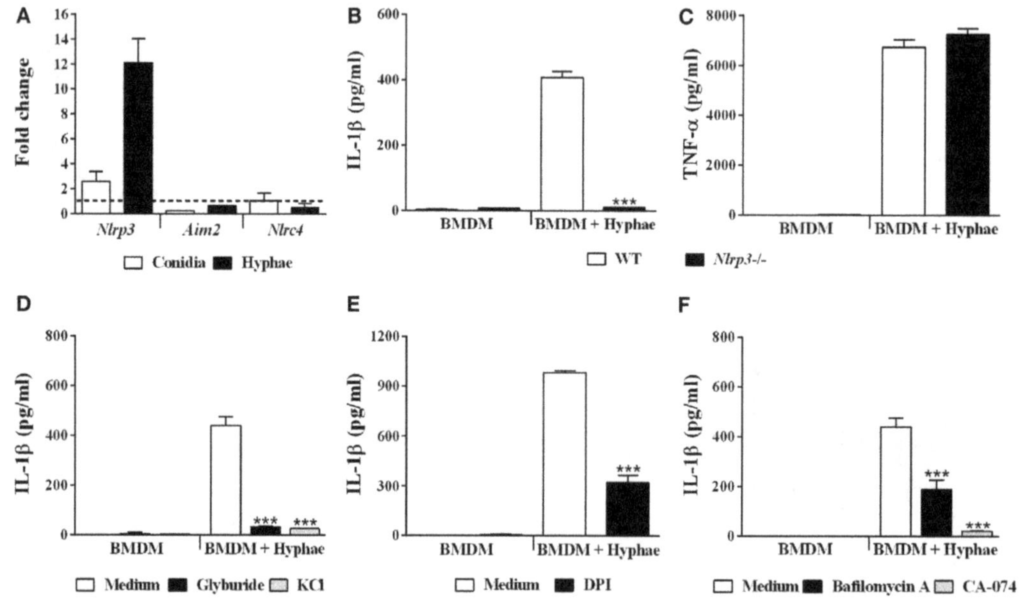

FIGURE 5 | *Fonsecaea pedrosoi* hyphae activate the NLRP3 inflammasome, which depends on K^+ efflux, ROS production, phagolysosomal acidification, and cathepsin B release. Bone marrow-derived macrophages (BMDMs) were infected with conidia or hyphae for 6 h and, thereafter, were lysed for RT-qPCR analysis to quantify gene expression of indicated genes **(A)**. BMDMs obtained from wild-type (WT) or *NLRP3*$^{-/-}$ mice were infected with *F. pedrosoi* hyphae for 24 h **(B,C)**. WT BMDMs were pretreated for 2 h with glyburide (150 μM) or KCl (50 mM) **(D)**, DPI (20 μM) **(E)**, and bafilomycin A (250 nM) or CA-074 (50 μM) **(F)**. Then, cells were infected with *F. pedrosoi* hyphae for 24 h. The supernatant of 24 h cell culture assays **(B–F)** was evaluated for IL-1β by ELISA. Data shown are mean ± SEM and are representative of two to three independent experiments. $^{***}p < 0.001$, compared to WT-infected untreated cells.

acidification (**Figure 5F**). Furthermore, since cathepsin B release requires phagolysosome membrane permeabilization, we incubated BMDMs with FITC-dextran and evaluated whether it leaks into the cytosol (Figure S2 in Supplementary Material). Internalized FITC-dextran diffused into the cytosol after *F. pedrosoi* challenge, as previously described for *C. neoformans* infection (35), which suggests that disruption of the phagolysosome caused by *F. pedrosoi* preceded cathepsin B release in order to induce IL-1β secretion. Altogether, our data show that *F. pedrosoi* hyphae activate the NLRP3 inflammasome in BMDMs, which depends on K^+ efflux, ROS production, phagolysosomal acidification, and disruption followed by cathepsin B release. All cell treatments used above were previously successfully tested (27) to exclude the reduction of IL-1β due to cytotoxic effects.

Inflammasome Activation Does Not Promote *In Vitro* Fungicidal Activity of BMDMs Challenged with *F. pedrosoi* Conidia or Hyphae

Some studies have demonstrated that inflammasome activation drives host protective immune responses against fungal pathogens, such as *C. albicans*, *C. neoformans*, and *P. brasiliensis* (36). Thus, after clarifying the mechanisms of inflammasome activation in BMDMs infected with *F. pedrosoi*, we aimed to verify whether this is reflected in enhanced fungicidal activity by BMDMs against *F. pedrosoi* conidia and hyphae. To this end, we infected WT, *Caspase-1/11*$^{-/-}$ and *Nlrp3*$^{-/-}$ BMDMs for 24 h and thereafter performed the CFU assay. We observed no differences in fungal burden among experimental groups (**Figures 6A,E**), which we already expected for infection with conidia, since this morphotype alone is unable to activate the inflammasome in BMDMs, as demonstrated in the present study (**Figure 2A**). We did not observe NO production in these groups (**Figures 6C,G**). Therefore, we went further and co-stimulated infected BMDMs with nigericin to promote strong inflammasome activation, as shown in **Figure 2A**, and then performed the CFU assay. Nevertheless, the inducible burst in inflammasome activity was not accompanied by diminished recovery of viable fungus from BMDMs infected with conidia or hyphae (**Figures 6B,F**). Interestingly, a control group treated simultaneously with LPS and IFN-γ showed no difference in fungal killing (**Figures 6B,F**), despite the induced NO production (**Figures 6D,H**). This can be explained in part because *F. pedrosoi* morphotypes, especially hyphae, inhibited NO production (**Figures 6D,H**).

NLRP3 Inflammasome Does Not Contribute to Fungal Clearance in a Murine CBM Model

In order to verify whether *F. pedrosoi* could activate the inflammasome *in vivo*, and to further investigate the functional role

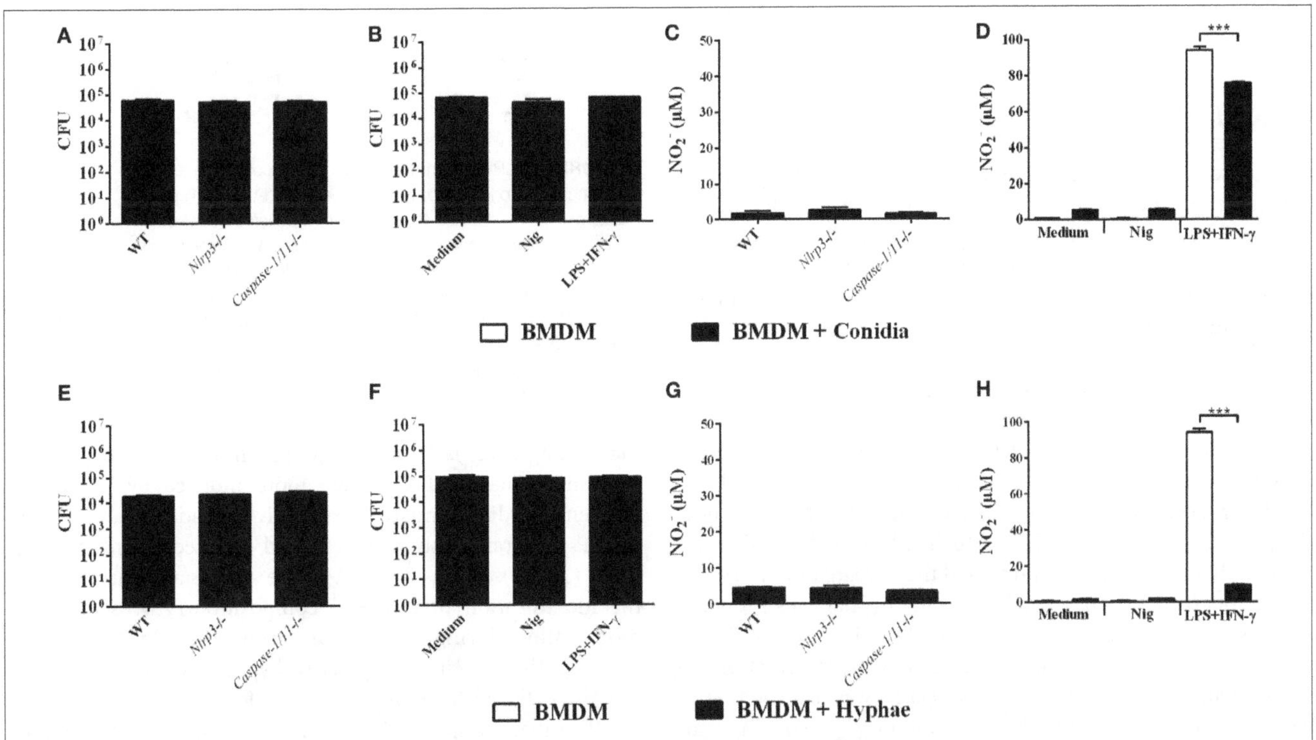

FIGURE 6 | Inflammasome activation does not promote *in vitro* fungicidal activity of bone marrow-derived macrophages (BMDMs) challenged with *Fonsecaea pedrosoi* conidia or hyphae. BMDMs were infected for 24 h with *F. pedrosoi* conidia **(A–D)** or hyphae **(E–H)**. Then, culture supernatant was collected for nitrite measurement by Griess reagent, whereas infected cells were lysed to perform colony-forming unit (CFU) analysis. CFU **(A,E)** and NO_2^- **(C,G)** values of an assay with infected wild-type (WT), *NLRP3*$^{-/-}$ and *Caspase-1*$^{-/-}$ BMDMs. CFU **(B,F)** and NO_2^- **(D,H)** values of an assay with non-infected (white bars) and infected (black bars) WT BMDMs co-stimulated (or not) with both LPS and IFN-γ (500 and 20 ng/mL added 3 h before fungal infection, respectively) or nigericin (20 µM during the last 60 min of incubation). Data shown are mean ± SEM and are representative of three independent experiments. ***$p < 0.001$, between groups indicated by brackets.

of the inflammasome in an experimental model of CBM, we infected WT, *Nlrp3* and *Caspase-1/11*-deficient mice subcutaneously in the footpad with a mixed inoculum of fungal propagules consisting of conidia and hyphae. WT-infected mice showed a sustained production of IL-1β at all the time points analyzed, which was reduced at 21 and 28 days postinfection (d.p.i.) in *Nlrp3*$^{-/-}$ mice (**Figure 7A**). In addition, we observed significant levels of IL-18 only in an advanced stage of remission of the disease, at 28 d.p.i., with defective cytokine production in *Nlrp3*$^{-/-}$ mice (**Figure 7B**). There was no difference in the production of both cytokines between WT and *Caspase-1/11*$^{-/-}$ mice (**Figures 7A,B**). Interestingly, the production of IL-1β and IL-18, regulated by NLRP3 and Caspase-1/11 in response to *F. pedrosoi* hyphae (**Figures 4** and **5**), did not affect the fungal load of the footpad, as we did not observe statistical differences in CFU assays among WT and both groups of knockout mice, at any of the times analyzed (**Figure 7C**). Histological examination of infected tissues from all groups show similar features as indicated by the presence of exudative areas and inflammatory infiltrates early as 14 d.p.i., which diminished over time and was accompanied by tissue remodeling and repair (Figure S3A in Supplementary Material). Consistently with CFU and histological analysis, there was no difference in morphometric measurements of the injured footpad among experimental groups (Figure S3B in Supplementary Material).

These data indicate that *F. pedrosoi* induces the production of IL-1β and IL-18 in the course of a subcutaneous experimental infection model, but this production does not affect the fungal clearance.

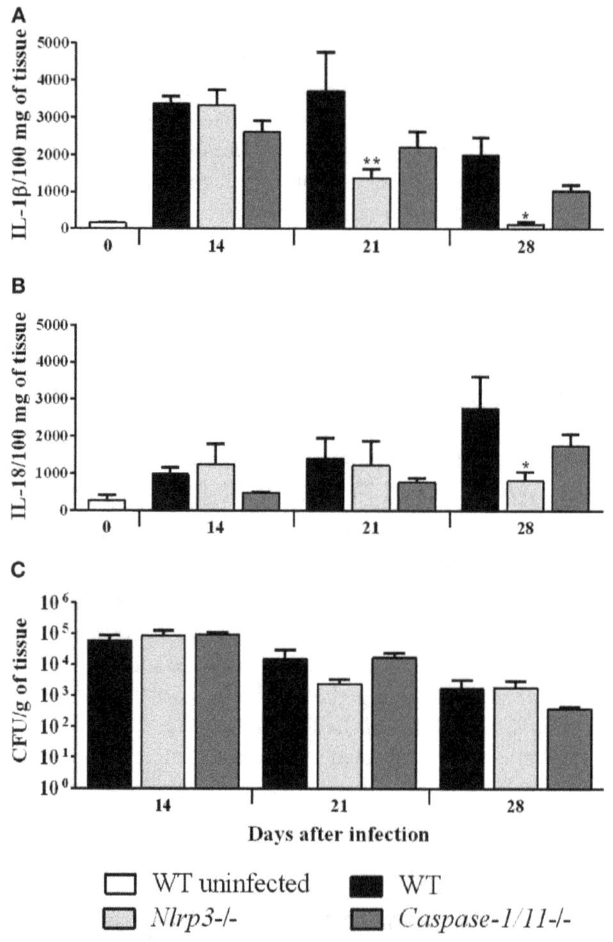

FIGURE 7 | NLRP3 inflammasome does not contribute to fungal clearance in a murine chromoblastomycosis model. Wild-type (WT), *Nlrp3*$^{-/-}$ and *Caspase-1/11*$^{-/-}$ C57BL/6 mice ($n = 4$) were infected in both hind footpads with 1×10^6 *Fonsecaea pedrosoi* propagules. WT uninfected mice were used as control. Mice were euthanized at the indicated days postinfection, and the footpad tissue homogenate was assessed for both cleaved and uncleaved IL-1β **(A)** and interleukin-18 **(B)** by ELISA, and plated for colony-forming unit analysis **(C)**. Data shown are mean ± SEM and are representative of two independent experiments. $^*p < 0.05$; $^{**}p < 0.01$, compared to WT infected.

DISCUSSION

Studies examining innate immune cell recognition of *F. pedrosoi* are scarce. Although the involvement of CLRs and TLRs in this process is relatively well known, cytoplasmic NLRs had never been considered. In this study, we demonstrate that the main agent of CBM, *F. pedrosoi*, activates NLRP3 inflammasome-dependent secretion of IL-1β and IL-18 in phagocytes and *in vivo*. Moreover, the mechanisms underlying this process encompass Syk-coupled CLR receptors, caspase-1 and caspase 8 proteolytic activity and several DAMPs.

One key aspect shown to determine NLRP3 inflammasome activation during fungal infection is morphogenesis. We show here that live *F. pedrosoi* hyphae, and not conidia, were able to induce the production of mature IL-1β and IL-18 in BMDMs, despite the fact that both cell types prompted the upregulation of IL-1β transcripts (pro-IL-1β). In addition, only hyphal cells induced IL-1β secretion in human monocytic THP-1 cells. Similarly, activation of NLRP3 inflammasome and cytokine secretion in macrophages challenged with *A. fumigatus* was achieved only with hyphae. This suggests that an invading aggressive hyphal form may be necessary to trigger the inflammatory response (23). Actually, in lung tissues of NLRP3-deficient mice, minimal inflammatory reaction to *Aspergillus* hyphae infection is observed (19). Further, *F. pedrosoi* swollen conidia, an intermediate stage of conidia-into-hyphae germination, were not able to induce mature IL-1β production, as also shown in *A. fumigatus*-infected macrophages (23). Interestingly, inflammasome-independent cytokines, such as TNF-α, are more induced by *Aspergillus* swollen conidia compared to inactive conidia, and cell wall PAMPs are transiently displayed and detected by macrophage PRRs (38, 39). In this context, future studies are warranted for the identification of cell wall composition/PAMPs exposure modification during *F. pedrosoi* germination. In *C. albicans*, although the switch from yeast to hyphal morphogenesis was initially believed to be indispensable for the activation of the NLRP3 inflammasome (17), recent studies have showed that the remodeling of its cell wall leading to PAMPs exposure during phagocytosis is the main factor associated with inflammasome activation (40, 41).

Another important aspect that influences NLRP3 inflammasome activation during infectious processes is the host cell type. Indeed, differently from what is shown in macrophages,

F. pedrosoi conidia alone were able to induce mature IL-1β production in dendritic cells. In addition, when nigericin (bacterial pore formation toxin) was added to macrophage cell culture, a significant amount of IL-1β secretion was observed, corroborating the fact that conidia induce pro-IL-1β production but fail to provide inflammasome-activating second signal in macrophages. Consistent with this observation, our group previously showed that *P. brasiliensis* can trigger pro-IL-1β production in macrophages and dendritic cells, but it was only in the latter that infection resulted in IL-1β maturation and release (27). Also, activation of NLRP3 inflammasome and production of mature IL-1β in macrophages infected with *C. albicans* yeast occurred only after a priming step with LPS (17, 42) whereas the fungus alone induced mature cytokine release in the dendritic cell (16). These results are in line with the fact that NLRP3 concentration is critical to the efficacy of inflammasome activation (31), and NLRP3 protein levels under steady-state conditions and after PRR engagement are higher in dendritic cells when compared with macrophages (43, 44). Furthermore, *in vivo* murine splenic conventional dendritic cells reveal constant high *Nlrp3* transcript levels (45). Thus, both fungal form and phagocyte type are critical factors that dictate NLRP3 inflammasome activation in fungal infections.

Priming is the first step required for inflammasome activation, and this process is generally associated with PRRs engagement by PAMPs leading to pro-IL-1β, pro-IL-18, and NLRP3 production. CLRs are the major PRRs family for the recognition of fungal carbohydrate residues and have been associated with the priming step of inflammasome activation in several fungal infections (46). For instance, the dectin-1 receptor is necessary for the production of pro-IL-1β and IL-1 β in murine and human macrophages and dendritic cells infected with *Microsporum canis*, *C. albicans*, and *Malassezia* spp. (42, 47, 48). Also, signaling mediated by dectin-2 is required for the production of IL-1β in dendritic cells infected with both hyphae and conidia of *C. albicans* (49). Interestingly, dectin-1 and dectin-2 have been associated with the induction of cytokine secretion, including inflammasome-dependent IL-1β, in a collaborative manner. Dectin-1 and dectin-2 double-deficient dendritic cells infected with *Trichophyton rubrum* or *H. capsulatum* have impaired secretion of IL-1β when compared to WT cells and cells with either receptor deficiency alone (21, 50). Moreover, using blocking antibodies for dectin-1 or dectin-2 in single or double dectin-1/dectin-2 deficient cells, Chang et al. (21) elegantly demonstrated that dectin-2 was the major receptor for inflammasome activation in *H. capsulatum*-infected dendritic cells. Although we did not employ double deficient cells, our results using cells lacking dectin-1 or dectin-2 clearly show that these CLRs play a significant role in inducing the secretion of IL-1β by macrophages infected with *F. pedrosoi* hyphae. This is in line with the fact that dectin-1 and dectin-2 are required for the development of Th17 cells in mice subcutaneously infected with *F. pedrosoi*, since IL-1β associated with IL-23 favors a Th17 response (11, 51).

Besides dectin-1 and dectin-2, we also demonstrated a role for dectin-3 in the induction of IL-1β secretion by BMDMs infected with *F. pedrosoi* hyphae. It is noteworthy that dectin-3 can form heterodimers with dectin-2 for sensing and mediation of host protective anti-*C. albicans* defense (32). In addition, dectin-3 is necessary for the development of vaccine-induced Th17 cells that are associated with protection against the fungal pathogen *Blastomyces dermatitidis* (52). The role of dectin-3 in the recognition of *F. pedrosoi* conidia has been evaluated using lacZ activity measurement in reporter cells coexpressing dectin-2/dectin-3 or expressing dectin-2 or dectin-3 alone (11). Only a weak response was detected in dectin-3 expressing cells, and cells coexpressing dectin-2/dectin-3 did not show an enhanced dectin-2 induced reporter activity. Furthermore, IL-6 production was not significantly altered in dectin-3-deficient cells. In this context, our results suggest that, contrary to conidia, *F. pedrosoi* hyphae may expose dectin-3 ligands leading to recognition and pro-inflammatory cytokine production by macrophages.

Upon PAMP binding, all three aforementioned CLRs initiate intracellular signaling pathways, and the Syk-CARD9-NFkB pathway is the best characterized and the most common during fungal infections (36, 46). For instance, Syk-dependent NLRP3 priming occurs in *C. albicans*, *A. fumigatus*-, *C. neoformans*- and *P. brasiliensis*-infected cells (16, 18, 23, 27). Indeed, a significant reduction in IL-1β secretion was shown here in macrophages infected with *F. pedrosoi* and treated with chemical inhibitors of Syk kinase and NFkB activity. This result parallels those showing *Syk* and *Nfkb1* upregulated transcripts induced by *F. pedrosoi* hyphae. It was noted that *Myd88* transcripts were also significantly induced by hyphae in macrophages, but their inhibition did not affect the production of IL-1β. Conversely, the secretion of the inflammasome-independent cytokine TNF-α relied upon dectin-1 and both Syk- and Myd88-mediated signaling, which is in accordance with previous studies showing that TNF-α production in macrophages treated with β-glucans (i.e., dectin-1 ligand) requires that Syk-dependent signaling synergizes with the Myd88 pathway (53).

Followed by priming, the proteolytic cleavage of pro-IL-1β into its mature form is canonically performed by the protease caspase-1, and this process is largely dependent on the assembly of the NLRP3 inflammasome in fungal infections (36, 54). Using a fluorescence-based assay, we demonstrated that only *F. pedrosoi* hyphae were directly able to activate caspase-1 in macrophages. In addition, caspase-1/11-deficient macrophages and macrophages treated with caspase-1 peptide inhibitor produced a significant, but not total, impairment in mature IL-1β secretion, suggesting that caspase-1-independent processes may also be involved. In fact, non-canonical processing of IL-1β has been shown to operate in phagocytes infected with fungal pathogens. *C. albicans* triggers caspase-8-mediated cleavage of pro-IL-1β independently of a NLR-containing inflammasome. This occurs *via* assembly of the CARD9–Bcl-10–MALT1 scaffold mediated by Syk signaling, followed by the recruitment of caspase-8 into this scaffold for direct IL-1β processing (34). Caspase-8 can also function in a NLRP3-dependent inflammasome activation manner, as demonstrated in phagocytes infected with *A. fumigatus* and *C. neoformans* (19, 35). The use of a specific caspase-8 peptide inhibitor shows here that this protease has a role in the processing of IL-1β in *F. pedrosoi*-infected macrophages. Given the fact that NLRP3-deficient macrophages completely failed to produce IL-1β upon *F. pedrosoi* challenge, the function of caspase-8 in our model probably relies on the NLRP3 inflammasome assembly instead of a direct processing activity.

Along with NLRP3, NLRC4 and AIM2-containing-inflammasomes have been implicated in the antifungal response (36, 54). Specifically, *C. albicans* triggers NLCR4 inflammasome exclusively in mucosal cells, and deficiency in this NLR results in impaired neutrophil infiltration in the mucosa in a murine model of oral infection (55). Conversely, the NLRP3 inflammasome is strictly required in phagocytes infected with *C. albicans* (16). Regarding *A. fumigatus*, this fungus induces cooperative and synergistic activation of the NLRP3 and AIM2 inflammasomes in phagocytes and in an experimental murine model of intranasal infection (19). Similarly, NLRP3 and AIM2 inflammasomes are activated by plasmodium hemozoin and DNA (56). In this context, we evaluated the transcript levels of *Nlrp3*, *Nlrc4*, and *Aim2* genes in BMDMs infected with the infective forms of *F. pedrosoi*. Hyphae induced the upregulation of *Nlrp3* transcripts only. These data, coupled with the fact that NLRP3-deficient infected macrophages do not produce IL-1β, as mentioned above, indicate that multiple inflammasome activation is probably not in use in our fungal model. At the same time, these results also suggest that, unlike in *A. fumigatus*, there is a poor availability of *F. pedrosoi* dsDNA (the main AIM2 ligand) in the cytosol of infected cells. Nevertheless, the use of mice deficient in NLRC4 and AIM2 would shed light on this issue.

Although not fully characterized, cellular stresses that induce endogenous DAMPs have been associated with NLRP3 assembly and inflammatory caspase activation. Among them, K^+ efflux due to stimulation of the ATP-sensitive K^+ channel, ROS generation, and lysosome rupture are usually presented (15). Using chemical inhibitors, we demonstrated that *F. pedrosoi* hyphae promote these intracellular disturbances in macrophages, leading to inflammasome activation. Both K^+ efflux and ROS are the main cellular disturbances associated with NLRP3 activation in phagocytes infected with diverse fungi, encompassing those causing dermathophytoses (47, 48, 57), and invasive mycosis (16, 18, 21, 27). Specifically, potassium efflux is considered a common unifying pathway for NLRP3 inflammasome complex activation triggered by numerous NLRP3 stimuli (58). As such, we tested two inhibitors of K^+ efflux, glyburide and KCl. Both treatments resulted in a significant impairment of IL-1β secretion by macrophages, reinforcing the central role of intracellular K^+ level reduction in the regulation of NLRP3 inflammasome activation. Similarly, the use of DPI, an inhibitor of NADPH oxidase-dependent and mitochondria-derived ROS production, also led to diminished IL-1β production. It is noteworthy that ROS generation is apparently not directly associated with the NLRP3 activation (i.e., inflammasome assembly) step. Instead, it may affect the priming step, as several inhibitors of ROS generation or scavengers of ROS have been shown to inhibit NFκB-mediated transcription of NLRP3 and pro-IL-1β (16, 59). Indeed, besides IL-1β, the production of the inflammasome-independent NFκB-dependent TNF-α was abrogated with the treatment with DPI in macrophages infected with *F. pedrosoi* (data not shown). In addition to ROS and K^+ efflux, disruption of the phagolysosomal membrane, leading to impairment of phagolysosomal acidification and leakage of enzymes such as cathepsin B into the cytoplasm results in NLRP3 activation (15). Therefore, macrophages infected with *F. pedrosoi* were treated with bafilomycin, which inhibits the vacuolar H^+ ATPase, or CA-074, which in turn inhibits cathepsin B activity. The treatments resulted in a significant reduction in IL-1β secretion, similar to the activation of the inflammasome by several bacteria and particulate matter (15, 36). Regarding fungi, cathepsin B is not required for IL-1β production in dendritic cells infected with *C. albicans* or *A. fumigatus* (16, 19). Conversely, the production of this cytokine in macrophages infected with *C. albicans* is dependent on cathepsin B (17). In phagocytes infected with *P. brasiliensis*, dendritic cells, but not macrophages, require phagolysosomal disruption for NLRP3 inflammasome activation (27, 60). Thus, the requirement for phagolysosomal disruption in the assembly of NLRP3 inflammasome is not universal, as it is dependent on the cell type and fungal pathogen.

Macrophages are essential innate immunity cells that are critical for direct antifungal response. Macrophages, along with neutrophils and lymphocytes, are regularly observed within the chronic granulomatous lesions of CBM patients, displaying different degrees of maturation and activation, and they also form multinucleated giant cells that harbor fungi (29, 30). In addition, *F. pedrosoi* cells can be detected in intracytoplasmic vacuoles of skin macrophages (61). Thus, we investigated whether NLRP3 inflammasome activation would play a part in the microbicidal capacity of macrophages infected with *F. pedrosoi*. In BMDMs lacking NLRP3 or Caspase-1 and infected with hyphae or conidia, no significant difference in the fungal burden was observed. Since conidia alone are not able to induce inflammasome activation, we treated macrophages with nigericin for the induction of the second signal for inflammasome activation and consequently production of mature IL-1β. Macrophages infected with hyphae were also treated with nigericin, leading to enhanced IL-1β secretion. Again, fungal viability was not affected, reinforcing the supposition that the NLRP3 inflammasome has no role in modulating the ability of macrophages to kill *F. predosoi*. In fact, the killing process of *F. pedrosoi* by macrophages is rarely efficient, and it is neutrophils that are considered the main phagocyte cell with microbicidal activity against this fungus (62, 63). Several studies have demonstrated that *F. pedrosoi* is able to survive and proliferate in murine macrophages, and activated macrophages are only fungistatic (62, 64–66). One important factor associated with the inability of macrophages to kill *F. pedrosoi* is the inhibition of NO production by macrophages (66). In line with this finding, no significant levels of nitrite were detected in the supernatant of macrophage cultures infected with *F. pedrosoi* cells. Furthermore, macrophages infected with either conidia or hyphae and treated with IFN-γ and LPS were not fungicidal and their nitrite production was significantly impaired. Lack of properly activated macrophages may serve *F. pedrosoi* intracellular parasitism, leading to disease establishment and progression in susceptible hosts.

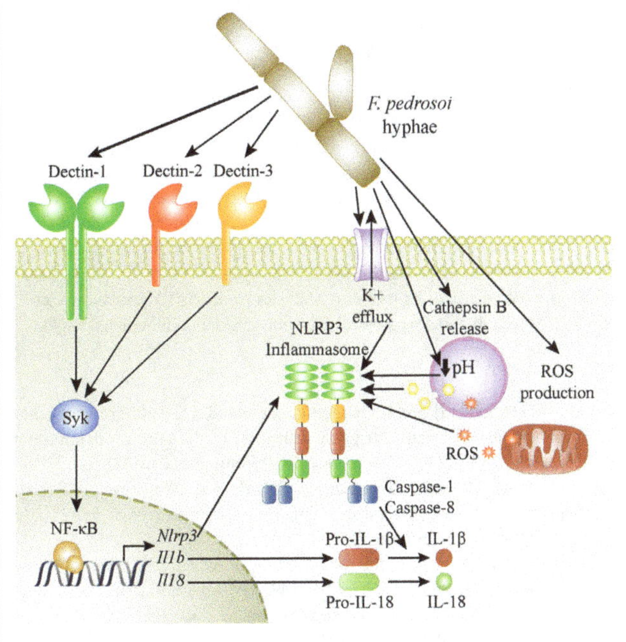

FIGURE 8 | Suggested model of activation of the NLRP3 inflammasome by *Fonsecaea pedrosoi* hyphae in macrophages. *F. pedrosoi* hyphae induce macrophage priming by a canonical Syk-NF-kB signaling pathway coupled to dectin-1, dectin-2, and dectin-3 recognition of the fungus. This leads to NLRP3, pro-IL-1β, and pro-IL-18 production. Then, the NLRP3-inflammasome is activated as a result of potassium efflux, phagolysosome acidification, cathepsin B release, and ROS production, which subsequently leads to IL-1β and IL-18 processing and secretion by caspase-1 and caspase-8 dependent cleavage.

Since *F. pedrosoi* activates the NLRP3 inflammasome *in vitro*, we investigated whether *in vivo* activation occurs and the possible role of this process in controlling fungal infection. Employing a mouse model of subcutaneous *F. pedrosoi* infection (24, 67), WT-infected mice showed a sustained production of IL-1β at all the time points analyzed, which was significantly reduced in mice lacking NLRP3. In addition, the NLRP3 inflammasome was also required for the production of IL-18, as assessed in the footpad macerate at 28 d.p.i. These results suggest that NLRP3 sensing is required for the maturation of IL-1β and IL-18 in mice infected with *F. pedrosoi*. Surprisingly, the production of these cytokines was not significantly different in the footpad of caspase-1/11-deficient mice, although there was a tendency for IL-1β and IL-18 to be lower than in control mice. In macrophages infected with *F. pedrosoi*, caspase-1, and caspase-8 were required for the production of IL-1β. It is possible that *in vivo*, caspase-8 compensates for the lack of caspase-1. For instance, *C. neoformans* activates NLRP3-caspase-8 inflammasome in the absence of caspase-1 (35). Also, caspase-independent cleavage of pro-IL-1β may ensue, especially *via* neutrophil-derived serine proteases (68). This is in line with the fact that the chronic inflammatory response observed in murine and human CBM is characterized by a mononuclear granuloma modified by the influx of neutrophils, giving rise to a suppurative neutrophilic infiltrate (5, 24). In this context, in disseminated candidiasis where neutrophils are the main component of the infiltrates in inflammatory organs, IL-1β processing is probably mainly achieved by neutrophil-derived protease, rather than by caspase-1 (69, 70).

Differently from several models of systemic mycosis where NLRP3 inflammasome activation is associated with host protection and impairment of fungal growth (16–22), NLRP3 and caspase-1 deficient mice subcutaneously infected with *F. pedrosoi* developed to be self-healing in 30–40 days with a progressive fungal clearance. This finding is in accordance with the fact that infected mice lacking NLRP3 or Caspase-1 had similar histological and morphometric analyses of the footpad tissue when compared with control mice.

In conclusion, we revealed here the mechanisms of NLRP3 inflammasome activation in macrophages and in mice infected with the most important CBM etiologic agent *F. pedrosoi*, as depicted in our proposed model in **Figure 8**. Future studies employing other causative agents of CBM will contribute to a better understanding on the role of inflammasome activation in the pathogenesis of this neglected disease.

AUTHOR CONTRIBUTIONS

Conceived and designed the experiments: RJAC, IMS, PHB, AHT, and ALB. Performed the experiments: RJAC, IMS, MSJ, AMMB, PHHVJ, SAMO, and LCL. Analyzed the data: RJAC, IMS, AHT, and ALB. Contributed to reagents/material/analysis tools: AHT and ALB. Contributed to Caspase-1 and NLRP3 KO mice: KGM. Wrote the paper: RJAC, AHT, and ALB.

FUNDING

Funding for this research was provided by Fundação de Apoio à Pesquisa do Distrito Federal (FAPDF Project 193.00805/2015), Conselho Nacional de Pesquisa (CNPq Project 302752/2015-3) for financial support and Coordenação de Aperfeiçoamento de Pessoal de Nível Superior (CAPES) for graduate students' grants.

SUPPLEMENTARY MATERIAL

FIGURE S1 | *Fonsecaea pedrosoi* conidia reaches the swelling stage of germination. Flow cytometry analysis of *F. pedrosoi* conidia incubed for 6 h with phosphate-buffered saline, RPMI supplemented with 20% of SBF (R20 medium) or bone marrow-derived macrophages (BMDMs) for 6 and 24 h. Infected BMDMs were washed to discard nonphagocyted fungus and lysed to release intracellular fungi. After, conidia were fixed and evaluated by flow cytometry analysis. Commercial 2 and 3 μm sized-cytometry-beads were used as control. Dot plot side scatter (FSC) vs forward scatter (FSC) analysis of conidia **(A)**. Histogram analyses of conidia size **(B)**. Average conidia size using the median FSC and expressed as arbitrary units (au) **(C)**. Data shown are mean ± SEM and are representative of three independent experiments. ***$p < 0.001$, between groups indicated by brackets; n.s., not significantly.

FIGURE S2 | *Fonsecaea pedrosoi* hyphae infection cause phagolysosome membrane permeabilization contributing to inflammasome activation. Bone marrow-derived macrophages were seeded on glass bottom culture dishes with RPMI for 1 h for cell adhesion. After wash of unbound cells with warm RPMI, cells were incubated with 70 kDa FITC-dextran (Sigma-Aldrich; 2 mg/mL) in RPMI with 10% FBS for 2 h. The cells were washed and infected or not (medium) with *F. pedrosoi* hyphae (MOI 1) or *Cryptococcus neoformans* yeasts (MOI 2) opsonized with anti-GXM Ab. After 4 h of infection, non-phagocytosed fungi were washed and infection proceeded up to 20 h. After infection, cells were washed again, incubated with RPMI medium without phenol red supplemented with 10% FBS and stained with DAPI. Cells were washed, incubated with medium, and visualized by fluorescence microscopy. White arrowhead indicates internalized fungi.

FIGURE S3 | NLRP3 or caspase-1/11 absence do not affect tissue response to *Fonsecaea pedrosoi* infection. Wild-type, *Nlrp3*$^{-/-}$ and *Caspase-1/11*$^{-/-}$ mice were injected subcutaneously with 1×10^6 *F. pedrosoi* propagules into the hind footpad. For histology evaluation, infected mice were euthanized at the indicated days after infection and fragments of tissues were fixed with 10% phosphate-buffered formalin and embedded in paraffin. Paraffin-sectioned samples were stained with Hematoxilin and Eosin (H&E) and analyzed under a Zeiss inverted microscope **(A)**. During infection, the injured tissue was measured every 3 days with a caliper for morphometric examination **(B)**. Data shown are mean ± SEM (n = 4) and are representative of two independent experiments.

REFERENCES

1. McGinnis MR, Hilger AE. Infections caused by black fungi. *Arch Dermatol* (1987) 123:1300–2. doi:10.1001/archderm.1987.01660340062020
2. López Martínez R, Méndez Tovar LJ. Chromoblastomycosis. *Clin Dermatol* (2007) 25:188–94. doi:10.1016/j.clindermatol.2006.05.007
3. Queiroz-Telles F. Chromoblastomycosis: a neglected tropical disease. *Rev Inst Med Trop São Paulo* (2015) 57(Suppl 1):46–50. doi:10.1590/S0036-46652015000700009
4. Santos ALS, Palmeira VF, Rozental S, Kneipp LF, Nimrichter L, Alviano DS, et al. Biology and pathogenesis of *Fonsecaea pedrosoi*, the major etiologic agent of chromoblastomycosis. *FEMS Microbiol Rev* (2007) 31:570–91. doi:10.1111/j.1574-6976.2007.00077.x
5. Queiroz-telles F, de Hoog S, Santos WCL, Salgado CG, Vicente VA, Bonifaz A, et al. Chromoblastomycosis. *Clin Microbiol Rev* (2017) 30: 233–76. doi:10.1128/CMR.00032-16
6. Bonifaz A, Carrasco-Gerard E, Saúl A. Chromoblastomycosis: clinical and mycologic experience of 51 cases. *Mycoses* (2001) 44:1–7. doi:10.1046/j.1439-0507.2001.00613.x
7. Salgado CG, da Silva JP, Diniz JAP, da Silva MB, da Costa PF, Teixeira C, et al. Isolation of *Fonsecaea pedrosoi* from thorns of *Mimosa pudica*, a probable natural source of chromoblastomycosis. *Rev Inst Med Trop Sao Paulo* (2004) 46:33–6. doi:10.1590/S0036-46652004000100006
8. Queiroz-Telles F, Esterre P, Perez-Blanco M, Vitale RG, Salgado CG, Bonifaz A. Chromoblastomycosis: an overview of clinical manifestations, diagnosis and treatment. *Med Mycol* (2009) 47:3–15. doi:10.1080/13693780802538001
9. Teixeira de Sousa MDG, Ghosn EEB, Almeida SR. Absence of CD4+ T cells impairs host defence of mice infected with *Fonsecaea pedrosoi*. *Scand J Immunol* (2006) 64:595–600. doi:10.1111/j.1365-3083.2006.01846.x
10. Wevers BA, Kaptein TM, Zijlstra-Willems EM, Theelen B, Boekhout T, Geijtenbeek TBH, et al. Fungal engagement of the C-type lectin mincle suppresses dectin-1-induced antifungal immunity. *Cell Host Microbe* (2014) 15:494–505. doi:10.1016/j.chom.2014.03.008
11. Wüthrich M, Wang H, Li M, Lerksuthirat T, Hardison SE, Brown GD, et al. *Fonsecaea pedrosoi*-induced Th17-cell differentiation in mice is fostered by dectin-2 and suppressed by mincle recognition. *Eur J Immunol* (2015) 45:2542–52. doi:10.1002/eji.201545591
12. Sousa MDG, Reid DM, Schweighoffer E, Tybulewicz V, Ruland J, Langhorne J, et al. Restoration of pattern recognition receptor costimulation to treat chromoblastomycosis, a chronic fungal infection of the skin. *Cell Host Microbe* (2011) 9:436–43. doi:10.1016/j.chom.2011.04.005
13. Schroder K, Tschopp J. The inflammasomes. *Cell* (2010) 140:821–32. doi:10.1016/j.cell.2010.01.040
14. Wen H, Miao EA, Ting JP. Review mechanisms of NOD-like receptor-associated inflammasome activation. *Immunity* (2013) 39:432–41. doi:10.1016/j.immuni.2013.08.037
15. Jo EK, Kim JK, Shin DM, Sasakawa C. Molecular mechanisms regulating NLRP3 inflammasome activation. *Cell Mol Immunol* (2016) 13:148–59. doi:10.1038/cmi.2015.95
16. Gross O, Poeck H, Bscheider M, Dostert C, Hannesschläger N, Endres S, et al. Syk kinase signalling couples to the Nlrp3 inflammasome for anti-fungal host defence. *Nature* (2009) 459:433–6. doi:10.1038/nature07965
17. Joly S, Ma N, Sadler JJ, Soll DR, Cassel SL, Sutterwala FS. Cutting edge: *Candida albicans* hyphae formation triggers activation of the Nlrp3 inflammasome. *J Immunol* (2009) 183:3578–81. doi:10.4049/jimmunol.0901323
18. Guo C, Chen M, Fa Z, Lu A, Fang W, Sun B, et al. Acapsular *Cryptococcus neoformans* activates the NLRP3 inflammasome. *Microbes Infect* (2014) 16:845–54. doi:10.1016/j.micinf.2014.08.013
19. Karki R, Man SM, Malireddi RKS, Gurung P, Vogel P, Lamkanfi M, et al. Concerted activation of the AIM2 and NLRP3 inflammasomes orchestrates host protection against *Aspergillus* infection. *Cell Host Microbe* (2015) 17:357–68. doi:10.1016/j.chom.2015.01.006
20. Feriotti C, de Araújo EF, Loures FV, da Costa TA, de Lima GNA, Zamboni DS, et al. NOD-like receptor P3 inflammasome controls protective Th1/Th17 immunity against pulmonary paracoccidioidomycosis. *Front Immunol* (2017) 8:1–15. doi:10.3389/fimmu.2017.00786
21. Chang TH, Huang JH, Lin HC, Chen WY, Lee YH, Hsu LC, et al. Dectin-2 is a primary receptor for NLRP3 inflammasome activation in dendritic cell response to *Histoplasma capsulatum*. *PLoS Pathog* (2017) 13:e1006485. doi:10.1371/journal.ppat.1006485
22. Lei G, Chen M. Biofilm from a clinical strain of *Cryptococcus neoformans* activates the NLRP3 inflammasome. *Cell Res* (2013) 23:965–8. doi:10.1038/cr.2013.49
23. Saïd-Sadier N, Padilla E, Langsley G, Ojcius DM. *Aspergillus fumigatus* stimulates the NLRP3 inflammasome through a pathway requiring ROS production and the Syk tyrosine kinase. *PLoS One* (2010) 5:e10008. doi:10.1371/journal.pone.0010008
24. Siqueira IM, de Castro RJA, Leonhardt LCdM, Jerônimo MS, Soares AC, Raiol T, et al. Modulation of the immune response by *Fonsecaea pedrosoi* morphotypes in the course of experimental chromoblastomycosis and their role on inflammatory response chronicity. *PLoS Negl Trop Dis* (2017) 11:e0005461. doi:10.1371/journal.pntd.0005461
25. Lutz MB, Kukutsch N, Ogilvie ALJ, Roßner S, Koch F, Romani N, et al. An advanced culture method for generating large quantities of highly pure dendritic cells from mouse bone marrow. *J Immunol Methods* (1999) 223:77–92. doi:10.1016/S0022-1759(98)00204-X
26. Livak KJ, Schmittgen TD. Analysis of relative gene expression data using real-time quantitative PCR and the $2^{-\Delta\Delta CT}$ method. *Methods* (2001) 408:402–8. doi:10.1006/meth.2001.1262
27. Tavares AH, Magalhães KG, Almeida RDN, Correa R, Burgel PH, Bocca AL. NLRP3 inflammasome activation by *Paracoccidioides brasiliensis*. *PLoS Negl Trop Dis* (2013) 7:e2595. doi:10.1371/journal.pntd.0002595
28. Erwig LP, Gow NAR. Interactions of fungal pathogens with phagocytes. *Nat Rev Microbiol* (2016) 14:163–76. doi:10.1038/nrmicro.2015.21
29. Esterre P, Peyrol S, Sainte-Marie D, Pradinaud R, Grimaud JA. Granulomatous reaction and tissue remodelling in the cutaneous lesion of chromomycosis. *Virchows Arch A Pathol Anat Histopathol* (1993) 422:285–91. doi:10.1007/BF01608337
30. Minotto R, Edelweiss MIA, Scroferneker ML. Study on the organization of cellular elements in the granulomatous lesion caused by chromoblastomycosis. *J Cutan Pathol* (2017) 44:915–8. doi:10.1111/cup.13014
31. Bauernfeind FG, Horvath G, Stutz A, Alnemri ES, MacDonald K, Speert D, et al. Cutting edge: NF-kappaB activating pattern recognition and cytokine receptors license NLRP3 inflammasome activation by regulating NLRP3 expression. *J Immunol* (2009) 183:787–91. doi:10.4049/jimmunol.0901363

32. Zhu L-L, Zhao X-Q, Jiang C, You Y, Chen X-P, Jiang Y-Y, et al. C-type lectin receptors dectin-3 and dectin-2 form a heterodimeric pattern-recognition receptor for host defense against fungal infection. *Immunity* (2013) 39:324–34. doi:10.1016/j.immuni.2013.05.017
33. Gringhuis SI, den Dunnen J, Litjens M, van der Vlist M, Wevers B, Bruijns SCM, et al. Dectin-1 directs T helper cell differentiation by controlling noncanonical NF-kappaB activation through Raf-1 and Syk. *Nat Immunol* (2009) 10:203–13. doi:10.1038/ni.1692
34. Gringhuis SI, Kaptein TM, Wevers BA, Theelen B, van der Vlist M, Boekhout T, et al. Dectin-1 is an extracellular pathogen sensor for the induction and processing of IL-1β via a noncanonical caspase-8 inflammasome. *Nat Immunol* (2012) 13:246–54. doi:10.1038/ni.2222
35. Chen M, Xing Y, Lu A, Fang W, Sun B, Chen C, et al. Internalized *Cryptococcus neoformans* activates the canonical caspase-1 and the noncanonical caspase-8 inflammasomes. *J Immunol* (2015) 195:4962–72. doi:10.4049/jimmunol.1500865
36. Tavares AH, Bürgel PH, Bocca AL. Turning up the heat: inflammasome activation by fungal pathogens. *PLoS Pathog* (2015) 11:e1004948. doi:10.1371/journal.ppat.1004948
37. Bauernfeind F, Hornung V. Of inflammasomes and pathogens – sensing of microbes by the inflammasome. *EMBO Mol Med* (2013) 5:814–26. doi:10.1002/emmm.201201771
38. Hohl TM, Van Epps HL, Rivera A, Morgan LA, Chen PL, Feldmesser M, et al. *Aspergillus fumigatus* triggers inflammatory responses by stage-specific beta-glucan display. *PLoS Pathog* (2005) 1:e30. doi:10.1371/journal.ppat.0010030
39. Luther K, Torosantucci A, Brakhage AA, Heesemann J, Ebel F. Phagocytosis of *Aspergillus fumigatus* conidia by murine macrophages involves recognition by the dectin-1 beta-glucan receptor and toll-like receptor 2. *Cell Microbiol* (2007) 9:368–81. doi:10.1111/j.1462-5822.2006.00796.x
40. Wellington M, Koselny K, Krysan DJ. *Candida albicans* morphogenesis is not required for macrophage interleukin 1β production. *MBio* (2012) 4:e00433-12. doi:10.1128/mBio.00433-12
41. Wellington M, Koselny K, Sutterwala FS, Krysan DJ. *Candida albicans* triggers NLRP3-mediated pyroptosis in macrophages. *Eukaryot Cell* (2014) 13:329–40. doi:10.1128/EC.00336-13
42. Hise AG, Tomalka J, Ganesan S, Patel K, Hall BA, Brown GD, et al. An essential role for the NLRP3 inflammasome in host defense against the human fungal pathogen *Candida albicans*. *Cell Host Microbe* (2009) 5:487–97. doi:10.1016/j.chom.2009.05.002
43. Bauernfeind F, Rieger A, Schildberg FA, Knolle A, Schmid-burgk JL, Hornung V, et al. NLRP3 inflammasome activity is negatively controlled by miR-223. *J Immunol* (2012) 189:4175–81. doi:10.4049/jimmunol.1201516
44. He Y, Franchi L, Núñez G. TLR agonists stimulate Nlrp3-dependent IL-1β production independently of the purinergic P2X7 receptor in dendritic cells and in vivo. *J Immunol* (2013) 190:334–9. doi:10.4049/jimmunol.1202737
45. Guarda G, Zenger M, Yazdi AS, Ferrero I, Menu P, Tardivel A, et al. Differential expression of NLRP3 among hematopoietic cells. *J Immunol* (2011) 186:2529–34. doi:10.4049/jimmunol.1002720
46. Hardison SE, Brown GD. C-type lectin receptors orchestrate anti-fungal immunity. *Nat Immunol* (2012) 13:817–22. doi:10.1038/ni.2369
47. Mao L, Zhang L, Li H, Chen W, Wang H, Wu S, et al. Pathogenic fungus *Microsporum canis* activates the NLRP3 inflammasome. *Infect Immun* (2014) 82:882–92. doi:10.1128/IAI.01097-13
48. Kistowska M, Fenini G, Jankovic D, Feldmeyer L, Kerl K, Bosshard P, et al. Malassezia yeasts activate the NLRP3 inflammasome in antigen-presenting cells via Syk-kinase signalling. *Exp Dermatol* (2014) 23:884–9. doi:10.1111/exd.12552
49. Saijo S, Ikeda S, Yamabe K, Kakuta S, Ishigame H, Akitsu A, et al. Dectin-2 recognition of α-mannans and induction of Th17 cell differentiation is essential for host defense against *Candida albicans*. *Immunity* (2010) 32:681–91. doi:10.1016/j.immuni.2010.05.001
50. Yoshikawa FSY, Yabe R, Iwakura Y, De Almeida SR, Saijo S. Dectin-1 and dectin-2 promote control of the fungal pathogen *Trichophyton rubrum* independently of IL-17 and adaptive immunity in experimental deep dermatophytosis. *Innate Immun* (2016) 22:316–24. doi:10.1177/1753425916645392
51. Dong B, Li D, Li R, Chen SC, Liu W, Liu W, et al. A chitin-like component on sclerotic cells of *Fonsecaea pedrosoi* inhibits dectin-1-mediated murine Th17 development by masking β-glucans. *PLoS One* (2014) 9:e114113. doi:10.1371/journal.pone.0114113
52. Wang H, Li M, Lerksuthirat T, Klein B. The C-type lectin receptor MCL mediates vaccine-induced immunity against infection with *Blastomyces dermatitidis*. *Infect Immun* (2016) 84:635–42. doi:10.1128/IAI.01263-15
53. Gantner BN, Simmons RM, Canavera SJ, Akira S, Underhill DM. Collaborative induction of inflammatory responses by dectin-1 and toll-like receptor 2. *J Exp Med* (2003) 197:1107–17. doi:10.1084/jem.20021787
54. Van De Veerdonk FL, Joosten LAB, Netea MG. The interplay between inflammasome activation and antifungal host defense. *Immunol Rev* (2015) 265:172–80. doi:10.1111/imr.12280
55. Tomalka J, Ganesan S, Azodi E, Patel K, Majmudar P, Hall BA, et al. A novel role for the NLRC4 inflammasome in mucosal defenses against the fungal pathogen *Candida albicans*. *PLoS Pathog* (2011) 7:e1002379. doi:10.1371/journal.ppat.1002379
56. Kalantari P, Deoliveira RB, Chan J, Corbett Y, Rathinam V, Stutz A, et al. Dual engagement of the NLRP3 and AIM2 inflammasomes by plasmodium-derived hemozoin and DNA during malaria. *Cell Rep* (2013) 6:196–210. doi:10.1016/j.celrep.2013.12.014
57. Li H, Wu S, Mao L, Lei G, Zhang L, Lu A, et al. Human pathogenic fungus *Trichophyton schoenleinii* activates the NLRP3 inflammasome. *Protein Cell* (2013) 4:529–38. doi:10.1007/s13238-013-2127-9
58. Muñoz-Planillo R, Kuffa P, Martínez-Cólon G, Smith BL, Rajendiran TM, Kuffa P, et al. K+ efflux is the common trigger of NLRP3 inflammasome activation by bacterial toxins and particulate matter. *Immunity* (2013) 38:1142–53. doi:10.1016/j.immuni.2013.05.016
59. Bauernfeind F, Bartok E, Rieger A, Franchi L, Núñez G, Hornung V. Cutting edge: reactive oxygen species inhibitors block priming, but not activation, of the NLRP3 inflammasome. *J Immunol* (2011) 187:613–7. doi:10.4049/jimmunol.1100613
60. Ketelut-Carneiro N, Silva GK, Rocha FA, Milanezi CM, Cavalcanti-Neto FF, Zamboni DS, et al. IL-18 triggered by the Nlrp3 inflammasome induces host innate resistance in a pulmonary model of fungal infection. *J Immunol* (2015) 194:4507–17. doi:10.4049/jimmunol.1402321
61. Walter P, Garin Y, Richard-Lenoble D. Chromoblastomycosis. A morphological investigation of the host-parasite interaction. *Virchows Arch A Pathol Anat Histol* (1982) 397:203–14. doi:10.1007/BF00442390
62. Rozental S, Alviano CS, de Souza W. The in vitro susceptibility of *Fonsecaea pedrosoi* to activated macrophages. *Mycopathologia* (1994) 126:85–91. doi:10.1007/BF01146200
63. Rozental S, Alviano CS, de Souza W. Fine structure and cytochemical study of the interaction between *Fonsecaea pedrosoi* and rat polymorphonuclear leukocyte. *J Med Vet Mycol* (1996) 34:323–30. doi:10.1080/02681219680000551
64. Farbiarz SR, de Carvalho TU, Alviano C, De Souza W. Fine structure and cytochemistry of the interaction between *Fonsecaea pedrosoi* and mouse resident macrophages. *J Med Vet Mycol* (1990) 28:373–83. doi:10.1080/02681219080000481
65. Hayakawa M, Ghosn EEB, da Gloria Teixeria de Sousa M, Ferreira KS, Almeida SR. Phagocytosis, production of nitric oxide and pro-inflammatory cytokines by macrophages in the presence of dematiaceous [correction of dematiaceus] fungi that cause chromoblastomycosis. *Scand J Immunol* (2006) 64:382–7. doi:10.1111/j.1365-3083.2006.01804.x
66. Bocca AL, Brito PPMS, Figueiredo F, Tosta CE. Inhibition of nitric oxide production by macrophages in chromoblastomycosis: a role for *Fonsecaea pedrosoi* melanin. *Mycopathologia* (2006) 161:195–203. doi:10.1007/s11046-005-0228-6
67. Ahrens J, Graybill JR, Abishawl A, Tio FO, Rinaldi MG. Experimental murine chromomycosis mimicking chronic progressive human disease. *Am J Trop Med Hyg* (1989) 40:651–8. doi:10.4269/ajtmh.1989.40.651
68. Netea MG, Joosten LAB. Inflammasome inhibition: putting out the fire. *Cell Metab* (2015) 21:513–4. doi:10.1016/j.cmet.2015.03.012
69. Vonk AG, Netea MG, Van Krieken JH, Iwakura Y, Van Der Meer JWM, Kullberg BJ. Endogenous interleukin (IL)-1α and IL-1β are crucial for host defense against disseminated candidiasis. *J Infect Dis* (2006) 193:1419–26. doi:10.1086/503363

2

Leucine-Rich Repeat Kinase 2 Controls the Ca^{2+}/Nuclear Factor of Activated T Cells/IL-2 Pathway during *Aspergillus* Non-Canonical Autophagy in Dendritic Cells

*Alicia Yoke Wei Wong[1,2], Vasilis Oikonomou[3], Giuseppe Paolicelli[3], Antonella De Luca[3], Marilena Pariano[3], Jan Fric[1,4], Hock Soon Tay[1], Paola Ricciardi-Castagnoli[1,5] and Teresa Zelante[1,3]**

[1]Singapore Immunology Network, Agency for Science, Technology and Research, Singapore, Singapore, [2]National University of Singapore Graduate School for Integrative Sciences and Engineering, National University of Singapore, Singapore, Singapore, [3]Department of Experimental Medicine, University of Perugia, Perugia, Italy, [4]Center for Translational Medicine (CTM), International Clinical Research Center (ICRC), St. Anne's University Hospital Brno, Brno, Czechia, [5]Toscana Life Sciences Foundation, Siena, Italy

***Correspondence:**
Teresa Zelante
teresa.zelante@unipg.it

The Parkinson's disease-associated protein, Leucine-rich repeat kinase 2 (LRRK2), a known negative regulator of nuclear factor of activated T cells (NFAT), is expressed in myeloid cells such as macrophages and dendritic cells (DCs) and is involved in the host immune response against pathogens. Since, the Ca^{2+}/NFAT/IL-2 axis has been previously found to regulate DC response to the fungus *Aspergillus*, we have investigated the role played by the kinase LRRK2 during fungal infection. Mechanistically, we found that in the early stages of the non-canonical autophagic response of DCs to the germinated spores of *Aspergillus*, LRRK2 undergoes progressive degradation and regulates NFAT translocation from the cytoplasm to the nucleus. Our results shed new light on the complexity of the Ca^{2+}/NFAT/IL-2 pathway, where LRRK2 plays a role in controlling the immune response of DCs to *Aspergillus*.

Keywords: leucine-rich repeat kinase 2, nuclear factor of activated T cells, NRON, dendritic cell, *Aspergillus*, autophagy

INTRODUCTION

Leucine-rich repeat kinase 2 (LRRK2) was first discovered in genome-wide linkage studies of patients of Parkinson's disease (1, 2). Since then, the majority of studies on LRRK2 have been focused on linking various point mutations in the various domains of LRRK2 with Parkinson's disease (3), and the contribution of mutated LRRK2 protein to neuronal toxicity (4–6). Studies have also shown a possible involvement of the immune system in Parkinson's disease pathogenesis. Inflammation is thought to lead to the neurodegeneration and neurotoxicity seen in Parkinson's disease (7, 8). Also, it is known that patients of Parkinson's disease are often hospitalized for various types of infections, such as urinary tract infection and pneumonia (9). The involvement of LRRK2 in response to inflammatory stimulus (10), as well as microbes, and pathogen-associated molecular patterns (PAMPs) (11–14), have also been seen in several studies.

Leucine-rich repeat kinase 2 has been reported to negatively regulate the nuclear factor of activated T cells (NFAT) pathway in bone marrow-derived macrophages (BMDMs) *via* the NRON complex. LRRK2 was found to bind 5 of the 11 proteins associated with the NRON complex, and overexpression of LRRK2 increases binding of NFAT with NRON complex members, in particular IQGAP, chromosome segregation 1-like (CSE1L), and transportin-1 (15). This regulation of NFAT by LRRK2 was found to be independent of its kinase function. Given the importance of the NFAT pathway in the regulation of T cell development and function [as reviewed in Ref. (16)], it is of notice that LRRK2 expression is lower in T cells than in BMDMs and bone marrow-derived dendritic cells (BMDCs) (15), underlining a possible role of LRRK2 in innate immunity during infection as supported by other studies (10, 17).

It has been established that the Ca^{2+}/NFAT/IL-2 pathway is activated in DCs in response to live *Candida albicans* and zymosan binding to Dectin-1 leading to the production of cytokines, including IL-2 (18). To this end, we have also shown that NFAT signaling regulates cytokine IL-2 expression in DCs stimulated *in vitro* with *Saccharomyces cereviseae*-derived whole glucan particles (19), and that DC-derived IL-2 expression in lung $CD103^+$ DCs is important for eliciting the appropriate Th17 cell response to *Aspergillus fumigatus* infection (20). In this study, we report that LRRK2 localizes to lysosomic and endosomic structures in DCs at steady state, as well as after *Aspergillus* exposure, and that autophagy is able to influence LRRK2 expression, and subsequently, the activation of Ca^{2+}/NFAT/IL-2 axis in DCs differently from the other NRON complex components. In conclusion, our findings suggest a role for LRRK2 and the NRON complex in the early phases of the immune response to *Aspergillus*.

MATERIALS AND METHODS

Mice

Eight-week-old wild-type C57BL/6 mice used for experiments were bred and kept under specific pathogen-free conditions in the Biomedical Resource Centre, Singapore. All experiments and procedures were approved by the Institutional Animal Care and Use Committee (IACUC) of A*STAR (Biopolis, Singapore) (Authorization No.: IACUC 110626) in accordance with the guidelines of the Agri-Food and Veterinary Authority (AVA) and the National Advisory Committee for Laboratory Animal Research (NACLAR) of Singapore. Z. Liu of Institute of Biophysics Chinese Academy of Sciences provided LRRK2 $^{-/-}$ mice bone marrows.

Fungal Cells

Aspergillus fumigatus isolate AF293 (MYA-4609, ATCC, Manassas, VA, USA) was used for cultures. *A. fumigatus* was cultivated for 5 days on potato dextrose agar (Sigma-Aldrich, St. Louis, MO, USA) before conidia were harvested by washing with PBS 0.05% Tween 20. Swollen conidia were obtained by incubating conidia in liquid yeast extract peptone dextrose at 37°C for 4 h on a rotary shaker at 300 rpm. In addition, a red fluorescent protein (RFP)-expressing *A. fumigatus* AF293 strain used in this study was obtained from Prof. Eric Pearlman (Case Western Reserve University, Cleaveland, OH, USA).

Cell Cultures

Bone marrow-derived dendritic cells were generated by culturing mouse bone marrow extracted by flushing the femurs and tibias. The collected bone marrow was treated with ammonium-chloride-potassium lysing buffer. The remaining cells post-lysis were cultured in suspension plates with Iscove's Modified Dulbeccos Medium (IMDM) (HyClone, Thermo Fisher Scientific, Waltham, MA, USA) containing 10% fetal bovine serum (FBS) (Euroclone, Milan, Italy), 2 mM L-glutamine (Gibco, Life Technologies, Carlsbad, CA, USA), 100 U/mL Penicillin/Streptomycin (Gibco, Life Technologies, Carlsbad, CA, USA), supplemented with 10% supernatant from a GM-CSF-producing B16 melanoma cell line to a final concentration of 20 ng/mL GM-CSF to generate BMDCs.

The long-term GM-CSF cytokine-dependent DC cell line, D1 (21), was grown in suspension plates with IMDM containing 10% FBS (Australian origin, Gibco, Life Technologies, Carlsbad, CA, USA) 2 mM L-glutamine, 100 U/mL Penicillin/Streptomycin, and 55 μM β-mercaptoethanol (Gibco, Life Technologies, Carlsbad, CA, USA), supplemented with 30% supernatant from NIH/3T3 cells transfected to produce GM-CSF to a final concentration of 10 ng/mL.

In all stimulation experiments, cells were stimulated with *A. fumigatus* swollen conidia in a 1:10 (fungi:cell) ratio. Pharmaceuticals used in these experiments include 3-methyladenine (3MA) (Sigma-Aldrich, St. Louis, MO, USA), Bafilomycin A (Baf) from *Streptomyces griseus* (Calbiochem, Merck Millipore, Billerica, MA, USA), Cytochalasin D (CytoD) (Sigma-Aldrich, St. Louis, MO, USA), leupeptin hemisulfate (Sigma-Aldrich, St. Louis, MO, USA), and ammonium chloride (Leu/A) (Sigma-Aldrich, St. Louis, MO, USA).

NFAT Nuclear Translocation

D1 nuclear factor of activated T cells translocation-firefly luciferase reporter cells were generated by transducing the D1 cells with Cignal Lenti NFAT Reporter with firefly luciferase (SABiosciences, Qiagen, Venlo, Limburg, Netherlands). NFAT nuclear translocation was detected by ONE-Glo™ Luciferase assay System (Promega, Madison, WI, USA) and the luminescence signal quantified with the GloMax®-Multi Detection System Luminometer module (Promega, Madison, WI, USA).

shRNA Knockdown

MISSION® Lentiviral Particles (Sigma-Aldrich, St. Louis, MO, USA) with the pLKO.1-puro vector containing shRNA sequences targeting NRON, CSE1L, sperm-associated antigen 9 (SPAG9), LRRK2 shRNA, PPP2R1A were used.

Below details includes the gene reference identification number (NM ID) and The RNAi Consortium (TRC) clone identification number (clone ID) for the shRNA-lentiviral particles for targeting these genes (**Table 1**).

NRON shRNA lentiviral particles were custom designed and packaged into lentiviral particles (ACGGTGGGTTTATGACAAATT and ACGGGTGCTGGATGACATATT) by Sigma-Aldrich

TABLE 1 | Details of commercially purchased MISSION® lentiviral particles.

Gene target	NM ID	The RNAi Consortium (TRC) clone ID
Chromosome segregation 1-like	NM_023565	TRCN0000174506 TRCN0000174691
Sperm-associated antigen 9	NM_027569	TRCN0000176696 TRCN0000177089
Ppp2r1a	NM_016891	TRCN0000012624 TRCN0000012626
Leucine-rich repeat kinase 2	NM_025730	TRCN0000022656 TRCN0000022657

(St. Louis, MO, USA). MISSION® pLKO.1-puro non-target shRNA control transduction particles (Sigma-Aldrich, St. Louis, MO, USA) were used as a transduction control.

For the transduction, D1 cells were seeded and rested overnight in antibiotic-free D1 medium. The next day, the medium was replaced with antibiotic-free D1 medium containing 2 µg/mL SureEntry™ transduction reagent (SABiosciences, Qiagen, Venlo, Limburg, Netherlands). The D1 cells were then transduced with MISSION® lentiviral particles at multiplicity of infection (MOI) 10 and allowed to incubate for 20 h at 37°C in 5% CO_2. After 20 h incubation, the medium containing the lentivirus particles was aspirated out, replaced with complete D1 medium, and allowed to rest for 48 h at 37°C in 5% CO_2. After being allowed to rest, successfully transduced cells were selected 4 days by replacing the medium with D1 medium containing 0.5 µg/mL of puromycin dihydrochloride (Calbiochem, Merck Millipore, Billerica, MA, USA).

For *in vitro* silencing of *Rubcn*, *Nox2*, and *Atg7*, D1 were transfected with 40 nM of the following siRNAs: *Rubcn* (Duplex name mm.Ri.1700021K19Rik.13.1; sense, 5′-GUACUUGACC GCUAGUAAAAUCATT-3′; antisense, 5′-GACAUGAACUGGC GAUCAUUUUAGUAA-3′), Nox2 (Duplex name mm.Ri.Cybb.13.1; sense, 5′-GUUCAAGGUCAGUUUAUUGAAUGAA-3′; antisense, 5′-CACAAGUUCCAGUCAAAUAACUUACUU-3′), Atg7 (Duplex name mm.Ri.Atg7.13.1; sense, 5′CUUGAUCAGUACGAGCGA GAAGGAT-3′; antisense, 5′-AAGAACUAGUCAUGCUCGCU CUUCCUA-3′) (all from IDT). Silencing was performed using TransIT-TKO® Transfection Reagent (Mirus) and incubated for 24 h (as indicated by preliminary experiments performed at 12, 24, or 48 h) at 37°C in 5% CO_2. Transfected cells were exposed to A-sw.

Cytotoxicity Assay

The sensitivity of cells to different inhibitors was determined by 3-(4,5-dimethylthiazol-2-yl)-2,5-diphenyltetrazolium bromide (MTT; Trevigen) assay. Briefly, 2,500 D1 cells were seeded in 180 µL medium in quadruplicate in 96-well tissue culture plates and following overnight incubation with A-sw in a 1:10 (fungi:cell) ratio with or without inhibitors. After 24 h MTT was added and the absorbance of the formazan product was measured on a microplate reader TECAN infinite m200 together with the i-control™ software (Mannedorf, Switzerland) at 600 nm.

Lysosome Isolation

Lysosomes were isolated from D1 cells as described by Graham (22). Briefly, D1 cells were harvested from suspension plates and washed with PBS. The cell pellet was then resuspended in ice cold homogenization medium (0.25 M sucrose, 1 mM EDTA, 10 mM HEPES, pH 7) and homogenized in a Wheaton type Dounce tissue grinder (Wheaton, Millville, NJ, USA) on ice until above 90% cell breakage was observed under the microscope by staining with PBS containing 0.04% v/v Tryphan blue (Sigma-Aldrich, St. Louis, MO, USA). The homogenate was then centrifuged at 800 *g* for 10 min to pellet nuclei and cell debris. The resulting supernatant from the centrifuge was mixed with bovine serum albumin (final proportion of 4% v/v) and Percoll (final proportion of 22% v/v). The mixture was then ultracentrifuged for 30 min at 36,000 × *g* without brake activation. After centrifugation, a visible band of the enriched lysosomes was seen near the bottom of the tube. 400 µL fractions, containing the enriched lysosomes were collected, and Igepal CA-630 (final proportion of 0.5% v/v) was used to solubilize the lysosome membranes. Solubilized fractions were centrifuged at 100,000 × *g* for 2 h to pellet the Percoll, and the resulting supernatants were obtained for analysis by western blotting.

Cytokine Detection

Cell culture medium was assayed for cytokine production by sandwich enzyme-linked immunosorbent assay (ELISA) for IL-2, IL-12/IL-23p40, and IL-23. IL-2 and IL-12/IL-23p40 were assayed using commercially available antibody pairs and standards from BioLegend (San Diego, CA, USA) and eBioscience (San Diego, CA, USA), respectively. Measurements were detected using the TECAN infinite m200 together with the i-control™ software (Mannedorf, Switzerland; measurement wavelength 450 nm, reference wavelength 570 nm). IL-23 was assayed using mouse IL-23 ELISA Ready-SET-Go!® (Second-generation assay) (Affymetric eBioscience, San Diego, CA, USA) according to manufacturer's instructions. In addition, selected supernatant samples were analyzed using the Milliplex Multi Analyte Panels Mouse TH17 Magnetic Bead Panel Immunology Multiplex assay (MTH17MAG-47K) in conjunction with the Luminex MAGPIX® system (Merck Millipore, Billerica, MA, USA).

Western Blot

Whole cell lysates were obtained by lysing cells in radioimmunoprecipitation assay buffer containing 1× cOmplete, EDTA-free Protease Inhibitor Cocktail (Roche, Basel, Switzerland), 1× PhosSTOP Phosphatase Inhibitor Cocktail (Roche, Basel, Switzerland), and 1 mM phenylmethanesulfonylfluoride. The protein concentration in the cell lysates were measured using the Pierce™ 660 nm Protein assay kit (Thermo Scientific, Waltham, MA, USA), and colorimetric readings were obtained by measuring the wavelength at 660 nm using the TECAN infinite m200 together with the i-control™ software (Mannedorf, Switzerland). Protein lysates were diluted with Laemmli buffer containing 2.5% v/v β-mercaptoethanol (Sigma-Aldrich, St. Louis, MO, USA) and heated at 95°C for 10 min prior to separation on sodium dodecyl sulfate (SDS)-polyacrylamide gel electrophoresis (PAGE) in

Tris-glycine-SDS buffer, along side the Precision Plus Protein Dual Color standards protein ladder (Bio-Rad, Hercules, CA, USA). Up to 50 μg of protein was loaded into each well for separation. The SDS-PAGE gel was run at 60 V till all samples entered the resolving gel, before increasing the running voltage to 110 V until the dye front had traveled to the end of the gel. The separated proteins were then transferred to polyvinylidene fluoride membrane in Tris-glycine buffer containing 10% v/v methanol at either 240 mA for 2 h or 200 mA for 4 h. For LRRK2, lysates were first concentrated using the Vivaspin 500 molecular weight cut off 100,000 columns (Sartorius, Goettingen, Germany), and the NuPAGE® large protein analysis system (Life Technologies, Carlsbad, CA, USA) was adopted. Antibodies used for western blot include: LRRK2 rabbit monoclonal antibody, clone: MJFF2 (Epitomics, Abcam, Cambridge, UK), LC3B antibody (cell Signaling Technology, Danvers, MA, USA), Purified anti-mouse CD107a (LAMP-1), clone: 1D4B (Biolegend, San Diego, CA, USA), anti-TATA binding protein (TBP), clone: 1TBP18 (Abcam, Cambridge, UK), Rab5 (C8B1) Rabbit mAb (cell Signaling Technology, Danvers, MA, USA), JIP4/SPAG9 (D72F4) XP® Rabbit mAb (cell Signaling Technology, Danvers, MA, USA), Anti-PPP2R1A antibody [6F9] (Abcam, Cambridge, UK), GAPDH antibody, clone: 6C5 (Merck Millipore, Billerica, MA, USA), DAPK1 mouse polyclonal antibody, clone: RB3033 (antibodies-online.com). For DAPK1, normalization was performed by probing the membrane with mouse monoclonal β-actin antibody, clone: AC-40 (Sigma-Aldrich). Band pixel density was analyzed from the film scans by ImageJ software (NIH, Bethesda, MD, USA).

RNA Extraction, Real-time Quantitative PCR

Cells were lysed with 1 mL of TRIzol® reagent (Ambion, Life Technologies, Carlsbad, CA, USA) and flash frozen on dry ice prior to storage at −80°C. To extract RNA, 200 μL (20% v/v) of chloroform (Merck, Kenilworth, NJ, USA) was added to each sample. Each sample was then shaken vigorously, and then centrifuged at 15,000 rpm, 4°C for 15 min. This separated the sample into a top organic phase containing the RNA, a thin interface containing DNA and a bottom organic phase containing protein. The top supernatant was aspirated and transferred to a new tube. An equal volume of 70% v/v ethanol was added and mixed to the sample. RNA was extracted from this mixture using the RNeasy mini kit (Qiagen, Venlo, Limburg, Netherlands) according to the manufacturer's instructions. Extracted RNA samples were then treated with DNase using the TURBO DNA-free™ kit (Ambion, Life Technologies, Carlsbad, CA, USA) according to manufacturer's instructions. The RNA content of each sample was then quantified using the Nanodrop™ 1000 (Thermo Scientific, Waltham, MA, USA). 2 μg of RNA was retro-transcribed into cDNA using the High Capacity Reverse Transcription Kit (Applied Biosystems, Life Technologies, Carlsbad, CA, USA) according to manufacturer's instruction. The obtained cDNA was then used for real-time quantitative PCR. The Brilliant SYBR® Green QPCR Mastermix and Reference Dye (Stratagene, Agilent Technologies, Santa Clara, CA, USA) was used to set up the real-time quantitative PCR reaction, and the samples were run in the MX3000P instrument (Stratagene, Agilent Technologies, Santa Clara, CA, USA). Gene expression data was analyzed using the MxPro QPCR software (Stratagene, Agilent Technologies, Santa Clara, CA, USA). Primer sequences targeting mouse genes used in this study are listed in **Table 2**.

Immunofluorescence Confocal Microscopy

D1 cells were seeded and stimulated in μ-slide 8-well chambers (Ibidi, Martinsried, Germany). Post-stimulation cells were fixed in 2% paraformaldehyde (Sigma-Aldrich, St. Louis, MO, USA), and permeabilized in PBS containing 0.1% saponin (Sigma-Aldrich, St. Louis, MO, USA), 0.2% gelatin (Fluka Analytical, Sigma-Aldrich, St. Louis, MO, USA), and 5% bovine serum albumin (Merck Millipore, Darmstadt, Germany). Cells were stained and washed using PBS containing 0.01% saponin and 0.2% gelatin. Cells were stained with a primary LC3B antibody (Cell Signaling Technology, Danvers, MA, USA) and a secondary goat α-rabbit IgG antibody conjugated to Alexa Fluor® 488 (Invitrogen, Life Technologies, Carlsbad, CA, USA). In addition, 4',6-diamidino-2-phenylindole (Invitrogen, Life Technologies, Carlsbad, CA, USA) was used to stain the cell nuclei. Images were acquired on an Olympus FV1000 confocal microscope in conjunction with the Fluorview FV1000 software (Olympus, Tokyo, Japan).

For DAPK1 staining, DAPK1 mouse polyclonal antibody, clone: RB3033 (antibodies-online.com) and Alexa Fluor® 488 phalloidin was used for selective labeling of F-actin. After overnight staining with primary antibody, slides were washed and incubated with Rabbit IgG-TRITC antibody (Sigma-Aldrich).

TABLE 2 | List of real-time quantitative PCR primers.

Gene	Forward primer (5′–3′)	Reverse primer (5′–3′)
Chromosome segregation 1-like	GTGGGAAAGGACAGGAAACA	AAACCTTGGTGATCGTTTGC
Gapdh	TTGAGGTCAATGAAGGGGTC	TCGTCCCGTAGACAAAATGG
Leucine-rich repeat kinase 2	GATGTCAGTACGCCCCTGAT	CTGCCAGCGCTATGATGTTA
Nron	CAGTAAAGGAGCAGTAGTGGAAACAG	TGGGGGGAGCGAATGGCATCGGGAAC
Ppp2r1a	CAACCTGGATTGGTGGAACG	GATCCACTAGCCAGGCCATA
Sperm-associated antigen 9	AAACCTCAGGGACTCCAGGT	CCCCACCACTGCTACTTTGT
Rubcn	GUACUUGACCGCUAGUAAAAUCATT	GACAUGAACUGGCGAUCAUUUUAGUAA
Atg7	CUUGAUCAGUACGAGCGAGAAGGAT	AAGAACUAGUCAUGCUCGCUCUUCCUA
Nox2	GUUCAAGGUCAGUUUAUUGAAUGAA	CACAAGUUCCAGUCAAAUAACUUACUU
Dapk1	CGAGUUUGGAUAUGACAAGGAUACA	UGUAUCCUUGUCAUAUCCAAACUCGCC

Images were acquired using a Zeiss Axio Observer. Z1 inverted microscope, equipped with Apotome filter and Axiocam MRm camera detection system Zeiss using a 63×/1.25 oil Plan/neofluar objective.

Transmission Electron Microscopy

Stimulated D1 cells were harvested from the suspension plate with 2 mM EDTA in PBS and washed with 0.2 M sodium cacodylate buffer (pH 7.4). Cells were then fixed in cacodylate fixative buffer (0.1 M sodium cacodylate, 2% paraformaldehyde, and 3% gluteraldehyde) overnight at 4°C. The cells were then washed with 0.2 M sodium cacodylate buffer and dehydrated on an alcohol series (30, 50, 70, 80, 90, and 100%) for 15 min each. Specimens were then embedded into acrylic resin. Ultrafine sections were obtained by cutting into the resin specimens with a glass blade on an ultramicrotome, and mounted on nickel grids. The grids were then washed with PBS and then stained with antibodies LRRK2 rabbit monoclonal antibody clone: MJFF2 (Epitomics, Abcam, Cambridge, UK) and purified anti-mouse CD107a (LAMP-1) clone: 1D4B (Biolegend, San Diego, CA, USA), followed by secondary antibodies that have been conjugated with either 5 or 15 nm gold particles (Cytodiagnostics, Burlington, ON, Canada). All antibody incubations were done in PBS containing 1% bovine serum albumin. After antibody staining, grids were post-fixed with cacodylate fixative buffer for 15 min, and then stained with 2% uranyl acetate. Micrographs were taken with an EM 208 transmission electron microscope (Phillips, Amsterdam, Netherlands).

Graphs and Statistics

Statistical significance of experiments was determined either by Student's *t*-test, one-way ANOVA, or two-way ANOVA as indicated. For statistics generated by one-way ANOVA, the differences between individual groups were compared using the Bonferroni's Multiple Comparison post-test. All graphs and statistics were generated using the Graphpad Prism® software version 6.0 (Graphpad Software, La Jolla, CA, USA).

Flow Cytometry Analysis

At 16 h post-silencing, BMDCs were treated with *Aspergillus* RFP swollen conidia (ratio of 1:1) for 1 h. BMDCs were collected, washed twice with FACS buffer, stained with CD11c-Alexa Fluor 700® (BD) and analyzed by flow cytometry. Data (mean ± SD) represent three independent experiments in which technical triplicates of 100,000 cells per sample were acquired using a Fortessa cytometer (BD). Phagocytosis was calculated using flow cytometry analysis (described above). The percentage of phagocytosis equals the number of BMDCs that have engulfed RFP *A. fumigatus*.

Time Lapse Video

Bone marrow-derived dendritic cells grown in 48-well plates were exposed with shRNA RUBICON or scramble overnight. Cells were then treated with *Aspergillus* swollen conidia for 1 h. Time-lapse imaging was performed over a period of 1 h with a 40× objective using the time-lapse function of the EVOS FL Auto Imaging System with the Invitrogen™ EVOS™ Onstage Incubator.

RESULTS

LRRK2 Is Expressed in DCs and Is Regulated during *A. fumigatus* Infection

Leucine-rich repeat kinase 2 is known to regulate NFAT translocation in response to TLR ligands (15). Since, we have previously shown that *A. fumigatus* swollen conidia, more than ungerminated conidia, induces Ca^{2+}/NFAT/IL-2 pathway in DCs (20), here we went to study the regulation of LRRK2 in response to fungal infection. First, we measured LRRK2 expression at the mRNA and protein level in D1 cells at resting state as well as in D1 cells stimulated with swollen conidia. We found that at resting state, DCs express LRRK2 on both the mRNA (**Figure 1A**) and the protein level (**Figure 1B**). Upon stimulation with swollen conidia, LRRK2 levels were found to be downregulated on both the mRNA as well as the protein level. At 8 h post-stimulation, downregulation of LRRK2 on the gene level was found to be statistically significant, while LRRK2 protein levels decreased further significantly (8 h 0.217 ± 0.1). The downregulation of LRRK2 was further maintained on protein level at 18 h (0.373 ± 0.2), and on gene expression at 24 h post-stimulation, showing that *Aspergillus* is able to influence *Lrrk2* gene expression on both transcriptional and translational level. Interestingly, the downregulation of LRRK2 in DCs responding to *Aspergillus* swollen conidia corresponded to the upregulation of NFAT1 translocation (Figure S1A in Supplementary Material) and IL-2 production (Figure S1B in Supplementary Material).

LRRK2 Intracellular Localization

It has been reported that LRRK2 is degraded in lysosomes (23). In order to understand the subcellular localization of LRRK2 in DCs, lysosomes and early endosomes were enriched from D1 cells by gradient centrifugation protocol (22), and the protein content of the fractions enriched with these organelles were analyzed by western blot (**Figure 2A**). Fraction (lane 1) was harvested and further centrifuged (lane 2), which was negative for the nuclear marker, TBP, indicating that there was no contamination with nuclear material. We found that LRRK2 was present in fractions that expressed lysosomal-associated membrane protein 1 (LAMP-1) and Rab5, which are markers for lysosomes and early endosomes, respectively. This is in line with what was already reported (24, 25). In addition, by electron microscopy, lysosomes were LAMP-1 positive, spherical, enclosed by one membrane, with a diameter of 70–150 nm, homogenous and electron-dense interior. Endosomes were LAMP-1 negative and poorly electron-dense (**Figure 2B**). Interestingly, LRRK2 (**Figure 2C**) was found localized also on endosomic structures. In addition, as endosomes have been proposed to be signaling hubs, where components of signaling pathways can localize and interact (26), the localization of LRRK2 on endosomes implies that the endosomes serve as a possible niche were NFAT signaling pathway is kept under control.

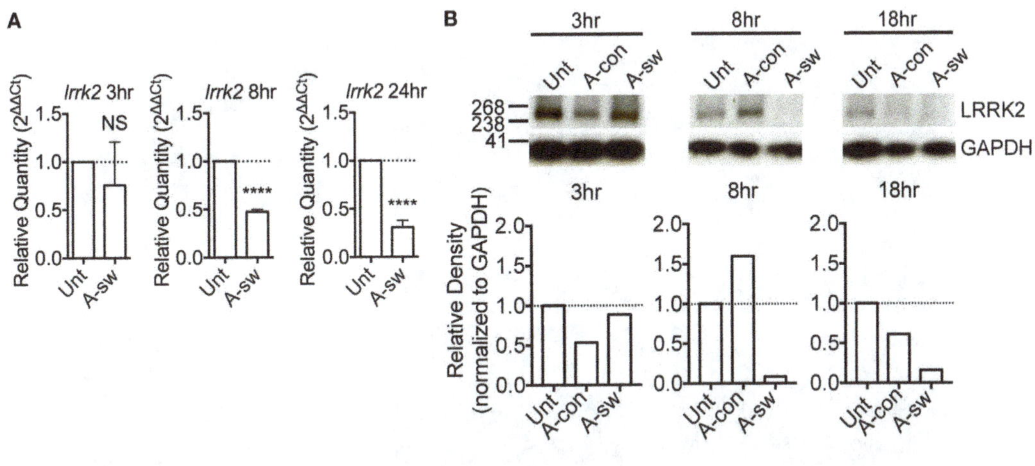

FIGURE 1 | Leucine-rich repeat kinase 2 (LRRK2) is expressed in dendritic cells and is downregulated by *Aspergillus fumigatus*. **(A)** LRRK2 mRNA in D1 cells. Data is displayed as the mean gene expression ± SD of two biological replicates and normalized to the housekeeping protein, GAPDH. Differences found to be statistically significant by one-way ANOVA with Bonferonni's Multiple Comparison post-test are indicated (NS, non-significant; ****, $p < 0.0001$). **(B)** Protein expression level of LRRK2 in whole cell lysates of D1 cells stimulated with *A. fumigatus* condia and swollen conidia. For densitometry analysis, band densities for LRRK2 were normalized to the band density of the housekeeping protein, GAPDH, after which the density of the LRRK2 band of the treated sample was compared with that of the untreated sample. Data is representative of three independent experiments. Abbreviations used: Untreated (Unt); *A. fumigatus* conidia (A-con); *A. fumigatus swollen conidia* (A-sw).

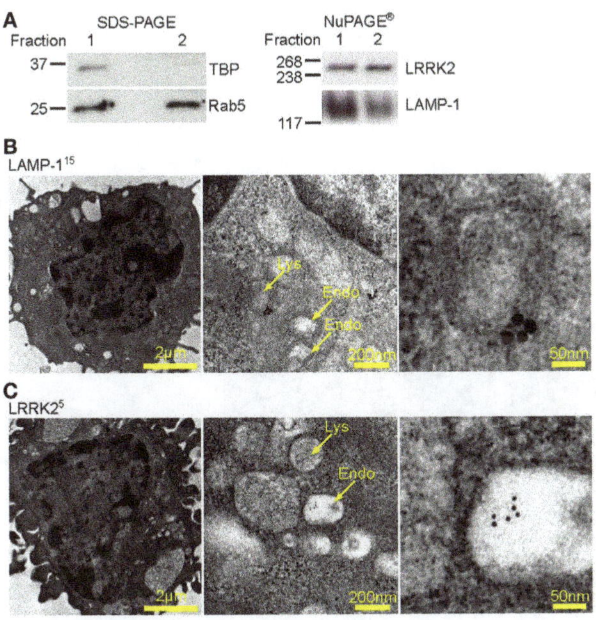

FIGURE 2 | Leucine-rich repeat kinase 2 (LRRK2) is localized on lysosomes and endosomes of dendritic cells. **(A)** Western blot analysis of presence of TATA binding protein, Rab5, LRRK2, and LAMP-1 in a representative protein fraction obtained from the enrichment of lysosomes from D1 cells. Lysate from the protein fraction was run on both sodium dodecyl sulfate-polyacrylamide gel electrophoresis (PAGE) and NuPAGE® to probe for the proteins indicated. Data are representative of three independent experiments **(B–C)**, D1 cells were processed for immune-electron microscopy, stained for LAMP-1 or LRRK2, and labeled with appropriate secondary antibodies conjugated with 5 or 15 nm gold particles (size of particles indicated in superscript). Lysosomic and endosomic structures are as indicated. Electron micrographs of D1 cells show LAMP-1 positive lysosome **(B)**, as well as endosomic structures positive for LRRK2 **(C)**. Size of scale bars are as indicated.

A. fumigatus Swollen Conidia Activate the Non-Canonical Autophagic Pathway in DCs

Lysosomes are known to be involved in the maturation of autophagic vesicles. Given that autophagy is activated by β-glucan (27) and *A. fumigatus* (28, 29), we investigated autophagy in D1 cells stimulated with *Aspergillus* swollen conidia in order to establish a possible role of the autophagic response in the regulation of the NFAT1 translocation. D1 cells stimulated with swollen conidia showed the formation of LC3-positive phagosomes [LC3 associated phagocytosis (LAPosome)] (**Figure 3A**) similar to that induced by β-glucan (27) and *A. fumigatus* (30) in other studies, although germinated A-sw conidia were only partially engulfed. Indeeed, by electron microscopy, it was clear that the resulting membrane cupping was not formed by the double-membranes characteristic of classical autophagy (**Figure 3B**) as previously shown (30). Although images (**Figure 3B**) show partial fungal internalization, time-lapse imaging of DCs demonstrates the bright field on the EVOS FL Auto Cell Imaging System a complete process of phagocytosis (Supplementary Video S1 in Supplementary Material). Taken together, the observations from immunofluorescent staining of LC3 and electron microscopy indicate that the autophagic response induced by *A. fumigatus* swollen conidia in DCs is non-canonical, as reported for conidia (31). LC3-I to LC3-II conversion and higher LC3-II turnover was indeed observed in *A. fumigatus*-stimulated DCs, and p62 was not degraded (**Figure 3C**; Figure S1C in Supplementary Material). Our results indicate that swollen conidia induce non-canonical autophagy in DCs. In addition, we found that there was an increase of subcellular multivesicular structures present in DCs stimulated with swollen conidia as revealed by electron microscopy. Multivesicular structures express LAMP-1 as well as

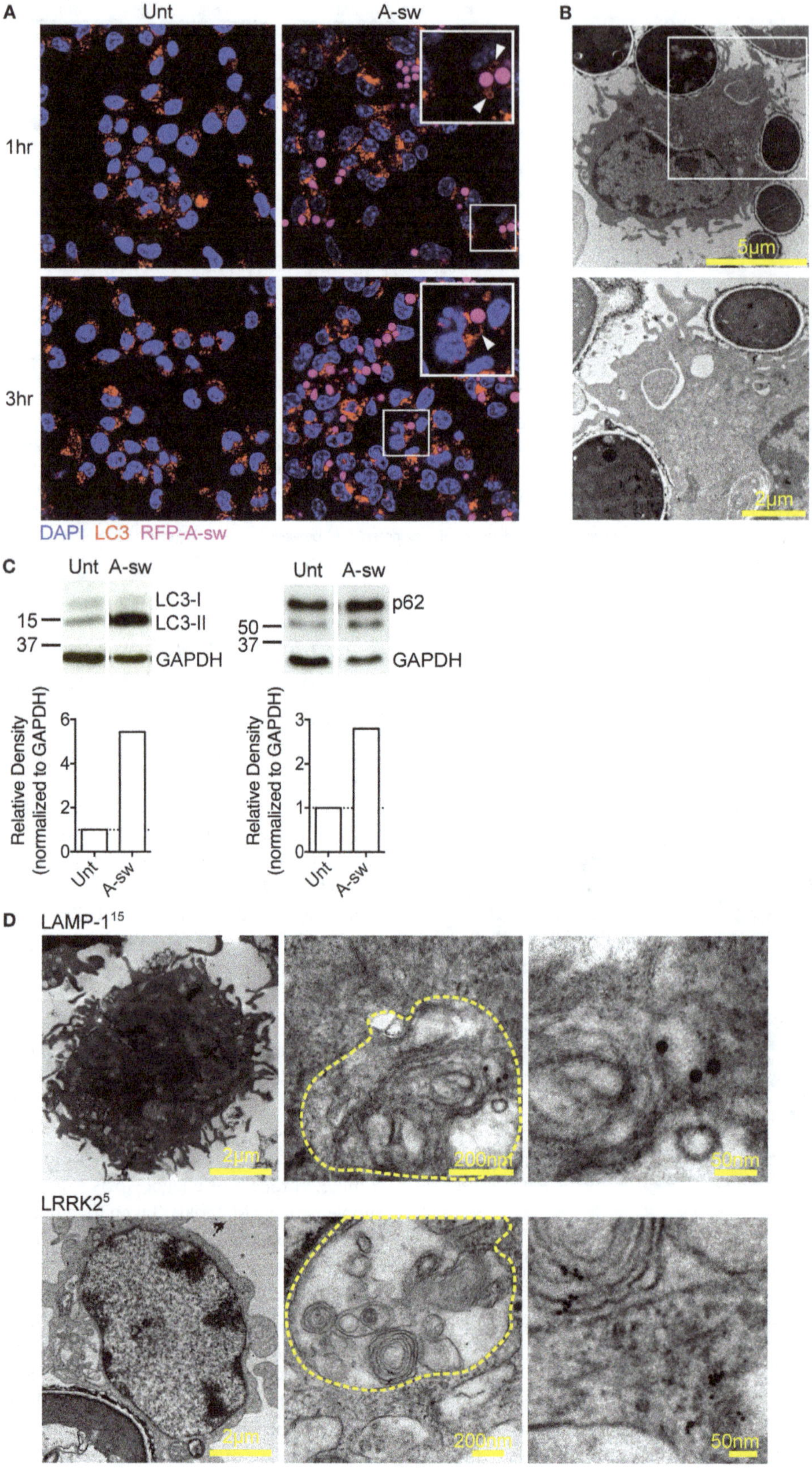

FIGURE 3 | Continued

FIGURE 3 | *Aspergillus fumigatus* swollen conidia activate non-canonical autophagy and the formation of multivesicular bodies in dendritic cells. D1 cells were stimulated with *A. fumigatus* swollen conidia for 3 h. **(A)** Immunofluorescent staining of LC3 (red). Data is representative of two independent experiments. **(B)** Electron micrograph of *Aspergillus* cupping. The bottom panel is zoomed in from the area indicated in the top panel. Data is representative of two independent experiments. **(C)** Expression of LC3 and p62 proteins by western blot in whole cell lysates of D1 cells stimulated for 24 h with *A. fumigatus* swollen conidia. Densitometry for LC3 was performed on the LC3-II band to measure LC3-II turnover, while densitometry analysis of p62 was done on the upper band corresponding to its expected molecular weight of 60kD. Data is representative of two biological replicates. **(D)** Multilamellar bodies (encircled in yellow dashed lines) observed by electron microscopy in *A. fumigatus* swollen conidia-stimulated D1 cells and labeled for LAMP-1 or Leucine-rich repeat kinase 2 with 5 nm or 15 nm gold particles (size of particles indicated in superscript). Cells were incubated with fungi for 3 h. Size of scale bars are as indicated. Abbreviations: Untreated (Unt); *A. fumigatus swollen conidia* (A-sw).

LRRK2 (**Figure 3D**). These structures are lysosomal organelles comprising of multiple concentric layers of membrane, that have been shown to require autophagy for its formation (32). Therefore, taking into account our findings, the germinated form of *Aspergillus* is able to trigger the non-canonical autophagic response together with formation of multivesicular structure formation LRRK2^{+} in DCs.

Ca^{2+}/NFAT/IL-2 Axis Is Affected by Early Autophagic Events, Phagocytosis, and Lysosomal Maturation

Based on the previous findings, two types of autophagy inhibitors, 3MA and Baf were used to investigate whether NFAT1 translocation is mediated by the autophagic response to *A. fumigatus*. As the initiation of autophagosome formation requires Class III PI3 kinase activity, 3MA, a PI3 kinase inhibitor, functions by inhibiting autophagy in the early stages of its initiation. Baf inhibits the last step of autophagosome cargo degradation by preventing the autophagosome–lysosome fusion as well as lysosome acidification (33). We found that NFAT1 translocation and IL-2 cytokine production in DCs stimulated with *Aspergillus* germinated conidia were significantly decreased upon inhibition of the early stages of autophagy by 3-MA, but not with an inhibitor of the late stage of autophagy, Baf (**Figure 4A**). In addition, NFAT pathway in stimulated DCs was also significantly decreased when cells were treated with the phagocytosis inhibitor, CytoD (**Figure 4B**). DCs were also treated with a combination of Leupeptin and ammonium chloride (Leu/A) to inhibit lysosomal maturation by preventing acidification, and it was observed that NFAT1 translocation increased, while IL-2 production unexpectedly decreased in drug-exposed DCs in response to fungi (**Figure 4C**). In order to understand whether those variations were due to a reduced cell viability, we performed the MTT proliferation assay on all the conditions tested above (**Figure 4D**). Pivotally, cells were not affected in terms of viability by the different treatments (**Figure 4D**).

Finally, since more recently, non-canonical autophagy, also defined as LAP, has been extensively described for infection with *A. fumigatus* (29, 31), we performed shRNA of the main key players (*Rubicon, Nox2, Atg7*) of LAP on D1 cells upon *Aspergillus* treatment and we went to analyze IL-2 transcription as a key response downstream of NFAT translocation (**Figure 4E**; Figure S2 in Supplementary Material). Results here indicate that shRNA of *Rubicon* and *Nox2* mRNA, lead to a significant decrease of IL-2 transcription upon A-sw stimulation. Together, the results show that early events that occur after fungal stimulation, such as phagocytosis and the early part of the autophagy pathway, are important in the activation of the NFAT pathway, but not late-stage autophagy. Moreover, inhibition of LAP is particularly interfering NFAT translocation in DCs although shRNA of *Rubicon* is not affecting the phagocytosis process (Figure S3 in Supplementary Material). Thus, the induction of non-canonical autophagy as well as the downregulation of LRRK2 expression in *A. fumigatus*-stimulated DCs raises the possibility of autophagy being responsible for the degradation of LRRK2, resulting in the activation of NFAT1. This is further supported by the presence of LRRK2 in lysosomic-endosomic structures (**Figure 2C**) and multilamellar bodies (**Figure 3D**).

LRRK2 Deficiency in DCs Leads to Increased NFAT/IL-2 Activation Axis in Response to *A. fumigatus*

Since LRRK2 has been reported as a negative regulator of the NFAT pathway (15), we used LRRK2 $^{-/-}$ BMDCs (Figure S4 in Supplementary Material) to measure IL-2 release as well as other two cytokine regulated by NFAT in DCs (34) upon *Aspergillus* germinated spore stimulation. LRRK2$^{-/-}$ BMDCs showed a significant increase in IL-2 production when stimulated with *Aspergillus* swollen conidia at 8, 18, and 24 h, while cytokine as IL-12/IL-23p40 was significantly increased only at 8 h and IL-23 did not show significant changes (**Figure 5A**). More interestingly, stimulated NFAT-luciferase reporter D1 cells, upon silencing with LRRK2 shRNA and exposed to A-sw showed that NFAT nuclear translocation was also significantly increased (**Figure 5B**). In these settings, IL-2 was also increased upon A-sw stimulation (data not shown). Therefore, LRRK2 regulates the NFAT pathway in response to the fungus *Aspergillus*. Consequently, LRRK2 deficiency may disentangle a possible dysregulation of the NFAT/IL-2 cascade in response to the germinated fungus *Aspergillus*.

The Independent Role of LRRK2 in Regulating the NFAT/IL-2 Axis in *Aspergillus*-Stimulated DCs

It has been reported that LRRK2 physically associates with the NRON complex, and that NRON was important for mediating the regulation of NFAT1 nuclear translocation by LRRK2 (15), hence the expression of four members of the NRON complex; NRON, PPP2R1A, CSE1L, and SPAG9 was investigated in DCs in response to *Aspergillus* swollen conidia. Gene expression analysis shows that components of the NRON complex are expressed in DCs, and are negatively regulated by fungal exposure (Figure S5A in Supplementary Material). On the protein level, the expression of the NRON complex components, including PPP2R1A, CSE1L

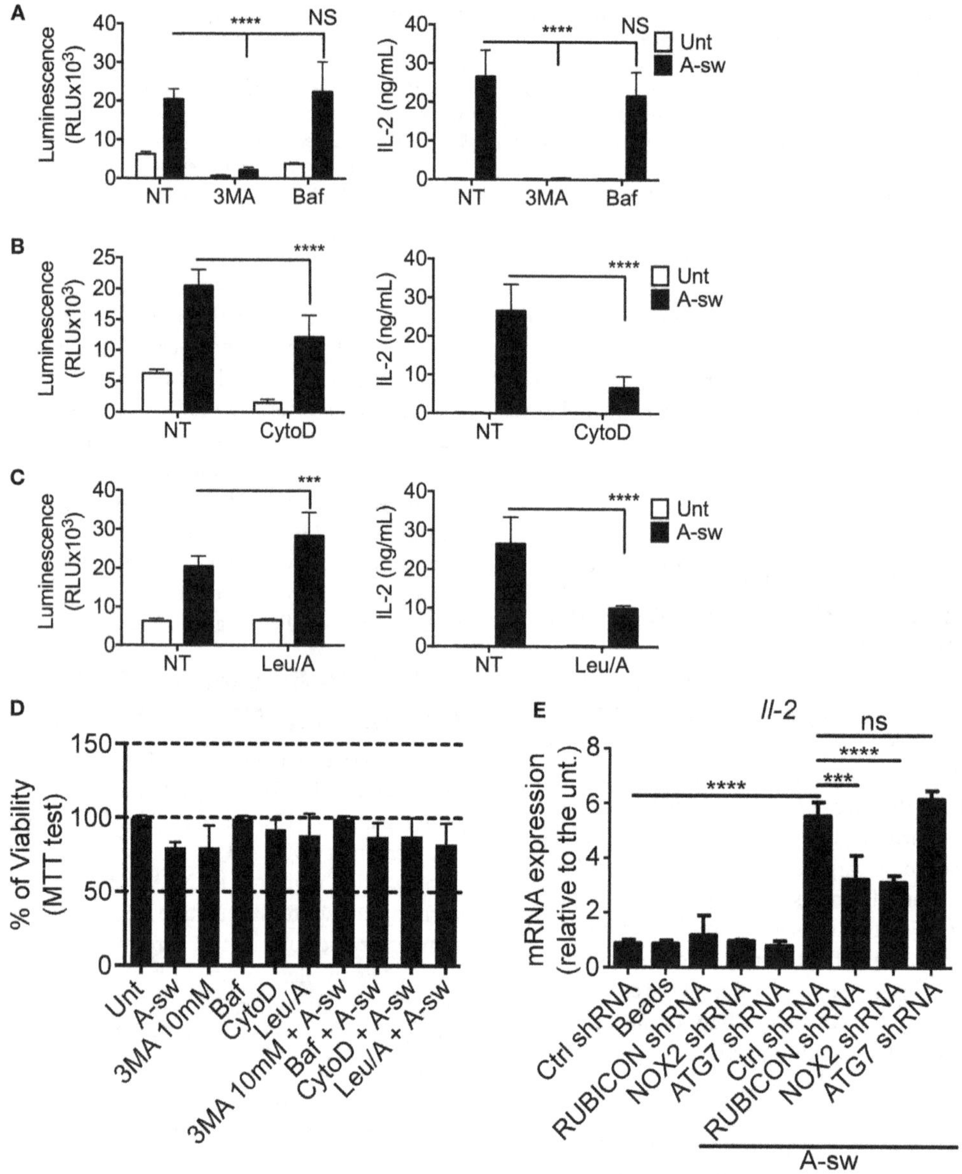

FIGURE 4 | Ca^{2+}-NFAT-IL-2 axis is affected by early autophagic events, phagocytosis and LAP. nuclear factor of activated T cells translocation and IL-2 production of NFAT-luciferase reporter D1 cells that have been stimulated with A-sw for 6 h in the presence and absence of drugs inhibiting specific cellular processes. **(A)** Fungus-stimulated D1 cells in the presence and absence of the type III Phosphatidylinositol 3-kinase inhibitor 3MA, 10 mM, or the vacuolar H + ATPase inhibitor, Baf (50 nM), which inhibits the early and late stage of autophagy respectively. **(B)** Fungus-stimulated D1 cells in the presence or absence of the phagocytosis inhibitor, CytoD (2 µg/mL). **(C)** D1 cells stimulated with fungi in the presence or absence of the lysosomal acidification inhibiting combination of Leu/A. Data is displayed as the mean ± SD of five (in the case of Leu/A) or eight biological replicates. **(D)** Viability of D1 cells treated with fungus, drugs, or a combination of the both. **(E)** mRNA expression of IL-2 in D1 cells silenced for various mRNA regulating LAP in the presence or absence of *A. fumigatus* swollen conidia. Data is displayed as means ± SD of three biological replicates. Differences found to be statistically significant by one-way ANOVA with Bonferroni's Multiple Comparison post-test are indicated (NS, non-significant; ***, $p < 0.001$; ****, $p < 0.0001$). Abbreviations: Untreated (Unt); *A. fumigatus swollen conidia* (A-sw); Vehicle non-treated control (NT); 3-methyladenine (3MA); Bafilomycin (Baf); Cytochalasin D (CytoD), combination of Leupeptin and ammonium chloride (Leu/A).

and SPAG9, could also be detected at basal level. Interestingly, *Aspergillus*-stimulated D1 cells showed marked downregulation of the PPP2R1A protein (Figure S5B in Supplementary Material). Altogether, this shows that *Aspergillus* by inducing phagocytosis and LAP may also influence the expression of other components of the NRON complex as for LRRK2 in DCs. In order to investigate whether the NRON complex in DCs was affecting the NFAT/IL-2 axis as shown for LRRK2, D1 cells were knocked down for NRON, IQGAP, CSE1L, and PPP2R1A (a subunit of the PPP2RA protein), or SPAG9 using shRNA-containing lentiviral particles. Silencing efficiency was investigated and the DC clone was selected accordingly (Figure S6 in Supplementary Material).

Surprisingly, no increase in IL-2 release in response to *Aspergillus* stimulation from silenced D1 cells was observed as we

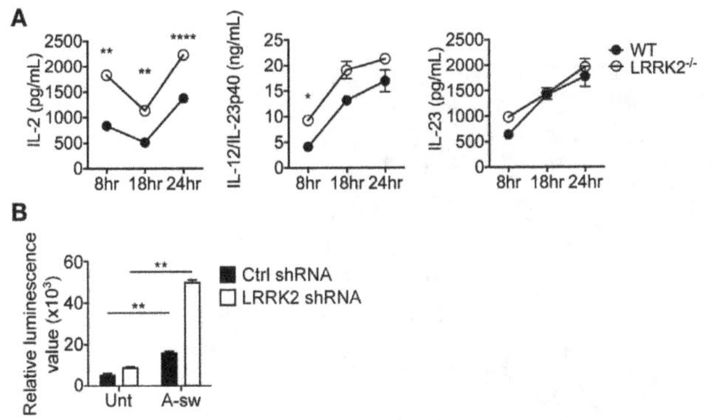

FIGURE 5 | Leucine-rich repeat kinase 2 (LRRK2) deficiency in dendritic cells (DCs) leads to increased IL-2 production and nuclear factor of activated T cells (NFAT) translocation in response to *Aspergillus fumigatus*. **(A)** IL-2, IL-12/IL-23p40, and IL-23 cytokine production of wild-type (closed circles) and LRRK2$^{-/-}$ (open circles) bone marrow-derived DCs in response to fungal stimulation with *A. fumigatus* swollen conidia. Data is displayed as the mean cytokine concentration ± SD of two biological replicates and statistical significance determined by one-way ANOVA with Bonferroni's Multiple Comparison post-test. **(B)** NFAT translocation measured by luminescence signal in A-sw-stimulated NFAT-luciferase reporter D1 cells upon LRRK2 silencing. Data is displayed as the mean luminescence signal ± SD of three biological replicates and statistical significance determined by Student's *t*-test. Differences found to be statistically significant are indicated (*, $p < 0.05$; **, $p < 0.01$; ****, $p < 0.0001$). Abbreviations: Untreated (Unt); *A. fumigatus swollen conidia* (A-sw).

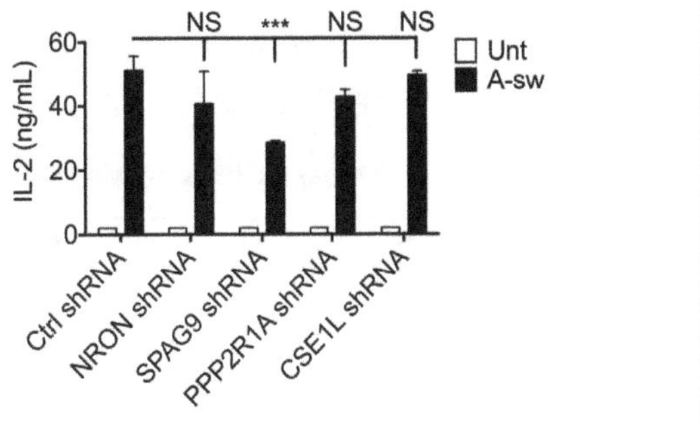

FIGURE 6 | Regulation of IL-2 by NRON complex components. IL-2 cytokine production at 8 h post-exposure from A-sw stimulated D1 cells that were knocked down for NRON, sperm-associated antigen 9, PPP2R1A, or chromosome segregation 1-like through the use of shRNA-lentiviral particles. Data are displayed as the mean ± SD of three replicates. Differences between *Aspergillus*-stimulated cells found to be statistically significant by one-way ANOVA with Bonferroni's Multiple Comparison post-test are indicated (NS, non-significant; ***, $p < 0.001$). Abbreviations: Untreated (Unt); *A. fumigatus swollen conidia* (A-sw).

found in LRRK2 deficiency. Interestingly, other cytokines involved in DC response to infections as IL-1β, IL-6, IL12/IL-23p40, IL-22, IL-23, and TNFα are differently affected by silencing the NRON complex components (Figure S7 in Supplementary Material). Regarding IL-2, only knocking down of SPAG9 led to a decrease of IL-2 production by DCs (**Figure 6**).

Finally, since recently, a mechanism by which inflammation is regulated during LAP through the death-associated protein kinase 1 (DAPK1) has been described in macrophages (31), we investigated a possible cross-regulation between these two proteins during LAP. Moreover, *Dapk1* and *Lrrk2* are both target genes of IFN-γ in myeloid cells (10, 35). Therefore, we have analyzed DAPK1 expression in DCs (**Figures 7A,B**), and we found that DAPK1 protein level increases in response to A-sw (**Figure 7A**) differently from LRRK2 in DCs (**Figure 1A**). However, DCs treated with LRRK2 shRNA (**Figure 7C**), do not show any significant differential expression of *Dapk1* (**Figure 7D**) as well as DAPK1 shRNA treated DCs show similar *Lrrk2* expression than Ctrl shRNA (data not shown). In conclusion, our results underline a more prominent and independent (from NRON components) role of LRRK2 in regulating the NFAT1 translocation to the nucleus and in regulating IL-2 cytokine release in DCs (Figure S8 in Supplementary Material).

DISCUSSION

Leucine-rich repeat kinase 2 was first discovered to play a role in Parkinson's disease (2), and it has been shown to be involved in various signaling pathways and cellular processes. In addition, LRRK2 is genetically associated with other inflammatory diseases (15, 36, 37) and modulated in inflammation by PAMPs (10, 15). Also, LRRK2 was reported to be a negative regulator of the NFAT pathway in BMDMs (15), activated downstream of Dectin-1 by fungi (18). Interestingly, LRRK2 has been investigated recently in immune response to pathogens (10, 17). However, as of now the role of LRRK2 protein in fungal immunity has not been explored.

In support of the observations of *Liu* et al. (15), our study here demonstrates that LRRK2 is indeed involved as a negative regulator of the NFAT pathway in DC response to fungi.

At resting state in DCs, we found that LRRK2 localizes to endosomes, accordingly to recent studies, where LRRK2 interaction with the endocytic network have been recently demonstrated (24, 38, 39). Liu et al. (15) reported LRRK2 to be bound to 5 of the 11 proteins of the NRON complex. In view of these reports, the localization of LRRK2 and possibly also other NRON complex components to endosomes at steady state could serve to regulate NFAT, and this is possibly accomplished by sequestering it at the endosomal membrane.

In this study, four components, including NRON, PPP2R1A, CSE1L, and SPAG9 of the NRON complex were also investigated, and it was found that expression levels of NRON and PPP2R1A in particular, were downregulated in DCs in response to *Aspergillus* stimulation as LRRK2. This is in line with what has been reported that the NRON complex, together with LRRK2, mediates NFAT translocation regulation (15) since a downregulation of NRON complex components would likely lead to a dissociation of this regulatory complex. A knockdown of these components was carried out to investigate whether other than LRRK2 other components may affect NFAT nuclear translocation in DCs. IL-2 production from *Aspergillus*-stimulated DCs knocked down for any of these components was found not to be significantly affected, or was decreased as in the case when SPAG9 was knocked down. This indicates that perhaps NRON, PPP2R1A, and CSE1L alone are not sufficient to regulate the NFAT/IL-2 axis. SPAG9, on the other hand, individually could be positively regulating the NFAT/IL-2 axis, rather than inhibiting it.

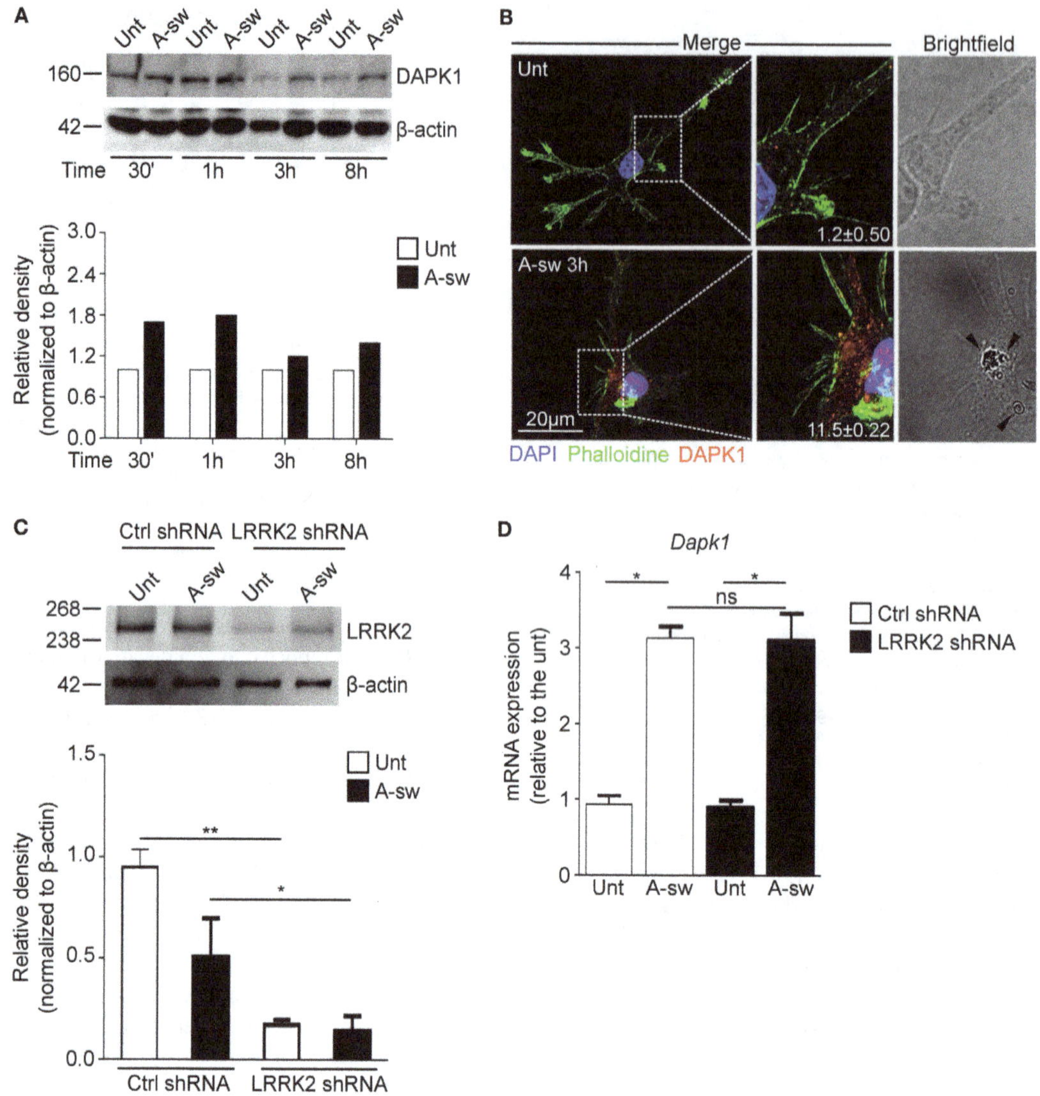

FIGURE 7 | Death-associated protein kinase 1 (DAPK1) expression during LAP is not controlled by Leucine-rich repeat kinase 2 (LRRK2). **(A)** Protein expression of DAPK1 in *A. fumigatus* swollen conidia-stimulated D1 cells. For densitometry analysis, band densities for DAPK1 were normalized to the band density of the housekeeping protein, β-actin, after which the density of the DAPK1 band of the treated sample was compared with that of the untreated sample. Data are representative of three independent experiments. **(B)** Immunofluorescent stanining of DAPK1 and brightfield microscopy of *Aspergillus fumigatus* swollen conidia-stimulated D1 cells. Signal intensity of the DAPK1 was quantified and displayed as mean fluorescence signal ± SD of three biological replicates. Brightfield imaging of the same cell is displayed with arrows indicating the presence of *A. fumigatus* swollen conidia in the cell. **(C)** Knockdown of LRRK2 in D1 cells was assessed by western blot. Data are represented as mean ± SD of three biological replicates and statistical significance determined by two way ANOVA **(D)** mRNA expression of DAPK1 in fungal-treated D1 cells that have been silenced for LRRK2. Data are displayed as the mean mRNA expression ± SD of three biological replicates and statistical significance determined by two way ANOVA. Differences found to be statistically significant are indicated (*, $p < 0.05$; **, $p < 0.01$). Abbreviations: *A. fumigatus swollen conidia* (A-sw); Untreated (Unt); D1 cells transduced with non-targeting control shRNA (Ctrl).

More interestingly, the individual components of the NRON complex were regulating DC cytokine response differently, implying that they may not work in concert.

For SPAG9, CSE1L, and PPP2R1A, besides being known to be part of the NRON complex (15, 40), their reported functions were not originally concerning the immune system. SPAG9 has been proposed as a biomarker for diagnosis in carcinoma of the breast (41), endometrium (42), cervix (43), thyroid (44), and colon (45), and has been proposed to be involved in the tumorogenesis and growth. CSE1L is a nuclear exportin protein that is involved in the cell cycle, and SPAG9 has also been associated with various carcinomas [as reviewed in Behrens et al. (46)]. PPP2R1A is a subunit of protein phosphatase 2A (PP2A). PP2A has been implicated in meiosis and mitosis in numerous studies (47, 48) and is currently being explored as a treatment target for pancreatic cancer (49). More related to the context of this study, PP2A proteins have been shown to interact with signaling pathways, such as the TLR-TRIF signaling (50), Ras signaling (51), as well as Ca^{2+}/Calmodulin-dependent protein kinase B/Akt (52). In relation to neurological disorders, PP2A has been suggested as a possible treatment target for neurological disorders Alzheimer's disease (53) and has been recently implicated in Tau pathology of Parkinson's disease (54). This study hints that the function of SPAG9, CSE1L, and PPP2R1A may also be related to the immune response to pathogens.

It has been shown that LRRK2 localizes to lysosomes and can be degraded by CMA in neurons (23). In a similar way, this study here shows that LRRK2 is localized to endosomes and lysosomes in steady state DCs, and that *Aspergillus* is able to induce a non-canonical type of autophagy in DCs that is reminiscent of LC3-positive phagosomes, previously reported (27, 30, 31, 55).

The use of transmission electron microscopy allowed the observation of LRRK2-positive multilamellar body formation in *Aspergillus*-stimulated DCs, further strengthening the connection of LRRK2 with lysosomes and autophagy. Multilamellar bodies are reported to be part of the lysosomal pathway and its formation is dependent on autophagy and lysosomal degradation (32), and the localization of LRRK2 to these structures is supported by what has been previously reported in cultured human cells (25).

Interestingly, GSK3-β, a protein involved in phosphorylating NFAT, has also been shown to localize to the endosomal membrane and this is thought to serve to isolate it from interaction with other signaling components (26).

How the NFAT pathway is influenced by the events following the engagement of Dectin-1 by *Aspergillus* in DCs was also investigated here. The dependency of phagocytosis on IL-2 production in response to particulate β-glucan in DCs has been previously demonstrated (19), hence in this study the finding that the NFAT/IL-2 axis in response to *Aspergillus* is also dependent on this cellular process was expected. What was interesting was that early, but not late autophagic events are also required to activate the NFAT/IL-2 pathway.

Autophagy also occurs in macrophages, and with this respect Ma et al. (27) and Kyrmizi et al. (30) have both demonstrated that the formation of LC3-positive phagosomes also occur in macrophages incubated with fungi, and that the recruitment of LC3 is important for macrophage signaling and function in response to fungi. In particular, Kyrmizi, Gresnigt (30) show that the recruitment of LC3 is needed for macrophage ROS production and killing of *Aspergillus* spores.

In this study, we have also evaluated whether DAPK1 may contribute to regulating LRRK2 function (and vice versa), since both are regulated during LAP and concur to the regulation of the inflammatory response during fungal LAP. To this purpose, we have resorted to shRNA of LRRK2 and analyzed DAPK1 expression.

To conclude, our study has shown that DCs express LRRK2 and that it negatively regulates the NFAT pathway activated in response to *Aspergillus*. Upon *Aspergillus* binding to Dectin-1 in DCs, non-canonical autophagy, as well as multilamellar body formation is triggered. Taking into account the findings of previously published reports, the sequestration of LRRK2 in the multilamellar bodies could lead to the dissociation of the NRON complex. Therefore, the role of the NRON complex in immune response of DCs to *Aspergillus* has been shown to be more complex than previously thought, and their interaction with other signaling pathways activated in the immune response will add a new dimension to their currently known cellular functions. Given that DCs have an important role in the immune system as antigen presenting cells and initiating the appropriate adaptive immune response, future *in vivo* studies could elucidate better the immunological function of LRRK2 and the NRON complex eventually in T cell priming. The knowledge obtained from such studies not only sheds light on the control of the NFAT pathway, but also could have implications in other diseases associated with LRRK2, such as Crohn's disease, IBD, and Parkinson's disease.

AUTHOR CONTRIBUTIONS

AW designed the study, conducted, analyzed experiments, and wrote the manuscript. VO performed western blotting and immunofluorescence experiments. GP performed qPCR data. AL performed ELISA; MP analyzed western blotting data. JF performed the LRRK2$^{-/-}$ bone marrow expansion experiments. HT generated the D1 NFAT translocation-firefly luciferase reporter cells. PR-C supervised the project. TZ conceived, coordinated the project, and wrote the manuscript.

ACKNOWLEDGMENTS

The authors wish to thank Z. Liu of Institute of Biophysics Chinese Academy of Sciences for LRRK2$^{-/-}$ mice bone marrow; A. Balachander (SIgN) for confocal microscopy; R. Iannitti of the Department of Experimental Medicine, University of Perugia, and P. Rondoni of the Centro Universitario di Microscopia Electtronica (CUME), University of Perugia, for transmission electron microscopy; Prof. A. Milani, S. Pasqua, A. Moriconi of the laboratory E-learning, University of Perugia, Italy for video editing.

FUNDING

This research was funded by the Biomedical Research Council, A*STAR, and the Italian grant "Programma per Giovani Ricercatori – Rita Levi Montalcini 2013." JF was supported by European Social Fund and European Regional Development Fund—Project MAGNET (No. CZ.02.1.01/0.0/0.0/15_003/0000492).

SUPPLEMENTARY MATERIAL

VIDEO S1 | BMDCs phagocytosis of Aspergillus swollen conidia. Representative example of time-lapse imaging data of in vitro mouse BMDCs. BMDCs were infected with Aspergillus swollen conidia and imaged over a period of 1 hour to identify the process of phagocytosis. Images were captured every 2 minutes in the bright field channel on the EVOS FL Auto Cell Imaging System. A movie was then generated from the images at rate of 4 frame/sec.

REFERENCES

1. Paisán-Ruíz C, Jain S, Evans E, Gilks W, Simón J, van der Brug M, et al. Cloning of the gene containing mutations that cause PARK8-linked Parkinson's disease. *Neuron* (2004) 44(4):595–600. doi:10.1016/j.neuron.2004.10.023
2. Funayama M, Hasegawa K, Kowa H, Saito M, Tsuji S, Obata F. A new locus for Parkinson's disease (PARK8) maps to chromosome 12p11.2-q13.1. *Ann Neurol* (2002) 51(3):296–301. doi:10.1002/ana.10113
3. Mata I, Wedemeyer W, Farrer M, Taylor J, Gallo K. LRRK2 in Parkinson's disease: protein domains and functional insights. *Trends Neurosci* (2006) 29(5):286–93. doi:10.1016/j.tins.2006.03.006
4. Jorgensen N, Peng Y, Ho CC-Y, Rideout H, Petrey D, Liu P, et al. The WD40 domain is required for LRRK2 neurotoxicity. *PLoS One* (2009) 4(12):e8463. doi:10.1371/journal.pone.0008463
5. Smith W, Pei Z, Jiang H, Moore D, Liang Y, West A, et al. Leucine-rich repeat kinase 2 (LRRK2) interacts with parkin, and mutant LRRK2 induces neuronal degeneration. *Proc Natl Acad Sci U S A* (2005) 102(51):18676–81. doi:10.1073/pnas.0508052102
6. West A, Moore D, Choi C, Andrabi S, Li X, Dikeman D, et al. Parkinson's disease-associated mutations in LRRK2 link enhanced GTP-binding and kinase activities to neuronal toxicity. *Hum Mol Genet* (2007) 16(2):223–32. doi:10.1093/hmg/ddl471
7. Liu B. Modulation of microglial pro-inflammatory and neurotoxic activity for the treatment of Parkinson's disease. *AAPS J* (2006) 8(3):21. doi:10.1208/aapsj080369
8. Whitton P. Inflammation as a causative factor in the aetiology of Parkinson's disease. *Br J Pharmacol* (2007) 150(8):963–76. doi:10.1038/sj.bjp.0707167
9. Gerlach OH, Winogrodzka A, Weber W. Clinical problems in the hospitalized Parkinson's disease patient: systematic review. *Mov Disord* (2011) 26(2):197–208. doi:10.1002/mds.23449
10. Gardet AS, Benita Y, Li C, Sands B, Ballester I, Stevens C, et al. LRRK2 is involved in the IFN-gamma response and host response to pathogens. *J Immunol* (2010) 185(9):5577–85. doi:10.4049/jimmunol.1000548
11. Hakimi M, Selvanantham T, Swinton E, Padmore R, Tong Y, Kabbach G, et al. Parkinson's disease-linked LRRK2 is expressed in circulating and tissue immune cells and upregulated following recognition of microbial structures. *J Neural Transm (Vienna)* (2011) 118(5):795–808. doi:10.1007/s00702-011-0653-2
12. Moehle M, Webber P, Tse T, Sukar N, Standaert D, DeSilva T, et al. LRRK2 inhibition attenuates microglial inflammatory responses. *J Neurosci* (2012) 32(5):1602–11. doi:10.1523/JNEUROSCI.5601-11.2012
13. Gillardon F, Schmid R, Draheim H. Parkinson's disease-linked leucine-rich repeat kinase 2(R1441G) mutation increases proinflammatory cytokine release from activated primary microglial cells and resultant neurotoxicity. *Neuroscience* (2012) 208:41–8. doi:10.1016/j.neuroscience.2012.02.001
14. Kim B, Yang MS, Choi D, Kim JH, Kim HS, Seol W, et al. Impaired inflammatory responses in murine Lrrk2-knockdown brain microglia. *PLoS One* (2012) 7(4):e34693. doi:10.1371/journal.pone.0034693
15. Liu Z, Lee J, Krummey S, Lu W, Cai H, Lenardo M. The kinase LRRK2 is a regulator of the transcription factor NFAT that modulates the severity of inflammatory bowel disease. *Nat Immunol* (2011) 12(11):1063–70. doi:10.1038/ni.2113
16. Macian F. NFAT proteins: key regulators of T-cell development and function. *Nat Rev Immunol* (2005) 5(6):472–84. doi:10.1038/nri1632
17. Liu W, Liu X, Li Y, Zhao J, Liu Z, Hu Z, et al. LRRK2 promotes the activation of NLRC4 inflammasome during *Salmonella typhimurium* infection. *J Exp Med* (2017) 214(10):3051–66. doi:10.1084/jem.20170014
18. Goodridge HS, Simmons RM, Underhill DM. Dectin-1 stimulation by *Candida albicans* yeast or zymosan triggers NFAT activation in macrophages and dendritic cells. *J Immunol* (2007) 178(5):3107–15. doi:10.4049/jimmunol.178.5.3107
19. Fric J, Zelante T, Ricciardi-Castagnoli P. Phagocytosis of particulate antigens – all roads lead to calcineurin/NFAT signaling pathway. *Front Immunol* (2014) 4:513. doi:10.3389/fimmu.2013.00513
20. Zelante T, Wong AY, Ping TJ, Chen J, Sumatoh HR, Viganò E, et al. CD103(+) dendritic cells control Th17 cell function in the lung. *Cell Rep* (2015) 12(11):1789–801. doi:10.1016/j.celrep.2015.08.030
21. Winzler C, Rovere P, Rescigno M, Granucci F, Penna G, Adorini L, et al. Maturation stages of mouse dendritic cells in growth factor-dependent long-term cultures. *J Exp Med* (1997) 185(2):317–28. doi:10.1084/jem.185.2.317
22. Graham JM. Isolation of lysosomes from tissues and cells by differential and density gradient centrifugation. *Curr Protoc Cell Biol* (2001) Chapter 3:Unit 3.6. doi:10.1002/0471143030.cb0306s07
23. Orenstein S, Kuo SH, Tasset I, Arias E, Koga H, Fernandez-Carasa I, et al. Interplay of LRRK2 with chaperone-mediated autophagy. *Nat Neurosci* (2013) 16(4):394–406. doi:10.1038/nn.3350
24. Schreij AM, Chaineau M, Ruan W, Lin S, Barker PA, Fon EA, et al. LRRK2 localizes to endosomes and interacts with clathrin-light chains to limit Rac1 activation. *EMBO Rep* (2015) 16(1):79–86. doi:10.15252/embr.201438714
25. Alegre-Abarrategui J, Christian H, Lufino M, Mutihac R, Venda L, Ansorge O, et al. LRRK2 regulates autophagic activity and localizes to specific membrane microdomains in a novel human genomic reporter cellular model. *Hum Mol Genet* (2009) 18(21):4022–34. doi:10.1093/hmg/ddp346
26. Pálfy M, Reményi A, Korcsmáros T. Endosomal crosstalk: meeting points for signaling pathways. *Trends Cell Biol* (2012) 22(9):447–56. doi:10.1016/j.tcb.2012.06.004
27. Ma J, Becker C, Lowell C, Underhill D. Dectin-1-triggered recruitment of light chain 3 protein to phagosomes facilitates major histocompatibility complex class II presentation of fungal-derived antigens. *J Biol Chem* (2012) 287(41):34149–56. doi:10.1074/jbc.M112.382812
28. De Luca A, Iannitti R, Bozza S, Beau R, Casagrande A, D'Angelo C, et al. CD4(+) T cell vaccination overcomes defective cross-presentation of fungal antigens in a mouse model of chronic granulomatous disease. *J Clin Invest* (2012) 122(5):1816–31. doi:10.1172/JCI60862
29. Martinez J, Malireddi RK, Lu Q, Cunha LD, Pelletier S, Gingras S, et al. Molecular characterization of LC3-associated phagocytosis reveals distinct roles for Rubicon, NOX2 and autophagy proteins. *Nat Cell Biol* (2015) 17(7):893–906. doi:10.1038/ncb3192
30. Kyrmizi I, Gresnigt MS, Akoumianaki T, Samonis G, Sidiropoulos P, Boumpas D, et al. Corticosteroids block autophagy protein recruitment in *Aspergillus fumigatus* phagosomes via targeting dectin-1/Syk kinase signaling. *J Immunol* (2013) 191(3):1287–99. doi:10.4049/jimmunol.1300132
31. Oikonomou V, Moretti S, Renga G, Galosi C, Borghi M, Pariano M, et al. Noncanonical fungal autophagy inhibits inflammation in response to IFN-gamma via DAPK1. *Cell Host Microbe* (2016) 20(6):744–57. doi:10.1016/j.chom.2016.10.012
32. Hariri M, Millane G, Guimond MP, Guay G, Dennis JW, Nabi IR. Biogenesis of multilamellar bodies via autophagy. *Mol Biol Cell* (2000) 11(1):255–68. doi:10.1091/mbc.11.1.255
33. Mizushima N, Yoshimori T, Levine B. Methods in mammalian autophagy research. *Cell* (2010) 140(3):313–26. doi:10.1016/j.cell.2010.01.028
34. Yu HB, Yurieva M, Balachander A, Foo I, Leong X, Zelante T, et al. NFATc2 mediates epigenetic modification of dendritic cell cytokine and chemokine responses to dectin-1 stimulation. *Nucleic Acids Res* (2015) 43(2):836–47. doi:10.1093/nar/gku1369
35. Gade P, Manjegowda SB, Nallar SC, Maachani UB, Cross AS, Kalvakolanu DV. Regulation of the death-associated protein kinase 1 expression and autophagy via ATF6 requires apoptosis signal-regulating kinase 1. *Mol Cell Biol* (2014) 34(21):4033–48. doi:10.1128/MCB.00397-14
36. Barrett J, Hansoul S, Nicolae D, Cho J, Duerr R, Rioux J, et al. Genome-wide association defines more than 30 distinct susceptibility loci for Crohn's disease. *Nat Genet* (2008) 40(8):955–62. doi:10.1038/ng.175
37. Törkvist L, Halfvarson J, Ong R, Lördal M, Sjöqvist U, Bresso F, et al. Analysis of 39 Crohn's disease risk loci in Swedish inflammatory bowel disease patients. *Inflamm Bowel Dis* (2010) 16(6):907–9. doi:10.1002/ibd.21105
38. Yun HJ, Kim H, Ga I, Oh H, Ho DH, Kim J, et al. An early endosome regulator, Rab5b, is an LRRK2 kinase substrate. *J Biochem* (2015) 157(6):485–95. doi:10.1093/jb/mvv005
39. Gómez-Suaga P, Rivero-Ríos P, Fdez E, Blanca Ramírez M, Ferrer I, Aiastui A, et al. LRRK2 delays degradative receptor trafficking by impeding late endosomal budding through decreasing Rab7 activity. *Hum Mol Genet* (2014) 23(25):6779–96. doi:10.1093/hmg/ddu395
40. Willingham A, Orth A, Batalov S, Peters E, Wen B, Aza-Blanc P, et al. A strategy for probing the function of noncoding RNAs finds a repressor of NFAT. *Science* (2005) 309(5740):1570–3. doi:10.1126/science.1115901

41. Kanojia D, Garg M, Gupta S, Gupta A, Suri A. Sperm-associated antigen 9, a novel biomarker for early detection of breast cancer. *Cancer Epidemiol Biomarkers Prev* (2009) 18(2):630–9. doi:10.1158/1055-9965.EPI-08-0629
42. Yu P, Yan L, Zhang H, Lin X, Zhao X. Expression and clinical significance of sperm-associated antigen 9 in patients with endometrial carcinoma. *Int J Gynecol Cancer* (2012) 22(1):87–93. doi:10.1097/IGC.0b013e3182370f2e
43. Garg M, Kanojia D, Salhan S, Suri S, Gupta A, Lohiya NK, et al. Sperm-associated antigen 9 is a biomarker for early cervical carcinoma. *Cancer* (2009) 115(12):2671–83. doi:10.1002/cncr.24293
44. Garg M, Kanojia D, Suri S, Gupta S, Gupta A, Suri A. Sperm-associated antigen 9: a novel diagnostic marker for thyroid cancer. *J Clin Endocrinol Metab* (2009) 94(11):4613–8. doi:10.1210/jc.2009-0703
45. Kanojia D, Garg M, Gupta S, Gupta A, Suri A. Sperm-associated antigen 9 is a novel biomarker for colorectal cancer and is involved in tumor growth and tumorigenicity. *Am J Pathol* (2011) 178(3):1009–20. doi:10.1016/j.ajpath.2010.11.047
46. Behrens P, Brinkmann U, Wellmann A. CSE1L/CAS: its role in proliferation and apoptosis. *Apoptosis* (2003) 8(1):39–44. doi:10.1023/A:1021644918117
47. Hu WW, Wang ZB, Jiang ZZ, Qi ST, Huang L, Liang QX, et al. Scaffold subunit Aalpha of PP2A is essential for female meiosis and fertility in mice. *Biol Reprod* (2014) 91(1):19. doi:10.1095/biolreprod.114.120220
48. Porter IM, Schleicher K, Porter M, Swedlow JR. Bod1 regulates protein phosphatase 2A at mitotic kinetochores. *Nat Commun* (2013) 4:2677. doi:10.1038/ncomms3677
49. Chien W, Sun QY, Lee KL, Ding LW, Wuensche P, Torres-Fernandez LA, et al. Activation of protein phosphatase 2A tumor suppressor as potential treatment of pancreatic cancer. *Mol Oncol* (2015) 9(4):889–905. doi:10.1016/j.molonc.2015.01.002
50. Woo CW, Kutzler L, Kimball SR, Tabas I. Toll-like receptor activation suppresses ER stress factor CHOP and translation inhibition through activation of eIF2B. *Nat Cell Biol* (2012) 14(2):192–200. doi:10.1038/ncb2408
51. Ory S, Zhou M, Conrads TP, Veenstra TD, Morrison DK. Protein phosphatase 2A positively regulates Ras signaling by dephosphorylating KSR1 and Raf-1 on critical 14-3-3 binding sites. *Curr Biol* (2003) 13(16):1356–64. doi:10.1016/S0960-9822(03)00535-9
52. Fedida-Metula S, Feldman B, Koshelev V, Levin-Gromiko U, Voronov E, Fishman D. Lipid rafts couple store-operated Ca2+ entry to constitutive activation of PKB/Akt in a Ca2+/calmodulin-, Src- and PP2A-mediated pathway and promote melanoma tumor growth. *Carcinogenesis* (2012) 33(4):740–50. doi:10.1093/carcin/bgs021
53. Sontag J-MM, Sontag E. Protein phosphatase 2A dysfunction in Alzheimer's disease. *Front Mol Neurosci* (2014) 7:16. doi:10.3389/fnmol.2014.00016
54. Arif M, Kazim SF, Grundke-Iqbal I, Garruto RM, Iqbal K. Tau pathology involves protein phosphatase 2A in parkinsonism-dementia of Guam. *Proc Natl Acad Sci U S A* (2014) 111(3):1144–9. doi:10.1073/pnas.1322614111
55. Nicola AM, Albuquerque P, Martinez LR, Dal-Rosso RA, Saylor C, Jesus M. De, et al. Macrophage autophagy in immunity to *Cryptococcus neoformans* and *Candida albicans*. *Infect Immun* (2012) 80(9):3065–76. doi:10.1128/IAI.00358-12

3

Host-Derived Leukotriene B_4 is Critical for Resistance against Invasive Pulmonary Aspergillosis

*Alayna K. Caffrey-Carr[1,2], Kimberly M. Hilmer[1], Caitlin H. Kowalski[2], Kelly M. Shepardson[1,2], Rachel M. Temple[2], Robert A. Cramer[2] and Joshua J. Obar[2]**

[1] Department of Microbiology and Immunology, Montana State University, Bozeman, MT, United States, [2] Department of Microbiology and Immunology, Geisel School of Medicine at Dartmouth, Lebanon, NH, United States

***Correspondence:**
Joshua J. Obar
joshua.j.obar@dartmouth.edu

Aspergillus fumigatus is a mold that causes severe pulmonary infections. Our knowledge of how immune competent hosts maintain control of fungal infections while constantly being exposed to fungi is rapidly emerging. It is known that timely neutrophil recruitment to and activation in the lungs is critical to the host defense against development of invasive pulmonary aspergillosis, but the inflammatory sequelae necessary remains to be fully defined. Here, we show that 5-Lipoxygenase (5-LO) and Leukotriene B_4 (LTB_4) are critical for leukocyte recruitment and resistance to pulmonary *A. fumigatus* challenge in a fungal-strain-dependent manner. 5-LO activity was needed in radiosensitive cells for an optimal anti-fungal response and *in vivo* LTB_4 production was at least partially dependent on myeloid-derived hypoxia inducible factor-1α. Overall, this study reveals a role for host-derived leukotriene synthesis in innate immunity to *A. fumigatus*.

Keywords: ***Aspergillus fumigatus*, leukotrienes, leukotriene B_4, neutrophils, eosinophils, hypoxia inducible factor-1α, respiratory tract infections, fungal infection**

INTRODUCTION

Aspergillus fumigatus is a ubiquitous mold that causes severe infections, such as invasive pulmonary aspergillosis (IPA), in the immunocompromised population. Due to a combination of (i) difficulty in diagnosis, (ii) limited efficacy of anti-fungal drugs coupled with the emergence of drug resistance, and (iii) a lack of an effective vaccine against *Aspergillus* spp., mortality rates of IPA are extremely high (1, 2). To this end, development of novel immunomodulatory strategies that can potentially be combined with current anti-fungal treatments is an active area of research.

On a day-to-day basis, inhaled spores are removed from the body through physical barriers encountered within the respiratory tract. If spores are deposited in the lung, resident alveolar macrophages and $CCR2^+$ monocytes, together with alveolar epithelial cells, phagocytose, and kill fungal conidia (3, 4). However, in individuals that lack this immune response, conidia are able to germinate and grow within the lung causing tissue damage and disease. These initial encounters are important in the recruitment and activation of neutrophils, inflammatory monocytes, NK cells, and CD4 T cells to further control fungal growth within the lung (5). Of these, neutrophils have long been recognized as one of the key effector cells necessary for resistance against *Aspergillus* infection and neutropenia is a key risk factor for patients that will develop IPA (6).

Neutrophil recruitment and activation is a highly controlled process that is regulated by a number of different inflammatory mediators including C5a, PAF, fMLP, Leukotriene B_4 (LTB_4), CXCR2 ligands, CCR1 ligands, TNFα, and IL-17 (7, 8). However, our understanding of the inflammatory mediators driving neutrophil accumulation and activation following *A. fumigatus* challenge remains incomplete. Following *A. fumigatus* challenge, IL-1RI/MyD88 signaling is essential for optimal production of CXCL1 that is necessary for early neutrophil recruitment through CXCR2 (6, 9, 10). In addition, an unknown CARD9-dependent pathway is critical for late neutrophil accumulation following *A. fumigatus* challenge (9). Additionally, a TLR9/Btk/calcineurin/NFAT-dependent pathway regulates neutrophil accumulation during aspergillosis through its regulation of TNFα (11). Moreover, further complexity exists in that *A. fumigatus* isolates with differing virulence depend on distinct inflammatory responses to maintain host resistance (12, 13). Thus, greater knowledge about the inflammatory pathways which contribute to the anti-*Aspergillus* neutrophil response is required.

Regulation of inflammatory responses by lipid mediators is an emerging area. Particularly, LTB_4 has a critical role in the early recruitment and activation of neutrophils in other inflammatory models (14). Additionally, lipid mediators have been shown to be critical regulators of the host immune response against pathogenic fungi. Following challenge of alveolar macrophages or resident mouse peritoneal macrophages with *Candida albicans* arachidonic acid is effectively mobilized by cPLA2 (15–17), which is necessary for production of both prostaglandins and leukotrienes. cPLA2 is critical for host resistance against *C. albicans* challenge, through the regulation of macrophage transcriptional responses and likely through increased anti-fungal activity of alveolar macrophages (17, 18). Moreover, exogenous LTB_4 and LTD_4 can enhance phagocytosis and killing of *C. albicans* by macrophages (19). Finally, LTB_4-mediated inflammation is critical for host resistance and neutrophil recruitment during *Histoplasma capsulatum* (20, 21), and *Paracoccidioides brasiliensis* (22, 23) infection. Moreover, LTB_4-mediated inflammation is critical for establishing memory T cells for the prevention of histoplasmosis (24). Thus, we asked whether LTB_4 was crucial in the neutrophil response following pulmonary *A. fumigatus* challenge. Here, we show that leukotrienes are produced rapidly after *A. fumigatus* challenge by host cells and play a critical role in the anti-fungal neutrophil response necessary for host resistance against pulmonary *A. fumigatus* challenge.

MATERIALS AND METHODS

Mice

C57BL/6J (Stock #000664), C57BL/6NJ (Stock #005304), B6.129S2-*Alox5*^{tm1Fun} (*Alox5*$^{-/-}$; Stock #004155), and B6.129S4-*Ltb4r1*^{tm1Adl} (*Ltb4r1*$^{-/-}$; Stock #008102) were purchased from Jackson Laboratories. Mice with a targeted deletion of *Hif1a* in myeloid cells were created via crosses into a background of lysozyme M-driven cre-recombinase (*Hif1a*$^{LysM/LysM}$), as previously done (30). All mice were 8–10 weeks of age at the time of infection. All animal experiments were approved by the Montana State University Institutional Animal Care and Use Committee or Dartmouth College Institutional Animal Care and Use Committee.

Preparation of *A. fumigatus* and Pulmonary Challenge Model

Aspergillus fumigatus strains CEA10 and Af293 were grown and harvested as previously described (10). For fungal inoculation, mice were anesthetized with isoflurane and challenged by the intratracheally (i.t.) route with 4–7 × 10^7 *A. fumigatus* conidia in 100 μl sterile PBS. At the indicated time after challenge, mice were euthanized using an overdose of pentobarbital. Samples were collected and analyzed for inflammatory cell recruitment, fungal growth, lung damage, and vascular/epithelial leakage as previously described (10). For survival studies, mice were challenged with 4–7 × 10^7 conidia of either CEA10 or Af293 and monitored daily using a humane endpoint scoring system. Mice were humanely euthanized once they met endpoint criteria.

Bone Marrow Chimeric Mice

Bone marrow chimeric mice were made by lethal irradiation of C57BL/6 mice followed by intravenous reconstitution with either C57BL/6 bone marrow or *Alox5*$^{-/-}$ bone marrow. Mice were rested 6–8 weeks prior to challenge with 4 × 10^7 conidia of CEA10 i.t. At the indicated time-points, mice were euthanized using an overdose of pentobarbital, and samples collected and analyzed for inflammatory cell recruitment and fungal growth as previously described (10).

Leukotriene Quantification

Lipids were extracted from bronchoalveolar lavage fluid (BALF) using a hot-methanol extraction. Briefly, three parts HPLC-grade methanol were added to one part BALF sample. Samples were then vortexed for 30 s and placed into an 80°C water bath for 2 min. Tubes were spun at 14,000 RPM for 15 min and supernatant was collected then dried using a vacuum concentrator. Pellets were resuspended in HPLC-grade water in a volume equal to the starting volume of BALF sample. Extracted samples were then analyzed using enzyme immunoassay kits for LTB_4, cysteinyl leukotrienes (cysLT) (Cayman Chemical). Plates were read using a SpectraMax® Paradigm® plate reader (Molecular Devices).

Statistical Analysis

Statistical significance between experimental groups was determined using a Mann–Whitney *U* test (comparison of two experimental groups that are not normally distributed) or an one-way ANOVA with a Dunn's post-test (comparison of greater than two experimental groups that are not normally distributed), using the GraphPad Prism 6 software. For survival studies, Mantel–Cox log-rank test was used to determine whether there were significant differences in survival between C57BL/6, Hif1a$^{LysM/LysM}$, *Ltb4r1*$^{-/-}$, and *Alox5*$^{-/-}$ mice for each *A. fumigatus* strain.

RESULTS

Leukotriene Production following Pulmonary Challenge with *A. fumigatus*

In order to determine whether leukotrienes are produced following *A. fumigatus* challenge, we challenged C57BL/6 wild-type mice with the CEA10 strain of *A. fumigatus*. Throughout a time course of 6–48 h post-infection (hpi), we collected BALF and measured leukotriene production. We found that LTB_4 and cysLT showed increased production after *A. fumigatus* CEA10 challenge. The production of these inflammatory lipid mediators followed a similar trend early after infection in which their expression peaked at 6 hpi, followed by decreased levels at 12 hpi. At 24 and 48 hpi LTB_4 increased from the 12 hpi levels, while the cysLT levels continue to decrease (**Figure 1**). These data demonstrate that both LTB_4 and cysLTs are synthesized following challenge of immunocompetent mice with *A. fumigatus*.

Ltb4r1$^{-/-}$ Mice Have a Defect in Inflammatory Cell Recruitment and Resistance to IPA

LTB_4 is known to be important in the recruitment of neutrophils in numerous inflammatory settings (14), but whether it is crucial in regulating the innate immune response following *A. fumigatus* challenge is unknown. To address whether LTB_4 was critical for neutrophil recruitment and resistance against IPA, we challenged *Ltb4r1*$^{-/-}$ and C57BL/6 mice with *A. fumigatus*. At 12 hpi, we analyzed BALF *via* differential cytospins stained with Diff-Quik™ to assess early inflammatory cell recruitment to the airways. Compared with the C57BL/6 mice, *Ltb4r1*$^{-/-}$ mice had a significant defect in neutrophil and eosinophil numbers, while macrophage numbers was similar (**Figure 2A**). Because the early recruitment of neutrophils is needed for host resistance to invasive *A. fumigatus* infection (6), we next addressed whether fungal growth was enhanced in the *Ltb4r1*$^{-/-}$ animals. At 24 hpi, Grocott-Gomori methenamine silver (GMS) staining of lung sections revealed the presence of an increased proportion of germinated *A. fumigatus* in *Ltb4r1*$^{-/-}$ mice compared with C57BL/6 mice (**Figure 2B**) demonstrating *Ltb4r1*$^{-/-}$ mice were impaired in their ability to clear the fungi (**Figure 2C**). Lastly, lung damage and endothelial/epithelial leakage induced by *A. fumigatus* challenge were assessed by quantifying lactate dehydrogenase (LDH) and albumin in the BALF, respectively. Albumin levels were significantly elevated in *Ltb4r1*$^{-/-}$ mice compared with C57BL/6 mice, indicating an increase in protein leakage from the vascular system (**Figure 2D**). In contrast, LDH levels were only mildly elevated suggesting induction of similar degrees of cell damage (**Figure 2D**). Taken together, these data demonstrate that LTB_4 signaling through its high-affinity receptor LTB4R1 is important in mediating neutrophil and eosinophil recruitment to the airways, which was ultimately necessary for host resistance to *A. fumigatus* growth.

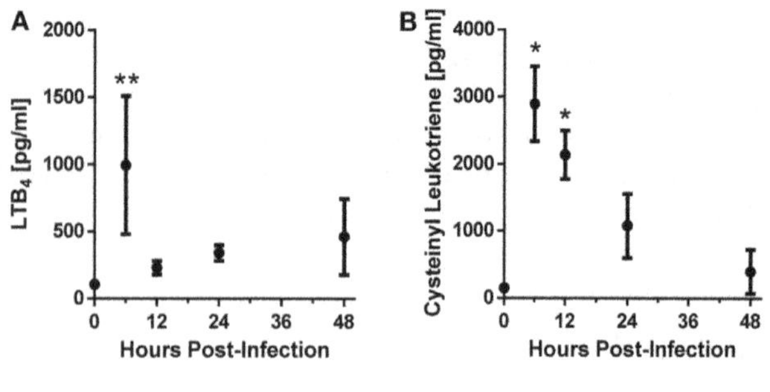

FIGURE 1 | C57BL/6 mice produce leukotrienes after pulmonary challenge with the CEA10 isolate of *Aspergillus fumigatus*. Mice were infected intratracheally with 5×10^7 CEA10 conidia and at indicated time-points, mice were euthanized and bronchoalveolar lavage fluid (BALF) collected. Lipids were then extracted from BALF using a hot-methanol extraction procedure, and LTB4 **(A)** and cysteinyl leukotriene **(B)** levels in the extracted BALF samples were measured using Cayman Chemical enzyme immunoassay kits. Data are representative of five mice per time-point. Each dot represents the mean ± 1 SEM. Statistically significant differences were determined using an one-way ANOVA with a Dunn's post-test ($^*p < 0.05$ and $^{**}p < 0.01$).

Alox5$^{-/-}$ Mice Are Impaired in Inflammatory Cell Recruitment and Resistance to IPA

Aspergillus fumigatus itself is known to be capable of producing eicosanoids (25), which results in an infection system in which both the mammalian and fungal cells could be the source of bioactive LTB_4. Thus, to address whether LTB_4 production coming from the murine cells was necessary for host resistance against *A. fumigatus*, we challenged 5-lipoxygenase (5-LO) (*Alox5*$^{-/-}$) deficient mice with *A. fumigatus*. *Alox5*$^{-/-}$ mice cannot convert arachidonic acid to LTA_4 and, therefore, lack all leukotriene synthesis (22). After *A. fumigatus* challenge, inflammatory cell recruitment to the airways was quantified at 12 hpi *via* cytospins and Diff-Quik™ staining. Similar to what we found with the *Ltb4r1*$^{-/-}$ mice, *Alox5*$^{-/-}$ mice had a significant defect in both neutrophil and eosinophil recruitment, while macrophage accumulation remained largely similar to C57BL/6 (**Figure 3A**). This defect in neutrophil and eosinophil recruitment correlated with an impairment in the ability of *Alox5*$^{-/-}$ mice to control fungal growth within the lung, demonstrated by a significantly higher germination rate (**Figures 3B,C**). We also measured LDH and albumin levels in the BALF of the *Alox5*$^{-/-}$ mice to assess lung damage and vascular/epithelial permeability, respectively. Interestingly, unlike the *Ltb4r1*$^{-/-}$ mice, LDH and albumin levels in BALF from *Alox5*$^{-/-}$ mice were not significantly different than C57BL/6 levels (**Figure 3D**). Together, these data indicate that leukotriene synthesis by host cells is critical for neutrophil and eosinophil recruitment, as well as host resistance against *A. fumigatus* growth.

Radiosensitive Cells Contribute to 5-LO Activity following Pulmonary *A. fumigatus* Challenge

To begin to determine the cells that contribute to 5-LO activity after *A. fumigatus* challenge, we utilized a bone marrow chimera approach. C57BL/6 mice were lethally irradiated then reconstituted with either C57BL/6 or *Alox5*$^{-/-}$ bone marrow intravenously to develop the following groups: C57BL/6 mice possessing C57BL/6 bone marrow and C57BL/6 mice possessing *Alox5*$^{-/-}$ bone marrow. Mice were then rested for 6–8 weeks prior to challenge with 4×10^7 conidia of CEA10. At 36 hpi, mice were euthanized, BAL collected for analysis of leukocyte recruitment to the airways, and lungs saved for histological analysis to assess fungal growth by GMS staining. Compared with C57BL/6 mice possessing C57BL/6 bone marrow, C57BL/6 mice possessing *Alox5*$^{-/-}$ bone marrow had a significant defect in neutrophil and eosinophil recruitment to the airways at 36 hpi, while macrophage accumulation was not significantly altered (**Figure 4A**). Moreover, at 36 hpi, C57BL/6

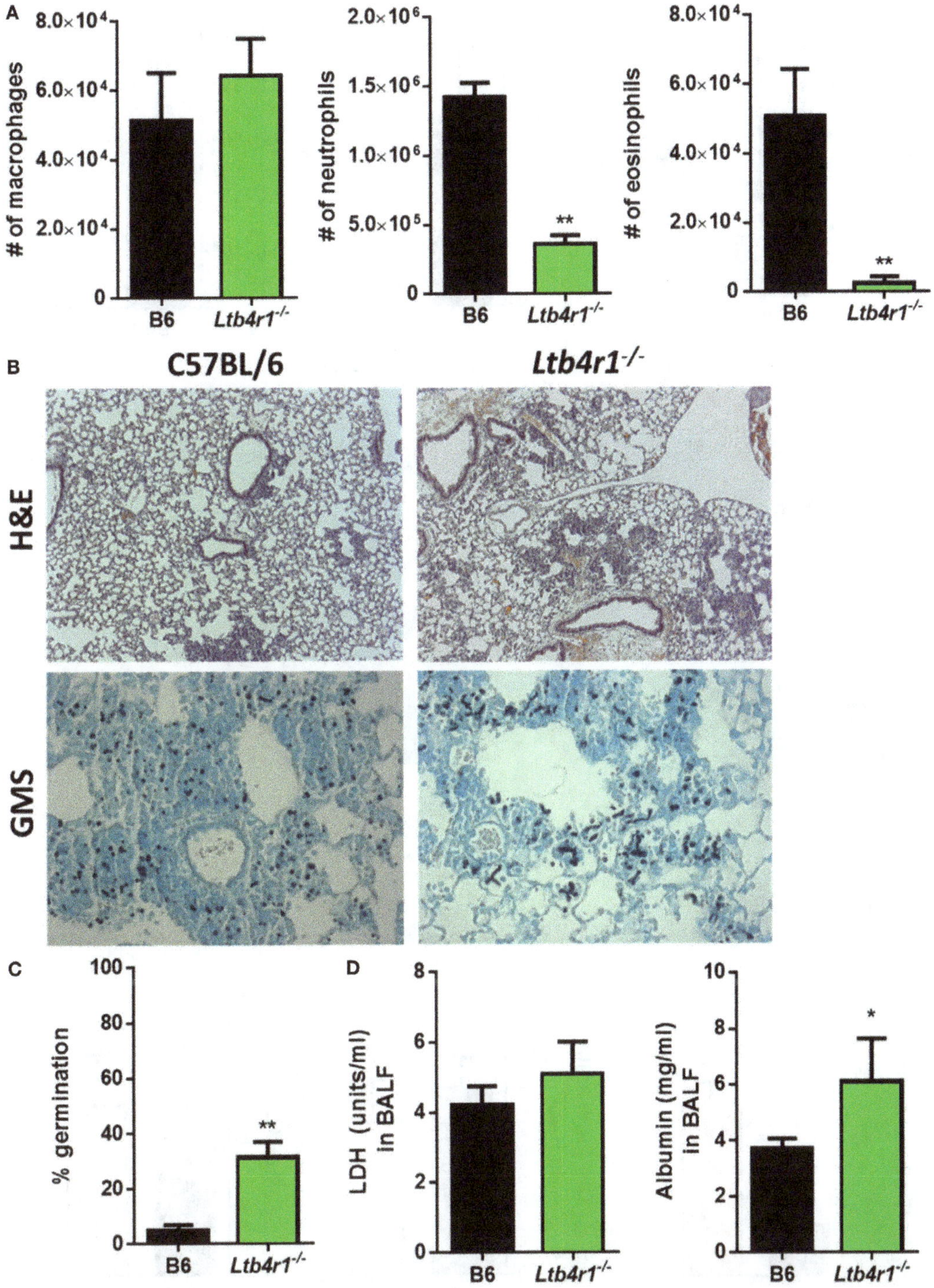

FIGURE 2 | *Ltb4r1*-deficient mice have a defect in neutrophil and eosinophil recruitment and increased fungal burden after pulmonary *Aspergillus fumigatus* challenge. Age-matched C57BL/6 or *Ltb4r1*-deficient mice were infected intratracheally with 5 × 10^7 CEA10 conidia and at indicated time-points, mice were euthanized, bronchoalveolar lavage fluid (BALF) collected, and lungs saved for histological analysis. **(A)** Total macrophage (left panel), neutrophil (middle panel), and eosinophil (right panel) numbers in the BALF was measured at 12 h post-infection (hpi). **(B)** Formalin-fixed lungs were paraffin embedded, sectioned, and stained with hematoxylin and eosin (H&E) (top) or Grocott-Gomori methenamine silver (GMS) (bottom) for analysis by microscopy. Representative lung sections from C57BL/6 and *Ltb4r1*-deficient mice infected with CEA10 are shown using the 10x objective for H&E staining or 40x objective for GMS staining. **(C)** *A. fumigatus* germination rates were assessed at 24 hpi by microscopically counting the number of conidia and germlings in GMS-stained sections from C57BL/6 and *Ltb4r1*-deficient mice. **(D)** Lung damage (left panel) and leakage (right panel) were assessed at 24 hpi by measuring lactate dehydrogenase (LDH) and albumin levels in the BALF, respectively. Data are representative of at least two independent experiments consisting of five to eight mice per group. Bar graphs show the group mean ± 1 SEM. Statistically significant differences were determined using Mann–Whitney *U* test (*$p < 0.05$, **$p < 0.01$).

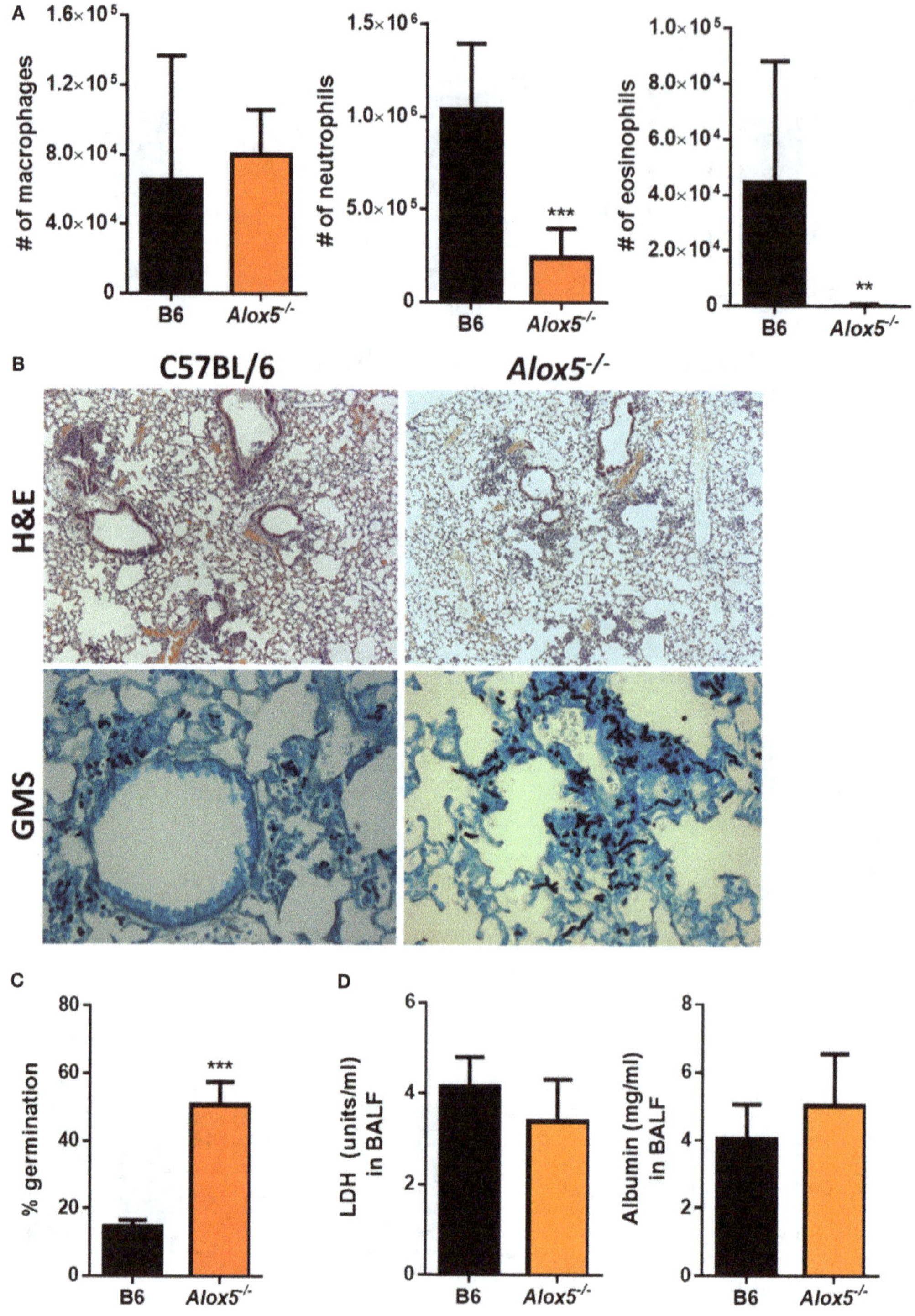

FIGURE 3 | *Alox5*-deficient mice have a defect in neutrophil and eosinophil recruitment and increased fungal burden after pulmonary *Aspergillus fumigatus* challenge. Age-matched C57BL/6J or *Alox5*-deficient mice were infected intratracheally with 5×10^7 CEA10 conidia and at indicated time-points, mice were euthanized [bronchoalveolar lavage fluid (BALF)] collected, and lungs saved for histological analysis. **(A)** Total macrophage (left panel), neutrophil (middle panel), and eosinophil (right panel) numbers in the BALF was measured at 12 hpi. **(B)** Formalin-fixed lungs were paraffin embedded, sectioned, and stained with hematoxylin and eosin (H&E) (top) or Grocott-Gomori methenamine silver (GMS) (bottom) for analysis by microscopy. Representative lung sections from C57BL/6J and *Alox5*-deficient mice infected with CEA10 are shown using the 10x objective for H&E staining or 40x objective for GMS staining. **(C)** *A. fumigatus* germination rates were assessed at 36 hpi by microscopically counting the number of conidia and germlings in GMS-stained sections from C57BL/6J and *Alox5*-deficient mice. **(D)** Lung damage (left panel) and leakage (right panel) were assessed at 36 hpi by measuring lactate dehydrogenase (LDH) and albumin levels in the BALF, respectively. Data are representative of at least two independent experiments consisting of five to eight mice per group. Bar graphs show the group mean ± 1 SEM. Statistically significant differences were determined using Mann–Whitney *U* test (**$p < 0.01$ and ***$p < 0.001$).

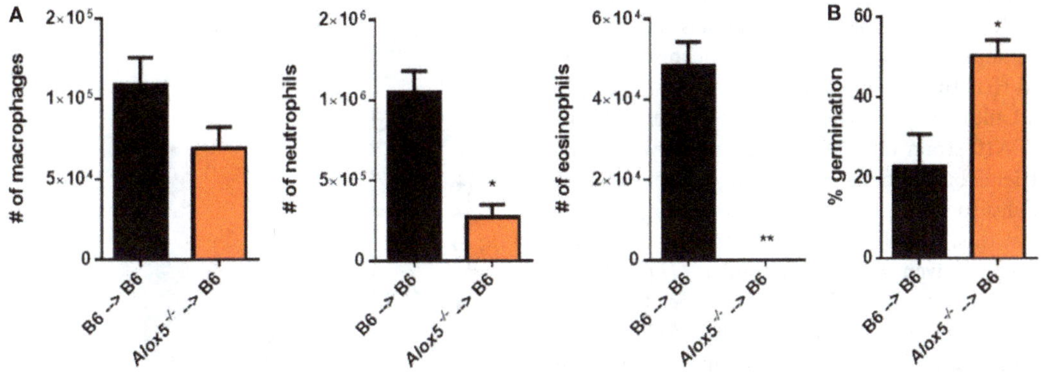

FIGURE 4 | Radiosensitive cells contribute to 5-lipoxygenase activity after pulmonary *Aspergillus fumigatus* challenge. Bone marrow chimeric mice were made by lethally irradiating C57BL/6 mice and reconstituting the mice with bone marrow from either C57BL/6 or *Alox5*$^{-/-}$ mice. These mice were challenged intratracheally with 4 × 10^7 conidia of CEA10 and at 36 hpi, mice were euthanized and **(A)** bronchoalveolar lavage fluid collected for quantification of leukocyte numbers to the airways and **(B)** lungs saved for histological analysis in which formalin-fixed lung were paraffin embedded, sectioned, and stained with Grocott-Gomori methenamine silver for analysis by microscopy. Data consist of four to five mice per group. Bar graphs show the group mean ± 1 SEM. Statistical significance was determined using a Mann–Whitney *U* test (*$p < 0.05$ and **$p < 0.01$).

mice possessing *Alox5*$^{-/-}$ bone marrow were impaired in their ability to control fungal germination compared with C57BL/6 mice possessing C57BL/6 bone marrow (**Figure 4B**). Taken together, these data suggest that radiosensitive cells contribute to 5-LO activity which is needed for neutrophil and eosinophil recruitment to the airways and control of fungal germination following pulmonary *A. fumigatus* challenge.

Leukotriene Synthesis Is Critical for Host Survival following Challenge with the CEA10 Strain of *A. fumigatus*, but Not the Af293 Strain

Thus far, we have shown that in response to the CEA10 strain of *A. fumigatus*, host-derived leukotriene synthesis is critical for timely neutrophil recruitment and control of fungal germination within the lung. Due to studies that demonstrate fungal-strain dependency on the host immune response, we next sought to determine if leukotriene-dependent immunity was reliant on the strain of *A. fumigatus* used for challenge (12, 13, 26). Inflammatory responses against the hypervirulent CEA10 isolate are highly inflammatory and heavily dependent on IL-1α for maintaining host resistance (12). Additionally, we showed that IL-1α release from macrophages following CEA10 challenge required calpain, which is a Ca^{2+}-dependent protease. Since, cPLA2 release of arachidonic acid is also a Ca^{2+}-dependent event, we hypothesized that strain-specific LTB_4 responses might be likely. To test this, we challenged C57BL/6 and *Alox5*$^{-/-}$ mice intratracheally with 5 × 10^7 conidia of either CEA10 or Af293. We monitored health and survival of mice in the 192 h following fungal challenge. *Alox5* (5-LO) was dispensable for survival of mice challenged with the Af293 strain of *A. fumigatus*, which is demonstrated by 100% survival of all mice challenged with Af293 (**Figure 5**). Conversely, *Alox5*$^{-/-}$ mice challenged with CEA10 displayed significantly higher mortality than C57BL/6 mice. Similar mortality trends were observed in the *Ltb4r1*$^{-/-}$ mice (data not shown). Overall, these data are in agreement with several other

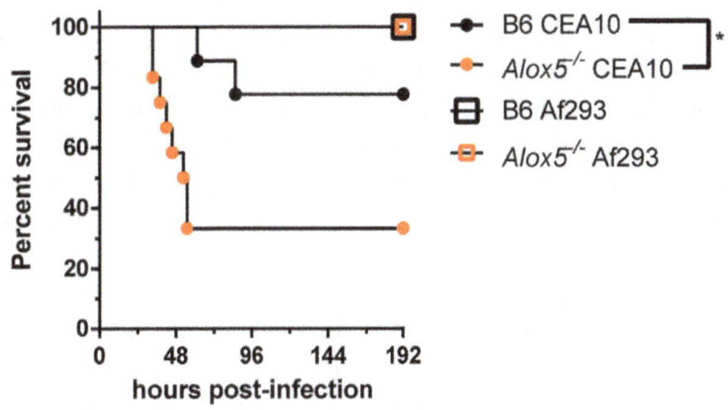

FIGURE 5 | Leukotriene-mediated immunity is fungal-strain dependent. C57BL/6 and *Alox5*-deficient were challenged with 5 × 10^7 conidia of CEA10 or Af293 intratracheal. Mice were monitored daily using a humane endpoint scoring system (based on weight loss, inactivity, ruffled fur, difficulty breathing, and neurological symptoms), and when the humane endpoint criteria was reached mice were humanely euthanized. Data are representative of 9–12 mice per group. Survival was plotted on Kaplan–Meier curves, and statistical significance between curves determined using the Mantel–Cox log rank (ns, not significant, *$p < 0.05$).

studies demonstrating that innate immune responses necessary for host resistance against *A. fumigatus* are highly dependent on the fungal strains used.

Hif1a-Deficient Mice Show a Defect in LTB4 Production following Challenge with CEA10, but Not with Af293

Under hypoxic conditions, the transcription factor hypoxia inducible factor-1α (HIF-1α) is activated, which allows translocation to the nucleus where it can bind to hypoxia response elements in the promoter region of target genes (27). HIF-1α is involved in controlling expression of 5-LO activating protein, a protein critical for the biosynthesis of LTB_4 and cysLTs, after hypoxic challenge

(28). Previous work has shown that hypoxic microenvironments form within the lung in multiple murine models of IPA (29). In an immune competent model of fungal bronchopneumonia, myeloid-derived HIF-1α was shown to be critical for neutrophil recruitment and ultimately, survival of mice challenged with *A. fumigatus* CEA10 strain (30). Given the link between HIF-1α and leukotriene biosynthesis, we sought to determine if HIF-1α contributes to LTB_4 production following *A. fumigatus* challenge. To test this, C57BL/6 or myeloid-specific lysozyme-M cre-recombinase driven HIF-1α null mice (*Hif1a*$^{LysM/LysM}$) mice were challenged with 5×10^7 conidia of either CEA10 or Af293, and LTB_4 protein levels measured in the BALF at 8 hpi. Following challenge with CEA10, there was a significant decrease in LTB_4 protein released into the airways of *Hif1a*$^{LysM/LysM}$ mice compared with C57BL/6 mice (**Figure 6A**). Interestingly, following Af293 challenge LTB_4 levels remained unchanged between C57BL/6 and *Hif1a*$^{LysM/LysM}$ mice (**Figure 6A**). Overall, this suggests that HIF-1α contributes to control of LTB_4 release following pulmonary *A. fumigatus* challenge in a fungal-strain-dependent manner.

Due to strain-specific release of LTB_4 in *Hif1a*$^{LysM/LysM}$ mice (**Figure 6A**), we next sought to determine if *Hif1a*$^{LysM/LysM}$ mice displayed a strain-specific susceptibility to *A. fumigatus* challenge. To test this, we challenged C57BL/6 and *Hif1a*$^{LysM/LysM}$ mice intratracheally with 7×10^7 conidia of either CEA10 or Af293. We monitored health and survival of mice in the 11 days following fungal challenge. HIF-1α expression in LysM-expressing cells was dispensable for survival of mice challenged with the Af293 strain of *A. fumigatus*, which is demonstrated by 90% survival of all mice challenged with Af293 (**Figure 6B**). Conversely, *Hif1a*$^{LysM/LysM}$ mice challenged with CEA10 displayed significantly higher mortality (10% survival), as previously reported (**Figure 6B**). Overall, these data are in agreement with the survival analysis of the *Alox5*$^{-/-}$ mice and reiterate that the innate immune responses necessary for host resistance against highly virulent *A. fumigatus* isolates, such as CEA10, are highly dependent on a robust inflammatory response.

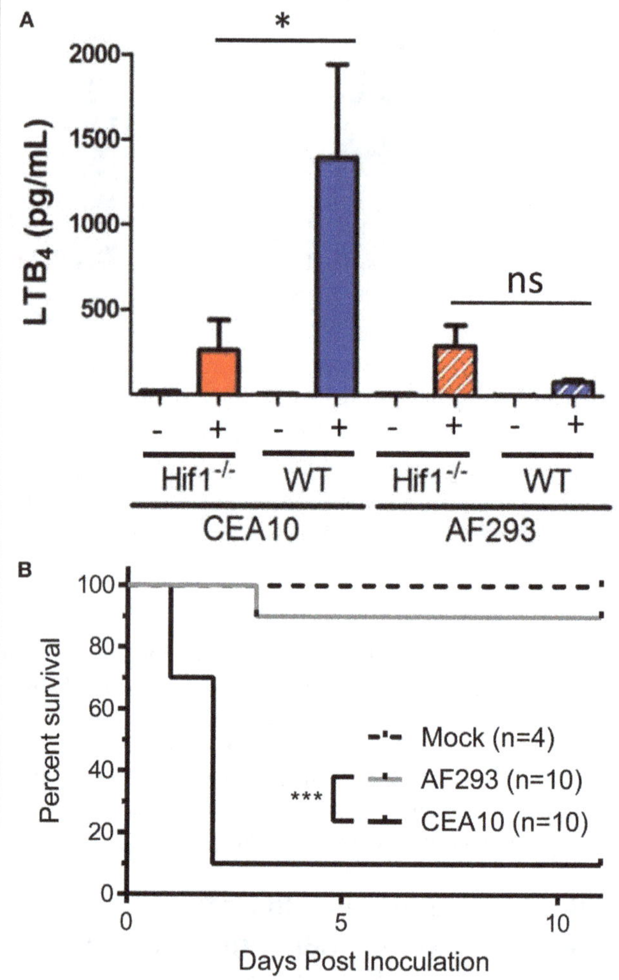

FIGURE 6 | LTB_4 production following *Aspergillus fumigatus* challenge is dependent on hypoxia inducible factor-1α (HIF-1α). **(A)** C57BL/6 or myeloid-specific lysozyme-M cre-recombinase driven HIF-1α null mice (Hif1$^{LysM/LysM}$) were challenged with either 5×10^7 CEA10 or Af293 by the intratracheal (i.t.) route. At 8 hpi, mice were euthanized, bronchoalveolar lavage fluid collected and LTB_4 measured. Data consist of four mice per group for *A. fumigatus*-challenged mice and one mouse per group challenged with PBS. Statistically significant differences were determined by a one-way ANOVA with a Dunn's post-test (ns, not significant, $^*p < 0.05$). **(B)** C57BL/6 or myeloid-specific lysozyme-M cre-recombinase driven HIF-1α null mice (Hif1$^{LysM/LysM}$) were challenged with either 7×10^7 CEA10 or Af293 by the i.t. route. Mice were monitored daily using a humane endpoint scoring system (based on weight loss, inactivity, ruffled fur, difficulty breathing, and neurological symptoms), and when the humane endpoint criteria was reached mice were humanely euthanized. Data are representative of 10 mice per experimental group or 4 mice in the uninfected control group. Survival was plotted on Kaplan–Meier curves, and statistical significance between curves determined using the Mantel–Cox log rank ($^{***}p < 0.0001$).

DISCUSSION

This study reveals an essential role for host-derived LTB_4 in the recruitment of both neutrophils and eosinophils through its high-affinity chemotactic receptor LTB4R1 following pulmonary challenge with high-virulent *A. fumigatus* strain CEA10. Ultimately, 5-LO and LTB_4 were crucial for host resistance to *A. fumigatus* challenge. In addition to recruitment of neutrophils, it was recently shown that LTB_4-treated neutrophils have enhanced anti-fungal activity against *A. fumigatus* (31). Thus, LTB_4 will not only recruit neutrophils to the site of *A. fumigatus* infection, but also simultaneously activates their anti-fungal armory. While our data are the first to demonstrate a critical role for LTB_4 in regulating neutrophil recruitment following challenge with a mold, others have reported leukotrienes are critical for leukocyte recruitment and activation following infection with the dimorphic fungi, *H. capsulatum* and *P. brasiliensis* (20, 22, 32). In these systems, it is unknown how leukotriene synthesis is initiated, but with the yeast *C. albicans* treatment of macrophages *in vitro* results in the synthesis of leukotrienes through a Dectin1-, Dectin2-, and MyD88-dependent pathway (16). Given that Dectin1, Dectin2, and MyD88 play a role in recognizing not only *A. fumigatus* (9, 10, 33, 34), but a range of fungal pathogens, it is likely this pathway will be important in the induction of the inflammatory eicosanoid pathway universally following challenge with fungal pathogens.

While it is well known that neutrophils are one of the most important effector cells against *A. fumigatus* (5), a recent study demonstrated a potential role for eosinophils in limiting the development of IPA (35). Our data demonstrate that LTB_4 is also critical for the recruitment of eosinophils to the airways of *A. fumigatus*-challenged mice. In immunocompetent mice, the absence of eosinophils resulted in a defect in *A. fumigatus* clearance *in vivo* which did not correlate with a defect in recruitment or function of other inflammatory cells, but rather the potential direct anti-fungal activity of eosinophils (35). In contrast, with repeated administration of *A. fumigatus* eosinophils were shown to have a detrimental effect on disease outcome and eosinophilia was associated with a decrease in neutrophil recruitment (36). Thus, more studies are needed to determine the exact role eosinophils play in different experimental models of IPA, and whether crosstalk between eosinophils and neutrophils regulate anti-fungal immunity.

Clinically, patients with chronic granulomatous disease have a higher risk of developing invasive *Aspergillus* infections, which is mirrored in mice lacking the NADPH oxidases. In these mice, IPA is characterized by excessive inflammation and tissue damage (37, 38). Interestingly, when *gp91*^{phox}-deficient mice were exposed subcutaneously to *A. fumigatus* there is an early neutrophilic response which is associated with elevated LTB_4 levels (38). Thus, it will be intriguing whether limiting LTB_4 signaling can ameliorate IPA in *gp91*^{phox}-deficient mice, similarly to what was observed with anakinra treatment to limit IL-1 signaling (37). This is plausible because in a *Mycobacterium tuberculosis* model, eicosanoid and IL-1 signaling regulate *M. tuberculosis* growth and pathogenicity (39). Furthermore, LTB_4 antagonism is an attractive treatment, because there are a number of clinically available inhibitors of this pathway. Another patient population at high risk of developing IPA is individuals receiving long-term corticosteroid treatment. Treatment with glucocorticoids leads to inhibition of cytosolic phospholipase A2α through the induction of lipocortin-1, blocking the conversion of phospholipids to arachidonic acid (40). Given this link between glucocorticoid treatment and the arachidonic acid pathway, it would be interesting to see the overall impact the presence or absence of leukotrienes has on the outcome of disease during a corticosteroid model of IPA. Moreover, in mice challenged with *A. fumigatus* corticosteroid treatment inhibited HIF-1α translocation to the nucleus, where it binds to target genes to regulate transcription (30). Due to the HIF-1α-dependent production of LTB_4 (**Figure 5**), it will be important to determine if the impaired HIF-1α translocation to the nucleus contributes to impaired LTB4 production, which results in enhanced susceptibility to IPA in those patients. Finally, these data suggest that the susceptibility of *Hif1α*-deficient mice to IPA may also be fungal-strain dependent, which warrants further dissection.

In conclusion, we have shown that during the inflammatory response of immunocompetent mice following pulmonary challenge with *A. fumigatus*, leukotriene production from hematopoietic cells is induced. In the absence of all leukotriene synthesis, and specifically in the absence of LTB4R1 signaling, there is a significant defect in neutrophil and eosinophil recruitment to the airways. This defect in leukocyte recruitment correlated with an elevated susceptibility of these mice to developing IPA, as measured by enhanced fungal germination in the lungs and enhanced mortality of mice devoid of leukotriene synthesis. Furthermore, the enhanced susceptibility of mice lacking leukotriene synthesis was fungal-strain dependent. Overall, these data reveal that the leukotriene pathway is critical in maintaining host resistance against *A. fumigatus* infection. Interestingly, prostaglandin E2 was recently shown to be involved in the anti-*Aspergillus* immune response (41), demonstrating a generally important role for arachidonic acid metabolites in regulating anti-fungal immunity.

AUTHOR CONTRIBUTIONS

AC-C, CK, KS, RC, and JO conceived and designed the experiments. AC-C, KH, CK, KS and RT performed the experiments. AC-C, KH, CK, KS, RT, RC, and JO analyzed the data. AC-C and JO wrote the paper. AC-C, RC, and JO edited the paper.

ACKNOWLEDGMENTS

The authors wish to thank Dr. David Leib for use of their microscope. Research in this study was funded in part by NIH R01 AI081838 (RC). JO and RC were supported in part by institutional startup funds and in part through the Dartmouth Lung Biology Center for Molecular, Cellular, and Translational Research grant P30 GM106394 (PI: Bruce A. Stanton) and Center for Molecular, Cellular, and Translational Immunological Research grant P30 GM103415 (PI: William R. Green). RC is an Investigators in the Pathogenesis of Infectious Diseases supported by the Burroughs Wellcome Fund. JO was partially supported by funding from National Institutes of Health NIGMS grant P20-GM1035000 (PI: Mark T. Quinn), the MSU Agricultural Experiment Station, and an equipment grant from the M. J. Murdock Charitable Trust. The funders had no role in study design, data collection and analysis, decision to publish, or preparation of the manuscript.

REFERENCES

1. Segal BH. Aspergillosis. *N Engl J Med* (2009) 360(18):1870–84. doi:10.1056/NEJMra0808853
2. Brown GD, Denning DW, Gow NA, Levitz SM, Netea MG, White TC. Hidden killers: human fungal infections. *Sci Transl Med* (2012) 4(165):165rv13. doi:10.1126/scitranslmed.3004404
3. Obar JJ, Hohl TM, Cramer RA. New advances in invasive aspergillosis immunobiology leading the way towards personalized therapeutic approaches. *Cytokine* (2016) 84:63–73. doi:10.1016/j.cyto.2016.05.015
4. Espinosa V, Rivera A. First line of defense: innate cell-mediated control of pulmonary aspergillosis. *Front Microbiol* (2016) 7:272. doi:10.3389/fmicb.2016.00272
5. Cramer RA, Rivera A, Hohl TM. Immune responses against *Aspergillus fumigatus*: what have we learned? *Curr Opin Infect Dis* (2011) 24(4):315–22. doi:10.1097/QCO.0b013e328348b159
6. Park SJ, Mehrad B. Innate immunity to *Aspergillus* species. *Clin Microbiol Rev* (2009) 22(4):535–51. doi:10.1128/CMR.00014-09
7. Kolaczkowska E, Kubes P. Neutrophil recruitment and function in health and inflammation. *Nat Rev Immunol* (2013) 13(3):159–75. doi:10.1038/nri3399
8. Williams M, Azcutia V, Newton G, Alcaide P, Luscinskas FW. Emerging mechanisms of neutrophil recruitment across endothelium. *Trends Immunol* (2011) 32(10):461–9. doi:10.1016/j.it.2011.06.009
9. Jhingran A, Kasahara S, Shepardson KM, Junecko BA, Heung LJ, Kumasaka DK, et al. Compartment-specific and sequential role of MyD88 and CARD9 in chemokine induction and innate defense during respiratory fungal infection. *PLoS Pathog* (2015) 11(1):e1004589. doi:10.1371/journal.ppat.1004589

10. Caffrey AK, Lehmann MM, Zickovich JM, Espinosa V, Shepardson KM, Watschke CP, et al. IL-1α signaling is critical for leukocyte recruitment after pulmonary *Aspergillus fumigatus* challenge. *PLoS Pathog* (2015) 11(1):e1004625. doi:10.1371/journal.ppat.1004625
11. Herbst S, Shah A, Mazon Moya M, Marzola V, Jensen B, Reed A, et al. Phagocytosis-dependent activation of a TLR9-BTK-calcineurin-NFAT pathway co-ordinates innate immunity to *Aspergillus fumigatus*. *EMBO Mol Med* (2015) 7(3):240–58. doi:10.15252/emmm.201404556
12. Caffrey-Carr AK, Kowalski CH, Beattie SR, Blaseg NA, Upshaw CR, Thammahong A, et al. IL-1α is critical for resistance against highly virulent *Aspergillus fumigatus* isolates. *Infect Immun* (2017) 85(12):e00661-17. doi:10.1128/IAI.00661-17
13. Rizzetto L, Giovannini G, Bromley M, Bowyer P, Romani L, Cavalieri D. Strain dependent variation of immune responses to *A. fumigatus*: definition of pathogenic species. *PLoS One* (2013) 8(2):e56651. doi:10.1371/journal.pone.0056651
14. Sadik CD, Luster AD. Lipid-cytokine-chemokine cascades orchestrate leukocyte recruitment in inflammation. *J Leukoc Biol* (2012) 91(2):207–15. doi:10.1189/jlb.0811402
15. Parti RP, Loper R, Brown GD, Gordon S, Taylor PR, Bonventre JV, et al. Cytosolic phospholipase A(2) activation by *Candida albicans* in alveolar macrophages: role of dectin-*1*. *Am J Respir Cell Mol Biol* (2010) 42(4):415–23. doi:10.1165/rcmb.2009-0110OC
16. Suram S, Gangelhoff TA, Taylor PR, Rosas M, Brown GD, Bonventre JV, et al. Pathways regulating cytosolic phospholipase A(2) activation and eicosanoid production in macrophages by *Candida albicans*. *J Biol Chem* (2010) 285(40):30676–85. doi:10.1074/jbc.M110.143800
17. Suram S, Silveira LJ, Mahaffey S, Brown GD, Bonventre JV, Williams DL, et al. Cytosolic phospholipase A(2)α and eicosanoids regulate expression of genes in macrophages involved in host defense and inflammation. *PLoS One* (2013) 8(7):e69002. doi:10.1371/journal.pone.0069002
18. Jayaraja S, Dakhama A, Yun B, Ghosh M, Lee H, Redente EF, et al. Cytosolic phospholipase A(2) contributes to innate immune defense against *Candida albicans* lung infection. *BMC Immunol* (2016) 17:27. doi:10.1186/s12865-016-0165-9
19. Morato-Marques M, Campos MR, Kane S, Rangel AP, Lewis C, Ballinger MN, et al. Leukotrienes target F-actin/cofilin-1 to enhance alveolar macrophage anti-fungal activity. *J Biol Chem* (2011) 286(33):28902–13. doi:10.1074/jbc.M111.235309
20. Secatto A, Soares EM, Locachevic GA, Assis PA, Paula-Silva FWG, Serezani CH, et al. The leukotriene B_4/BLT1 axis is a key determinant in susceptibility and resistance to histoplasmosis. *PLoS One* (2014) 9(1):e85083. doi:10.1371/journal.pone.0085083
21. Secatto A, Rodrigues LC, Serezani CH, Ramos SG, Dias-Baruffi M, Faccioli LH, et al. 5-lipoxygenase deficiency impairs innate and adaptive immune responses during fungal infection. *PLoS One* (2012) 7(3):e31701. doi:10.1371/journal.pone.0031701
22. Santos PC, Santos DA, Ribeiro LS, Fagundes CT, de Paula TP, Avila TV, et al. The pivotal role of 5-lipoxygenase-derived LTB(4) in controlling pulmonary paracoccidioidomycosis. *PLoS Negl Trop Dis* (2013) 7(8):e2390. doi:10.1371/journal.pntd.0002390
23. Balderramas HA, Ribeiro OG, Soares ÂMVC, Oliveira SL. The role of leukotriene B_4 in early stages of experimental paracoccidioidomycosis induced in phenotypically selected mouse strains. *Med Mycol* (2013) 51(6):625–34. doi:10.3109/13693786.2013.777163
24. Medeiros AI, Sá-Nunes A, Turato WM, Secatto A, Frantz FG, Sorgi CA, et al. Leukotrienes are potent adjuvant during fungal infection: effects on memory T cells. *J Immunol* (2008) 181(12):8544–51. doi:10.4049/jimmunol.181.12.8544
25. Noverr MC, Toews GB, Huffnagle GB. Production of prostaglandins and leukotrienes by pathogenic fungi. *Infect Immun* (2002) 70(1):400–2. doi:10.1128/IAI.70.1.400-402.2002
26. Kowalski CH, Beattie SR, Fuller KK, McGurk EA, Tang Y-W, Hohl TM, et al. Heterogeneity among isolates reveals that fitness in low oxygen correlates with *Aspergillus fumigatus* virulence. *MBio* (2016) 7(5):e1515-6. doi:10.1128/mBio.01515-16
27. Nizet V, Johnson RS. Interdependence of hypoxic and innate immune responses. *Nat Rev Immunol* (2009) 9(9):609–17. doi:10.1038/nri2607
28. Gonsalves CS, Kalra VK. Hypoxia-mediated expression of 5-lipoxygenase-activating protein involves HIF-1α and NF-κB and microRNAs 135a and 199a-5p. *J Immunol* (2010) 184(7):3878–88. doi:10.4049/jimmunol.0902594
29. Grahl N, Puttikamonkul S, Macdonald JM, Gamcsik MP, Ngo LY, Hohl TM, et al. *In vivo* hypoxia and a fungal alcohol dehydrogenase influence the pathogenesis of invasive pulmonary aspergillosis. *PLoS Pathog* (2011) 7(7):e1002145. doi:10.1371/journal.ppat.1002145
30. Shepardson KM, Jhingran A, Caffrey A, Obar JJ, Suratt BT, Berwin BL, et al. Myeloid derived hypoxia inducible factor 1-alpha is required for protection against pulmonary *Aspergillus fumigatus* infection. *PLoS Pathog* (2014) 10(9):e1004378. doi:10.1371/journal.ppat.1004378
31. Jones CN, Dimisko L, Forrest K, Judice K, Poznansky MC, Markmann JF, et al. Human neutrophils are primed by chemoattractant gradients for blocking the growth of *Aspergillus fumigatus*. *J Infect Dis* (2016) 213(3):465–75. doi:10.1093/infdis/jiv419
32. Medeiros AI, Sá-Nunes A, Soares EG, Peres CM, Silva CL, Faccioli LH. Blockade of endogenous leukotrienes exacerbates pulmonary histoplasmosis. *Infect Immun* (2004) 72(3):1637–44. doi:10.1128/IAI.72.3.1637-1644.2004
33. Steele C, Rapaka RR, Metz A, Pop SM, Williams DL, Gordon S, et al. The beta-glucan receptor dectin-1 recognizes specific morphologies of *Aspergillus fumigatus*. *PLoS Pathog* (2005) 1(4):e42. doi:10.1371/journal.ppat.0010042
34. Sun H, Xu X-Y, Shao H-T, Su X, Wu X-D, Wang Q, et al. Dectin-2 is predominately macrophage restricted and exhibits conspicuous expression during *Aspergillus fumigatus* invasion in human lung. *Cell Immunol* (2013) 284(1–2):60–7. doi:10.1016/j.cellimm.2013.06.013
35. Lilly LM, Scopel M, Nelson MP, Burg AR, Dunaway CW, Steele C. Eosinophil deficiency compromises lung defense against *Aspergillus fumigatus*. *Infect Immun* (2014) 82(3):1315–25. doi:10.1128/IAI.01172-13
36. O'Dea EM, Amarsaikhan N, Li H, Downey J, Steele E, Van Dyken SJ, et al. Eosinophils are recruited in response to chitin exposure and enhance Th2-mediated immune pathology in *Aspergillus fumigatus* infection. *Infect Immun* (2014) 82(8):3199–205. doi:10.1128/IAI.01990-14
37. de Luca A, Smeekens SP, Casagrande A, Iannitti R, Conway KL, Gresnigt MS, et al. IL-1 receptor blockade restores autophagy and reduces inflammation in chronic granulomatous disease in mice and in humans. *Proc Natl Acad Sci U S A* (2014) 111(9):3526–31. doi:10.1073/pnas.1322831111
38. Petersen JE, Hiran TS, Scott Goebel W, Johnson C, Murphy RC, Azmi FH, et al. Enhanced cutaneous inflammatory reactions to *Aspergillus fumigatus* in a murine model of chronic granulomatous disease. *J Invest Dermatol* (2002) 118(3):424–9. doi:10.1046/j.0022-202x.2001.01691.x
39. Mayer-Barber KD, Andrade BB, Oland SD, Amaral EP, Barber DL, Gonzales J, et al. Host-directed therapy of tuberculosis based on interleukin-1 and type I interferon crosstalk. *Nature* (2014) 511(7507):99–103. doi:10.1038/nature13489
40. Rhen T, Cidlowski JA. Antiinflammatory action of glucocorticoids—new mechanisms for old drugs. *N Engl J Med* (2005) 353(16):1711–23. doi:10.1056/NEJMra050541
41. Garth JM, Reeder KM, Godwin MS, Mackel JJ, Dunaway CW, Blackburn JP, et al. IL-33 signaling regulates innate IL-17A and IL-22 production via suppression of prostaglandin E2 during lung fungal infection. *J Immunol* (2017) 199(6):2140–8. doi:10.4049/jimmunol.1602186

4

Involvement of Dihydrolipoyl Dehydrogenase in the Phagocytosis and Killing of *Paracoccidioides brasiliensis* by Macrophages

Taise N. Landgraf[1], Marcelo V. Costa[2], Aline F. Oliveira[3], Wander C. Ribeiro[1], Ademilson Panunto-Castelo[2] and Fabrício F. Fernandes[3]*

[1] Department of Biochemistry and Immunology, Ribeirão Preto Medical School, University of São Paulo, Ribeirão Preto, Brazil, [2] Department of Biology, Faculty of Philosophy, Sciences and Letters of Ribeirão Preto, University of São Paulo, Ribeirão Preto, Brazil, [3] Department of Cell and Molecular Biology, Ribeirão Preto Medical School, University of São Paulo, Ribeirão Preto, Brazil

***Correspondence:**
Fabrício F. Fernandes
fabsff@yahoo.com.br

Paracoccidioides brasiliensis and *Paracoccidioides lutzii* are fungi causing paracoccidioidomycosis (PCM), an autochthonous systemic mycosis found in Latin America. These microorganisms contain a multitude of molecules that may be associated with the complex interaction of the fungus with the host. Here, we identify the enzyme dihydrolipoyl dehydrogenase (DLD) as an exoantigen from *P. brasiliensis* (Pb18_Dld) by mass spectrometry. Interestingly, the DLD gene expression in yeast form showed higher expression levels than those in mycelial form and transitional phases. Pb18_Dld gene was cloned, and the recombinant protein (rPb18_Dld) was expressed and purified for subsequent studies and production of antibodies. Immunogold labeling and transmission electron microscopy revealed that the Pb18_Dld is also localized in mitochondria and cytoplasm of *P. brasiliensis*. Moreover, when macrophages were stimulated with rPb18Dld, there was an increase in the phagocytic and microbicidal activity of these cells, as compared with non-stimulated cells. These findings suggest that Pb18_Dld can be involved in the pathogen-host interaction, opening possibilities for studies of this protein in PCM.

Keywords: *Paracoccidioides brasiliensis*, dihydrolipoyl dehydrogenase, exoantigen, subcellular localization, microbicidal activity

INTRODUCTION

Paracoccidioidomycosis (PCM) is a chronic granulomatous mycosis caused by thermally dimorphic fungi *Paracoccidioides lutzii* and *P. brasiliensis*, which contain a complex of at least four different cryptic species, S1, PS2, PS3, and PS4 (Matute et al., 2006; Carrero et al., 2008; Teixeira et al., 2009, 2014; Theodoro et al., 2012). PCM is the most important systemic mycosis in Latin America with high prevalence in Brazil, Colombia, Argentina, and Venezuela. The mean annual mortality rate is 1.65 per million inhabitants, the highest for any systemic mycosis, making PCM the eighth most important cause of mortality among chronic or recurrent infectious, parasitic diseases, and infectious diseases in Brazil (Coutinho et al., 2002; Colombo et al., 2011; Bocca et al., 2013).

Fungi of the genus *Paracoccidioides* are asexual and dimorphic, growing as mycelial forms at 25°C and as yeast form at 37°C (da Silva et al., 1994; de Almeida, 2005). Transformation of the fungus from mycelia to yeast is responsible for establishing the infectious process (Bagagli et al., 2008) as well as for the initial interaction of the fungus with the immune system, which determines the fate of the infecting forms. Secretion of antimicrobial proteins by the pulmonary epithelium and phagocytic activity of resident alveolar macrophages mediates the initial response to infection (Calich et al., 2008). Infections can stimulate different subsets of T cells and consequently induce the production of distinct patterns of cytokines that are responsible for the protection or susceptibility of the host to pathogens (Della Bella et al., 2017), including fungal infections (Calich and Kashino, 1998; Oliveira et al., 2002; Romani, 2004).

The ability of this pathogenic fungus to develop a multi-faceted response to a wide variety of stressors found in the host is extremely important for its virulence and pathogenesis. Many of these extracellular molecules are secreted by or are associated with the fungal wall (Casotto, 1990; Diniz et al., 1999, 2001). Numerous proteins or glycoproteins that are common to different strains of *P. brasiliensis* are secreted in culture, and these are recognized, to varying degrees, by the serum of the patients (Panunto-Castelo et al., 2003). The most studied exoantigen (ExoAg) of *P. brasiliensis* is the 43-kDa glycoprotein (gp43), which is a molecule involved in binding of *P. brasiliensis* to the extracellular matrix and surface of epithelial cells (Vicentini et al., 1994; Gesztesi et al., 1996). More recently, Torres et al. (2013) showed that *P. brasiliensis* cell lines in which gp43 was silenced were less internalized by macrophages.

Some studies have been carried out in order to elucidate the complex programs of gene expression that *Paracoccidioides* spp. uses to survive when exposed to conditions similar to those found in the host. Tavares et al. (2007) showed, for instance, that *P. brasiliensis* regulates expression of 119 genes during phagocytosis. These genes were first associated with glucose and amino acid limitation, cell wall building, and oxidative stress. Subsequent studies also elucidated the molecules involved in the adaptation of the fungus. In addition to the activation of enzymes involved in the defense against oxidative stress (Derengowski et al., 2008; de Arruda Grossklaus et al., 2013; Parente-Rocha et al., 2015), other metabolic modifications have been suggested to occur in yeast cells, such as gluconeogenesis, ethanol production, and degradation of fatty acids and amino acids (Lima et al., 2014).

In this study, we aimed to identify the proteins that were secreted/excreted by *P. brasiliensis*. We also attempted to evaluate whether these molecules could have any association with the phagocytosis and killing activity, contributing to the pathogenic process. Although *P. brasiliensis* secretes a number of different proteins into the basal medium, one protein in particular drew our attention because it was present in high amount. The protein was identified as dihydrolipoyl dehydrogenase (Pb18_Dld), which was expressed at high levels in the pathogenic form, and was located in and outside the mitochondria, which improved the macrophage-mediated phagocytic and microbicidal activity.

MATERIALS AND METHODS

Ethics Statement and Mice

This work was conducted according to the ethical principles of animal research adopted by the Brazilian Society of Laboratory Animal Science, and received approval from the Ethics Committee on Animal Use of the Ribeirão Preto Medical School, USP. The Protocol number is 105/2007. Male BALB/c mice, aged 6–8 weeks, were purchased from the Central Animal House of the Ribeirão Preto Campus of University de São Paulo (USP), and were maintained in the Animal Facilities of the Department of Biology, Faculty of Philosophy, Sciences and Letters of Ribeirão Preto, USP.

Growth Conditions of the *P. brasiliensis* Isolate

Virulent yeast cells of *P. brasiliensis* strain 18 (Pb18) were cultured for 15 days at 37°C in DMEM (Sigma-Aldrich, St Louis, USA), in a shaking incubator at 100 rpm. The yeast cells were maintained by culturing at 37°C, while the mycelial forms were obtained by culturing at 25°C. Both cultures were maintained under these conditions for 7 days. The transition phase from mycelium-to-yeast was induced by culturing the mycelia at 25°C for 72 h, changing the temperature to 37°C, and incubating for 24 h. The transition from yeast to mycelium was induced by growing yeast for 72 h at 37°C, changing the temperature to 25°C, and incubating for 24 h. One aliquot of each *P. brasiliensis* culture was treated with 50 μg/mL Calcofluor white stain (Sigma-Aldrich) for 30 min at 37°C to analyze the fungal morphological forms by fluorescence microscopy.

Preparation of Extracellular Extract and Total Soluble Antigen from *P. brasiliensis* and Pb18_Dld Identification

Supernatants of the cultures containing ExoAgs were recovered by centrifugation at 10,000 × g, concentrated and diafiltrated against 10 mM phosphate-buffered saline (PBS, pH 7.2) using centrifugal filtration devices with a molecular weight cut-off of 10,000 kDa (Millipore, Billerica, USA). The ExoAgs were analyzed using 12% sodium dodecyl sulfate-polyacrylamide gel electrophoresis (SDS-PAGE). The gels were stained with Coomassie brilliant blue G250 (USB Corporation, Cleveland, USA). The relative amount of the 60-kDa protein band was calculated with the ImageJ 1.37v software (National Institutes of Health, Bethesda, USA) and the values were normalized against the total amount of loaded proteins. Next, the 60-kDa band was excised from the gel, and mass spectrometry was performed at the FingerPrint Proteomics and Mass Spectrometry Facility, College of Life Sciences, University of Dundee. Mascot (version 2.3; Matrix, United Kingdom) analysis was performed to identify peptides and to search for proteins in the NCBI non-redundant (nr) database. Total soluble antigen derived from *P. brasiliensis* yeast cells was prepared according to reported by Fernandes et al. (Panunto-Castelo et al., 2003).

In Silico Analysis

The *in silico* analyses were performed based on Pb18_Dld amino acid sequence (GenBank accession no. EEH50415.1) that was submitted to NetOGlyc 3.1 Server (http://www.cbs.dtu.dk/services/NetOGlyc-3.1/), NetNGlyc 1.0 Server (http://www.cbs.dtu.dk/services/NetNGlyc/), SignalP 4.1 Server (http://www.cbs.dtu.dk/services/SignalP/), and TargetP v1.1 Server (http://www.cbs.dtu.dk/services/TargetP/). Protein conserved domains are available in the CDD NCBI's conserved domain database (https://www.ncbi.nlm.nih.gov/Structure/cdd/wrpsb.cgi).

Differential Expression of Dld mRNA from Different Morphological Forms of *P. brasiliensis*

The gene expression profile of *P. brasiliensis* was analyzed in mycelium, yeast, and transition forms from mycelium-to-yeast and yeast-to-mycelium, which were cultivated as described previously. The total RNA from the *P. brasiliensis* morphological forms was extracted using *TRIzol* (Thermo Fisher Scientific Inc., Waltham, USA). Briefly, cells were harvested, disrupted by grinding in liquid nitrogen, and mixed with TRizol, according to the manufacturer's instructions. Total RNA was treated with DNase I (Thermo Fisher Scientific Inc.). The concentration of RNA was measured with the help of a spectrophotometer at 260 nm and the quality of RNA was evaluated by the ratio of absorbance at 260 and 280 nm. In order to ensure RNA integrity, samples were electrophoresed in 1.5% agarose gel. In addition, the absence of contaminating chromosomal DNA was confirmed, after the treatment of the RNA with DNaseI, by the absence of the HSP60 gene amplification (Fernandes et al., 2016) after PCR. cDNA was synthesized using 1 μg of total RNA with oligo-dT_{12-18} primer (Thermo Fisher Scientific Inc.) and SuperScript III reverse transcriptase (Thermo Fisher Scientific Inc.), according to the manufacturer's instructions. Real-time PCR was performed using *Kit Platinum SYBR Green qPCR SuperMix-UDG with ROX* (Thermo Fisher Scientific Inc.), according to the manufacturer's instructions. Next, specific primers were used for Pb18_DLD: 5′-GGTTTGGACAAGGTCGG-3′ (sense) and 5′-CATGGCCGTAGCCCTTC-3′ (antisense). To measure the gene expression levels, we used CFX96 real-time PCR detection system (Bio-Rad, Hercules, USA). Fold changes in mRNA expression were calculated using the $2^{-\Delta Cq}$ formula, where ΔCq is the difference in the threshold cycle (*Cq*) between the DLD (target) gene and the β-actin (Sequence ID: ref |XM_010763641.1|) or α-tubulin references (housekeeping) genes (Goldman et al., 2003). The reaction of the genes β-actin and α-tubulin was done using a couple of primers: 5′-GGATGAGGAGATGGATTATGG-3′ (sense) and 5′-GAAACACTCGACGCACACGAC-3′ (antisense); and 5′-GTGGACCAGGTGATCGATGT-3′ (sense) and 5′-ACCCTGGAGGCAGTCACA-3′ (antisense), respectively. All experiments were performed using biological and experimental triplicates.

Cloning of the Pb18_Dld Gene Transcript

The cDNA obtained from the mRNA of yeast cells of *P. brasiliensis* was used to amplify the region encoding Pb18_Dld using oligonucleotide primers 5′-CATATGTTTCGGCCCCTTCTCCC-3′ (sense) and 5′-GGATCCCTAGAAATGAATCGCTTTCG-3′ (antisense), and high-fidelity Taq DNA polymerase (Thermo Fisher Scientific Inc.). The amplified fragment was cloned into pCR 2.1-TOPO vector (Thermo Fisher Scientific Inc.), and was sequenced at the Laboratory of Plant Molecular Biology from the *Faculty of Philosophy, Sciences, and Letters of Ribeirão* Preto—USP. Next, the fragment was removed from the pCR 2.1-TOPO vector using restriction enzymes *NdeI* and *BamHI* (Fermentas, Carlsbad, USA), and was sub-cloned into pET-28a vector (Addgene, Cambridge, USA).

Expression and Purification of rPb18_Dld

The pET-28a vector, containing the gene transcript of Pb18_Dld, was transformed into *Escherichia coli* BL21 cells for expression of the Pb18_Dld recombinant protein (rPb18_Dld). Briefly, cultures were grown in LB medium supplemented with kanamycin sulfate (50 μg/mL) at 37°C until an absorbance of 0.4–0.5 was observed at 600 nm. Then, rPb18_rDld expression was induced with 0.8 mM isopropyl-D-thiogalactopyranoside (IPTG) for 6 h. The bacterial cells were then harvested by centrifugation at 10,000 × g, at 25°C for 10 min, resuspended in buffer containing 50 mM NaH_2PO_4, 300 mM NaCl, and 20 mM imidazole (pH 8.0), and lysed by sonication. The pellet containing the insoluble fractions was washed five times with a washing buffer [50 mM NaH_2PO_4, 300 mM NaCl, 2 M urea, 2 mM 2-mercaptoethanol, 20 mM imidazole, and 1% Triton X-100 (pH 8.0)]. Then, the pellet was resuspended in solubilization buffer [50 mM NaH_2PO_4, 300 mM NaCl, 20 mM imidazole, 7 M urea (pH 8.0)], followed by incubation for 1 h at room temperature. The solubilized material was recovered by centrifugation at 10,000 × g at 4°C for 10 min, and was filtered through Millex-GV PVDF (pore size, 0.22 μm; Millipore). The rPb18_Dld was purified by performing metal chelate affinity chromatography with a Ni^{2+}–Sepharose affinity column (His-Trap; GE Healthcare, Piscataway, USA). Next, the rPb18_Dld was eluted using elution buffer (50 mM NaH_2PO_4, 300 mM NaCl, 300 mM imidazole, 7 M urea), refolded by dialysis against PBS, and concentrated by ultrafiltration. Protein concentration was determined using BCA kit (Pierce Chemical Co., Rockford, USA) and purity, size, and identity of the rPb18_Dld protein were evaluated using SDS-PAGE (12%). In addition, the recombinant protein samples were analyzed for endotoxin contamination by using Limulus amebocyte lysate (LAL) assay (Sigma-Aldrich), and were found to contain <0.05 ng/mL of bacterial endotoxin.

Mice Immunization

We used purified rPb18_Dld protein to generate specific anti-rPb18_Dld polyclonal antibody in mice serum. Male BALB/c mice were immunized by subcutaneous injection of 50 μL of purified protein (10 μg/mice) with 50 μL of complete Freund's adjuvant (CFA, Sigma-Aldrich) at first administration. Animals were boosted twice, at 1-week intervals, with the same amount of antigen emulsified in 50 μL of incomplete Freund's adjuvant. One week after the last boost, the serum containing polyclonal antibody to rPb18_rDld was aliquoted and stored at −20°C.

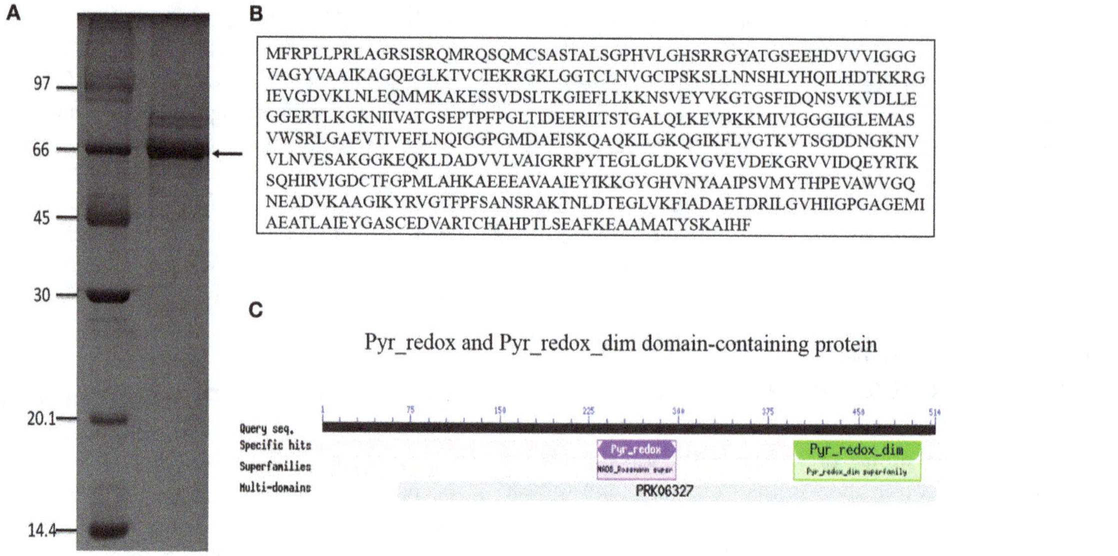

FIGURE 1 | Pb18_Dld identification. **(A)** SDS-PAGE result of *P. brasiliensis* exoantigens grown in DMEM, for 15 days at 37°C. After this period, cultures were centrifuged, and the supernatant was dialyzed and analyzed. The band indicated by the arrow was excised from the gel and analyzed by mass spectrometry. SDS-PAGE was stained with Coomassie brilliant blue. **(B)** Pb18_Dld amino acid sequence. **(C)** Conserved domains (available on CDD NCBI's conserved domain database).

Western Blotting

The electrophoresis analyses were performed on 12% SDS–PAGE, and transferred to polyvinylidene fluoride membranes (PVDF)—Hybond membranes Amersham 0.45 P PVDF (GE Healthcare). Thereafter, membranes were incubated with Tris-buffered saline (TBS-T) [20 mM Tris-HCl, 150 mM NaCl and 0.1% (v/v) Tween-20 (pH 7.6)] containing 3% gelatin for 1 h at 25°C, and incubated for 4 h at room temperature with anti-Pb18_rDld polyclonal antibody diluted 1:1,000 in TBS-T containing 1% gelatin. Thereafter, membranes were washed five times with TBS-T and incubated for 2 h at room temperature with the anti-mouse IgG rabbit secondary antibody conjugated to peroxidase (Sigma-Aldrich) diluted 1:500 in TBS-T containing 1% gelatin. Blots were washed five times with TBS-T and then immersed in a fresh mixture of 4-chloro-1-naphthol (4C1N) (Sigma-Aldrich) and 3/3-diaminobenzidine tetrahydrochloride (Sigma-Aldrich) or ECL reagent for 1 min to detection of protein using a ChemiDoc MP Imaging System (Bio-Rad, Hercules, USA).

Electron Microscopy

The Pb18_Dld subcellular localization was performed with yeast and mycelia washed with PBS and fixed in 3.7% formaldehyde buffered with PBS at 25°C for 1 h. After fixation, cells were washed with PBS and resuspended in 0.05% glutaraldehyde buffered with PBS and incubated at 25°C. After 15 min, the cells were centrifuged at 5,000 × g for 5 min at 25°C and washed three times with 1 mL of PBS. Then, the cells were resuspended in PBS containing 0.1% Triton X-100 and incubated at 25°C for 45 min. The cells were recovered by centrifugation at 5,000 × *g* for 5 min and washed with 1 mL PBS. Samples were incubated with 1 mL PBS-1% BSA at 25°C. After 45 min, anti-Pb18_rDld polyclonal antibody (1:500) was added for 1 h, followed by incubation at 25°C under gentle agitation. After washing with PBS-1% BSA, colloidal gold-conjugated anti-mouse IgG (Nanoprobes Inc., NY, USA) was added to the cells for 1 h at 25°C under gentle agitation. The cells were washed five times with PBS, with 5 min incubation for each wash and fixed with 2.5% glutaraldehyde in 100 mM cacodylate buffer (pH 7.4) (EM Sciences, Hatfield, USA) at 25°C for 1 h. Cells were washed with cacodylate buffer and incubated at 4°C for 18 h, followed by washing five times with ultrapure water. Further processing of cells was conducted as per the manufacturer's instructions of GoldEnhancement (Nanoprobes). Subsequently, the fixed cells were incubated in 1% OsO_4 (EM Sciences) for 2 h, rinsed in ultrapure water, and incubated with a solution of saturated thiocarbohydrazide (EM Sciences), followed by 1% OsO_4. Yeast cells were dehydrated with ethanol (30–100% v/v) and coated with gold in a BAL-TEC SCD 050 Sputter Coater (BAL-TEC AG, Balzers, Liechtenstein). Finally, the sections were observed with a transmission electron microscope Jeol JEM—100 CXII (JEOL, Peabody, MA, USA).

Macrophages Phagocytic and Microbicidal Activity Assays

Macrophages were obtained from the peritoneal cavity of BALB/c mice 72 h after an intraperitoneal injection of 1 mL of 3% sterile sodium thioglycollate medium (Sigma-Aldrich), according to the described protocol (Freitas et al., 2016). Peritoneal macrophages (1×10^6) were stimulated or not with 10 µg of rPb18_Dld and maintained in a 5% CO_2 humidified atmosphere incubator at 37°C. After 24 h, macrophages were infected with 3×10^5 yeast cells of *P. brasiliensis* and incubated for 4 h at 37°C.

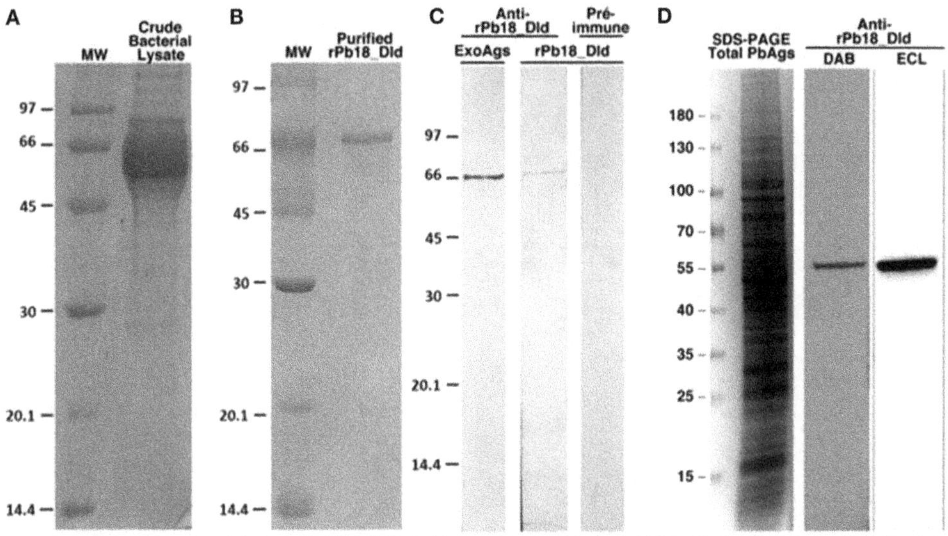

FIGURE 2 | Analysis of the expression and purification of rPb18_Dld, and production of anti-rPB18_Dld polyclonal antibody. SDS-PAGE results of **(A)** rPb18_Dld expression and **(B)** purified rPb18_Dld by affinity chromatography using a liquid chromatographic system, Akta Purifier in HisTrap Crude FF column. The purified protein was dialyzed against PBS. SDS-PAGE was stained with Coomassie brilliant blue. **(C)** Western blotting analysis of anti-rPb18_Dld polyclonal serum. Membranes containing rPb18_Dld or total exoantigens containing native Pb18_Dld (ExoAg) were incubated with serum containing polyclonal anti-rPb18_Dld antibodies. Negative control of the reaction was performed using the membrane containing rPb18_Dld incubated with preimmune serum. The membranes were visualized by peroxide substrate hydrogen and diaminobenzidine tetrahydrochloride. **(D)** SDS-PAGE stained with Coomassie brilliant blue of total soluble antigen from *P. brasiliensis* (Total PbAgs). Western blotting analysis of anti-rPb18_Dld polyclonal serum with membranes containing Total PbAgs were incubated with 1:1,000 containing polyclonal anti-rPb18_Dld antibodies. The membranes were visualized by peroxide substrate hydrogen and diaminobenzidine tetrahydrochloride (DAB) or by chemiluminescent with ECL reagent (ECL).

The cultures were washed with RPMI-incomplete medium. To evaluate the phagocytic activity, 1 mL of distilled water was added to the microplate wells to promote macrophage lysis. The samples were serially diluted and cultured for 10 days at 37°C in solid BHI medium supplemented with 1% glucose to determine the presence of colony forming units (CFU) of viable yeasts. To analyze microbicidal activity, the washed cultures were additionally incubated for 48 h. Macrophage lysis and yeast cultures were carried out as described above. The number of CFU were counted and expressed as CFU/well.

Statistical Analyses

Data are expressed as mean ± standard deviation from at least duplicate experiments. Statistical differences between the means of the experimental groups were determined using the Student's unpaired *t*-test (GraphPad Software, San Diego, USA). Differences with $P < 0.05$ were considered statistically significant.

RESULTS

Identification of Dihydrolipoyl Dehydrogenase (Pb18_Dld) as the Predominant Protein in the *P. brasiliensis* Culture Supernatant

Antigens secreted by *P. brasiliensis* could play an important role in fungus-host interactions. Therefore, we sought to identify new antigens from supernatants after centrifugation of *P. brasiliensis* cultured in DMEM, which is a basal medium that does not contain proteins. When the supernatants were analyzed by SDS-PAGE, we observed that a major band of 60 kDa was invariably present in all ExoAgs preparations (**Figure 1A**), comprising more than 85% of the total protein content. Some minor bands were observed in the supernatants, such as the proteins of 90-, 85-, and 43-kDa, the latter possibly being gp43. One-dimensional nano-LC-MS/MS analysis of tryptic fragments of the 60 kDa protein band revealed two unique peptides that matched the sequence of Pb18_Dld (GenBank accession number EEH50415.1). Pb18_Dld is a protein involved in fungal metabolism (Weber et al., 2012; Parente-Rocha et al., 2015), and is composed of 514 amino acids (**Figure 1B**), with a small NADH binding domain, a larger FAD-binding domain (Pyr_redox), and a dimerization domain (Pyr_redox_dim) (**Figure 1C**).

To confirm the presence of Pb18_DLD in the culture supernatant, we used anti-rPb18_Dld polyclonal antibody. First, we cloned the *Pb18_Dld* gene transcript in an expression plasmid, pET28-a, for the production of the recombinant protein in bacteria (rPb18_Dld) (**Figure 2A**). **Figure 2B** shows the recombinant protein, which was purified using a nickel column for the production of anti-rPb18_Dld polyclonal antibodies in mouse. Use of the anti-recombinant protein antibody revealed the presence of Dld in total soluble antigen from yeast cells, as well as, in *P. brasiliensis* DMEM culture supernatant (**Figures 2C,D**), suggesting that Pb18_Dld is a protein secreted by *P. brasiliensis*.

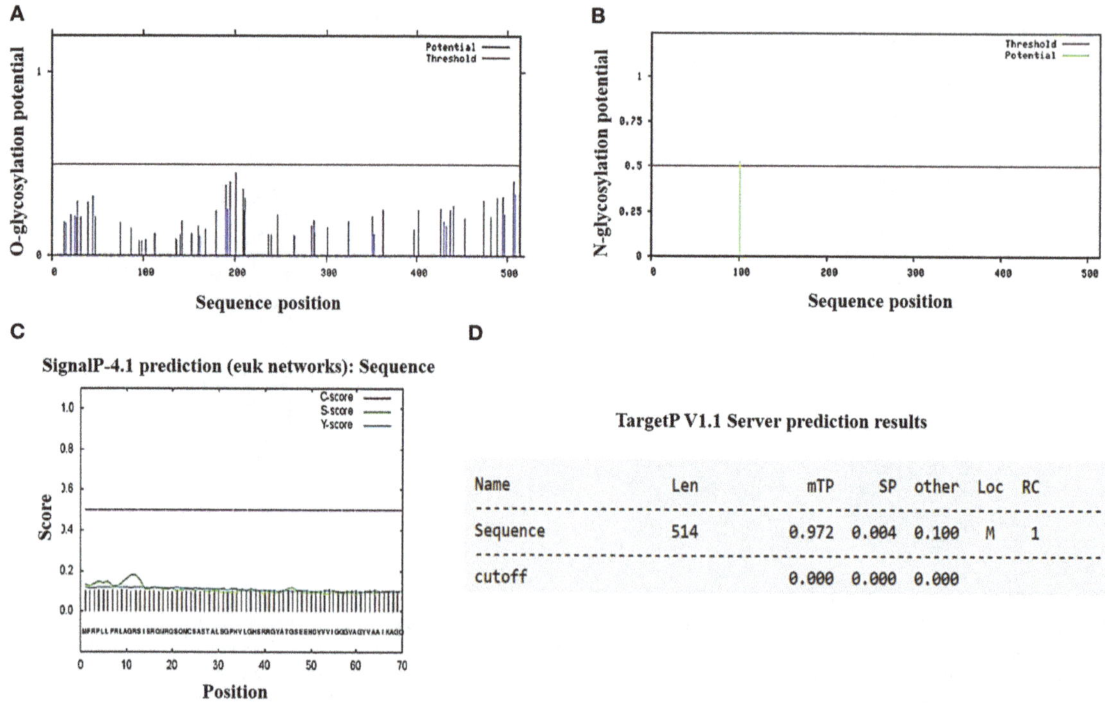

Name	Len	mTP	SP	other	Loc	RC
Sequence	514	0.972	0.004	0.100	M	1
cutoff		0.000	0.000	0.000		

FIGURE 3 | *In silico* analysis of the presence of glycosylation potential sites, signal peptide, and prediction analysis of subcellular location from Pb18_Dld. The amino acid sequence of Pb18_Dld protein was used for analysis in different programs **(A,B)** NetOGlyc 1.0 and NetNGlyc 3.11 show graphics with horizontal lines that represent the reliability limits of the results and vertical lines that indicate the potential sites of O- and N-glycosylation. **(C)** SignalP-4.1 shows graphic with dotted line, representing the reliability limits of results. The lines C, S, and Y-score indicate possible signal peptide cleavage positions and signal peptide regions. **(D)** TargetP v1.1 shows the length (Len), mitochondrial target peptide (mTP), secretory pathway (SP), localization (Loc), mitochondria (M), and reliability class (RC).

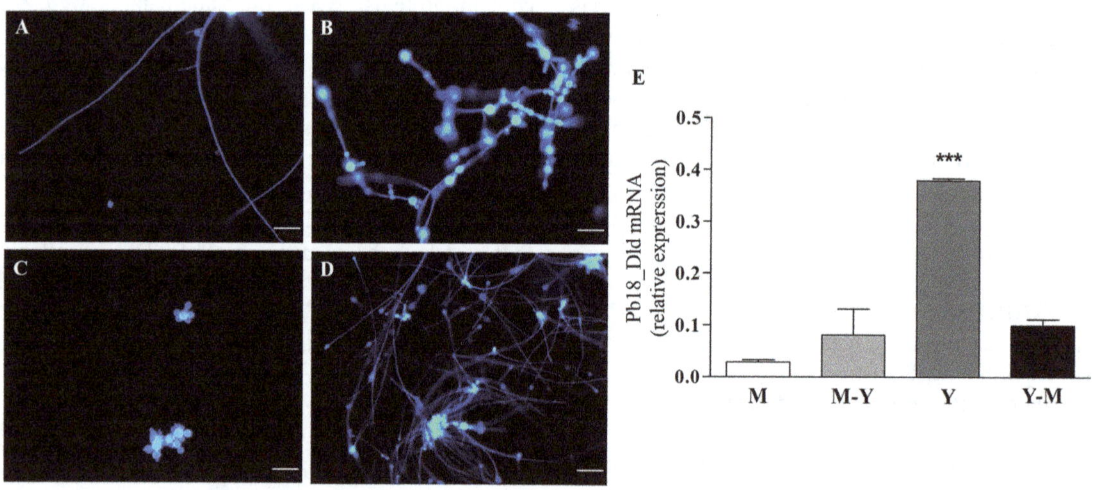

FIGURE 4 | Pb18_Dld mRNA differential expression in different morphological forms of *P. brasiliensis*. **(A–D)** Morphological analysis by fluorescence microscopy. An aliquot of each fungal culture was incubated with Calcofluor white stain solution (50 μg/mL) for labeling the fungal cells. The bars correspond to 20 μm. **(E)** Evaluation of Pb18_Dld mRNA differential expression by RT-qPCR using cDNA from mycelia **(A)**, mycelia-to-yeast **(B)**, yeast **(C)**, and yeast-to-mycelia **(D)**. The β-actin and α-tubulin reference genes were used as endogenous controls to normalize the relative Pb18_Dld mRNA expression.

In Silico Analysis of Pb18_Dld

As part of a complementary analysis to characterize Pb18_Dld, we conducted an *in silico* examination of the protein to check for the presence of putative N- and O-linked oligosaccharides and signal peptides in the amino acid sequence. The analysis revealed that this protein possessed only one putative N-glycosylation site

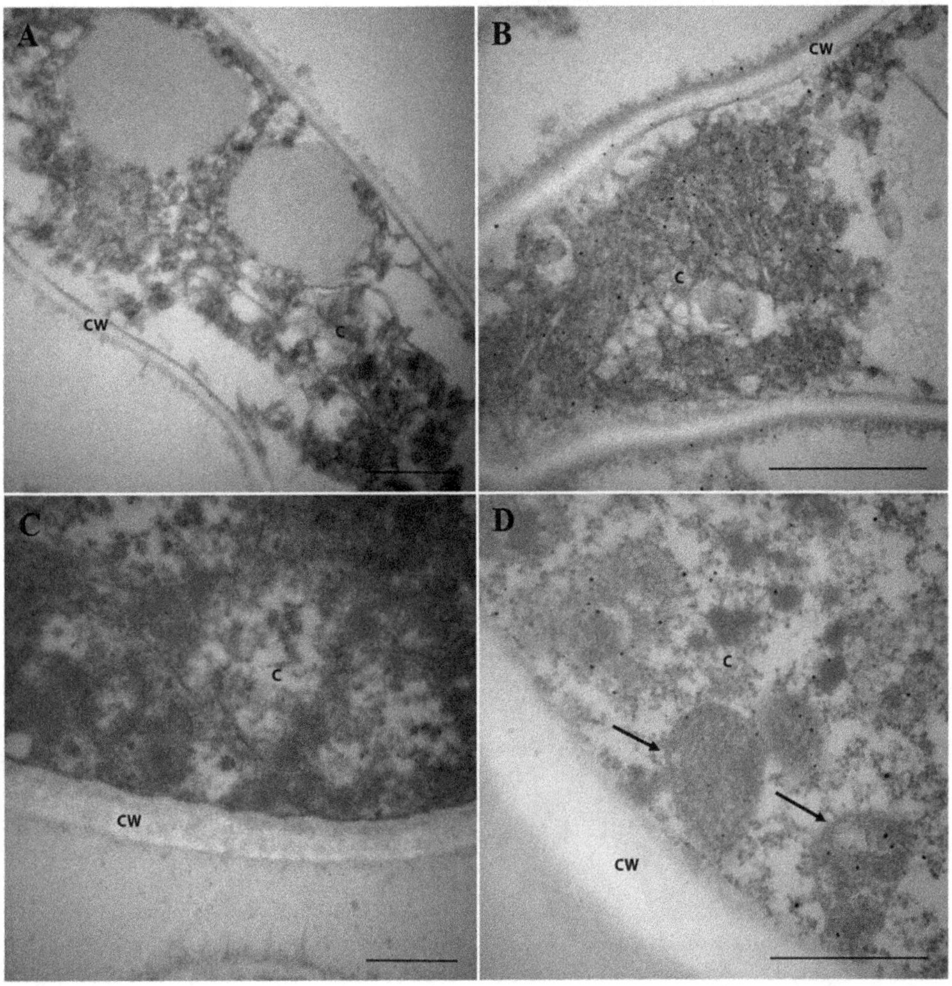

FIGURE 5 | Pb18_Dld localization in mycelia and yeast cells from *P. brasiliensis*, visualized by immunoelectron microscopy. **(A,B)** Mycelium and **(C,D)** yeast from *P. brasiliensis* were labeled with primary polyclonal antibody anti-rPb18_Dld **(B,D)** or pre-immune serum **(A,B)** and secondary antibody conjugated to colloidal gold. The staining of Pb18_Dld was analyzed by electron microscopy. Bars correspond to 2 μm. The C and CW identifications correspond to the cytoplasm and cell wall, respectively. The arrows indicate mitochondria.

in the asparagine residue at the 101 position, no potential site of O-glycosylation (**Figures 3A,B**) and no signal peptide that targeted the protein to the secretory pathway (**Figures 3C,D**). Moreover, the data obtained *in silico* by using TargetP predicted that Pb18_Dld was localized in mitochondria (**Figure 3D**), although it was also identified in the extracellular fraction. Together, these data suggest that Pb18_Dld is a mitochondrial protein that can be secreted via a non-conventional pathway.

Pb18_Dld from *P. brasiliensis* Is Expressed Primarily in Yeast Form

To determine if there were differences in expression levels of Pb18_Dld in yeast, mycelia, and transition forms, we compared normalized mRNA-expression levels among *in vitro* grown phases. Prior to mRNA extraction, we confirmed that the fungal morphology corresponded to expected forms by fluorescence microscopy of samples stained with Calcofluor white (**Figures 4A–D**). Pb18_Dld transcripts were detected in all evaluated morphological forms, although they showed higher expression in yeast, which is the pathogenic form, as compared with levels in transition phases (mycelium-to-yeast and yeast-to-mycelium) or the mycelial form (**Figure 4E**).

Pb18_Dld Subcellular Localization in *P. brasiliensis* Yeast and Mycelia

As Pb18_Dld was a component of ExoAgs and *in silico* analysis of its sequence did not show the signal peptide, we intended to investigate the localization of Pb18_Dld in fungal yeast. Yeast and mycelia of *P. brasiliensis* were fixed and incubated with anti-rPb18_Dld polyclonal mice antibody, and subsequently, incubated with secondary antibody, colloidal gold anti-mouse IgG conjugate, for immunodetection of the protein by electron microscopy. Control samples were obtained by incubation with pre-immune mice serum (**Figures 5A,C**). Electron microscopy assays revealed the ubiquitous distribution of gold particles in cytoplasm and mitochondria of both forms of *P. brasiliensis* (**Figures 5B,D**). In addition, the protein was also present in the mycelial cell wall (**Figure 5B**). Together, these results are in accordance with the mitochondrial localization predicted by *in silico* analysis, and suggest that Pb18_Dld could be secreted by an alternative secretion pathway.

Phagocytosis of Macrophages is Increased in the Presence of rPb18_Dld

Macrophages comprise one of the primary defense mechanisms against infection by *P. brasiliensis* (Brummer et al., 1988a,b). Additionally, Pb18_Dld showed higher expression in the pathogenic form. Therefore, we evaluated whether this protein could have some effect on the phagocytic and microbicidal activity of macrophages. Phagocytosis and killing assays were performed using peritoneal macrophages. Interestingly, when the cells were pretreated with rPb18_Dld, we observed a significant increase in the phagocytic activity, i.e., after 4 h of co-culture, from 3.98×10^3 CFU/mL $\pm$ 1.28 to 6.9×10^3 CFU/mL $\pm$ 0.30. We also observed an increase in the microbicidal activity i.e., after 48 h of co-culture, with a reduction from 4.18×10^3 CFU/mL $\pm$ 0.71 to 2.6×10^3 CFU/mL $\pm$ 0.78 at rDld-Pb18 stimulated-macrophages, representing relative killing of 62% of yeast cells (**Figure 6**). Together, our data suggest that this protein may be important to improve fungicidal process by macrophages during infection.

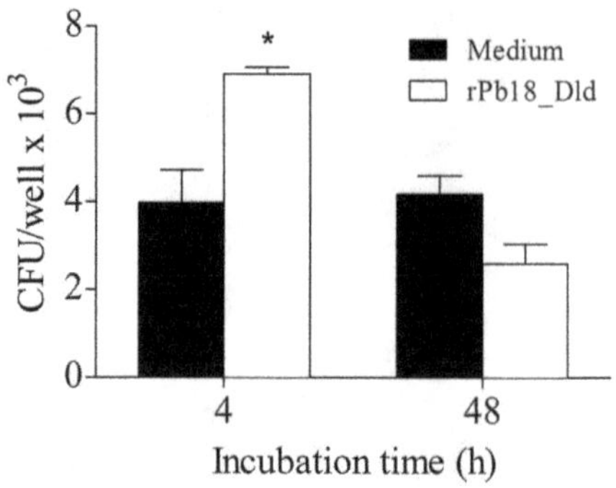

FIGURE 6 | Phagocytic and microbicidal activity of macrophages stimulated with rPb18_Dld. *P. brasiliensis* yeast cells were grown in DMEM medium at 37°C for 5 days and co-cultured with peritoneal macrophages, prestimulated or not with 10 μg of rPb18_rDld. Phagocytic and microbicidal activity were determined by counting the CFU of yeast recovered from the lysate of murine peritoneal macrophages after 4 and 48 h of incubation with yeast at 37°C, respectively. Results represent the mean $\pm$ standard deviation values of two independent experiments in triplicate. $^*P < 0.05$ in relation to the other experimental groups, as determined by Student *t*-test.

DISCUSSION

In this study, to identify new antigens from *P. brasiliensis* that could be associated with the host, we focused on ExoAgs preparations and isolated a highly expressed protein, identified by mass spectrometry as Pb18_Dld. The fact that Pb18_Dld could be detected in the extracellular extract suggested that it was an ExoAg released by the fungus. This is an intriguing observation because orthologs of this protein were typically detected in the mitochondria. It is part of the machinery responsible for aerobic respiration, in which the pyruvate produced by glycolysis and via the phosphate pentose pathway is mainly oxidized and decarboxylated to acetyl-CoA by the pyruvate dehydrogenase complex (Lehninger et al., 2005). In accordance with its function, our electron microscopy data showed that this enzyme is located in the mitochondria and, interestingly, in the cytoplasm of mycelia and yeast and in the mycelial cell wall. Corroborating our findings, work published by Weber et al. (2012) showed that Dld from *P. lutzii* is a component of extracellular proteomics of mycelial and yeast forms.

The presence of Pb18_Dld and other proteins at the cell surface or outside the fungal cell wall, in the absence of a conventional N-terminal signal sequence responsible for targeting the protein to classical secretory pathway, is an intriguing question. To explain this occurrence, non-conventional secretory pathways, as well as unusual signal sequences, had been described. An example of unusual transport is the extracellular vesicles produced by fungi (Straus et al., 1996). In fact, some enzymes involved in the glycolytic pathway and tricarboxylic acid cycle were identified in the contents of these vesicles (Vallejo et al., 2012).

Carbohydrates are the primary and preferred carbon source used by most organisms (Askew et al., 2009). For survival of pathogens in the hostile host microenvironment, expression of virulence factors and their ability to assimilate various carbon sources for energy production are important (Lorenz et al., 2004; Barelle et al., 2006; Askew et al., 2009; Romani, 2011). Some studies indicate that metabolic remodeling observed in *Paracoccidioides* spp. infection is a survival strategy (Lima et al., 2014). *P. lutzii*, when grown under copper deprivation, showed induction of the pyruvate dehydrogenase complex, suggesting that availability of acetyl-CoA by the generated pyruvate could be important for the survival of *P. lutzii* in inhospitable conditions (de Oliveira et al., 2014). Parente-Rocha et al. (2015) demonstrated that the fungi could modify their metabolism when subjected to conditions that mimic macrophage infection by *P. brasiliensis*. In this study, we observed that there is an increase in the Dld expression in yeast cells, which is the pathogenic form of *P. brasiliensis*.

High Dld expression in the ExoAgs preparation of *P. brasiliensis* raised the possibility that this protein might be a potential virulence factor, facilitating the infection. A common approach for recognition of virulence factors in dimorphic fungi is the correlation with increased expression of the possible factor in the pathogenic form of the fungus (Rappleye and Goldman, 2006). Our results have shown that the expression of Pb18_Dld mRNA is the highest in the yeast morphology, which is the fungal pathogenic form. Similar to Dld, glyceraldehyde-3-phosphate dehydrogenase (GAPDH), a glycolytic enzyme from *P. brasiliensis*, was shown to be present in larger amounts in the parasitic yeast phase than in the mycelia, suggesting a putative role for GAPDH in the parasitic phase of the fungus (Barbosa et al., 2004). Subsequently, it was demonstrated that GAPDH is located at the outermost layer in the cell wall of *P. brasiliensis* yeast forms, and has adhesive properties (Barbosa et al., 2006). The ability to perform biological functions unrelated to the protein canonical function is common for some metabolic enzymes of *Paracoccidioides* spp. that are frequently involved in virulence (Marcos et al., 2014). When we added rPb18_Dld to cultures of macrophages from the peritoneal cavity, it induced a higher phagocytosis rate. To date, there has been no report regarding the role of this metabolic protein in immune responses of the host. Although our results suggested that Pb18_Dld possibly displayed immunostimulatory effects in host cells, it was undeniable that many molecules induced the activation of macrophages and yet had a deleterious effect on the host (Medzhitov, 2008). Therefore, further experiments are needed before we reject the association of Pb18_Dld with *P. brasiliensis* virulence.

In summary, we demonstrated that Dld, a glycolytic enzyme, which is present in the mitochondria, cytoplasm, and cell wall and is secreted by *P. brasiliensis*, is more prominently expressed in the pathogenic form of the fungus. In addition, this protein stimulates the immune system by increasing the phagocytic and microbicidal activity of macrophages. Although the significance of this protein in disease progression has to be confirmed by virulence tests, for instance, using genetically Pb18_Dld deficient yeast, our work offers a new approach to studying Pb18_Dld as a potential therapeutic target in PCM.

AUTHOR CONTRIBUTIONS

Conceived and designed the experiments: TL, AP, and FF. Performed the experiments: TL, MC, AO, WR, and FF. Analyzed the data: TL, AP, and FF. Contributed reagents/materials/analysis tools: AP and FF. Wrote the paper: TL, AP, and FF.

FUNDING

This work was supported by Fundação de Amparo à Pesquisa de São Paulo (grant numbers 2012/08552-0, 2013/12278-3, and 2016/00629-4).

ACKNOWLEDGMENTS

We thank Andréa Carla Quiapim for technical support in sequencing. We thank Maria Dolores Seabra Ferreira and José Augusto Maulin for technical support in electron microscopy.

REFERENCES

1. Askew, C., Sellam, A., Epp, E., Hogues, H., Mullick, A., Nantel, A., et al. (2009). Transcriptional regulation of carbohydrate metabolism in the human pathogen *Candida albicans*. *PLoS Pathog.* 5:e1000612. doi: 10.1371/journal.ppat. 1000612
2. Bagagli, E., Theodoro, R. C., Bosco, S. M., and McEwen, J. G. (2008). *Paracoccidioides brasiliensis*: phylogenetic and ecological aspects. *Mycopathologia* 165, 197–207. doi: 10.1007/s11046-007-9050-7
3. Barbosa, M. S., Bao, S. N., Andreotti, P. F., de Faria, F. P., Felipe, M. S., dos Santos Feitosa, L., et al. (2006). Glyceraldehyde-3-phosphate dehydrogenase of *Paracoccidioides brasiliensis* is a cell surface protein involved in fungal adhesion to extracellular matrix proteins and interaction with cells. *Infect. Immun.* 74, 382–389. doi: 10.1128/IAI.74.1.382-389.2006
4. Barbosa, M. S., Cunha Passos, D. A., Felipe, M. S., Jesuino, R. S., Pereira, M., and de Almeida Soares, C. M. (2004). The glyceraldehyde-3-phosphate dehydrogenase homologue is differentially regulated in phases of *Paracoccidioides brasiliensis*: molecular and phylogenetic analysis. *Fungal Genet. Biol.* 41, 667–675. doi: 10.1016/j.fgb.2004.02.002
5. Barelle, C. J., Priest, C. L., Maccallum, D. M., Gow, N. A., Odds, F. C., and Brown, A. J. (2006). Niche-specific regulation of central metabolic pathways in a fungal pathogen. *Cell. Microbiol.* 8, 961–971. doi: 10.1111/j.1462-5822.2005. 00676.x
6. Bocca, A. L., Amaral, A. C., Teixeira, M. M., Sato, P. K., Shikanai-Yasuda, M. A., and Soares Felipe, M. S. (2013). Paracoccidioidomycosis: eco-epidemiology, taxonomy and clinical and therapeutic issues. *Future Microbiol.* 8, 1177–1191. doi: 10.2217/fmb.13.68
7. Brummer, E., Hanson, L. H., and Stevens, D. A. (1988a). Gamma-interferon activation of macrophages for killing of *Paracoccidioides brasiliensis* and evidence for nonoxidative mechanisms. *Int. J. Immunopharmacol.* 10, 945–952. doi: 10.1016/0192-0561(88)90041-0
8. Brummer, E., Hanson, L. H., Restrepo, A., and Stevens, D. A. (1988b). *In vivo* and *in vitro* activation of pulmonary macrophages by IFN-gamma for enhanced killing of *Paracoccidioides brasiliensis* or *Blastomyces dermatitidis*. *J. Immunol.* 140, 2786–2789.
9. Calich, V. L., and Kashino, S. S. (1998). Cytokines produced by susceptible and resistant mice in the course of *Paracoccidioides brasiliensis* infection. *Braz. J. Med. Biol. Res.* 31, 615–623. doi: 10.1590/S0100-879X1998000500003
10. Calich, V. L., da Costa, T. A., Felonato, M., Arruda, C., Bernardino, S., Loures, F. V., et al. (2008). Innate immunity to *Paracoccidioides brasiliensis* infection. *Mycopathologia* 165, 223–236. doi: 10.1007/s11046-007-9048-1
11. Carrero, L. L., Nino-Vega, G., Teixeira, M. M., Carvalho, M. J., Soares, C. M., Pereira, M., et al. (2008). New *Paracoccidioides brasiliensis* isolate reveals unexpected genomic variability in this human pathogen. *Fungal Genet. Biol.* 45, 605–612. doi: 10.1016/j.fgb.2008.02.002
12. Casotto, M. (1990). Characterization of the cellular antigens of *Paracoccidioides brasiliensis* yeast form. *J. Clin. Microbiol.* 28, 1188–1193.
13. Colombo, A. L., Tobon, A., Restrepo, A., Queiroz-Telles, F., and Nucci, M. (2011). Epidemiology of endemic systemic fungal infections in Latin America. *Med. Mycol.* 49, 785–798. doi: 10.3109/13693786.2011.577821
14. Coutinho, Z. F., Silva, D., Lazera, M., Petri, V., Oliveira, R. M., Sabroza, P. C., et al. (2002). Paracoccidioidomycosis mortality in Brazil (1980-1995). *Cad. Saúde Publica* 18, 1441–1454. doi: 10.1590/S0102-311X2002000500037
15. da Silva, A. M., Borba, C. M., and de Oliveira, P. C. (1994). Viability and morphological alterations of *Paracoccidioides brasiliensis* strains preserved under mineral oil for long periods of time. *Mycoses* 37, 165–169. doi: 10.1111/j.1439-0507.1994.tb00295.x
16. de Almeida, S. M. (2005). Central nervous system paracoccidioidomycosis: an overview. *Braz. J. Infect. Dis.* 9, 126–133. doi: 10.1590/S1413-86702005000200002
17. de Arruda Grossklaus, D., Bailao, A. M., Vieira Rezende, T. C., Borges, C. L., de Oliveira, M. A., Parente, J. A., et al. (2013). Response to oxidative stress in *Paracoccidioides* yeast cells as determined by proteomic analysis. *Microbes Infect.* 15, 347–364. doi: 10.1016/j.micinf.2012.12.002
18. de Oliveira, H. C., da Silva Jde, F., Matsumoto, M. T., Marcos, C. M., Peres da Silva, R., Moraes da Silva, R. A., et al. (2014). Alterations of protein expression in conditions of copper-deprivation for *Paracoccidioides lutzii* in the presence of extracellular matrix components. *BMC Microbiol.* 14:302. doi: 10.1186/s12866-014-0302-7
19. Della Bella, C., Benagiano, M., De Gennaro, M., Gomez-Morales, M. A., Ludovisi, A., D'Elios, S., et al. (2017). T-cell clones in human trichinellosis: evidence for a mixed Th1/Th2 response. *Parasite Immunol.* 39:e12412. doi: 10.1111/pim.12412
20. Derengowski, L. S., Tavares, A. H., Silva, S., Procopio, L. S., Felipe, M. S., and Silva- Pereira, I. (2008). Upregulation of glyoxylate cycle genes upon *Paracoccidioides brasiliensis* internalization by murine macrophages

and *in vitro* nutritional stress condition. *Med. Mycol.* 46, 125–134. doi: 10.1080/136937807016 70509
21. Diniz, S. N., Cisalpino, P. S., Freire, A. T., Silva-Teixeira, D. N., Contigli, C., Rodrigues Junior, V., et al. (2001). *In vitro* granuloma formation, NO production and cytokines profile from human mononuclear cells induced by fractionated antigens of *Paracoccidioides brasiliensis*. *Hum. Immunol.* 62, 799–808. doi: 10.1016/S0198-8859(01)00268-3
22. Diniz, S. N., Cisalpino, P. S., Koury, M. C., Andrade, G. M., Nogueira, M. G., and Goes, A. M. (1999). *In vitro* human immune reactivity of fast protein liquid chromatography fractionated *Paracoccidioides brasiliensis* soluble antigens. *Microbes Infect.* 1, 353–360. doi: 10.1016/S1286-4579(99) 80051-3
23. Fernandes, F. F., Oliveira, L. L., Landgraf, T. N., Peron, G., Costa, M. V., Coelho- Castelo, A. A., et al. (2016). A detrimental effect of fungal 60-kDa heat shock protein on experimental *Paracoccidioides brasiliensis* infection. *PLoS ONE* 11:e0162486. doi: 10.1371/journal.pone.0162486
24. Freitas, M. S., Oliveira, A. F., da Silva, T. A., Fernandes, F. F., Goncales, R. A., Almeida, F., et al. (2016). Paracoccin induces M1 polarization of macrophages via interaction with TLR4. *Front. Microbiol.* 7:1003. doi: 10.3389/fmicb.2016.01003
25. Gesztesi, J. L., Puccia, R., Travassos, L. R., Vicentini, A. P., de Moraes, J. Z., Franco, M. F., et al. (1996). Monoclonal antibodies against the 43,000 Da glycoprotein from *Paracoccidioides brasiliensis* modulate laminin-mediated fungal adhesion to epithelial cells and pathogenesis. *Hybridoma* 15, 415–422. doi: 10.1089/hyb.1996.15.415
26. Goldman, G. H., dos Reis Marques, E., Duarte Ribeiro, D. C., de Souza Bernardes, L. A., Quiapin, A. C., Vitorelli, P. M., et al. (2003). Expressed sequence tag analysis of the human pathogen *Paracoccidioides brasiliensis* yeast phase: identification of putative homologues of *Candida albicans* virulence and pathogenicity genes. *Eukaryotic Cell* 2, 34–48. doi: 10.1128/EC.2.1.34- 48.2003
27. Lehninger, A. L., Nelson, D. L., and Cox, M. M. (2005). *Lehninger Principles of Biochemistry, 4th Edn.* New York, NY: W. H. Freeman.
28. Lima P. S., Casaletti, L., Bailao, A. M., de Vasconcelos, A. T., Fernandes Gda, R., and Soares, C. M. (2014). Transcriptional and proteomic responses to carbon starvation in *Paracoccidioides*. *PLoS Negl. Trop. Dis.* 8:e2855. doi: 10.1371/journal.pntd.0002855
29. Lorenz, M. C., Bender, J. A., and Fink, G. R. (2004). Transcriptional response of *Candida albicans* upon internalization by macrophages. *Eukaryotic Cell* 3, 1076–1087. doi: 10.1128/EC.3.5.1076-1087.2004
30. Marcos, C. M., de Oliveira, H. C., da Silva Jde, F., Assato, P. A., Fusco-Almeida, A. M., and Mendes-Giannini, M. J. (2014). The multifaceted roles of metabolic enzymes in the Paracoccidioides species complex. *Front. Microbiol.* 5:719. doi: 10.3389/fmicb.2014.00719
31. Matute, D. R., McEwen, J. G., Puccia, R., Montes, B. A., San-Blas, G., Bagagli, E., et al. (2006). Cryptic speciation and recombination in the fungus *Paracoccidioides brasiliensis* as revealed by gene genealogies. *Mol. Biol. Evol.* 23, 65–73. doi: 10.1093/molbev/msj008
32. Medzhitov, R. (2008). Origin and physiological roles of inflammation. *Nature* 454, 428–435. doi: 10.1038/nature07201
33. Oliveira, S. J., Mamoni, R. L., Musatti, C. C., Papaiordanou, P. M., and Blotta, M. H. (2002). Cytokines and lymphocyte proliferation in juvenile and adult forms of paracoccidioidomycosis: comparison with infected and non-infected controls. *Microbes Infect.* 4, 139–144. doi: 10.1016/S1286-4579(01)01521-0
34. Panunto-Castelo, A., Freitas-da-Silva, G., Bragheto, I. C., Martinez, R., and Roque- Barreira, M. C. (2003). *Paracoccidioides brasiliensis* exoantigens: recognition by IgG from patients with different clinical forms of paracoccidioidomycosis. *Microbes Infect.* 5, 1205–1211. doi: 10.1016/j.micinf.2003.07.008
35. Parente-Rocha, J. A., Parente, A. F., Baeza, L. C., Bonfim, S. M., Hernandez, O., McEwen, J. G., et al. (2015). Macrophage interaction with *Paracoccidioides brasiliensis* yeast cells modulates fungal metabolism and generates a response to oxidative stress. *PLoS ONE* 10:e0137619. doi: 10.1371/journal.pone.0137619
36. Rappleye, C. A., and Goldman, W. E. (2006). Defining virulence genes in the dimorphic fungi. *Annu. Rev. Microbiol.* 60, 281–303. doi: 10.1146/annurev.micro.59.030804.121055
37. Romani, L. (2004). Immunity to fungal infections. *Nat. Rev. Immunol.* 4, 1–23. doi: 10.1038/nri1255
38. Romani, L. (2011). Immunity to fungal infections. *Nat. Rev. Immunol.* 11, 275–288. doi: 10.1038/nri2939
39. Straus, A. H., Freymuller, E., Travassos, L. R., and Takahashi, H. K. (1996). Immunochemical and subcellular localization of the 43 kDa glycoprotein antigen of *Paracoccidioides brasiliensis* with monoclonal antibodies. *J. Med. Vet. Mycol.* 34, 181–186. doi: 10.1080/02681219680000301
40. Tavares, A. H., Silva, S. S., Dantas, A., Campos, E. G., Andrade, R. V., Maranhao, A. Q., et al. (2007). Early transcriptional response of *Paracoccidioides brasiliensis* upon internalization by murine macrophages. *Microbes Infect.* 9, 583–590. doi: 10.1016/j.micinf.2007.01.024
41. Teixeira, M. M., Theodoro, R. C., de Carvalho, M. J., Fernandes, L., Paes, H. C., Hahn, R. C., et al. (2009). Phylogenetic analysis reveals a high level of speciation in the *Paracoccidioides* genus. *Mol. Phylogenet. Evol.* 52, 273–283. doi: 10.1016/j.ympev.2009.04.005
42. Teixeira, M. M., Theodoro, R. C., Nino-Vega, G., Bagagli, E., and Felipe, M. S. (2014). *Paracoccidioides* species complex: ecology, phylogeny, sexual reproduction, and virulence. *PLoS Pathog.* 10:e1004397. doi: 10.1371/journal.ppat.1004397
43. Theodoro, R. C., Teixeira Mde, M., Felipe, M. S., Paduan Kdos, S., Ribolla, P. M., San-Blas, G., et al. (2012). Genus paracoccidioides: species recognition and biogeographic aspects. *PLOS ONE* 7:e37694. doi: 10.1371/journal.pone.0037694
44. Torres, I., Hernandez, O., Tamayo, D., Munoz, J. F., Leitao, N. P. Jr., Garcia, A. M., et al. (2013). Inhibition of PbGP43 expression may suggest that gp43 is a virulence factor in *Paracoccidioides brasiliensis*. *PLoS ONE*8:e68434. doi: 10.1371/journal.pone.0068434
45. Vallejo, M. C., Nakayasu, E. S., Matsuo, A. L., Sobreira, T. J., Longo, L. V., Ganiko, L., et al. (2012). Vesicle and vesicle-free extracellular proteome of *Paracoccidioides brasiliensis*: comparative analysis with other pathogenic fungi. *J. Proteome Res.* 11, 1676–1685. doi: 10.1021/pr200872s
46. Vicentini, A. P., Gesztesi, J. L., Franco, M. F., de Souza, W., de Moraes, J. Z., Travassos, L. R., et al. (1994). Binding of *Paracoccidioides brasiliensis* to laminin through surface glycoprotein gp43 leads to enhancement of fungal pathogenesis. *Infect. Immun.* 62, 1465–1469.
47. Weber, S. S., Parente, A. F., Borges, C. L., Parente, J. A., Bailao, A. M., and de Almeida Soares, C. M. (2012). Analysis of the secretomes of *Paracoccidioides mycelia* and yeast cells. *PLoS ONE* 7:e52470. doi: 10.1371/journal.pone.0052470

5

Human and Murine Innate Immune Cell Populations Display Common and Distinct Response Patterns during their *In Vitro* Interaction with the Pathogenic Mold *Aspergillus fumigatus*

*Anna-Maria Hellmann[1†], Jasmin Lother[1†], Sebastian Wurster[1], Manfred B. Lutz[2], Anna Lena Schmitt[1], Charles Oliver Morton[3], Matthias Eyrich[4], Kristin Czakai[1], Hermann Einsele[1] and Juergen Loeffler[1]**

[1] Medizinische Klinik & Poliklinik II, Universitätsklinikum Würzburg, Würzburg, Germany, [2] Institute of Virology and Immunobiology, University of Würzburg, Würzburg, Germany, [3] School of Science and Health, Western Sydney University, Campbelltown, NSW, Australia, [4] Kinderklinik und Poliklinik, Universitätsklinikum Würzburg, Würzburg, Germany

***Correspondence:**
Juergen Loeffler
loeffler_j@ukw.de

[†] These authors have contributed equally to this work.

Aspergillus fumigatus is the main cause of invasive fungal infections occurring almost exclusively in immunocompromised patients. An improved understanding of the initial innate immune response is key to the development of better diagnostic tools and new treatment options. Mice are commonly used to study immune defense mechanisms during the infection of the mammalian host with *A. fumigatus*. However, little is known about functional differences between the human and murine immune response against this fungal pathogen. Thus, we performed a comparative functional analysis of human and murine dendritic cells (DCs), macrophages, and polymorphonuclear cells (PMNs) using standardized and reproducible working conditions, laboratory protocols, and readout assays. *A. fumigatus* did not provoke identical responses in murine and human immune cells but rather initiated relatively specific responses. While human DCs showed a significantly stronger upregulation of their maturation markers and major histocompatibility complex molecules and phagocytosed *A. fumigatus* more efficiently compared to their murine counterparts, murine PMNs and macrophages exhibited a significantly stronger release of reactive oxygen species after exposure to *A. fumigatus*. For all studied cell types, human and murine samples differed in their cytokine response to conidia or germ tubes of *A. fumigatus*. Furthermore, Dectin-1 showed inverse expression patterns on human and murine DCs after fungal stimulation. These specific differences should be carefully considered and highlight potential limitations in the transferability of murine host–pathogen interaction studies.

Keywords: murine model, humans, *Aspergillus fumigatus*, innate immune response, fungal infection

INTRODUCTION

Humans inhale hundreds of airborne fungal spores daily, including spores from the saprophytic mold *Aspergillus fumigatus*, which is ubiquitous in the environment. While the fungus rarely causes diseases in healthy individuals, disorders of the immune system are associated with a wide spectrum of *Aspergillus*-related diseases (1). Overshooting immune response to the fungus can lead to hypersensitivity syndromes such as allergic bronchopulmonary aspergillosis, whereas invasive aspergillosis (IA) is a major cause of morbidity and mortality in immunocompromised patients.

The mammalian immune system, evolving under continuous exposure to airborne fungal spores, possesses a vast arsenal of strategies to combat invading fungi including mediating tolerance to commensals and limiting hyperinflammation to prevent tissue damage. In the absence of an effective immune response, *Aspergillus* conidia swell and become invasive by germinating into the lung tissue and entering the blood stream. Alveolar macrophages act as the first line of defense in the airways by phagocytosis of conidia and secretion of pro-inflammatory cytokines and reactive oxygen species (ROS) (2). Neutrophil granulocytes [polymorphonuclear cells (PMNs)] also play a major role in the early immune defense against IA, as they are able to prevent germination and kill fungal hyphae through the release of ROS, phagocytosis, or formation of neutrophil extracellular traps. Dendritic cells (DCs) represent an important bridge between innate and adaptive immunity as they process fungal antigens and subsequently stimulate specific T-cells *via* antigen-presentation by major histocompatibility complex (MHC) I and II molecules. They also orchestrate the immune response by secreting an array of pro- and anti-inflammatory cytokines. Stimulation of pattern recognition receptors (PRRs), such as toll-like receptors (TLR)-2 and -4 (3) and the Dectin-1-receptor, is crucial to the activation of these immune cell subsets (4).

Detailed insights into the pathophysiology of the infection and mechanisms of the host–pathogen interaction are urgently needed to facilitate development of new prophylactic and therapeutic tools and strategies. Due to their easy accessibility, relatively short generation time, and availability of genetically defined strains, mouse models are commonly used to characterize the interaction of *A. fumigatus* with the mammalian host *in vivo* and to evaluate novel therapeutic strategies. There is, however, increasing evidence of major functional differences between the human and murine immune systems, indicating limited application of data obtained in studies employing murine cells or models (5, 6). On one hand, the composition of the murine leukocyte repertoire differs from that of humans; in mice only 7–28% of peripheral blood leukocytes are PMNs in contrast to 35–70% in human blood (7). On the other hand, functional differences, such as the sequence of participating immunological cells after antigen challenge as well as the dose of antigen needed to initiate immunological reaction in delayed type hypersensitivity have been described (5).

So far, little is known about functional differences in the human and murine immune defense against *A. fumigatus*. Thus, this study sought to provide a comparative functional assessment between human and murine innate immune cell subsets routinely employed in host–pathogen interaction studies (8–13). Our data demonstrate that mice and men which differ in their size, habitat, lifespan, genome size, and blood composition possess principle differences in how selected innate immune cell populations specifically interact with the pathogenic mold *A. fumigatus*.

MATERIALS AND METHODS

Fungal Strains and Cultivation Conditions

Aspergillus fumigatus strain American Type Culture Collection 46645 was incubated on beer wort agar (Institute of Hygiene and Microbiology, University of Wuerzburg, Germany) for 72 h at 37°C. Conidial suspensions were prepared by rinsing plates with sterile water and filtered through a 40-μm cell strainer (BD Falcon™ Cell Strainer, BD Biosciences). To generate germ tubes, 1×10^8 resting conidia were inoculated in Rosewell Park Memorial Institute (RPMI) 1640 Medium (Life technologies) and cultured at 37°C until the germ tubes reached a length of about 10–30 μm. To preserve fungal morphotypes during coculture experiments, conidia and germ tubes were inactivated with 100% ethanol (Sigma) for 30 min, washed five times with sterile water, and stored in RPMI at −20°C. For time-lapse microscopy red fluorescent *A. fumigatus* conidia and germ tubes were generated as described before (9).

Isolation and Culture of Human and Murine Immune Cells

Dendritic Cells

Peripheral blood mononuclear cells were isolated from leukocyte concentrates from healthy human donors (Institute of Transfusion Medicine, University Hospital of Wuerzburg) by Ficoll (Biochrome) density centrifugation. After positive magnetic selection of $CD14^+$ cells (CD14 MicroBeads, Miltenyi Biotec), monocytes were cultured for 5 days in RPMI 1640 medium supplemented with 10% fetal calf serum (FCS) (Sigma), rGM-CSF (100 ng/ml, Bayer), and rIL4 (10 ng/ml, Miltenyi Biotec) (9).

Murine bone marrow derived dendritic cells (BMDCs) were generated as described before (14). Briefly, bone marrow from healthy mice was harvested and cultured in R10-medium (RPMI 1640) (GIBCO BRL) with 100 U/ml Penicillin (Sigma), 100 μg/ml Streptomycin (Sigma), 2 mM L-glutamine (Sigma), 50 μM 2-mercaptoethanol (Sigma), 10% FCS (PAA), and 200 U/ml rmGM-CSF (Reprotech/Tebu) for 6 days. The non-adherent cells were harvested and cultured in R10-medium without cytokines.

Polymorphonuclear Cells

To isolate human PMNs anticoagulated blood from healthy human donors was layered on a polysaccharide gradient (Polymorphprep, Axis Shield). After 30 min of centrifugation (500*g*), the PMN interphase was harvested and pelleted for 5 min at 300*g*. Remaining erythrocytes were lysed with EL buffer (Qiagen). Isolation of murine PMNs, which were obtained from bone marrow of C57BL/6NCrl mice, was performed using the EasySep™ Mouse Neutrophil Enrichment Kit (Stem Cell Technologies) according to the manufacturer's protocol. Both murine and human PMNs were cultured in RPMI 1640 Medium with 5% FCS.

Macrophages

Human monocytes obtained from healthy subjects as described above were cultured in RPMI 1640 medium supplemented with 10% FCS and rM-CSF (Immunotools) for 6 days. Only adherent cells were used for experiments. To generate murine macrophages, bone marrow cells of healthy mice were cultured in R10-medium with M-CSF supernatant [mouse M-CSF (Immunotools) supernatant, L929] for 6 days. Adherent cells were harvested and suspended in R10-medium.

Time-Lapse Video Microscopy

3.5×10^4 human monocyte-derived immature dendritic cells (moDCs) or murine BMDCs were stimulated with 3.5×10^5 *A. fumigatus* (Afu-dTomato) conidia or germ tubes [multiplicity of infection (MOI) = 10]. Polystyrene beads (Sigma) were used as an unspecific stimulus. Image acquisition over a time period of 3 h was performed using a Leica AF6000 time-lapse microscope with a picture frequency of 5/min. Image analysis was conducted with LAS AF lite (Leica), ImageJ1.45s (Wayne Rasband), and Irfan View 4.32 (Irfan Skiljan) software. For each stimulus, phagocytosis activity was analyzed in six independent movies, respectively, following moDCs or BMDCs over a time period of 3 h by separately counting phagocytosed and extracellular particles or fungi, respectively.

Flow Cytometry

Dendritic cells were stimulated with inactivated *A. fumigatus* conidia and germ tubes (MOI = 1), 100 μg/ml zymosan depleted [a yeast cell wall preparation, which was treated with hot alkali to remove all TLR-stimulating properties to selectively activate Dectin-1 (dZym, InvivoGen)] or 1 mg/ml lipopolysaccharid (LPS, Sigma) for 24 h. Subsequently, cells were harvested, washed, and resuspended in cold Hank's balanced salt solution (HBSS, Sigma) containing 2 mM EDTA (Sigma). The following antibodies were used for extracellular staining: HLA-ABC-PE (BD Biosciences), HLA-DR-PE (BD Biosciences), CD1a-APC (BD Biosciences), CD14-FITC (BD Biosciences), CD80-APC (Miltenyi Biotec), CD86-PE (BD Biosciences), Dectin-1-PE (R&D) (human cells) and HLA-2K^b-FITC (BD Biosciences), HLA-Ia/I-E-PE (BioLegend), CD11c-APC (BioLegend), CD80-FITC (BioLegend), CD86-PE (BD Biosciences), and Dectin-1-PE (R&D) [murine cells]. 5×10^5 cells were stained for 15 min at 4°C. Subsequently, cells were washed twice and 10^4 viable cells according to FSC-SSC properties were acquired using a FACS Calibur (BD Biosciences) flow cytometer and CellQuest Pro software (version 5.2). Data were analyzed with FlowJo software (Tree Star Inc., Ashland, OR, USA).

ROS Quantification

Polymorphonuclear cells and macrophages were stimulated with inactivated *A. fumigatus* conidia and germ tubes (MOI = 1), 100 μg/ml zymosan depleted or 10 μg/ml phorbol-myristate-acetate [the major endogenous ROS inducer in PMNs and macrophages (PMA, Sigma-Aldrich)]. ROS-formation in human and murine PMNs and macrophages was determined by ROS-dependent CM-H_2DCF oxidation (dichlorfluorescein, Sigma-Aldrich). Excitation was performed at 485 nm, and fluorescence emission was detected at 535 nm (GENios microplate reader, TECAN). PMNs were stimulated at 37°C for 1 h and macrophages for 2.5 h before measuring fluorescence intensity.

Multiplex Cytokine Assays

Polymorphonuclear cells (2×10^6/ml), macrophages (8×10^5/ml), and DCs (1×10^6/ml) were stimulated with *A. fumigatus* conidia and germ tubes (MOI = 1), zymosan depleted (100 μg/ml), LPS (1 μg/ml), or plain culture medium (negative control). Supernatants were harvested after 3 h (PMNs), 12 h (macrophages), or 24 h (DCs) and stored at −20°C. Cytokine concentrations (IL1β, IL4, IL6, huIL8, muGroα, IL10, IL12p70, IL18, IL23, IP10, MCP1, MIP1α, MIP1β, TNFα) were quantified with a human and mouse 13-Plex panel assay (Affymetrix, eBioscience).

Fungicidal Activity of PMNs

Polymorphonuclear cell were isolated from whole blood of four healthy human donors and two mice as described above. PMNs were diluted in colorless RPMI + 10% FCS at a concentration of 2×10^6/ml. 5×10^5 PMNs were seeded per well of a 24-well plate and 5×10^5 vital *A. fumigatus* germ tubes were added (MOI = 1, ideal MOI was determined in a preceding experiment). Control wells containing only PNMs or fungal cells as well as blank wells containing culture medium without cells were prepared. After 2 and 4 h of coculture at 37°C, hypotonic lysis of PMNs was performed by washing wells twice with 1,000 μl cold distilled water, followed by 5 min incubation on ice. Supernatants were carefully removed, and 200 μl HBSS supplemented with 400 μg/ml of 2,3-bis-(2-methoxy-4-nitro-5-sulphenyl)-(2H)-tetrazolium-5-carboxanilide [XTT (Sigma)] and 50 μg/ml of coenzyme (Sigma) were added. After 90 min incubation at 37°C and centrifugation at 300*g* for 5 min, 100 μl supernatant of each well were transferred to a 96-well plate and OD_{450} was measured in a microplate reader. Fold changes of fungal XTT metabolism were calculated according to the following formula: Fold change $= (OD_{450}^{PMN+Fungus} - OD_{450}^{PMN}) / (OD_{450}^{Fungus} - OD_{450}^{Blank})$.

Statistics

Significance testing was performed using GraphPad Prism 7 (Graphpad Software, Inc.) using different statistical test which are noted in each figure legend. Statistical significance is denoted as follows: $^*p < 0.05$, $^{**}p < 0.01$, and $^{***}p < 0.001$.

RESULTS

Murine Neutrophils and Macrophages Show Stronger ROS Release upon Stimulation with *A. fumigatus* Germ Tubes and Depleted Zymosan (dZym)

Reactive oxygen species production by human and murine neutrophils and macrophages cocultured with *A. fumigatus* conidia or germ tubes was quantified and compared. No significant induction of oxidative burst in PMNs or macrophages of either species was observed upon conidial stimulation. *A. fumigatus* germ tubes and dZym (binding exclusively to dectin-1) led to significantly higher ROS release by murine PMNs (**Figure 1A**) and macrophages (**Figure 1B**). By contrast, human PMNs and

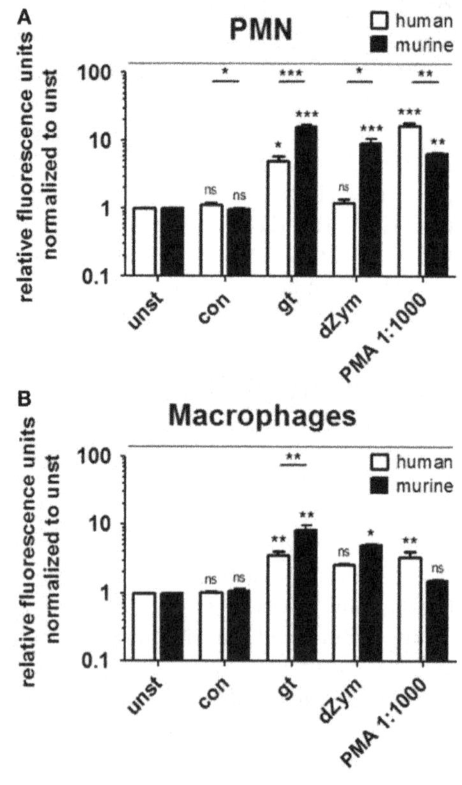

FIGURE 1 | Murine polymorphonuclear cells (PMNs) and macrophages exhibit a stronger reactive oxygen species (ROS) response to *Aspergillus fumigatus* germ tubes and depleted zymosan (dZym). Human and murine PMNs **(A)** or macrophages **(B)** were stimulated with *A. fumigatus* conidia (con), germ tubes (gt), dZym, or phorbol 12-myristate 13-acetate (PMA). ROS production was measured by a dichlorfluorescein-based assay. Mean fold changes of relative fluorescence units after 2 (PMNs) and 3 h (macrophages) are shown. Seven human and three murine samples were analyzed. Significance was calculated as difference to unstimulated with ANOVA and Tukey post-test (stars above of bars) as well as between human and mouse specimens with unpaired *t*-Test, Error bars indicate SDs.

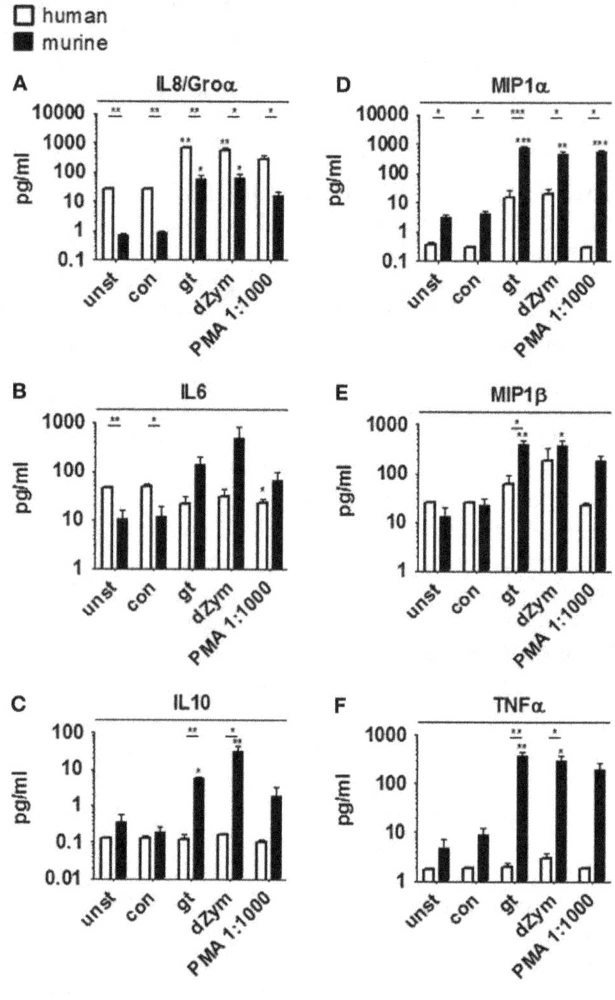

FIGURE 2 | *Aspergillus fumigatus* germ tubes and depleted zymosan (dZym) trigger strong pro-inflammatory cytokine release by murine neutrophils. Murine or human neutrophils were stimulated with *A. fumigatus* conidia, germ tubes, dZym or PMA for a period of 3 h. Subsequently, cytokine concentrations in the culture medium were determined by 13-plex cytokine assays. PMNs obtained from three human donors (white bars) and three mice (black bars) were assessed. Mean concentrations of IL8/Groα **(A)**, IL6 **(B)**, IL10 **(C)**, MIP1α **(D)**, MIP1β **(E)**, and TNFα **(F)** are shown. Error bars indicate standard deviations. Significance was calculated as difference to unstimulated with ANOVA and Tukey post-test (stars above of bars) as well as between human and mouse specimens with unpaired *t*-Test.

macrophages released significantly more ROS after stimulation with the major endogenous ROS inducer PMA.

Murine PMNs Exert Stronger and Broader Pro-inflammatory Cytokine Response to *A. fumigatus* Germ Tubes and dZym

Strong ROS response was paralleled by the secretion of pro-inflammatory cytokines Groα, IL6, MIP1α, MIP1β, and TNFα by murine PMNs after stimulation with *A. fumigatus* germ tubes or dZym, as well as the anti-inflammatory cytokine IL10 (**Figure 2**). Pro-inflammatory cytokine release was also significantly induced by PMA stimulation, whereas coculture with *A. fumigatus* conidia did not result in significant induction of MIP1β or TNFα secretion. Human PMNs showed strongly elevated IL8 release when stimulated with *A. fumigatus* germ tubes, dZym or PMA, while MIP1α and MIP1β secretion was weakly induced by *A. fumigatus* germ tubes and dZym.

Human and Murine Macrophages Release Distinct Cytokine Patterns When Cocultured with *A. fumigatus* or Stimulated with Synthetic Agonists

Pro- and anti-inflammatory cytokine secretion was strongly induced in both murine and human macrophages upon coculture with *A. fumigatus* germ tubes, dZym, or synthetic agonists LPS and Pam3CSK. While human macrophages released higher concentrations of MIP1α, IL8, and IL10 (**Figures 3B,D,E**), fold changes of IL8 and MIP1α were higher in murine samples due to differences in baseline levels. In comparison to murine cells stimulation of human macrophages by *A. fumigatus* germ tubes, dZym, and Pam3CSK resulted in significantly greater IL1β release (**Figure 3A**). Interestingly, a small but significant increase in MIP1α and TNFα (**Figures 3E,F**) secretion by macrophages of both species was observed upon conidial stimulation. In human macrophages, this was paralleled by an even more pronounced upregulation of IL8 release and minor elevations of IL1β and IL6 (**Figures 3A,C,D**).

Human moDCs Show Higher Phagocytosis Rates of *A. fumigatus* Conidia and Germ Tubes

Live imaging was performed to visualize the interaction between human (**Figure 4A**) or murine DCs (**Figure 4B**) with *A. fumigatus* conidia or germ tubes. Analyzing the number of touches of DCs and fungal cells or the unspecific polystyrene bead control revealed no significant differences between human and murine cells over 3 h (**Figure 4C**). Assessing the percentage of phagocytosed *A. fumigatus* conidia or germ tubes after 3 h, however, human moDCs showed higher phagocytosis rates than murine BMDCs, whereas the internalization of polystyrene beads by human and murine DCs did not differ significantly (**Figure 4D**).

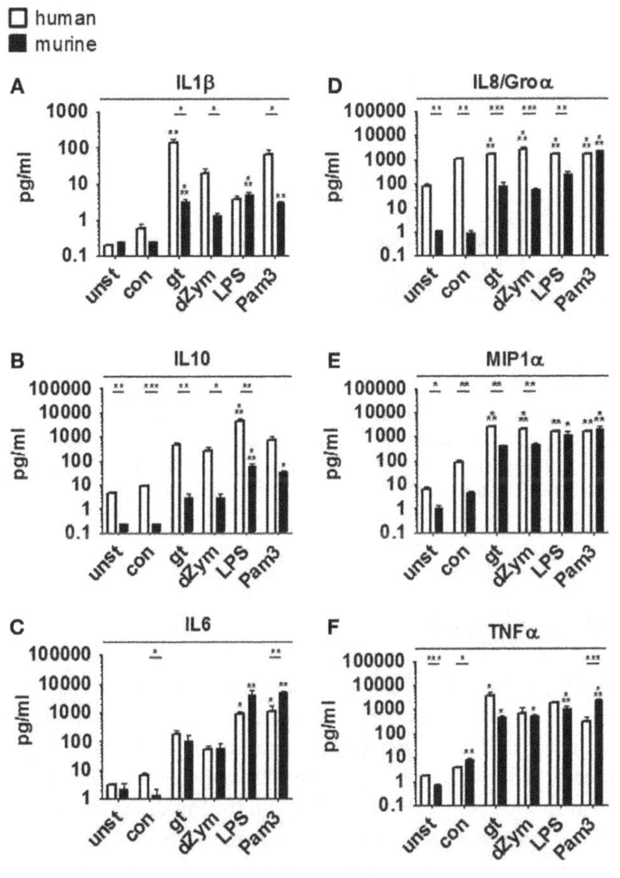

FIGURE 3 | Distinct cytokine response pattern to *Aspergillus fumigatus* by human and murine macrophages. Cytokine patterns in culture supernatants of human and murine macrophages were studied by a 13-plex cytokine assay upon 12 h stimulation with *A. fumigatus* conidia or germ tubes as well as depleted zymosan (dZym), LPS, or Pam3CSK. Four human (white bars) and four murine (black bars) samples were assessed. Mean concentrations of IL1β **(A)**, IL10 **(B)**, IL6 **(C)**, IL8/Groα **(D)**, MIP1α **(E)**, and TNFα **(F)** are shown. Error bars indicate standard deviations. Significance was calculated as difference to unstimulated with ANOVA and Tukey post-test (stars above of bars) as well as between human and mouse specimens with unpaired *t*-test.

Dectin-1 Is Inversely Regulated on Human and Murine DCs after Stimulation with *A. fumigatus* Conidia and Germ Tubes

The transmembrane glycoprotein Dectin-1, also known as C-type lectin domain family member 7A, plays an important role as an *A. fumigatus* phagocytosis receptor (4). Thus, Dectin-1 expression on DCs cocultured with ethanol-inactivated conidia and germ tubes for different periods was assessed and compared with unstimulated DCs. After only 1 h of coculture with both fungal morphotypes, surface expression of Dectin-1 started to decline on human moDCs, with a more pronounced effect after stimulation with germ tubes (**Figure 5A**). By contrast, increased Dectin-1 expression was observed on murine BMDCs stimulated with *A. fumigatus* germ tubes (**Figure 5B**). For each of the coculture periods studied, a significant difference in Dectin-1 surface expression was detected between human and murine DCs stimulated with *A. fumigatus* germ tubes, whereas prolonged exposure (18 h) to inactivated conidia was necessary to observe significantly different expression (**Figures 5C,D**).

Human and Murine DCs Cocultured with *A. fumigatus* Show Distinct Surface Antigen and Cytokine Response Patterns

To further characterize the response patterns of human and murine DCs confronted with resting and germinated stages of *A. fumigatus*, we analyzed the expression of maturation markers (CD80 and CD86) and MHC molecules (MHC-I and MHC-II) on the cell surface. 24 h of stimulation with inactivated *A. fumigatus* germ tubes, dZym, and LPS led to 1.3-fold upregulation of CD80, CD86, MHC-I, and MHC-II on both human and murine DCs (**Figure 6**). Upon coculture with all studied stimuli, significantly greater levels of CD80 and CD86 were observed on human moDCs (**Figures 6A,B**). Coculture with *A. fumigatus* germ tubes led to a significantly higher MHC-I and MHC-II surface expression on human moDCs, whereas conidial stimulation resulted in stronger upregulation of MHC-I in murine BMDCs (**Figures 6C,D**).

Further, cytokine profiles were studied by bead-based multiplex cytokine assays after 24 h coculture of DCs with *A. fumigatus* conidia, germ tubes, dZym, or LPS. Stimulation with *A. fumigatus* germ tubes or LPS led to release of a broad range of pro-inflammatory cytokines by both human moDCs and murine BMDCs. Human moDCs showed significantly stronger TNFα release in response to these stimuli and a trend toward stronger IL12p70 and IL23 induction. By contrast, murine BMDCs released significantly greater amounts of IL6 and IL18 (**Figure 7**).

Conidial stimulation resulted in the release of fewer cytokines and lower concentrations than other stimuli. Murine BMDCs

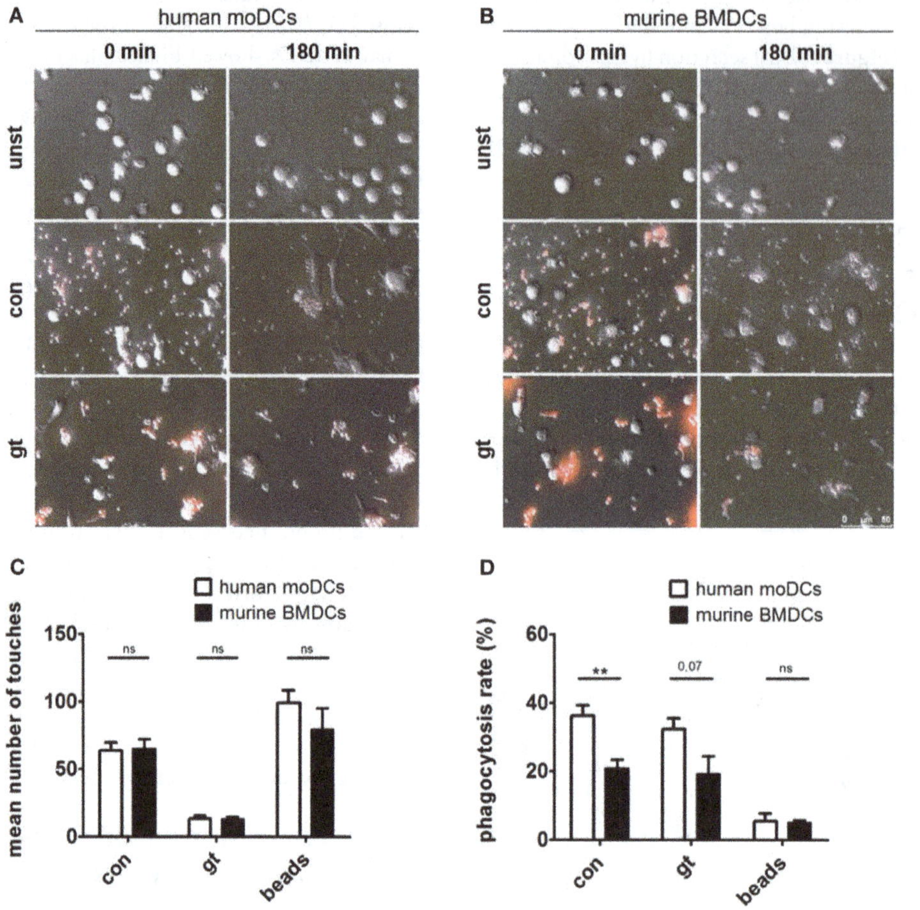

FIGURE 4 | Human dendritic cells (DCs) contact and phagocytose *Aspergillus fumigatus* conidia and germ tubes more effectively. Representative images show phagocytosis of red fluorescent conidia and germ tubes by human **(A)** and murine **(B)** DCs at the indicated time points (duration of coculture). Number of touches **(C)** of human and murine DCs with *A. fumigatus* conidia (con), germ tubes (gt), and polystyrene beads (beads) and phagocytosis rates **(D)** were determined by live imaging analysis. Mean values of touched **(C)** or mean percentage of phagocytosed **(D)** fungal cells or beads after 3 h of coculture are given in the figure. Six human and murine donors were assessed. Significance was calculated with unpaired *t*-Test and error bars indicate SDs.

showed strong and significant induction of the pro-inflammatory cytokines IL1β, IL6, TNFα, but also increased IL10 release after coculture with conidia. Stimulation of murine BMDCs with dZym led to significantly greater release of IL6, IL10, and IL18, whereas a tendency toward greater TNFα release by human moDCs was observed.

Taken together, these results highlight different response patterns of human moDCs and murine BMDCs confronted with *A. fumigatus*, with distinct cytokine profiles and stronger expression of maturation markers and MHC molecules on human moDCs.

Fungicidal Activity of PMNs

Colorimetric analysis of the fungal metabolism revealed that 2 h of *A. fumigatus* germ tube–PMN co-cultivation led to markedly increased fungal metabolism while fungal metabolic activity was decreased again after 4 h, compared to unstimulated control samples. No major difference was observed between human and murine PMNs (Figure S2 in Supplementary Material).

DISCUSSION

Aspergillus fumigatus is the most important cause of invasive fungal infections occurring almost exclusively in immunocompromised patients. A key to understanding *A. fumigatus* pathogenicity is knowledge of the interplay between the fungus and the immune system, in particular with the initial innate immune defense consisting of neutrophils, macrophages, and DCs.

In recent decades, several hundred studies characterized the functions of innate immune cells directed against *A. fumigatus* thereby improving the management and treatment of aspergillosis (15). This intensive work was based on *in vitro* studies involving culturing of primary human immune cells, and cell lines and a large variety of animal models including mice, which are frequently used to model human disease and to mimic scenarios of immunocompromised patients.

This study, the first to our knowledge, provides a comparative functional assessment of murine innate immune cell subsets routinely employed in *A. fumigatus in vitro* interaction studies with

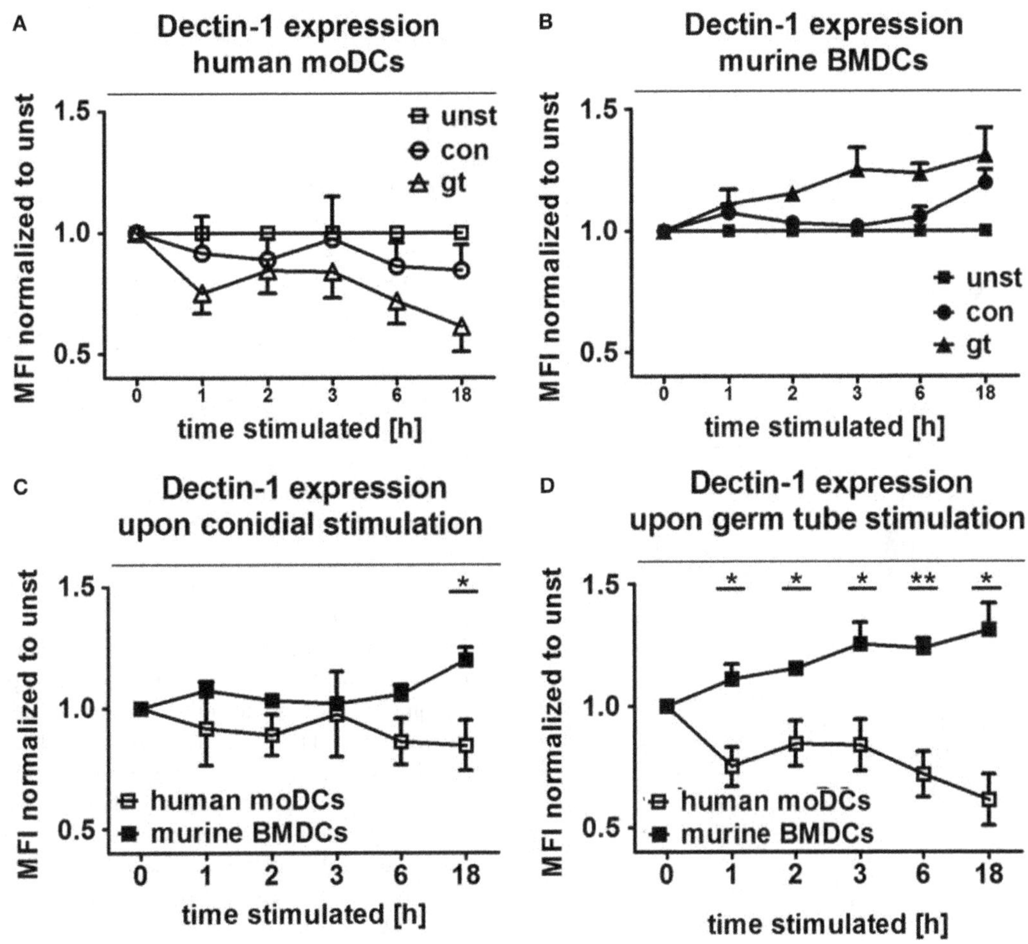

FIGURE 5 | Human and murine dendritic cells show inverse Dectin-1 surface expression patterns after exposure to *Aspergillus fumigatus*. Dectin-1 expression on the cell surface of human moDCs **(A)** and murine bone marrow derived dendritic cells (BMDCs) **(B)** was analyzed by flow cytometry after coculture with *A. fumigatus* conidia and germ tubes for different periods. Mean fold changes (±SDs) of mean fluorescence intensity (MFI) compared to unstimulated cells are given in the figure. Two murine and four human samples were analyzed. The lower panels directly compare Dectin-1 expression following exposure of human moDCs and murine BMDCs to *A. fumigatus* germ tubes **(C)** and conidia **(D)**. Human and murine samples were compared with unpaired *t*-Test, error bars show SDs.

their human counterparts. Humans and mice differ greatly in their size, lifespan, living conditions, and ecological niches. Even the blood composition between different mouse strains varies widely, while C57BL/6 mice contain 10–25% PMNs and 75–90% lymphocytes (16), CD-1 mice exhibit 15–20% PMNs (300–2,000 cells/μl) and 50–70% lymphocytes (1,000–7,000 cells/μl) (17). In contrast, human blood contains 50–70% PMNs (3,500–7,000 cells/μl) and 20–40% lymphocytes (1,400–4,000 cells/μl) (17). In consequence, a direct translation of murine *in vivo* experimental data to human pathological events often fails due to insufficient similarities in the organization of the immune system of both species (18).

In our study, we isolated and cultivated PMNs, macrophages, and DCs from both mammals and challenged them *in vitro* with *A. fumigatus* using standardized and reproducible working conditions, laboratory protocols and readout assays. We are aware that this *in vitro* comparison is restricted due to the isolated use of single immune cell types while well-established murine models allow a complex view of the pathogenesis of IA. However, the chosen comparative *in vitro* study design nicely illustrates the substantial parallel organization of the human and murine immune response against *A. fumigatus* but also provides examples for functional heterogeneity in the defense against the fungus.

Polymorphonuclear cells are among the first line response against *A. fumigatus*. When attracted by chemokines they leave the blood stream and migrate to the site of infection using a large number of PRRs to recognize and respond to the fungus. This includes the release of soluble antimicrobials, reactive metabolites, cytokines, and phagocytosis of conidia (19). In our experiments, murine and human neutrophils were directly isolated from anticoagulated blood using similar protocols (polysaccharide gradient for human blood and the commercial neutrophil enrichment kit for mice). Murine PMNs exhibited a significantly stronger ROS response to *A. fumigatus* and dZym,

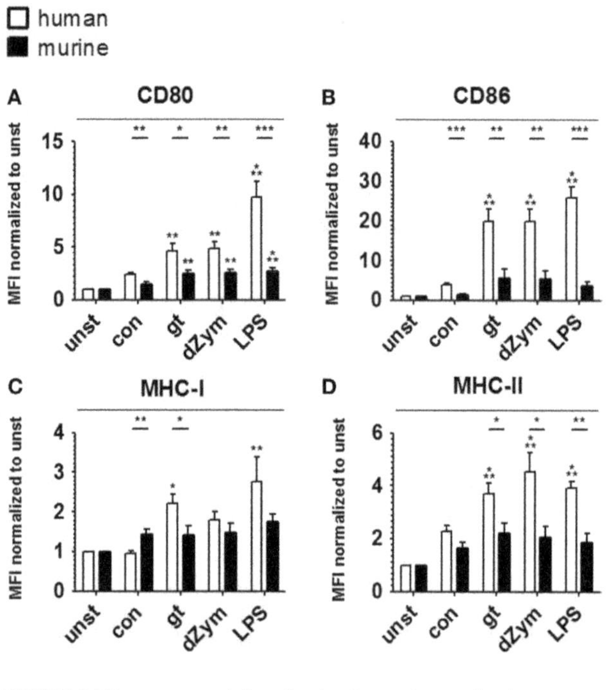

FIGURE 6 | Stronger upregulation of maturation markers and major histocompatibility complex (MHC) molecules upon *Aspergillus fumigatus* stimulation is observed in human moDCs. Surface expression of CD80 **(A)**, CD86 **(B)**, MHC-I **(C)**, and MHC-II **(D)** was analyzed by flow cytometry in human moDCs and murine bone marrow derived dendritic cells after 24 h stimulation with *A. fumigatus* conidia (con) and germ tubes (gt) as well as depleted zymosan (dZym) and LPS. Six human and murine dendritic cell samples were assessed. Mean fold changes of MFI values compared to unstimulated cells (unst) and SDs are shown. Significance between human and mouse specimen was calculated with the unpaired *t*-Test, the comparison to unstimulated specimens is shown as stars above bars and was calculated with ANOVA and Tukey post-test.

a pure dectin-1 agonist, than human PMNs (**Figure 1**). The role of ROS in the immune defense against *A. fumigatus* is rather unclear. While text-book knowledge indicates that ROS is used by PMNs to kill *A. fumigatus*, more recent reports state that they play a regulatory role as signaling molecules and in the activation of antimicrobial enzymes in the phagolysosome (20). Furthermore, it could be demonstrated only recently that murine lung PMNs trigger programmed cell death with apoptosis-like features in *A. fumigatus* conidia (21).

Furthermore, human PMNs showed strongly elevated IL8 release when stimulated with *A. fumigatus* germ tubes and dZym while murine PMNs secreted a much larger variety of cytokines and chemokines, including Groα, IL6, MIP1α, MIP1β, and TNFα, as well as the anti-inflammatory cytokine IL10. While IL8 is the most important chemoattractant for human neutrophil recruitment, an orthologous counterpart is absent in mice (22). In contrast, mice express CXCL15 as an attractant and other functional homologs of IL8, such as Groα (23).

Interestingly, in a preliminary experiment analyzing PMNs from four healthy human donors and two mice by an XTT metabolic assay, we revealed no major differences quantifying fungal metabolism after 2 and 4 h, respectively. We hypothesize that the increase of fungal metabolism after 2 h of co-cultivation with human and murine PMNs might reflect temporarily higher fungal metabolic activity due to early defense mechanisms of *A. fumigatus*.

Human moDCs were generated from $CD14^+$ monocytes using rGM-CSF and rIL4 while murine DCs were derived from bone marrow cultured in R10-medium supplemented with rmGM-CSF. While murine $Ly6C^{high}$ monocytes fail to proliferate (24), proliferating cells mostly represent macrophage-DC progenitors and common monocyte progenitor (25). This observation was described for human $CD14^+$ monocytes undergoing moDC differentiation as well (26). Thereby, GM-CSF has major effects on myelomonocytic cells leading to a massive expansion of macrophage–DC-restricted precursors, but very low effects on common dendritic cell precursors (24). In both, humans and mice, $Ly6C^{high}$ monocytes and moDCs are recruited into tissue under inflammatory and infectious conditions thereby initiating T cell priming in the draining lymph nodes, e.g., in the synovia of rheumatoid arthritis patients (27, 28). Thus, murine BMDCs and human moDCs are highly similar and thus can be considered as functional homologs (29, 30).

Both, human and murine DCs were able to phagocytose *A. fumigatus* conidia and germ tubes. Efficient phagocytosis is a prerequisite for adequate antigen processing and presentation to lymphocytes (31). This characteristic property of DCs in the interplay with *A. fumigatus* underlines their relevance in bridging innate and adaptive immunity during mold infections. The more efficient phagocytosis of *A. fumigatus* conidia in human moDCs might be due to the differential size of human and murine DCs or due to mouse-strain specific variabilities in phagocytosic capacity (32).

Human moDCs secreted substantially more of the pro-inflammatory mediators TNFα, MCP1, IL12p70, and IL1β, indicating their profound role in the broad activation of the innate and adaptive immune response. Murine BMDCs released significantly greater amounts of IL6 and IL18. Cenci et al. showed that IL6(−/−) mice were more susceptible to aspergillosis than the wild-type. Susceptibility was associated with increased inflammatory pathology, decreased antifungal effector functions of phagocytes, and impaired development of protective type 1 responses. Exposure to exogenous IL6 restored antifungal effector activity (33). Similarly, simultaneous neutralization of IL18 and IL12 resulted in a significant increase in *A. fumigatus* CFU in murine lung tissue demonstrating its key role in murine defense against *Aspergillus* infection (34).

Secretion of IL10, which suppresses proliferation, cytokine secretion, and costimulatory molecule expression of pro-inflammatory immune cells, differed markedly between human and murine cells. While *A. fumigatus* germ tubes and dZym led to a 100- and 60-fold induction of the IL10 secretion of human macrophages compared to unstimulated control cells, stimulation of murine macrophages led to lower increases (with germ tubes 14-fold, with dZym 14-fold). Interestingly, basal secretion of IL10 from unstimulated macrophages into the culture medium was over 20-fold higher in human cells than in their murine counterparts. Human and mouse IL10 have roughly 73% sequence homology and are secreted as 178-amino acid proteins (35). It is

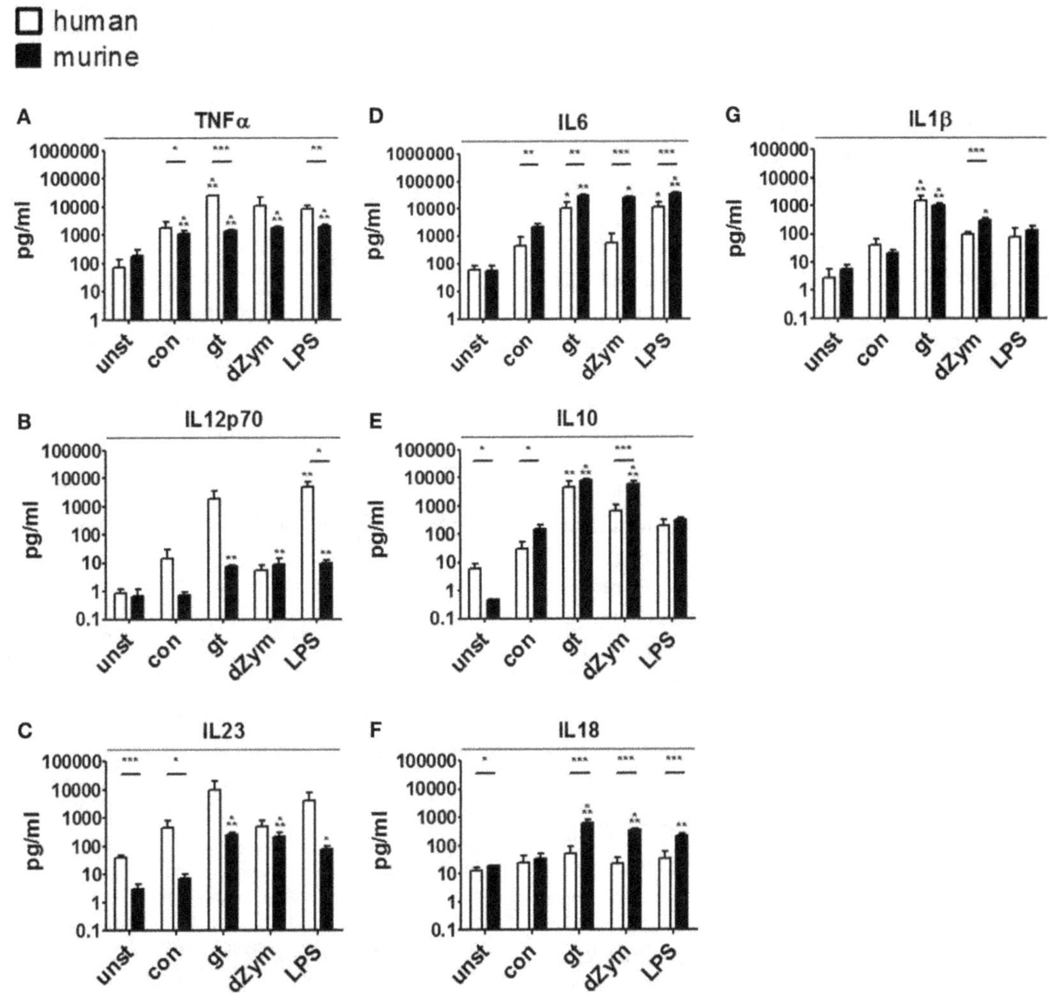

FIGURE 7 | Distinct cytokine response patterns to *Aspergillus fumigatus* are observed in human and murine dendritic cells (DCs). Cytokine concentrations (picograms/milliliter) in culture supernatants of human moDCs and murine bone marrow-derived dendritic cells stimulated with ethanol-inactivated *A. fumigatus* conidia or germ tubes, depleted zymosan (dZym) or LPS were quantified by 13-plex cytokine assays. Four human (white bars) and four murine (black bars) DC samples were assessed. Mean concentrations of TNFα **(A)**, IL12p70 **(B)**, IL23 **(C)**, IL6 **(D)**, IL10 **(E)**, IL18 **(F)**, and IL1β **(G)** are shown. Error bars indicate standard deviations. Significance was calculated as difference to unstimulated specimens with ANOVA and Tukey post-test (stars above of bars) as well as between human and mouse specimens with unpaired *t*-test.

unknown whether both cytokines have identical binding capacity to their receptors, stability, and degradation behavior.

Dectin-1, a β-glucan receptor, is expressed on monocytes, macrophages, DCs, neutrophils, and eosinophils (36). Brown et al. demonstrated that dZym, which was treated with hot alkali to remove its TLR-stimulating properties, triggers expression of pro-inflammatory cytokines *via* Dectin-1 signaling (37). In mice, sensing of *C. albicans* by Dectin-1 results in ingestion and killing of the fungus and the induction of an early inflammatory response, which results in the recruitment and activation of other immune cells to the infection site. Dectin-1 deficiency leads to increased susceptibility to systemic and mucosal candidiasis (38). In contrast, human Dectin-1 deficiency causes diminished cytokine responses, while alternative receptors are then responsible for fungal uptake and subsequent killing. Our results demonstrate inverse Dectin-1 surface expression after exposure to *A. fumigatus*. After 1 h of coculture, surface expression of Dectin-1 decreased on human moDCs, with a more pronounced effect after stimulation with germ tubes (**Figure 5A**). By contrast, increased Dectin-1 expression was observed on murine BMDCs stimulated with *A. fumigatus* germ tubes (**Figure 5B**). We hypothesize that downregulation of Dectin-1 exposure on human moDCs prevents severe and uncontrolled inflammatory reactions while on murine BMDCs, Dectin-1 expression is required for continuous ingestion and killing of the fungus. This is consistent with our previous data showing that anti-Dectin-1 antibody treatment of human moDCs as well as *ex vivo* myeloid DCs subsequently inhibited secretion of pro-inflammatory cytokines after contact with *A. fumigatus*, *C. albicans*, or zymosan (4, 39). This is also consistent with the observation that naïve mice lacking Dectin-1 show reduced killing of conidia and a higher mortality rate than wild-type mice (40).

Taken together, after 65 million years of independent evolution (5), immune systems of both species differ substantially. Mice are perfectly adapted to their relatively short lifespan of 2–3 years and their natural habitat on the ground. In the defense against invading fungi, resistance mechanisms and an efficient control over pathogens dominate in humans, while tolerance determines the immune response in mice (41). Our comparative functional assessment of selected human and murine innate immune cell subsets using standardized and reproducible working conditions, laboratory protocols, and readout assays underlined this hypothesis. We were able to provide examples for functional heterogeneity of mammalian innate immune cell populations in their *in vitro* response against the pathogenic mold *A. fumigatus*. These specific differences should be carefully considered in future comparative discovery and validation studies. Furthermore, they highlight potential limitations in the direct transferability of murine host–pathogen interaction studies. Additional studies are highly warranted comparatively employing murine and human cell populations to further study mold immunopathology and to evaluate new diagnostic and therapeutic strategies. Moreover, work on humanized mouse models or the development of synthetic human models might help to avoid difficulties in translating and harmonizing data across different mammalian species.

ETHICS STATEMENT

Use of whole blood specimens from healthy volunteers was approved by the University Hospital of Wuerzburg Ethical Committee (#302/15). Written informed consent was obtained and data analysis was performed anonymously. Mouse husbandry and experimental procedures were conducted in accordance with institutional guidelines and with the approval of the Committee on Animal Research of the regional government (Regierung von Unterfranken, Wuerzburg, Germany).

AUTHOR CONTRIBUTIONS

A-MH and JaL designed the study, performed experiments, performed data analyzes, and wrote the manuscript. AS performed experiments. SW and ML analyzed the data and contributed to the manuscript. CM, ME, and KC provided discussions, technical assistance and contributed to the manuscript. HE and JuL developed concepts, supervised the study, and wrote the manuscript.

FUNDING

This study was supported by the Deutsche Forschungsgemeinschaft (DFG) within the Collaborative Research Center CRC124 FungiNet "Pathogenic fungi and their human host: Networks of interaction" (project A2 to HE and JuL, A4 to JaL and funding for travel to CM) and by the Interdisciplinary Centre for Clinical Research Wuerzburg (grant Z-3/56 to SW). The authors thank all blood donors for their voluntary donation.

SUPPLEMENTARY MATERIAL

FIGURE S1 | Comparison of cytokine response patterns to *Aspergillus fumigatus* germ tubes. Cytokine secretion into the culture medium was analyzed by multiplex bead-based assay upon stimulation of murine or human dendritic cells (DCs), neutrophils [polymorphonuclear cells (PMNs)], or macrophages with *A. fumigatus* germ tubes. Fold changes compared to unstimulated samples are indicated by gray scale. OOR (out of range) indicates that >50% of samples did not meet the limits of detection and thus fold changes could not be calculated reliably.

FIGURE S2 | Impact of human and murine polymorphonuclear cells (PMNs) on fungal XTT metabolism. PMNs were isolated from whole blood of four healthy human donors and two mice as described in the Section "Materials and Methods." After 2 and 4 h of coculture at 37°C, hypotonic lysis of PMNs was performed. Supernatants were carefully removed and 200 µl HBSS supplemented with 400 µg/ml of 2,3-bis-(2-methoxy-4-nitro-5-sulphenyl)-(2 H)-tetrazolium-5-carboxanilide (XTT) and 50 µg/ml of coenzyme were added. After 90 min incubation at 37°C and centrifugation at 300*g* for 5 min, 100 µl supernatant of each well were transferred to a 96-well plate and OD_{450} was measured in a microplate reader. Fold changes of fungal XTT metabolism due to the presence of PMNs was calculated according to the following formula: Fold change $= (OD_{450}^{PMN+Fungus} - OD_{450}^{PMN}) / (OD_{450}^{Fungus} - OD_{450}^{Blank})$. Individual results for each human and murine PMN sample and mean values (black horizontal bars) are shown in the figure.

REFERENCES

1. Segal BH. Aspergillosis. *N Engl J Med* (2009) 360:1870–84. doi:10.1056/NEJMra0808853
2. Grimm MJ, D'Auria AC, Segal BH. Assessing anti-fungal activity of isolated alveolar macrophages by confocal microscopy. *J Vis Exp* (2014) (89):e51678. doi:10.3791/51678
3. Braedel S, Radsak M, Einsele H, Latge JP, Michan A, Loeffler J, et al. *Aspergillus fumigatus* antigens activate innate immune cells via toll-like receptors 2 and 4. *Br J Haematol* (2004) 125:392–9. doi:10.1111/j.1365-2141.2004.04922.x
4. Mezger M, Kneitz S, Wozniok I, Kurzai O, Einsele H, Loeffler J. Proinflammatory response of immature human dendritic cells is mediated by Dectin-1 after exposure to *Aspergillus fumigatus* germ tubes. *J Infect Dis* (2008) 197:924–31. doi:10.1086/528694
5. Mestas J, Hughes CC. Of mice and not men: differences between mouse and human immunology. *J Immunol* (2004) 172:2731–8. doi:10.4049/jimmunol.172.5.2731
6. Reynolds G, Haniffa M. Human and mouse mononuclear phagocyte networks: a tale of two species? *Front Immunol* (2015) 6:330. doi:10.3389/fimmu.2015.00330
7. Relle M, Thomaidis T, Galle PR, Schwarting A. Comparative aspects of murine proteinase 3. *Rheumatol Int* (2011) 31:1105–11. doi:10.1007/s00296-010-1672-2
8. Park SJ, Burdick MD, Mehrad B. Neutrophils mediate maturation and efflux of lung dendritic cells in response to *Aspergillus fumigatus* germ tubes. *Infect Immun* (2012) 80:1759–65. doi:10.1128/IAI.00097-12
9. Lother J, Breitschopf T, Krappmann S, Morton CO, Bouzani M, Kurzai O, et al. Human dendritic cell subsets display distinct interactions with the pathogenic mould *Aspergillus fumigatus*. *Int J Med Microbiol* (2014) 304:1160–8. doi:10.1016/j.ijmm.2014.08.009
10. Moretti S, Bozza S, Massi-Benedetti C, Prezioso L, Rossetti E, Romani L, et al. An immunomodulatory activity of micafungin in preclinical aspergillosis. *J Antimicrob Chemother* (2014) 69:1065–74. doi:10.1093/jac/dkt457
11. Prufer S, Weber M, Stein P, Bosmann M, Stassen M, Kreft A, et al. Oxidative burst and neutrophil elastase contribute to clearance of *Aspergillus fumigatus* pneumonia in mice. *Immunobiology* (2014) 219:87–96. doi:10.1016/j.imbio.2013.08.010
12. Liu C, Wang M, Sun W, Cai F, Geng S, Su X, et al. PU.1 serves a critical role in the innate defense against *Aspergillus fumigatus* via dendritic cell-associated C-type lectin receptor-1 and toll-like receptors-2 and 4 in THP-1-derived macrophages. *Mol Med Rep* (2017) 15:4084–92. doi:10.3892/mmr.2017.6504

13. Wiemann P, Perevitsky A, Lim FY, Shadkchan Y, Knox BP, Landero Figueora JA, et al. *Aspergillus fumigatus* copper export machinery and reactive oxygen intermediate defense counter host copper-mediated oxidative antimicrobial offense. *Cell Rep* (2017) 19:2174–6. doi:10.1016/j.celrep.2017.05.075
14. Lutz MB, Kukutsch N, Ogilvie AL, Rossner S, Koch F, Romani N, et al. An advanced culture method for generating large quantities of highly pure dendritic cells from mouse bone marrow. *J Immunol Methods* (1999) 223:77–92. doi:10.1016/S0022-1759(98)00204-X
15. Sales-Campos H, Tonani L, Cardoso CR, Kress MR. The immune interplay between the host and the pathogen in *Aspergillus fumigatus* lung infection. *Biomed Res Int* (2013) 2013:693023. doi:10.1155/2013/693023
16. Doeing DC, Borowicz JL, Crockett ET. Gender dimorphism in differential peripheral blood leukocyte counts in mice using cardiac, tail, foot, and saphenous vein puncture methods. *BMC Clin Pathol* (2003) 3:3. doi:10.1186/1472-6890-3-3
17. Haley PJ. Species differences in the structure and function of the immune system. *Toxicology* (2003) 188:49–71. doi:10.1016/S0300-483X(03)00043-X
18. Zschaler J, Schlorke D, Arnhold J. Differences in innate immune response between man and mouse. *Crit Rev Immunol* (2014) 34:433–54. doi:10.1615/CritRevImmunol.2014011600
19. Arnhold J, Flemmig J. Human myeloperoxidase in innate and acquired immunity. *Arch Biochem Biophys* (2010) 500:92–106. doi:10.1016/j.abb.2010.04.008
20. Brakhage AA, Bruns S, Thywissen A, Zipfel PF, Behnsen J. Interaction of phagocytes with filamentous fungi. *Curr Opin Microbiol* (2010) 13:409–15. doi:10.1016/j.mib.2010.04.009
21. Shlezinger N, Irmer H, Dhingra S, Beattie SR, Cramer RA, Braus GH, et al. Sterilizing immunity in the lung relies on targeting fungal apoptosis-like programmed cell death. *Science* (2017) 357:1037–41. doi:10.1126/science.aan0365
22. Zlotnik A, Yoshie O, Nomiyama H. The chemokine and chemokine receptor superfamilies and their molecular evolution. *Genome Biol* (2006) 7:243. doi:10.1186/gb-2006-7-12-243
23. Rossi DL, Hurst SD, Xu Y, Wang W, Menon S, Coffman RL, et al. Lungkine, a novel CXC chemokine, specifically expressed by lung bronchoepithelial cells. *J Immunol* (1999) 162:5490–7.
24. Helft J, Bottcher J, Chakravarty P, Zelenay S, Huotari J, Schraml BU, et al. GM-CSF mouse bone marrow cultures comprise a heterogeneous population of CD11c(+)MHCII(+) macrophages and dendritic cells. *Immunity* (2015) 42:1197–211. doi:10.1016/j.immuni.2015.05.018
25. Hettinger J, Richards DM, Hansson J, Barra MM, Joschko AC, Krijgsveld J, et al. Origin of monocytes and macrophages in a committed progenitor. *Nat Immunol* (2013) 14:821–30. doi:10.1038/ni.2638
26. Romani N, Gruner S, Brang D, Kampgen E, Lenz A, Trockenbacher B, et al. Proliferating dendritic cell progenitors in human blood. *J Exp Med* (1994) 180:83–93. doi:10.1084/jem.180.1.83
27. Randolph GJ, Beaulieu S, Lebecque S, Steinman RM, Muller WA. Differentiation of monocytes into dendritic cells in a model of transendothelial trafficking. *Science* (1998) 282:480–3. doi:10.1126/science.282.5388.480
28. Cheong C, Matos I, Choi JH, Dandamudi DB, Shrestha E, Longhi MP, et al. Microbial stimulation fully differentiates monocytes to DC-SIGN/CD209(+) dendritic cells for immune T cell areas. *Cell* (2010) 143:416–29. doi:10.1016/j.cell.2010.09.039
29. Xu Y, Zhan Y, Lew AM, Naik SH, Kershaw MH. Differential development of murine dendritic cells by GM-CSF versus Flt3 ligand has implications for inflammation and trafficking. *J Immunol* (2007) 179:7577–84. doi:10.4049/jimmunol.179.11.7577
30. Segura E, Touzot M, Bohineust A, Cappuccio A, Chiocchia G, Hosmalin A, et al. Human inflammatory dendritic cells induce Th17 cell differentiation. *Immunity* (2013) 38:336–48. doi:10.1016/j.immuni.2012.10.018
31. Steinman RM, Hemmi H. Dendritic cells: translating innate to adaptive immunity. *Curr Top Microbiol Immunol* (2006) 311:17–58.
32. Maree AF, Komba M, Finegood DT, Edelstein-Keshet L. A quantitative comparison of rates of phagocytosis and digestion of apoptotic cells by macrophages from normal (BALB/c) and diabetes-prone (NOD) mice. *J Appl Physiol (1985)* (2008) 104:157–69. doi:10.1152/japplphysiol.00514.2007
33. Cenci E, Mencacci A, Casagrande A, Mosci P, Bistoni F, Romani L. Impaired antifungal effector activity but not inflammatory cell recruitment in interleukin-6-deficient mice with invasive pulmonary aspergillosis. *J Infect Dis* (2001) 184:610–7. doi:10.1086/322793
34. Brieland JK, Jackson C, Menzel F, Loebenberg D, Cacciapuoti A, Halpern J, et al. Cytokine networking in lungs of immunocompetent mice in response to inhaled *Aspergillus fumigatus*. *Infect Immun* (2001) 69:1554–60. doi:10.1128/IAI.69.3.1554-1560.2001
35. Windsor WT, Syto R, Tsarbopoulos A, Zhang R, Durkin J, Baldwin S, et al. Disulfide bond assignments and secondary structure analysis of human and murine interleukin 10. *Biochemistry* (1993) 32:8807–15. doi:10.1021/bi00085a011
36. Willment JA, Marshall AS, Reid DM, Williams DL, Wong SY, Gordon S, et al. The human beta-glucan receptor is widely expressed and functionally equivalent to murine Dectin-1 on primary cells. *Eur J Immunol* (2005) 35:1539–47. doi:10.1002/eji.200425725
37. Brown GD, Herre J, Williams DL, Willment JA, Marshall AS, Gordon S. Dectin-1 mediates the biological effects of beta-glucans. *J Exp Med* (2003) 197:1119–24. doi:10.1084/jem.20021890
38. Reid DM, Gow NA, Brown GD. Pattern recognition: recent insights from Dectin-1. *Curr Opin Immunol* (2009) 21:30–7. doi:10.1016/j.coi.2009.01.003
39. Hefter M, Lother J, Weiß E, Schmitt AL, Fliesser M, Einsele H, et al. Human primary myeloid dendritic cells interact with the opportunistic fungal pathogen *Aspergillus fumigatus* via the C-type lectin receptor Dectin-1. *Med Mycol* (2016) 55:573–8. doi:10.1093/mmy/myw105
40. Werner JL, Metz AE, Horn D, Schoeb TR, Hewitt MM, Schwiebert LM, et al. Requisite role for the Dectin-1 beta-glucan receptor in pulmonary defense against *Aspergillus fumigatus*. *J Immunol* (2009) 182:4938–46. doi:10.4049/jimmunol.0804250
41. Raberg L, Sim D, Read AF. Disentangling genetic variation for resistance and tolerance to infectious diseases in animals. *Science* (2007) 318:812–4. doi:10.1126/science.1148526

6

The Syk-Coupled C-Type Lectin Receptors Dectin-2 and Dectin-3 are Involved in *Paracoccidioides brasiliensis* Recognition by Human Plasmacytoid Dendritic Cells

Nycolas Willian Preite, Claudia Feriotti, Dhêmerson Souza de Lima, Bruno Borges da Silva, Antônio Condino-Neto, Alessandra Pontillo, Vera Lúcia Garcia Calich and Flávio Vieira Loures*†

Departamento de Imunologia, Instituto de Ciências Biomédicas, Universidade de São Paulo, São Paulo, Brazil

***Correspondence:**
Flávio Vieira Loures
loures@unifesp.br

†Present address:
Flávio Vieira Loures,
Instituto de Ciência e Tecnologia,
Universidade Ferderal de São Paulo,
São José dos Campos, Brazil

Plasmacytoid dendritic cells (pDCs), which have been extensively studied in the context of the immune response to viruses, have recently been implicated in host defense mechanisms against fungal infections. Nevertheless, the involvement of human pDCs during paracoccidioidomycosis (PCM), a fungal infection endemic to Latin America, has been scarcely studied. However, pDCs were found in the cutaneous lesions of PCM patients, and in pulmonary model of murine PCM these cells were shown to control disease severity. These findings led us to investigate the role of human pDCs in the innate phase of PCM. Moreover, considering our previous data on the engagement of diverse Toll-like receptors and C-type lectin receptors receptors in *Paracoccidioides brasiliensis* recognition, we decided to characterize the innate immune receptors involved in the interaction between human pDCs and yeast cells. Purified pDCs were obtained from peripheral blood mononuclear cells from healthy donors and they were stimulated with *P. brasiliensis* with or without blocking antibodies to innate immune receptors. Here we demonstrated that *P. brasiliensis* stimulation activates human pDCs that inhibit fungal growth and secrete pro-inflammatory cytokines and type I IFNs. Surprisingly, *P. brasiliensis*-stimulated pDCs produce mature IL-1β and activate caspase 1, possibly *via* inflammasome activation, which is a phenomenon not yet described during pDC engagement by microorganisms. Importantly, we also demonstrate that dectin-2 and dectin-3 are expressed on pDCs and appear to be involved (*via* Syk signaling) in the pDC-*P. brasiliensis* interaction. Moreover, *P. brasiliensis*-stimulated pDCs exhibited an efficient antigen presentation and were able to effectively activate $CD4^+$ and $CD8^+$ T cells. In conclusion, our study demonstrated for the first time that human pDCs are involved in *P. brasiliensis* recognition and may play an important role in the innate and adaptive immunity against this fungal pathogen.

Keywords: paracoccidioidomycosis, plasmacytoid dendritic cells, C-type lectin receptors, dectin-2, dectin-3, type I IFNs, inflammasome

INTRODUCTION

Paracoccidioidomycosis (PCM), the most prevalent and endemic deep mycosis in Latin America, is caused by the thermally dimorphic fungus *Paracoccidioides brasiliensis.* The resistance to this disease was linked to the secretion of Th1 cytokines in humans and murine models of PCM, while reduced Th1 immunity and the predominant secretion of Th2 cytokines associate with systemic and progressive illness (1, 2). The role of Th17 immunity is poorly defined. Nevertheless, in PCM patients, IL-17-expressing cells have been observed in cutaneous and mucosal lesions and they have been associated with the development of granulomas (3). Moreover, the varied patterns of T cell responses in patients with PCM lead to diverse clinical manifestations. In infected asymptomatic individuals, the resistance to infection was shown to be mediated by the Th1 response, which is essential for macrophage activation and fungal killing, while the juvenile form, the most severe form of the disease, presents a dominant Th2/Th9 response and an elevated antibody response. In adult form of the disease, a chronic inflammatory response involving Th1 and Th17-mediated immunity was also described (2).

Plasmacytoid dendritic cells (pDCs) are a DC subset largely involved in immune responses against viruses (4, 5). Following Toll-like receptors (TLRs) stimulation, the pDCs mature and become potent antigen-presenting cells (APCs), upregulating MHC and costimulatory molecules, and secreting high levels of cytokines such as IFN-α and TNF-α. Activated mature pDCs prime naive T cells for Th1 or Th17 differentiation (6, 7). Outside of viral infections, important roles for pDCs have been described in the immune response against fungal infections (8–12). A pioneer study showed that human pDCs interact to and inhibit the growth of *Aspergillus fumigatus*-hyphae. Moreover, *in vivo* depletion of pDC confers hyper-susceptibility to aspergillosis in mice. In addition, it was also demonstrated that dectin-2, a C-type lectin receptor (CLR) expressed by human pDCs, acts in collaboration with the FcRγ chain to recognize hyphae of *A. fumigatus*. This interaction induces the synthesis of TNF-α and IFN-α, and facilitates efficient antifungal activity. Additionally, pDCs stimulated by *A. fumigatus* hyphae exhibit a characteristic gene expression signature, leading to the formation of extracellular traps (pETs) (10). *P. brasiliensis* was also shown to be recognized by murine pDCs. *In vitro* stimulation of bone marrow-derived DCs (BMDCs) from susceptible (B10.A) mice induces a prevalent inflammatory myeloid phenotype characterized by the secretion of high levels of IL-12, TNF-α, and IL-1β. In contrast, in BMDCs from the resistant (A/J) mice a varied population of myeloid cells and pDCs secreting inflammatory cytokines and expressing high levels of secreted and membrane-bound TGF-β were observed following BMDCs stimulation with fungal cells (8). Importantly, in 24 of 46 PCM patients, the presence of pDCs was verified when their cutaneous lesions were immunostained with anti-pDC specific antibodies (11). In addition, peripheral blood pDCs appeared in lower numbers in PCM patients compared to the number of blood pDCs found in health donors, suggesting that pDCs migrate to the lymph nodes, spleen, and target organs during a *P. brasiliensis* infection (12). Taking in account these findings and the fact that human innate immunity against *P. brasiliensis* infection is poorly defined, we aimed to investigate the interaction of human pDCs with *P. brasiliensis* yeast cells. Moreover, considering our previous data on the engagement of TLRs, complement receptor-3, and CLRs in *P. brasiliensis* recognition (13–17), we considered that it would be important to define the class of innate receptors involved in fungal recognition by human pDCs. Here, we show that when stimulated by *P. brasiliensis* yeast cells human pDCs are activated, produce inflammatory cytokines, and acquire enhanced fungicidal activity. In addition, we demonstrate that *P. brasiliensis* recognition by human pDCs is mediated by dectin-2 and dectin-3, and is regulated by Syk signaling. Our study of the secretion of mature IL-β and caspase-1 activation has also indicated that *P. brasiliensis* recognition triggers inflammasome activation in human pDC, a finding that, as far we know, has not been described previously. Finally, our data also suggested that *P. brasiliensis* activated pDCs can prime the activation of $CD4^+$ and $CD8^+$ T cells, and may participate in the acquired immunity to this pathogen.

MATERIALS AND METHODS

Ethics Statement

All research involving human participants was approved by the Institute of Biomedical Science Institutional Ethics Committee. Written informed consent was obtained from all human participants and all clinical investigations were conducted according to the principles expressed in the Declaration of Helsinki.

Isolation of Human pDCs, mDCs, and $CD3^+$ Cells

The human pDCs were isolated from healthy donors using magnetic beads as previously described (10). About 120 mL of the peripheral blood was collected by venipuncture. The blood samples was anticoagulated with heparin, and the peripheral blood mononuclear cells (PBMCs) were purified by Ficoll-Hypaque density gradient centrifugation. The PBMCs were stained with CD304-coated magnetic beads (Miltenyi Biotec) and the pDCs were isolated after two rounds of positive selection. For flow cytometric experiments in which pDCs were gated using an anti-CD123 antibody, only one round of positive selection was run. For some experiments, the flow-through cells (here called pDC^- cells), which consisted of PBMCs depleted of $CD304^+$ cells, were also collected. For coculture experiments, purified human myeloid dendritic cells (mDCs) and CD3 cells were obtained from PBMCs by positive selection using magnetic beads (Miltenyi Biotec). mDCs were also used in qPCR experiments. The purity of the cell populations was confirmed by assessing the expression of CD123, CD1c, and CD3 as pDC, mDC, and lymphocyte markers, respectively, by flow cytometry. The purity of pDCs, mDCs, and $CD3^+$ cells always exceeded 95%.

P. brasiliensis Yeast Cells and pDC Stimulation

Paracoccidioides brasiliensis yeast cells were maintained by weekly cultivation in Fava Netto culture medium at 37°C and used on day 7 of culture. The highly virulent *P. brasiliensis*

18 isolate was used in this study. To determine the viability of fungal cell suspensions we used Janus Green B vital dye (Merck), and the viability was always greater than 95%. For colony-forming units (CFU) and ELISA experiments, pDC (1×10^5) or flow through-cells (pDC⁻) were challenged overnight with *P. brasiliensis* in different ratios of pDC:*P. brasiliensis*, such as 10:1, 25:1, and 50:1 (1×10^4, 4×10^3, and 2×10^3 yeasts, respectively) as indicated in the figure legends.

Reagents and Cell Culture

The RPMI-1640 media was obtained from GIBCO (Invitrogen) and was supplemented with 100 U/mL penicillin, 100 U/mL streptomycin, and 2 mM L-glutamine. IgG Rat monoclonal anti-dectin-1 (Biolegend), dectin-2 (R&D System), dectin-3 (Biolegend), and antimincle (InvivoGen) blocking antibodies were used in the concentration indicated in the figure legends. The TLR-9 antagonist (A151, TTAGGG oligonucleotide sequence,

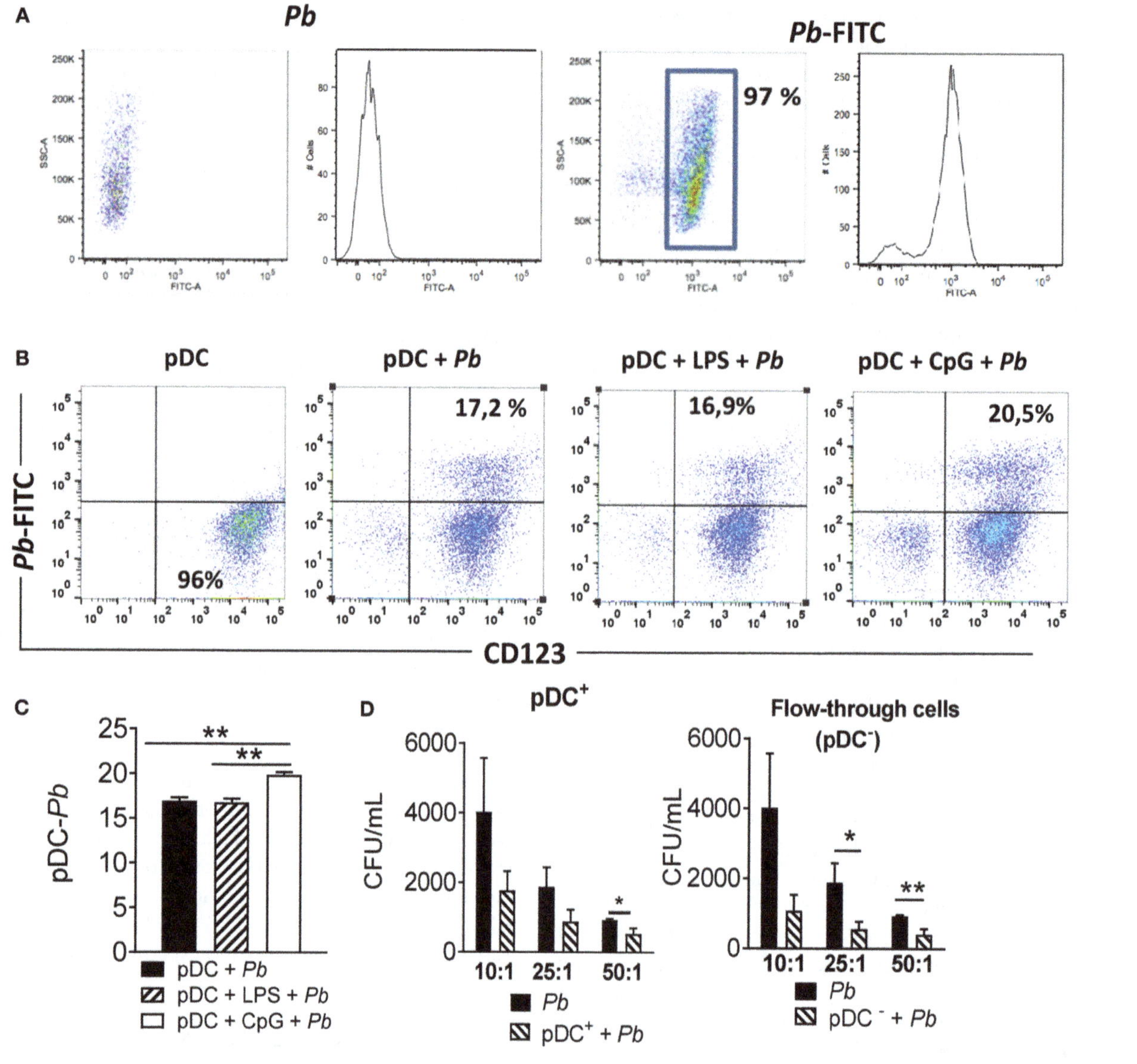

FIGURE 1 | Plasmacytoid dendritic cells (pDCs) interact with and control *Paracoccidioides brasiliensis* growth. **(A,B)** Peripheral blood mononuclear cells (PBMCs) were separated into pDC positive (pDCs+) using magnetic beads conjugated to an anti-CD304 antibody. The cells (2×10^5/well) were challenged for 4 h with *P. brasiliensis* yeast cells (2×10^5/well) previously labeled with FITC. Some wells were treated with CpG (100 ng/mL) or LPS (10 ng/mL) before the challenge. After 4 h of culture, the cells were labeled with an anti-CD123 antibody (specific to human pDCs) in the appropriate titration, and then 50,000 events were acquired by flow cytometry. **(B)** Dot plots are representative results for an experiment from three independents experiments. **(C)** Data represent means ± SE of the pDC–*P. brasiliensis* interaction from three donors, tested in triplicate **$p < 0.01$. **(D)** For CFU analysis, PBMCs were separated into pDC-positive (pDCs⁺) and pDC-negative (pDC⁻) fractions using CD304-coated magnetic beads. The pDCs⁺ and flow through-cells (1×10^5/well) were then challenged with *P. brasiliensis* yeast cells in different ratios of pDC: *Pb*, such as 10:1, 25:1 and 50:1 (1×10^4, 4×10^3, and 2×10^3 yeasts, respectively). After 18 h of culture, the plates were centrifuged and the supernatant was collected for cytokine measurements by ELISA. The pellet was lysed and suspended in 200 µL of phosphate-buffered saline. Next, 100 µL was transferred to BHI medium and the colonies (CFU) counted for 15 days. Data represent means ± SE of CFU from four donors, tested in triplicate. *$p < 0.05$, **$p < 0.01$, and ***$p < 0.001$.

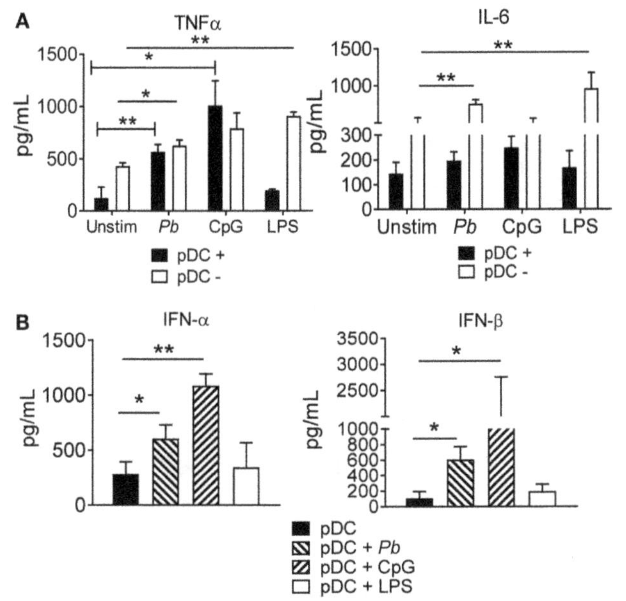

FIGURE 2 | Proinflammatory and type I IFNs cytokines released by plasmacytoid dendritic cells (pDCs) stimulated with *Paracoccidioides brasiliensis* yeast cells. Peripheral blood mononuclear cells (PBMCs) were separated into pDC-positive (pDCs$^+$) and pDC-negative (pDCs$^-$) populations using magnetic beads conjugated to anti-CD304 antibodies. The cells (1×10^5/well) were left without stimulation or challenged overnight with of *P. brasiliensis* yeast cells (2×10^3), CpG (100 ng/mL), or LPS (10 ng/mL). The supernatant was removed and the levels of IL-6, TNF-α **(A)**, and type I IFNs **(B)** were analyzed by ELISA. Data are represented as the mean ± SE of the average cytokine concentrations from five donors, tested in duplicate. ***$p < 0.001$ by comparing the data indicated by the bar.

10 μg/mL), TLR-7/9 inhibitor Bafilomycin A1 (10 μg/mL), and the immunostimulatory CpG 2336 oligonucleotide (100 ng/mL) were purchased from InvivoGen. Ultrapure *Escherichia coli* LPS (10 ng/mL) and the Syk inhibitor piceatannol (10 μM) was purchased from Sigma.

P. brasiliensis–pDC Interaction

Paracoccidioides brasiliensis yeast cells were labeled with fluorescein isothiocyanate (FITC) as previously described (18). Briefly, the yeasts were washed in phosphate-buffered saline (PBS, pH = 7.4) and heat-killed at 60°C for 1 h. To eliminate the aggregates, the yeast cells suspension was subjected to three cycles of sonication for 10 s each (21% amplitude) with Sonics (Vibra Cell VCX 750, Sonics & Materials). The yeasts were washed twice with PBS, counted and adjusted to 1×10^6 cells/mL, and then incubated with FITC (100 μg/mL, Sigma) for 25–30 min at 36°C. The yeast suspension was then washed with PBS twice. The pDCs (2×10^5) were challenged for 4 h with *P. brasiliensis*-FITC (1×10^5) at a ratio of 2:1 at 36°C in 5% CO_2 to permit fungi adhesion and ingestion. The cells were then harvested and the pDCs were labeled with anti-CD123 (eBioscience) antibody for 25 min at 4°C. Because *P. brasiliensis* yeast cells are highly variable in size and granularity (different sizes, number of buds, and number of nuclei), the granulocyte gates defined by size (FSC) and granularity (SSC) in order to determine the pDC population were not used. A minimum of 50,000 events were acquired on a FACScanto II flow cytometer (BD Biosciences) using the FACSDiva software (BD Biosciences). The data were analyzed using the FlowJo software (Tree Star).

Cytokine Measurements

The pDCs were cultured in 96-well plates in pDC media. The cells were left untreated or incubated with anti-dectin-1, dectin-2, dectin-3, or antimincle antibodies (100 μg/mL) for 30 min at 37°C. The pDCs were then challenged with *P. brasiliensis* yeast cells at a final volume of 200 μL in pDC media at the ratios indicated in the figure legends. Control wells contained pDCs only, pDCs and antibodies, pDCs and CpG, or pDCs and LPS. For the inhibition of TLR-9, pDCs were left untreated or incubated for 30 min with either 10 μg/mL of bafilomycin A1 or 10 μg/mL of the TLR-9 antagonist A151. After 18 h of incubation at 37°C, the supernatants were removed and the levels of TNF-α, IL-6, IL-1β, IFN-α, and IFN-β were measured by ELISA according to the manufacturers' protocols (eBioscience for TNF-α and IL-6; Biolegend for IL-1β; PBL Assay Science for IFN-α and IFN-β).

CFU Assays

The number of viable microorganisms in cell cultures was performed by counting the number of CFU as previously described (19). Briefly, after 18 h of coculture, the plates were centrifuged (400 *g*, 10 min, 4°C), and the supernatant was collected for cytokine measurements by ELISA. The wells were lysed with 200 μL of distilled water. The suspensions were collected in individual tubes and centrifuged (400 *g*, 10 min, 4°C). The pellet was suspended in 1 mL of PBS, and 100 μL of each lysate was spread onto BHI medium. The colonies (CFU) were counted for 15 days.

pDC Flow Cytometric Analysis

The pDC$^+$ populations (2×10^5/well) were either left unstimulated or challenged overnight with *P. brasiliensis* yeast cells (4×10^3). For cell-surface staining, the pDCs were washed and suspended at 2×10^5 cells/mL in staining buffer (PBS, 2% fetal calf serum, and 0.1% NaN_3) and then stained in the dark for 20 min at 4°C with the optimal dilution of anti-123, CD86, MHC-II antibodies. The cells were then washed twice with staining buffer, suspended in 200 μL of paraformaldehyde (PFA) to fix the cells. To measure caspase-1 activity, the pDCs were adjusted to 2×10^5 viable cells in 20 μL of apoptosis wash buffer. Cells were stained with FLICA probe according to the manufacturer's protocol (Immunochemistry Technologies) for 1 h at 37°C in 5% CO_2. Control wells contained untreated pDCs, pDC and CpG, or pDC and LPS. In some experiments, cells were treated with 1 mM ATP (Sigma-Aldrich) for 15 min and then stained with FLICA probe. Active caspase-1 was then measured by flow cytometry as previously described (16). To exclude dead cells, the Live/Dead Fixable Violet Cell Stain Kit (Life Technologies) was used according to the manufacturer's instructions. A minimum of 50,000 events were acquired on a FACScanto II flow cytometer (BD Biosciences) using the FACSDiva software (BD Biosciences). The pDCs were gated based upon their forward and side light scatter. The cell surface expression of pDC markers was analyzed using FlowJo software (Tree Star).

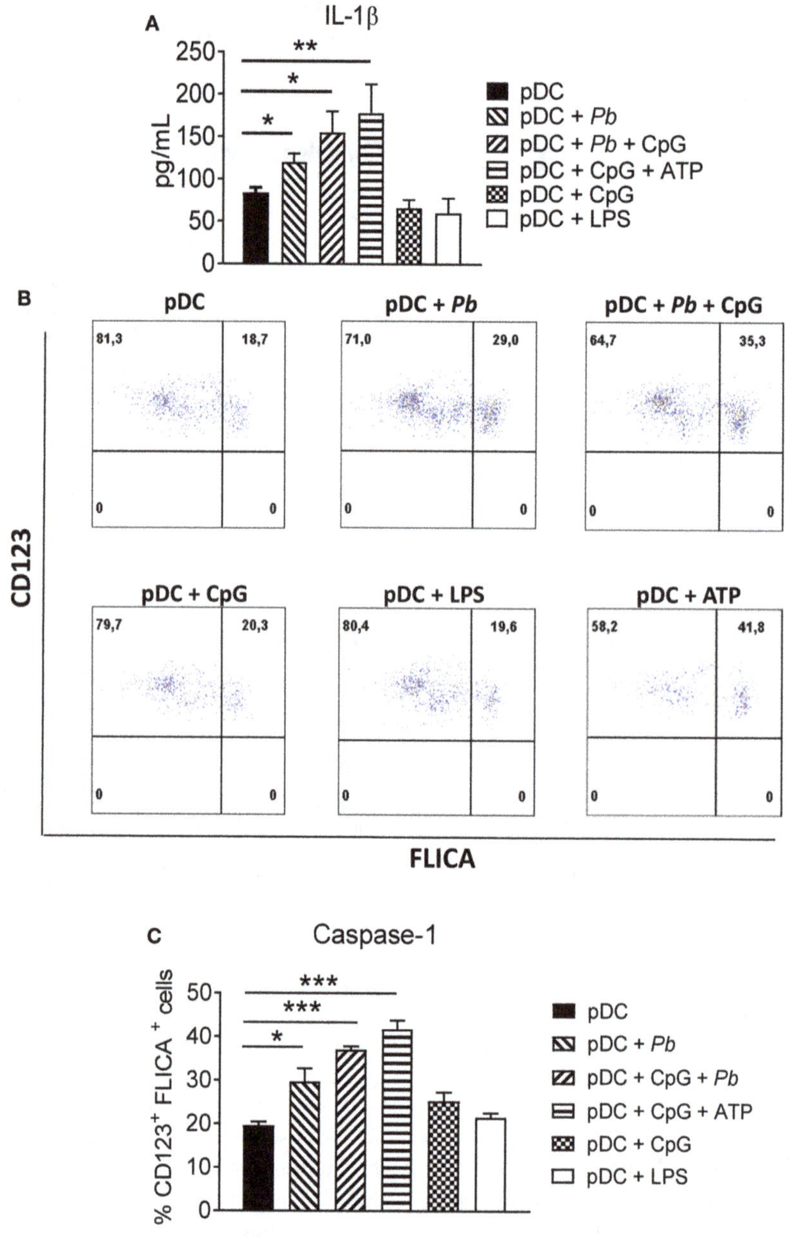

FIGURE 3 | Plasmacytoid dendritic cell (pDC) exposed to *Paracoccidioides brasiliensis* yeast cells secretes mature IL-1β and express activated caspase-1. **(A)** Peripheral blood mononuclear cells (PBMCs) were separated into pDC positive (pDCs+) cells using magnetic beads conjugated to anti-CD304 antibodies. The cells (1×10^5/well) were then left without stimulation or challenged overnight with *P. brasiliensis* yeast cells (2×10^3), CpG (100 ng/mL), or LPS (10 ng/mL). The supernatant was removed and the levels of IL-1β were analyzed by ELISA. Data are represented as the mean ± SE of the average cytokine concentrations from three donors, tested in duplicate. $^*p < 0.05$ by comparing the data indicated by the bar. **(B,C)** Caspase-1 activity was evaluated by flow cytometry. PBMCs were separated into pDC positive (pDCs$^+$) populations using magnetic beads conjugated to anti-CD304 antibodies. The cells (2×10^5/well) were left without stimulation or challenged overnight with *P. brasiliensis* yeast cells (4×10^3), CpG (100 ng/mL), or LPS (10 ng/mL). Cells were stained with FLICA probe for 1 h and the percentage of CD123$^+$FLICA$^+$ cells were determined by flow cytometry. **(B)** Dot plots are representative results of an experiment from two independent experiments. **(C)** Data are represented as the mean ± SE of CD123$^+$FLICA$^+$ cells from two donors, tested in duplicate. $^*p < 0.05$, $^{**}p < 0.01$, $^{***}p < 0.001$ by comparing the data indicated by the bars.

RNA Isolation and Relative Gene Expression Analysis

Total RNA was isolated and converted into cDNA from 2×10^5 purified pDC$^+$ and mDC$^+$, unstimulated or challenged overnight with *P. brasiliensis* yeast cells (4×10^3), using the TaqMan Gene Expression Cells-to-CT kit according to manufacturer's protocol (Applied Biosystems, Thermofisher Scientific). The expression of *CLEC7A/DECTIN1, CLEC6A/DECTIN2, CLEC4D/DECTIN3,*

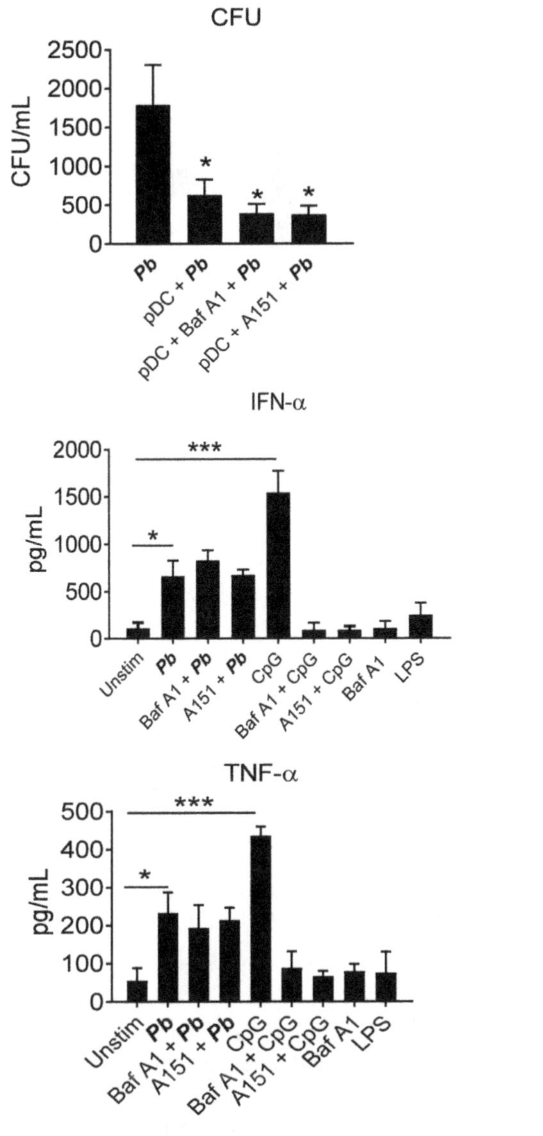

FIGURE 4 | Toll-like receptor (TLR)-9 is not used by plasmacytoid dendritic cells (pDCs) to sense *Paracoccidioides brasiliensis* yeast cells. peripheral blood mononuclear cells were separated into pDC-positive populations (pDCs+) using magnetic beads conjugated to anti-CD304 antibody. The cells (1×10^5/well) were challenged overnight with *P. brasiliensis* yeast cells (2×10^3). Some wells were kept unstimulated, with only the yeasts, and LPS (100 ng/mL). Some cultures were treated with an TLR-9 antagonist (A151, TTAGGG, 10 μg/mL) or with the TLR-9 inhibitor Bafilomycin A1 (10 μg/mL) before challenging either with the yeasts or with the positive control for TLR-9 activation CpG (100 ng/mL). After 18 h of culture, the plates were centrifuged and the supernatant was collected for cytokine measurements by ELISA. The pellet was lysed and suspended in 200 μL of phosphate-buffered saline. Next, 100 μL was transferred to BHI medium, and the colonies (CFU) were counted for 15 days. Data represent the means ± SE of the CFU and cytokine concentrations from three donors, tested in triplicate. $^*p < 0.05$ comparing the group maintained only with the fungus with the others.

CLEC4E/MINCLE was evaluated using gene-specific TaqMan assays (Applied Biosystems) and qPCR on a MxP3000P Real-Time PCR System (Stratagene). Raw expression data (Ct) were normalized with the expression of the housekeeping gene glyceraldehyde-3-phosphate dehydrogenase/*GAPDH* (ΔCt). Relative expression of the target genes was calculated as $2^{-\Delta Ct}$ according to Schmittgen and Livak (20), comparing stimulated and unstimulated cells ($\Delta\Delta Ct = \Delta Ct_{Pb} - \Delta Ct_{Unstimulated}$).

pDC/mDC and Lymphocyte Coculture

The pDCs+ or mDCs+ populations (1×10^5/well) were challenged with *P. brasiliensis* yeast cells (1×10^4) for 2 h and cocultured with CD3+ cells (1×10^6) for 5 days at 37°C in 5% CO_2. All cells populations were isolated from the same donor. The ratio DCs to lymphocytes (1:10) was determined in a previous study (15). For cell-surface staining, the cocultured cells were washed and suspended at a concentration of 5×10^5 cells/mL in staining buffer (PBS, 2% fetal calf serum and 0.1% NaN_3). They were then stained in the dark for 20 min at 4°C with the optimal dilution of anti-CD4, CD8, CD25, and anti-CD69 antibodies. The cells were then washed twice with staining buffer, and suspended in 200 μL of PFA to fix the cells. A minimum of 50,000 events were acquired on FACScanto II flow cytometer (BD Biosciences) using the FACSDiva software (BD Biosciences). The lymphocytes were gated based upon forward and side light scatter. The cell surface expression of lymphocyte markers was analyzed using FlowJo software (Tree Star).

Statistical Analysis

For comparisons of two groups, the means ± SE were analyzed using the two-tailed unpaired Student's *t*-test with the Bonferroni correction applied when making multiple comparisons. For comparisons of more than two groups, significance was determined using the one- or two-way analysis of variance with the Tukey multiple corrections. Kruskal–Wallis test was applied in RT-PCR experiments. All data were collected and analyzed from at least three independent experiments. The levels of significance were $p < 0.05$ ($^*p < 0.05$, $^{**}p < 0.01$, and $^{***}p < 0.001$). Calculations were performed using a statistical software package (GraphPad Prism 6.0).

RESULTS

The *P. brasiliensis*–pDC Interaction and Fungicidal Activity

Initially, we investigated the ability of human pDCs to interact and phagocytose *P. brasiliensis* yeast cells. PBMC-isolated pDCs were challenged with FITC-conjugated *P. brasiliensis* (**Figure 1A**) for 4 h, and the frequency of adhered or ingested *P. brasiliensis* yeast cells by pDCs was determined by counting the number of labeled pDC (CD123+ cells) containing *Pb*-FITC (CD123+ *Pb*-FITC+). **Figure 1B** shows that about 17% of the total pDCs were double-positive for CD123 and *Pb*-FITC, suggesting that pDCs interacted with *P. brasiliensis* yeast cells. Considering that human pDCs are TLR-9+ and TLR-4− (21, 22), the TLR-4 bacterial LPS agonist and the TLR-9 CpG agonist were used in some experiments to specifically prime pDCs to enhance their phagocytic ability. As expected, the ability of pDCs to interact with the yeasts did not significantly change in the presence of LPS. However, the addition of CpG enhanced the *P. brasilienis*–pDC interaction (**Figures 1B,C**).

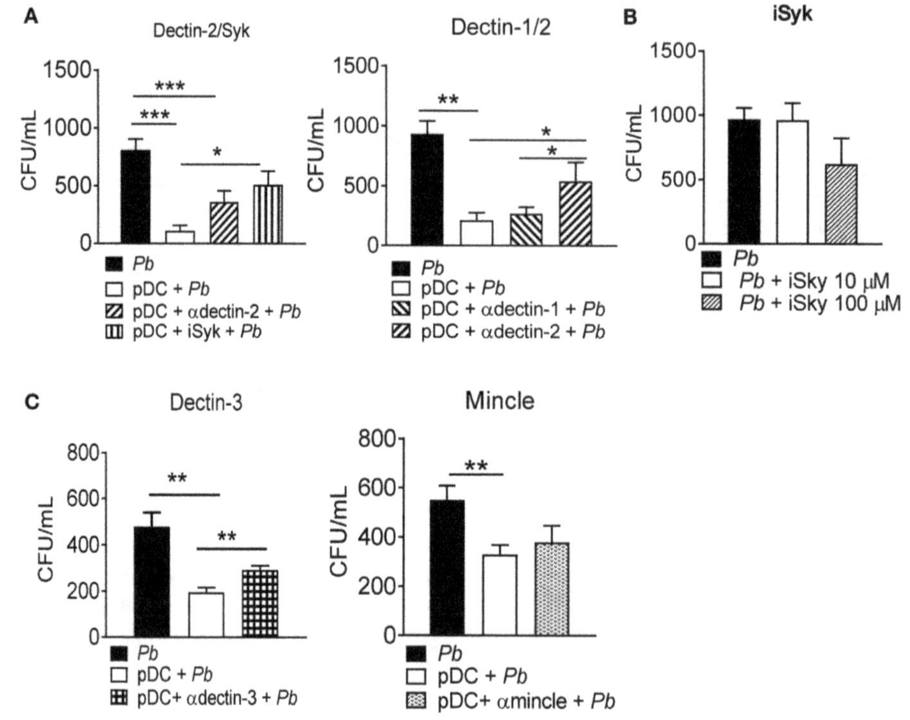

FIGURE 5 | Dectin2, dectin-3, and Syk signaling activate the fungicidal activity of plasmacytoid dendritic cells (pDCs). Peripheral blood mononuclear cells were separated into pDC-positive populations (pDCs+) using magnetic beads conjugated to anti-CD304 antibody. The cells (1 × 10^5/well) were challenged overnight with *P. brasiliensis* yeast cells (2 × 10^3). **(A)** Some cultures were treated with anti-dectin-1, dectin-2, or with a Syk pathway inhibitor, piceatannol (10 μM). **(B)** The Syk inhibitor (10 or 100 μM) was also cultured with *P. brasiliensis* yeast cells only. **(C)** Futher, anti-mincle and anti-dectin-3 antibodies (100 μg/mL) were also used, before challenging with *P. brasiliensis* yeast cells. After 18 h of culture, the plates were centrifuged, and the supernatant was collected for cytokine measurements by ELISA. The pellet was lysed and suspended in 200 μL of phosphate-buffered saline. Next, 100 μL was transferred to BHI medium, and the colonies (CFU) were counted for 15 days. Data represent the means ± SE of the CFU from three donors, tested in triplicate. *$p < 0.05$, **$p < 0.01$, ***$p < 0.001$ by comparing the data indicated by the bars.

To analyze the fungicidal ability of human pDCs, the PBMCs were separated into pDC$^+$ or pDC$^-$ populations. The pDC$^-$ fraction is composed of the flow-through cells resulting from the pDC isolation. This fraction, used as a control in some assays, contains mostly non-pDC PBMCs such as conventional DCs, monocytes, lymphocytes and small fractions of other cell subpopulations. The depletion of pDC was able to reduce the frequency of pDC on the PBMCs in about 90% (Figure S1 in Supplementary Material) resulting in less than 0.2% of pDC in the PBMCs. The cells were challenged overnight with *P. brasiliensis* yeast cells in different pDC: *Pb* ratios (10:1, 25:1, and 50:1). **Figure 1D** shows that only in the 50:1 ratio were pDCs able to control fungal growth. The pDC$^-$ fractions, however, showed fungicidal activity at ratios of 25:1 and 50:1.

Cytokine Release by Human pDCs Stimulated by *P. brasiliensis* Yeast Cells

Next, we examined whether the interaction between the pDCs and *P. brasiliensis* yeast cells could induce the secretion of inflammatory cytokines. The pDCs were challenged with *P. brasiliensis* for 18 h, and the levels of TNF-α and IL-6 in the culture supernatants were determined. Both cytokines were secreted by pDCs, but only TNF-α levels were increased by *P. brasiliensis*-stimulated pDCs. The TLR-9 ligand, CpG, strongly stimulated the pDCs, whereas the TLR-4 ligand, LPS, failed to stimulate these cells to produce either TNF-α or IL-6. As expected, LPS stimulated the pDC$^-$ fraction (which contained LPS-responsive monocytes) to release TNF-α and IL-6 (**Figure 2A**).

Next, we examined whether the interaction of pDCs with *P. brasiliensis* yeast cells could increase type I IFN release. Both IFN-α and IFN-β were secreted by pDCs$^+$ following stimulation with *P. brasiliensis* yeast cells. Once again, CpG strongly stimulated the pDCs, while LPS failed to activate these cells (**Figure 2B**).

P. brasiliensis Induces Production of IL-1β and Increases Caspase-1 Activity in Human pDCs

An emerging area of investigation examines the participation of the inflammasome in fungal infections (16, 23). The inflammasome is a multiprotein cytoplasmic complex assembled after an innate immune receptor [e.g., NOD-like receptor family, pyrin domain-containing (NLRP) 1, NLRP3, or absent in melanoma 2 (AIM2)] is activated by a pathogen-associated molecular pattern (PAMPs) or damage-associated molecular pattern. This results in a multi-protein platform that activates caspase-1, which processes pro-IL-1β and pro-IL-18 into their biologically active or mature forms (24).

In our experiments, *P. brasiliensis* yeast cells induced a significant production of IL-1β by pDCs. Importantly, treatment with CpG or LPS alone did not significantly increase IL-1β production by these cells (**Figure 3A**). Accordingly, caspase-1 activation was strongly induced in *P. brasiliensis*-stimulated pDCs, more than in LPS-treated or CpG-treated pDCs (**Figures 3B,C**). However, when pDCs received both signals (CpG and yeasts), enhancement in the activity of caspase-1 was observed. Importantly, the addition of 1 mM ATP to the cultures increased caspase-1 activity and IL-1β production, suggesting that a purinergic signaling could be involved in inflammasome activation by *P. brasiliensis*. To our knowledge, increased extracellular ATP activates NLRP3-inflammasome through the binding on P2 × 7 purinergic receptor inducing a K^+ efflux which in turn activates NLRP3 (25). Deeper investigations are needed to confirm the involvement of ATP-P2 × 7-NLRP3 axis in pDC response to *P. brasiliensis*, although the involvement of P2 × 7 receptor in the immunoprotection of murine PCM was demonstrated in our previous studies (26).

The Role of TLR-9 in the *P. brasiliensis*–pDC Interaction

Several studies have demonstrated that TLR-9 is an important PRR used by pDCs during their interaction with microorganisms. We have assessed the role of TLR-9 in the sensing of *P. brasiliensis* by human pDCs using two reagents that inhibit this receptor. Thus, the influence of bafilomycin A1, an endosomal acidification inhibitor known to interfere with TLR-9 signaling (27), and the TLR-9 antagonist A151 (28), on the ability of pDCs to kill *P. brasiliensis* and release cytokines was determined. Both TLR-9 inhibitors showed no effects on *P. brasiliensis* growth or IFN-α secretion. Furthermore, bafilomycin A1 did not affect TNF-α production. As expected, both inhibitors abrogated CpG-stimulated type I IFN release (**Figure 4**). These data suggest that *P. brasiliensis* is recognized by human pDCs in a TLR-9-independent manner.

The Role of CLRs in the *P. brasiliensis*–pDC Interaction

Since *P. brasiliensis* recognition was observed to be TLR-9-independent, we assessed the role of some CLRs in fungal recognition by pDCs. CLRs are a large family of calcium-dependent carbohydrate binding molecules expressed by macrophages, DCs and other leukocytes (29). The mannose receptor (MR), dectin-1, dectin-2, dectin-3, and mincle receptors are examples of CLRs involved in antifungal immunity, although their function and signaling mechanisms are still being clarified (30). Anti-dectin-1, dectin-2, dectin-3, and mincle antibodies were used to block these receptors during the interaction of pDCs with *P. brasiliensis* yeast cells. We also used piceatannol (10 μM), which blocks the activity of the Syk enzyme, involved in CLR signaling. The specific blockade of dectin 2 and Syk, but not dectin 1, reduced the fungicidal ability of pDCs. This indicated the involvement of dectin-2/Syk signaling during fungal

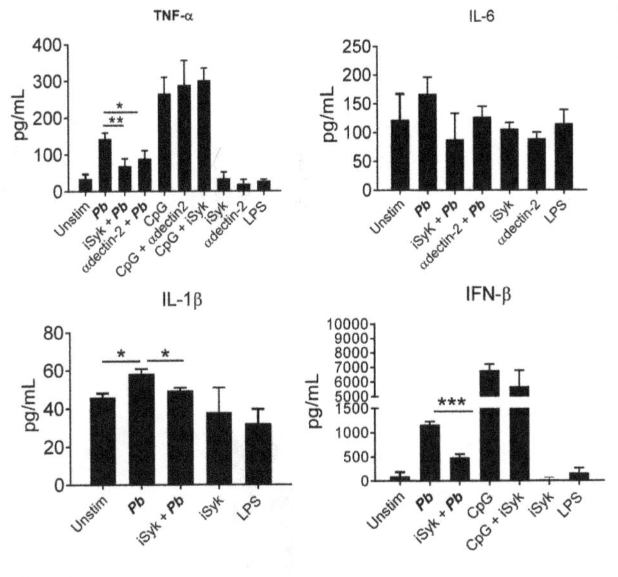

FIGURE 6 | Dectin-2/Syk signaling controls the secretion of cytokines by *Paracoccidioides brasiliensis* stimulated plasmacytoid dendritic cells (pDCs). Peripheral blood mononuclear cells were separated into pDC-positive populations (pDCs+) using magnetic beads conjugated to anti-CD304 antibodies. The pDCs (1 × 10^5/well) were challenged overnight with of *P. brasiliensis* yeast cells (2 × 10^3). Some wells were kept only with the yeasts, CpG (100 ng/mL), or LPS (10 ng/mL). Some cultures were treated with anti-dectin-2 antibody (100 μg/mL) or with a Syk pathway inhibitor, piceatannol (10 μM), before challenging with *P. brasiliensis* yeast cells. After 18 h of culture, the plates were centrifuged and the supernatant was collected for cytokines measurements by ELISA. Data are represented by the means ± SE of the average cytokine concentrations from four donors, tested in duplicate. $^{***}p < 0.001$ and $^{*}p < 0.05$ comparing the data indicated by the bars.

recognition and activation of pDCs (**Figure 5A**). Importantly, the Syk inhibitor piceatannol did not compromise fungal growth even when a high concentration (100 μM) was used in the *P. brasiliensis* culture (**Figure 5B**). We also investigated the role of dectin-3 and mincle receptors during the recognition of *P. brasiliensis* yeast cells by pDCs, because both CLRs were not previously studied in innate immunity against *P. brasiliensis* infection. Interestingly, dectin-3 but not mincle blocked by specific antibodies prior to *P. brasiliensis* stimulation, improved the recovery of yeast cells from the pDC-*P. brasiliensis* cocultures (**Figure 5C**).

Regarding cytokines released, an impaired production of TNF-α, IL-1β, and IFN-β was observed when dectin-2 or Syk were inhibited. No inhibition of IL-6 production was observed when the Syk pathway or dectin-2 were blocked (**Figure 6**). We also observed a reduction in the production of TNF-α and IL-1β following treatment with anti-dectin-3 antibody (**Figure 7A**). In line with the CFU results, treatment with the anti-mincle antibody did not influence cytokine production by *P. brasiliensis*-stimulated pDCs (**Figure 7B**). Again, treatment with both anti-dectin-3 and mincle antibodies did not alter IL-6 production. Importantly, in contrast with the absence of blocking activity on pDC, the anti-mincle antibody blocked mDC (Figure S2 in Supplementary Material).

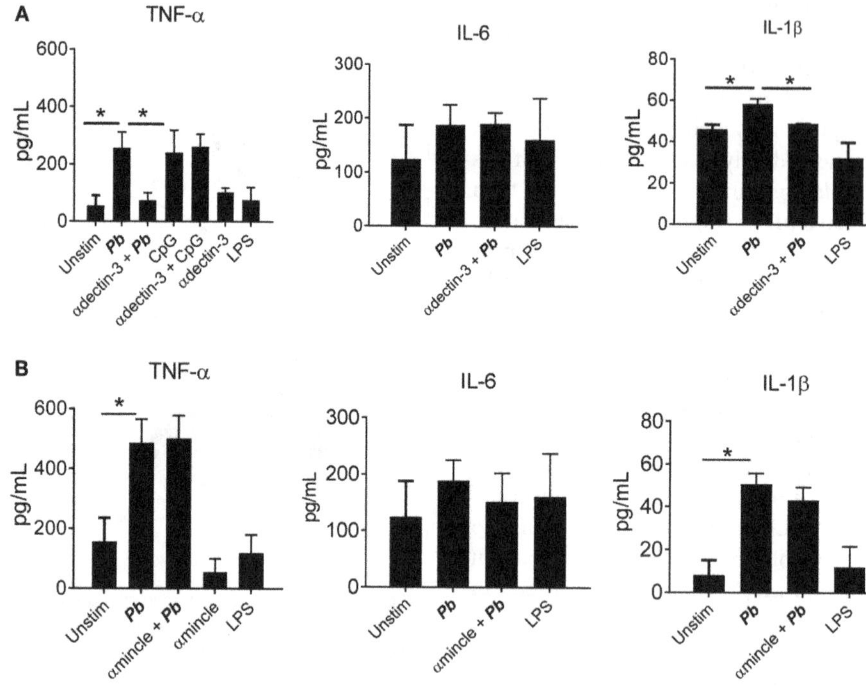

FIGURE 7 | Dectin-3, but not mincle, controls cytokine secretion by *Paracoccidioides brasiliensis* stimulated plasmacytoid dendritic cells (pDCs). Peripheral blood mononuclear cells were separated into pDC-positive populations ($pDCs^+$) using magnetic beads conjugated to anti-CD304 antibodies. The pDCs (1×10^5/well) were challenged overnight with *P. brasiliensis* yeast cells (2×10^3). Some wells were treated only with the yeasts or with LPS (10 ng/mL). Some cultures were treated with **(A)** anti-mincle (100 µg/mL) or **(B)** anti-dectin-3 antibody (100 µg/mL). After 18 h of culture, the plates were centrifuged, and the supernatant was collected for cytokine measurements by ELISA. Data are represented as the mean ± SE of the average of cytokine concentrations from four donors, tested in duplicate. $^{***}p < 0.001$ and $^{*}p < 0.05$ comparing the data indicated by the bar.

When the expression of *DECTIN1*, *DECTIN2*, *DECTIN3* and *MINCLE* genes was investigated in mDCs and pDCs, we observed that while all genes were expressed in mDCs, only *DECTIN2* and *DECTIN3* were found on human pDCs, therefore explaining the previously mentioned lack of effect of blocking antibodies for dectin-1 and mincle in pDC activation. The basal expression of *DECTIN2* resulted significantly higher in pDC compared to mDC ($p = 0.005$) (**Figure 8A**). When DCs where stimulated by *P. brasiliensis* yeast cells, the expression of *DECTIN2* and *DECTIN3* resulted downregulated compared to unstimulated resting cells ($FC < 1$) (**Figure 8B**). Of note *P. brasiliensis* induced a statistically significant downregulation of *DECTIN2* in mDCs ($FC = 0.10 \pm 0.08$; $logFC = -1.49 \pm 0.36$; $p = 0.025$), and of *DECTIN2* ($FC = 0.07 \pm 0.02$; $logFC = -1.24 \pm 0.17$; $p = 0.005$) and *DECTIN3* ($FC = 0.05 \pm 0.02$; $logFC = -1.51 \pm 0.24$; $p = 0.009$) in pDCs. These results highlight the importance of CLRs in *P. brasiliensis* recognition by human pDCs.

pDC–Lymphocyte Interaction

Additional studies demonstrated that *P. brasiliensis*-challenged pDCs showed an increased expression of membrane molecules typically found in activated APCs. *P. brasiliensis*-stimulated pDCs presented a higher expression of both MHC-class II and the costimulatory molecule CD86 when compared with unstimulated counterparts (**Figures 9A,B**). Since this result indicated that the pDCs transitioned to a mature status upon *P. brasiliensis* stimulation, we investigated the role of pDCs as APCs. In this regard, we explored the priming of antigen-specific $CD4^+$ and $CD8^+$ T lymphocytes *in vitro*. The $pDCs^+$ and $mDCs^+$ populations were each challenged with *P. brasiliensis* yeast cells and cocultured with $CD3^+$ cells for 5 days. The mDC-CD3 coculture was used as a positive control because the priming ability of mDCs to specific T lymphocytes was previously described (15). We verified that both pDCs and mDCs recognized, processed, and presented *P. brasiliensis* antigens to the T lymphocytes. A higher frequency of activated $CD4^+$ T lymphocytes ($CD4^+CD25^+$) was observed in both cultures maintained with mDCs and pDCs compared to the group of lymphocytes cultured without *P. brasiliensis* stimulation. A similar response was found for $CD8^+$ T lymphocytes; however, the sensitized mDCs expanded a higher frequency of activated $CD8^+$ T lymphocytes ($CD8^+CD69^+$) compared to the pDCs (**Figures 9C,D**, right panel). Importantly, the $CD3^+$ cells did not respond to the DC stimulation in the absence of *P. brasiliensis* in the coculture (**Figure 9D**, left panel).

DISCUSSION

The involvement of pDCs has been prominently described in viral infections (5). However, recent studies have opened new roles of pDCs to other types of pathogens, indicating an important

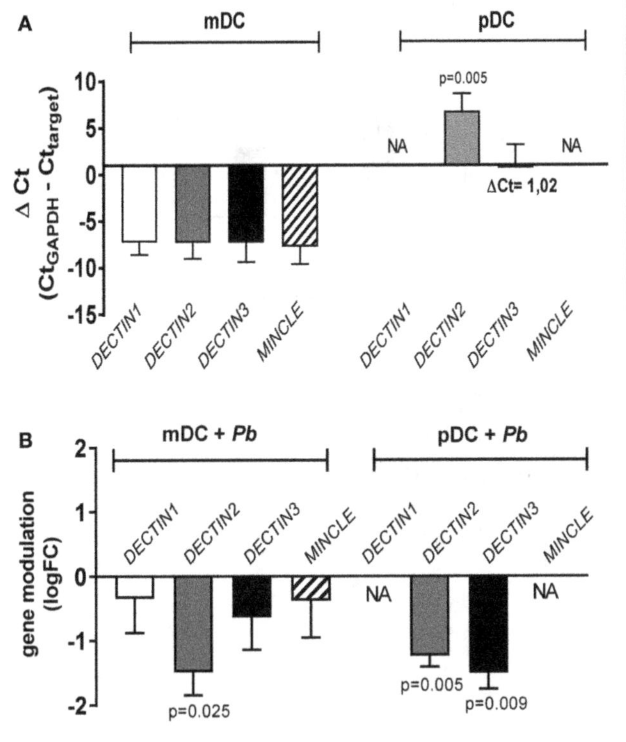

FIGURE 8 | DECTIN1/2/3 and MINCLE gene expression in myeloid dendritic cell (mDC) and plasmacytoid dendritic cell (pDC) stimulated with *Paracoccidioides brasiliensis*. mDCs and pDCs from four healthy individuals were either left unstimulated or challenged overnight with *P. brasiliensis* yeast cells. Then RNA was isolated from each condition and used to evaluate the expression of DECTIN1/2/3 and MINCLE genes by qPCR. GAPDH was used as housekeeping gene for raw data normalization. **(A)** Basal genes expression in mDC and pDC was calculated as ΔCt ($\Delta Ct = Ct_{GAPDH} - Ct_{target}$) as previously reported (31). Data are represented as mean (ΔCt) ± SE. Kruskal–Wallis test was applied to verify the significance of the difference between basal gene expression in mDC and pDC. When significant, the ΔCt of mDC versus pDC genes is indicated at the top of each bar (*p*). NA, not amplified. **(B)** The modulation of expression by *P. brasiliensis* was (20) calculated using the 2−ΔΔCt (fold-change, FC) method comparing stimulated and unstimulated cells (ΔΔCt = ΔCtPb − ΔCtUnstimulated). Data are represented as mean (logFC) ± SE. Student's *t*-test was applied to verify the significance of the FC. When significant, the fold-change of stimulated versus unstimulated cells is indicated at the top of each bar (*p*).

role for these cells in bacterial (32, 33) and fungal infections (8–12, 34). However, to our knowledge, no data are available regarding the role of human pDCs in innate and adaptive immunity against *P. brasiliensis*. Here, we show that human pDCs inhibit the growth of *P. brasiliensis* yeast cells. They also mature and produce cytokines upon stimulation with the yeasts. In addition, we have also demonstrated that dectin-2 and dectin-3 (*via* Syk signaling) are pattern receptors involved in *P. brasiliensis* sensing by human pDCs.

Studies with FITC labeled yeasts showed that about 15% of pDCs interact with yeast cells. As flow cytometric assays can not distinguish between adherent and ingested yeasts we can not guarantee that the yeasts were phagocytosed by the pDCs. However, our further experiments showed that the lymphocytes activation promoted by the pDCs was *P. brasiliensis*-specific indicating that pDCs can phagocytose, process and present fungal antigens to the lymphocytes. In addition, CpG, a TLR-9 agonist, has moderately increased the adhesion/engulfment of *P. brasiliensis* by pDCs. Although TLR-9 is not a phagocytic receptor, it is possible that the activation of pDCs *via* TLR-9 activates the cells and triggers mechanisms that promote the ability of pDCs to recognize the fungus. More importantly, we show in this study that human pDCs control fungal growth. Ramirez-Ortiz et al. (9) were the first authors to describe a non-redundant role for human pDCs during host defense against a human fungal pathogen. Human pDCs spread over *A. fumigatus* hyphae, inhibited their growth and released inflammatory cytokines (9). A recent report has also shown that mouse and human pDCs have cytotoxic activity against the opportunistic fungal pathogen *Cryptococcus neoformans*. The mechanism involves reactive oxygen species activity, which is distinct from that engaged by pDCs to control *A. fumigatus* infections (35).

The recognition of *P. brasiliensis* by human pDCs leads to TNF-α secretion. Although the pDCs were able to produce IL-6 in response to an infection (36), the levels of this cytokine did not increase following *P. brasiliensis* stimulation. The release of TNF-α by human pDCs is in agreement with the previous report regarding *A. fumigatus* hyphae stimulation (9, 10). In addition, in a mouse model of PCM, our group verified that *P. brasiliensis* infection induced BMDCs of resistant A/J mice to generate a population of pDCs that secreted inflammatory cytokines, including TNF-α (8). This was the first evidence that pDCs were involved in the host response to *P. brasiliensis*. We have also demonstrated that mouse pDCs release TNF-α and type I IFNs in response to *P. brasiliensis* yeast cells (34), a finding confirmed in the current study of human pDCs. Although the roles of type I IFN and pDCs are well known in DNA and RNA viral infections (36), their function in fungal infections is poorly defined. Romani et al. did not observed IFN-α secretion by pDCs stimulated by *A. fumigatus* resting conidia (37) but the tissue invasive hyphal morphotype was shown to stimulate human pDCs to release IFN-α (9, 10).

Our previous studies showed that dectin-1 and Syk signaling activate the NLRP3 inflammasome in *P. brasiliensis* stimulated macrophages (16). Furthermore, type I IFNs were shown to induce the expression of inflammasome components such as those of the NLRP3, retinoic acid-inducible gene 1, and AIM2 (38). This was in addition to the up-regulation of caspase-11, an enzyme required for the non-canonical activation of the NLRP3 inflammasome (39). These findings led us to investigate whether pDCs were able to activate the inflammasomes, activate caspase-1 and release IL-1β after *P. brasiliensis* stimulation. Our results showed that pDCs are capable of IL-1β release and caspase-1 activation, indicating that *P. brasiliensis* activates the pDCs inflammasome. This is a finding never described previously with regard to this DC subset during a host–microbe interaction.

Several PRRs, including dectin-1 (15, 17, 40), TLR-2 (13, 40), TLR-4 (14, 15, 40) and TLR-9 (41, 42) have been reported to recognize *P. brasiliensis* components. Human pDCs express several PPRs such as DC immunoreceptor, dectin-2, and siglec-H, but do not express TLR-2, TLR-4, and the CLRs dectin-1, MR, and

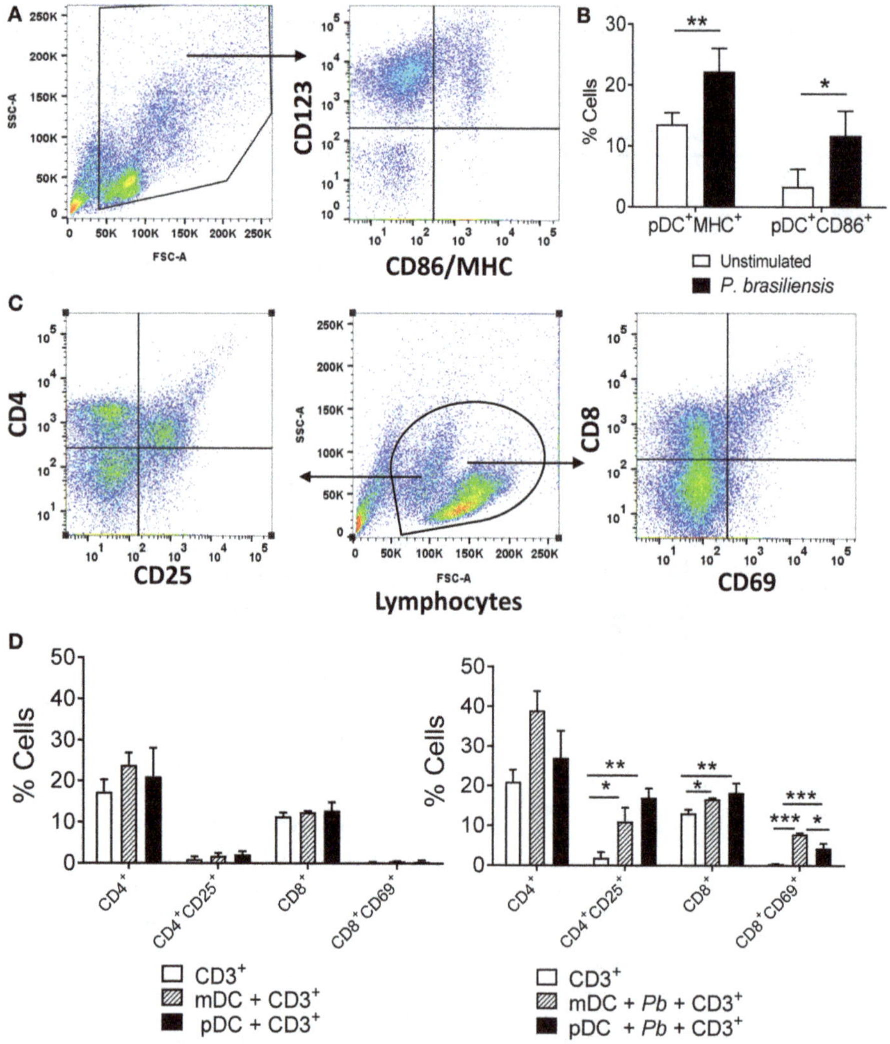

FIGURE 9 | *Paracoccidioides brasiliensis* stimulation induces a mature phenotype in plasmacytoid dendritic cells (pDCs) that become able to promote the activation of $CD4^+$ and $CD8^+$ T lymphocytes. Peripheral blood mononuclear cells (PBMCs) were separated into pDC-positive ($pDCs^+$) and myeloid dendritic cell (mDC)-positive (mDC^+) population using magnetic beads conjugated to anti-CD304 and anti-CD1c antibodies, respectively. **(A,B)** For characterization of pDCs activation, the cells were labeled with appropriate titers of anti-CD123, MHC-class II, and CD86 antibodies and then 50,000 events were acquired in the flow cytometer and gated as indicated in the dot plots **(A)**. As the pDC^+ population was stained with an specific pDC marker (anti-CD123), the characterization of cell maturation was performed by obtaining the pDCs from the PBMCs following one round of positive selection. Data are the means ± SE of the frequency of double-positive cells from three donors, tested in triplicate **(B)**. **(C,D)** For coculture experiments, the pDCs and mDCs (1×10^5/well) were cultured with or without *P. brasiliensis* yeast cells (1×10^4) and after 2 h they were then placed in cocultured with lymphocytes (1×10^6), which were previously obtained from PBMCs of the same donor and separated with anti-CD3 magnetic beads. After 5 days of coculture, the lymphocytes were analyzed by flow cytometry using anti-CD4, CD8, CD25, and anti-CD69 antibodies. The control wells contained only $CD3^+$ cells. The lymphocyte population was gated by FSC/SSC analysis and the gated cells were then analyzed for expression of lymphocyte activation markers **(C)**. Data are the means ± SE of the frequency of single positive ($CD4^+$/$CD8^+$) double-positive cells ($CD4^+CD25^+$ and $CD8^+CD69^+$) from three donors, tested in triplicate in cultures with [**(D)**, right panel] or without *P. brasiliensis* yeast cells [**(D)**, left panel]. $^*p < 0.05$, $^{**}p < 0.01$, $^{***}p < 0.001$ by comparing the data indicated by the bars.

DC-SIGN (43–46). In a previous study, we verified that dectin-2 participates in the interaction of pDC and *A. fumigatus*-hyphae and that this recognition leads to TNF-α and IFN-α release by the pDCs as well as improved antifungal resistance (10). In this study, we have also investigated the role of some PRRs in *P. brasiliensis* recognition by pDCs. Our studies show that TLR-9 does not play a role in the *P. brasiliensis*–pDC interaction. These results are similar to those found during the studies with *A. fumigatus* hyphae in which, the hyphae–pDC interaction was also TLR-9 independent (9). Although TLR-9 was reported as an important PRR in the control of murine PCM (41, 42), our data indicate that TLR-9 expressed by other innate immune cells was possibly responsible for this effect.

The cytoplasmic moieties of CLRs have an immunoreceptor tyrosine-based activation motif. These moieties engage the Syk tyrosine kinase, which transduces signals that activate the transcription factor NF-kB and downstream gene expression. This results in increased phagocytosis and cytokine production by innate immune cells (47). During *C. albicans*-hyphae recognition, dectin-3 forms heterodimers with dectin-2, compared with their respective homodimers, the dectin-3-dectin-2 heterodimers bind α-mannans more effectively, leading to potent inflammatory responses (48). Our results showed the involvement of dectin-2/dectin-3/Syk signaling during *P. brasiliensis* recognition by human pDCs.

As studies regarding the expression of CLRs on human pDC are scarce and sometimes conflicting (49), we have decided to investigate the gene expression for the dectin-1, dectin-2, dectin-3, and mincle receptors on human pDC upon *P. brasiliensis* stimulation. While all genes studied were expressed on human mDCs, only *DECTIN2* and *DECTIN3* were found on human pDCs. Although some studies have demonstrated the expression of dectin-1 on human pDCs (50) the expression of this receptor was not observed in our study. The absent expression of *DECTIN1* and *MINCLE* explained the lack of effect of blocking antibodies during pDC activation by *P. brasiliensis* yeast cells. Importantly, a limitation of our study is that we did not analyze the expression of these receptors on cell membrane of DCs after stimulation with the fungus. However, it is known that the endocytosis of plasma membrane-localized PRRs after a microbial encounter hinders their detection (51, 52). Notably, our findings are in agreement with a previous study of *A. fumigatus* in which fungal hyphae were recognized by human pDCs through dectin-2 rather than dectin-1 or TLR-7/9 (9, 10). Although yeasts of *P. brasiliensis* and *A. fumigutus*-hyphae are composed of different PAMPs (53–56), the involvement of dectin-2 and dectin-3 receptors in triggering pDCs responses following fungal stimulation indicates that these receptors play an important role in the innate immune response to fungal infections. Importantly, dectin-3 has also been shown to participate in the inhibition of *C. neoformans* growth by human and mouse pDCs (35). These previous findings and those reported here highlight the importance of some CLRs (mainly dectin-2 and dectin-3) in the fungal recognition response by human pDCs. However, mincle, another receptor belonging to the dectin-2 family of CLRs (57) was not observed to participate in *P. brasiliensis* sensing by human pDCs even though it is involved in fungal recognition by conventional DCs (44).

Importantly, curdlan (an agonist of dectin-1) was previously shown to induce the production and secretion of mature IL-1β by activating the cytosolic NLRP3 inflammasome and this process requires the phosphorylation of Syk kinase (58, 59). However, as our study indicated that human pDCs do not express dectin-1, it is possible that other CLRs *via* Syk signaling can be used by *P. brasiliensis*-stimulated pDCs to activate the inflammasomes pathway.

Although the fungicidal activity of pDCs observed in this study occurred only at very high concentrations of pDCs relative to the fungus, our results of pDC–yeast interaction and cytokine production brought original clues to elucidate the biological function of human pDCs in the immune response against *P. brasiliensis*. In addition, using the pDC-lymphocyte coculture experiments, we could demonstrate that this cell population can trigger an antigen-specific adaptive immune response. Mittelbrunn et al. were the first to show that mature pDCs form canonical immune synapses that involve the relocation of the microtubule-organizing center, F-actin and protein kinase C to the contact site, in addition to the activation of early signaling molecules in T cells (60). In pulmonary PCM, our group previously demonstrated that mouse pDCs exert an important regulatory function during the host defense process by preferentially expanding regulatory T lymphocytes in a mechanism dependent on the enzyme indolamine 2,3-dioxygenase-1, which confers a tolerogenic profile to pDCs (34). To our knowledge, the current work is in agreement with previous data showing the presence of pDC in cutaneous lesions and in the blood of PCM patients (11, 12), and this is the first study describing the ability of human pDCs to trigger adaptive immune responses in a context of non-viral infectious disease. However, additional studies are necessary to elucidate the patterns of T cell immunity induced by fungi-sensitized pDCs.

In conclusion, our data show for the first time that *P. brasiliensis* activates human pDCs that inhibit fungal growth and secrete pro-inflammatory cytokines such as TNF-α and type I IFNs. Surprisingly, *P. brasiliensis*-stimulated pDCs activate caspase 1 and produce mature IL-1β, possibly *via* inflammasome activation. This phenomenon has not been previously described during pDC engagement by a microorganism. Importantly, dectin-2 and dectin-3 (acting *via* Syk signaling) are PRRs expressed on pDC and are involved in the pDC–*P. brasiliensis* interaction that results in pDCs activation. Therefore, our data support an important role for CLRs in *P. brasiliensis* recognition by pDCs, indicating that this DC subset actively participate in the mechanisms of innate and adaptive immunity against this primary fungal pathogen.

AUTHOR CONTRIBUTIONS

Conceived and designed experiments: NP, ACN, AP, VC, and FL. Contributed with reagent: AP. Performed the experiments: NP, CF, DSL, BS, and FL. Analyzed the data: NP, BS, and FL. Wrote the article: NP, DSL, AP, ACN, VC, and FL.

ACKNOWLEDGMENTS

We are grateful to Eliseu Frank de Araujo and Tânia A. Costa and for invaluable technical assistance.

FUNDING

This project was supported by Fundação de Amparo à Pesquisa do Estado de São Paulo (FAPESP) research grant 2014/04783-2 to FL and 2016/23189-0 to VLGC; FAPESP felowship 2017/00711-5 to NP and 2013/02396-9 to CF. The funders had no role in this study design, data collection and analysis, decision to publish, or preparation of the manuscript.

REFERENCES

1. Kashino SS, Fazioli RA, Cafalli-Favati C, Meloni-Bruneri LH, Vaz CA, Burger E, et al. Resistance to *Paracoccidioides brasiliensis* infection is linked to a preferential Th1 immune response, whereas susceptibility is associated with absence of IFN-gamma production. *J Interferon Cytokine Res* (2000) 20:89–97. doi:10.1089/107999000312766
2. De Castro LF, Ferreira MC, da Silva RM, Blotta MH, Longhi LN, Mamoni RL. Characterization of the immune response in human paracoccidioidomycosis. *J Infect* (2013) 67:470–85. doi:10.1016/j.jinf.2013.07.019
3. Pagliari C, Fernandes ER, Stegun FW, da Silva WL, Seixas Duarte MI, Sotto MN. Paracoccidioidomycosis: cells expressing IL17 and Foxp3 in cutaneous and mucosal lesions. *Microb Pathog* (2011) 50:263–7. doi:10.1016/j.micpath.2010.12.008
4. Banchereau J, Steinman RM. Dendritic cells and the control of immunity. *Nature* (1998) 392:245–52. doi:10.1038/32588
5. Cao W, Liu YJ. Innate immune functions of plasmacytoid dendritic cells. *Curr Opin Immunol* (2007) 19:24–30. doi:10.1016/j.coi.2006.11.004
6. Yu CF, Peng WM, Oldenburg J, Hoch J, Bieber T, Limmer A, et al. Human plasmacytoid dendritic cells support Th17 cell effector function in response to TLR7 ligation. *J Immunol* (2010) 184:1159–67. doi:10.4049/jimmunol.0901706
7. Mouriès J, Moron G, Schlecht G, Escriou N, Dadaglio G, Leclerc C. Plasmacytoid dendritic cells efficiently cross-prime naive T cells in vivo after TLR activation. *Blood* (2008) 112:3713–22. doi:10.1182/blood-2008-03-146290
8. Pina A, de Araujo EF, Felonato M, Loures FV, Feriotti C, Bernardino S, et al. Myeloid dendritic cells (DCs) of mice susceptible to paracoccidioidomycosis suppress T cell responses whereas myeloid and plasmacytoid DCs from resistant mice induce effector and regulatory T cells. *Infect Immun* (2013) 81:1064–77. doi:10.1128/IAI.00736-12
9. Ramirez-Ortiz ZG, Lee CK, Wang JP, Boon L, Specht CA, Levitz SM. A nonredundant role for plasmacytoid dendritic cells in host defense. *Cell Host Microbe* (2011) 9:415–24. doi:10.1016/j.chom.2011.04.007
10. Loures FV, Röhm M, Lee CK, Santos E, Wang JP, Specht CA, et al. Recognition of *Aspergillus fumigatus* hyphae by human plasmacytoid dendritic cells is mediated by dectin-2 and results in formation of extracellular traps. *PLoS Pathog* (2015) 11:e1004643. doi:10.1371/journal.ppat.1004643
11. Pagliari C, Kanashiro-Galo L, Silva AA, Barboza TC, Criado PR, Duarte MI, et al. Plasmacytoid dendritic cells in cutaneous lesions of patients with chromoblastomycosis, lacaziosis, and paracoccidioidomycosis: a comparative analysis. *Med Mycol* (2014) 52:397–402. doi:10.1093/mmy/myt026
12. Venturini J, Cavalcante RS, Moris DV, Golim MA, Levorato AD, Reis KHD, et al. Altered distribution of peripheral blood dendritic cell subsets in patients with pulmonary paracoccidioidomycosis. *Acta Trop* (2017) 173:185–90. doi:10.1016/j.actatropica.2017.06.007
13. Loures FV, Pina A, Felonato M, Calich VL. TLR2 is a negative regulator of Th17 cells and tissue pathology in a pulmonary model of fungal infection. *J Immunol* (2009) 183:1279–90. doi:10.4049/jimmunol.0801599
14. Loures FV, Pina A, Felonato M, de Araújo EF, Leite KR, Calich VL. Toll-like receptor 4 signaling leads to severe fungal infection associated with enhanced proinflammatory immunity and impaired expansion of regulatory T cells. *Infect Immun* (2010) 78:1078–88. doi:10.1128/IAI.01198-09
15. Loures FV, Araújo EF, Feriotti C, Bazan SB, Calich VL. TLR-4 cooperates with dectin-1 and mannose receptor to expand Th17 and Tc17 cells induced by *Paracoccidioides brasiliensis* stimulated dendritic cells. *Front Microbiol* (2015) 6:261. doi:10.3389/fmicb.2015.00261
16. Feriotti C, Bazan SB, Loures FV, Araújo EF, Costa TA, Calich VL. Expression of dectin-1 and enhanced activation of NALP3 inflammasome are associated with resistance to paracoccidioidomycosis. *Front Microbiol* (2015) 6:913. doi:10.3389/fmicb.2015.00913
17. Loures FV, Araújo EF, Feriotti C, Bazan SB, Costa TA, Brown GD, et al. Dectin-1 induces M1 macrophages and prominent expansion of CD8+IL-17+ cells in pulmonary paracoccidioidomycosis. *J Infect Dis* (2014) 210:762–73. doi:10.1093/infdis/jiu136
18. Ribeiro LR, Loures FV, de Araújo EF, Feriotti C, Costa TA, Serezani CH, et al. Lipoxin inhibits fungal uptake by macrophages and reduces the severity of acute pulmonary infection caused by *Paracoccidioides brasiliensis*. *Mediators Inflamm* (2015) 2015:852574. doi:10.1155/2015/852574
19. Singers-Vermes LM, Ciavaglia MC, Kashino SS, Burguer E, Calich VL. The source of the growth-promoting factor(s) affects the plating efficiency of *Paracoccidioides brasiliensis*. *J Med Vet Mycol* (1992) 30:261–4. doi:10.1080/02681219280000331
20. Schmittgen TD, Livak KJ. Analyzing real-time PCR data by the comparative C(T) method. *Nat Protoc* (2008) 3:1101–8. doi:10.1038/nprot.2008.73
21. Gilliet M, Cao W, Liu YJ. Plasmacytoid dendritic cells: sensing nucleic acids in viral infection and autoimmune diseases. *Nat Rev Immunol* (2008) 8:594–606. doi:10.1038/nri2358
22. Pietras EM, Saha SK, Cheng G. The interferon response to bacterial and viral infections. *J Endotoxin Res* (2006) 12:246–50. doi:10.1179/096805106X118799
23. van de Veerdonk FL, Joosten LA, Netea MG. The interplay between inflammasome activation and antifungal host defense. *Immunol Rev* (2015) 265:172–80. doi:10.1111/imr.12280
24. Broz P, Dixit VM. Inflammasomes: mechanism of assembly, regulation and signalling. *Nat Rev Immunol* (2016) 16:407–20. doi:10.1038/nri.2016.58
25. Adinolfi E, Lisa Giuliani A, De Marchi E, Pegoraro A, Orioli E, Di Virgilio F. The P2X7 receptor: a main player in inflammation. *Biochem Pharmacol* (2017) 17:30733–5. doi:10.1016/j.bcp.2017.12.021
26. Feriotti C, de Araújo EF, Loures FV, da Costa TA, Galdino NAL, Zamboni DS, et al. NOD-like receptor P3 inflammasome controls protective Th1/Th17 immunity against pulmonary paracoccidioidomycosis. *Front Immunol* (2017) 8:786. doi:10.3389/fimmu.2017.00786
27. Rutz M, Metzger J, Gellert T, Luppa P, Lipford GB, Wagner H, et al. Toll-like receptor 9 binds single-stranded CpG-DNA in a sequence- and pH-dependent manner. *Eur J Immunol* (2004) 34:2541–50. doi:10.1002/eji.200425218
28. Krieg AM, Wu T, Weeratna R, Efler SM, Love-Homan L, Yang L, et al. Sequence motifs in adenoviral DNA block immune activation by stimulatory CpG motifs. *Proc Natl Acad Sci U S A* (1998) 95:12631–6. doi:10.1073/pnas.95.21.12631
29. Willment JA, Brown GD. C-type lectin receptors in antifungal immunity. *Trends Microbiol* (2008) 16:27–32. doi:10.1016/j.tim.2007.10.012
30. Drummond RA, Brown GD. Signalling C-type lectins in antimicrobial immunity. *PLoS Pathog* (2013) 9:e1003417. doi:10.1371/journal.ppat.1003417
31. Ostrop J, Jozefowski K, Zimmermann S, Hofmann K, Strasser E, Lepenies B, et al. Contribution of MINCLE-SYK signaling to activation of primary human APCs by mycobacterial cord factor and the novel adjuvant TDB. *J Immunol* (2015) 195:2417–28. doi:10.4049/jimmunol.1500102
32. Parcina M, Miranda-Garcia MA, Durlanik S, Ziegler S, Over B, Georg P, et al. Pathogen-triggered activation of plasmacytoid dendritic cells induces IL-10-producing B cells in response to *Staphylococcus aureus*. *J Immunol* (2013) 190:1591–602. doi:10.4049/jimmunol.1201222
33. Wu V, Smith AA, You H, Nguyen TA, Ferguson R, Taylor M, et al. Plasmacytoid dendritic cell-derived IFNα modulates Th17 differentiation during early *Bordetella pertussis* infection in mice. *Mucosal Immunol* (2016) 9:777–86. doi:10.1038/mi.2015.101
34. Araújo EF, Medeiros DH, Galdino NA, Condino-Neto A, Calich VL, Loures FV. Tolerogenic plasmacytoid dendritic cells control *Paracoccidioides brasiliensis* infection by inducting regulatory T cells in an IDO-dependent manner. *PLoS Pathog* (2016) 12:e1006115. doi:10.1371/journal.ppat.1006115
35. Hole CR, Leopold Wager CM, Mendiola AS, Wozniak KL, Campuzano A, Lin X, et al. Antifungal activity of plasmacytoid dendritic cells against *Cryptococcus neoformans* in vitro requires expression of dectin-3 (CLEC4D) and reactive oxygen species. *Infect Immun* (2016) 84:2493–504. doi:10.1128/IAI.00103-16
36. Lederle A, Su B, Holl V, Penichon J, Schmidt S, Decoville T, et al. Neutralizing antibodies inhibit HIV-1 infection of plasmacytoid dendritic cells by an FcγRIIa independent mechanism and do not diminish cytokines production. *Sci Rep* (2014) 4:5845. doi:10.1038/srep05845
37. Romani L, Bistoni F, Gaziano R, Bozza S, Montagnoli C, Perruccio K, et al. Thymosin alpha 1 activates dendritic cells for antifungal Th1 resistance through toll-like receptor signaling. *Blood* (2004) 103:4232–9. doi:10.1182/blood-2003-11-4036
38. Malireddi RK, Kanneganti TD. Role of type I interferons in inflammasome activation, cell death, and disease during microbial infection. *Front Cell Infect Microbiol* (2013) 3:77. doi:10.3389/fcimb.2013.00077
39. Case CL, Kohler LJ, Lima JB, Strowig T, de Zoete MR, Flavell RA, et al. Caspase-11 stimulates rapid flagellin-independent pyroptosis in response to *Legionella pneumophila*. *Proc Natl Acad Sci U S A* (2013) 110:5851–6. doi:10.1073/pnas.1211521110
40. Bonfim CV, Mamoni RL, Blotta MH. TLR-2, TLR-4 and dectin-1 expression in human monocytes and neutrophils stimulated by *Paracoccidioides brasiliensis*. *Med Mycol* (2009) 47:722–33. doi:10.3109/13693780802641425

41. Menino JF, Saraiva M, Gomes-Alves AG, Lobo-Silva D, Sturme M, Gomes-Rezende J, et al. TLR-9 activation dampens the early inflammatory response to *Paracoccidioides brasiliensis*, impacting host survival. *PLoS Negl Trop Dis* (2013) 7:e2317. doi:10.1371/journal.pntd.0002317
42. Morais EA, Chame DF, Melo EM, de Carvalho Oliveira JA, de Paula AC, Peixoto AC, et al. TLR 9 involvement in early protection induced by immunization with rPb27 against paracoccidioidomycosis. *Microbes Infect* (2016) 18:137–47. doi:10.1016/j.micinf.2015.10.005
43. Lande R, Gilliet M. Plasmacytoid dendritic cells: key players in the initiation and regulation of immune responses. *Ann N Y Acad Sci* (2010) 1183:89–103. doi:10.1111/j.1749-6632.2009.05152.x
44. Graham LM, Brown GD. The dectin-2 family of C-type lectins in immunity and homeostasis. *Cytokine* (2009) 48:148–55. doi:10.1016/j.cyto.2009.07.010
45. Meyer-Wentrup F, Benitez-Ribas D, Tacken PJ, Punt CJ, Figdor CG, de Vries IJ, et al. Targeting DCIR on human plasmacytoid dendritic cells results in antigen presentation and inhibits IFN-alpha production. *Blood* (2008) 111:4245–53. doi:10.1182/blood-2007-03-081398
46. Gavino AC, Chung JS, Sato K, Ariizumi K, Cruz PD Jr. Identification and expression profiling of a human C-type lectin, structurally homologous to mouse dectin-2. *Exp Dermatol* (2005) 14:281–8. doi:10.1111/j.0906-6705.2005.00312.x
47. Kerscher B, Willment JA, Brown GD. The dectin-2 family of C-type lectin-like receptors: an update. *Int Immunol* (2013) 25:271–7. doi:10.1093/intimm/dxt006
48. Zhu LL, Zhao XQ, Jiang C, You Y, Chen XP, Jiang YY, et al. C-type lectin receptors dectin-3 and dectin-2 form a heterodimeric patternrecognition receptor for host defense against fungal infection. *Immunity* (2013) 39:324–34. doi:10.1016/j.immuni.2013.05.017
49. Maldonado S, Fitzgerald-Bocarsly P. Antifungal activity of plasmacytoid dendritic cells and the impact of chronic HIV infection. *Front Immunol* (2017) 8:1705. doi:10.3389/fimmu.2017.01705
50. Joo H, Upchurch K, Zhang W, Ni L, Li D, Xue Y, et al. Opposing roles of dectin-1 expressed on human plasmacytoid dendritic cells and myeloid dendritic cells in Th2 polarization. *J Immunol* (2015) 195:1723–31. doi:10.4049/jimmunol.1402276
51. Zanoni I, Ostuni R, Marek LR, Barresi S, Barbalat R, Barton GM, et al. CD14 controls the LPS-induced endocytosis of toll-like receptor 4. *Cell* (2011) 147:868–80. doi:10.1016/j.cell.2011.09.051
52. Jiang W, Swiggard WJ, Heufler C, Peng M, Mirza A, Steinman RM, et al. The receptor DEC-205 expressed by dendritic cells and thymic epithelial cells is involved in antigen processing. *Nature* (1995) 375:151–5. doi:10.1038/375151a0
53. Latge JP, Beauvais A. Functional duality of the cell wall. *Curr Opin Microbiol* (2014) 20:111–7. doi:10.1016/j.mib.2014.05.009
54. Tomazett PK, Cruz AH, Bonfim SM, Soares CM, Pereira M. The cell wall of *Paracoccidioides brasiliensis*: insights from its transcriptome. *Genet Mol Res* (2005) 4:309–25.
55. Puccia R, Vallejo MC, Matsuo AL, Longo LV. The *Paracoccidioides* cell wall: past and present layers toward understanding interaction with the host. *Front Microbiol* (2011) 2:257. doi:10.3389/fmicb.2011.00257
56. de Oliveira HC, Assato PA, Marcos CM, Scorzoni L, de Paula E Silva AC, Da Silva Jde L, et al. *Paracoccidioides*-host interaction: an overview on recent advances in the paracoccidioidomycosis. *Front Microbiol* (2015) 6:1319. doi:10.3389/fmicb.2015.01319
57. Ishikawa T, Itoh F, Yoshida S, Saijo S, Matsuzawa T, Gonoi T, et al. Identification of distinct ligands for the C-type lectin receptors mincle and dectin-2 in the pathogenic fungus *Malassezia*. *Cell Host Microbe* (2013) 13:477–88. doi:10.1016/j.chom.2013.03.008
58. Kankkunen P, Teirilä L, Rintahaka J, Alenius H, Wolff H, Maitikainen S. (1,3)-beta-glucans activate both dectin-1 and NLRP3 inflammasome in human macrophages. *J Immunol* (2010) 184:6335–42. doi:10.4049/jimmunol.0903019
59. Gross O, Poeck H, Bscheider M, Dostert C, Hannesschläger N, Endres S, et al. Syk kinase signaling couples to the Nlrp3 inflammasome for anti-fungal host defense. *Nature* (2009) 459:433–6. doi:10.1038/nature07965
60. Mittelbrunn M, Martínez del Hoyo G, López-Bravo M, Martín-Cofreces NB, Scholer A, Hugues S, et al. Imaging of plasmacytoid dendritic cell interactions with T cells. *Blood* (2009) 113:75–84. doi:10.1182/blood-2008-02-139865

7

Natural Killer Cells in Antifungal Immunity

Stanislaw Schmidt, Lars Tramsen and Thomas Lehrnbecher*

Division for Pediatric Hematology and Oncology, Hospital for Children and Adolescents, Johann Wolfgang Goethe-University, Frankfurt, Germany

***Correspondence:**
Thomas Lehrnbecher
thomas.lehrnbecher@kgu.de

Invasive fungal infections are still an important cause of morbidity and mortality in immunocompromised patients such as patients suffering from hematological malignancies or patients undergoing hematopoietic stem cell transplantion. In addition, other populations such as human immunodeficiency virus-patients are at higher risk for invasive fungal infection. Despite the availability of new antifungal compounds and better supportive care measures, the fatality rate of invasive fungal infection remained unacceptably high. It is therefore of major interest to improve our understanding of the host–pathogen interaction to develop new therapeutic approaches such as adoptive immunotherapy. As experimental methodologies have improved and we now better understand the complex network of the immune system, the insight in the interaction of the host with the fungus has significantly increased. It has become clear that host resistance to fungal infections is not only associated with strong innate immunity but that adaptive immunity (e.g., T cells) also plays an important role. The antifungal activity of natural killer (NK) cells has been underestimated for a long time. *In vitro* studies demonstrated that NK cells from murine and human origin are able to attack fungi of different genera and species. NK cells exhibit not only a direct antifungal activity *via* cytotoxic molecules but also an indirect antifungal activity *via* cytokines. However, it has been show that fungi exert immunosuppressive effects on NK cells. Whereas clinical data are scarce, animal models have clearly demonstrated that NK cells play an important role in the host response against invasive fungal infections. In this review, we summarize clinical data as well as results from *in vitro* and animal studies on the impact of NK cells on fungal pathogens.

Keywords: natural killer cell, invasive fungal infection, *Aspergillus*, *Candida*, mucormycete, *Cryptococcus*, antifungal host response

INTRODUCTION

Invasive fungal infections are still associated with significant morbidity and mortality. For example, a retrospective cohort study in the US demonstrated that as compared to patients without

---

Abbreviations: ADCC, antibody-dependent cell-mediated cytotoxicity; CD, cluster of differentiation; SRIR, self-recognizing inhibitory receptors; EBV, Epstein–Barr virus; CMV, cytomegalovirus; ALL, acute lymphoblastic leukemia; AML, acute myeloid leukemia; IFN, interferon; ILC, innate lymphoid cell; DCs, dendritic cells; RANTES, regulated upon activation, normal T-cell expressed, and secreted; CCL5, chemokine ligand 5; GM-CSF, granulocyte-macrophage colony-stimulating factor; TNF-α, tumor necrosis factor alpha; HSCT, hematopoietic stem cell transplantation; ROS, reactive oxygen species; CMCC, chronic mucocutaneous candidiasis; SLE, systemic lupus erythematosus; HIV, human immunodeficiency virus; IL, interleukin; TRAIL, tumor necrosis factor related apoptosis inducing ligand; IgG, immunoglobulin G; NADPH, nicotinamide adenine dinucleotide phosphate; Hsp, heat shock protein; NCR, natural cytotoxicity receptors; Gr-MDSC, granulocyte myeloid-derived suppressor cell; ITAM, immunoreceptor tyrosine-based activation motif.

invasive aspergillosis, patients suffering from the infection had a significant longer hospital stay, caused significantly higher costs, and, most importantly, had a significant higher mortality (1). A population-based analysis of invasive fungal infections in France revealed that between 2001 and 2010, the incidence of invasive fungal disease due to *Candida* spp., *Aspergillus* spp., and mucormycetes increased by 7.8, 4.4, and 7.3% per year, respectively, which was highly significant for each pathogen (2). In contrast to cryptococcosis, which often occurs in human immunodeficiency virus (HIV)-patients, the population at high risk for candidemia, invasive aspergillosis, and mucormycosis includes in particular patients with hematological malignancies, patients undergoing hematopoietic stem cell transplantation (HSCT) and solid organ recipients (2–6). These patient populations are characterized by the impairment of multiple arms of the immune system (7, 8), such as of natural barriers, the phagocyte system, innate immunity, and lymphocytes, all of which may increase the risk for an invasive fungal infection. Therefore, it is not surprising that the mortality rate of invasive fungal disease is extremely high in these patient populations, exceeding 70% in HSCT recipients suffering from invasive aspergillosis or mucormycosis (4).

It is well known that the recovery of the immune system has a major impact on the outcome of invasive fungal infection in an immunocompromised patient (9, 10). Unfortunately, to date, immunomodulation using cytokine and growth factor therapies, as well as adoptive immunotherapeutic strategies such as granulocyte transfusions or the administration of *Aspergillus*-specific T-cells did not significantly improve the prognosis of immunocompromised patients with invasive fungal disease (11). It is therefore of major interest to improve our understanding of the host–pathogen interaction to develop new therapeutic strategies for immunocompromised individuals suffering from fungal infection. This review will summarize available clinical data as well as results from *in vitro* and animal studies on the impact of natural killer (NK) cells on fungal pathogens.

THE HOST RESPONSE TO FUNGAL INFECTION

Over the last decades, we could witness major advances not only in the understanding of the complexity of the immune system but also in our knowledge on the immunopathogenesis of invasive fungal infections. The host response to a fungal pathogen includes, but is not restricted to various cells of the innate and adaptive immunity such as monocytes, neutrophils, dendritic cells (DCs), T and B lymphocytes, as well as multiple soluble molecules such as collectins, defensins, cytokines including interferons (IFNs) (12, 13). Although it is known for a long time that severe and prolonged neutropenia (e.g., absolute neutrophil count $\leq 500/\mu l$ and duration of neutropenia ≥ 10 days) is the single most important risk factor for invasive aspergillosis, invasive *Candida* infection, and mucormycosis in patients receiving cytotoxic chemotherapy or undergoing allogeneic HSCT (9, 14), recent studies refined our understanding how neutrophils are controlling in particular the early stages of invasive fungal infection. Neutrophils are attracted by cytokines released by endothelial cells and macrophages and are able to quickly migrate to a focus of infection. In addition to recruiting and activating other immune cells by the production of pro-inflammatory cytokines, neutrophils may attack as front-line defense invading pathogens by phagocytosis, the production of reactive oxygen intermediates, and the release antimicrobial enzymes to the formation of complex extracellular traps (NETs) that help in the elimination of the fungus (15). DCs transport fungal antigens to the draining lymph nodes, where they orchestrate T cell activation and differentiation (16). A number of lymphocyte subsets have an important impact in the antifungal immunity, such as Th1 cells (important for inflammation and fungal clearance), Th17 cells (neutrophil recruitment, defensins), Th22 cells (defensins, tissue homeostasis), and Treg cells (immunosuppression). In addition, a number of cytokines play important roles in the complex crosstalk between different cells of the immune system, which modify and regulate innate and adaptive immune responses, such as the induction of proliferation and differentiation, as well as the activation or suppression of different target cells (11–13). Still, many open questions have to be resolved, including the influence of the genetic background in the delicate interplay of immune cells, the interaction of the innate and adaptive immune system in balancing protection and immunopathology in fungal infections (12), and the influence of fungal microbiota or "mycobiota" on health and disease (17). More importantly, we have to learn how to modify the immune system in the combat against invasive fungal infections, in particular in the immunocompromised host, which includes not only the activation of the immune response to eliminate the pathogen but also its suppression to avoid collateral tissue damage.

NK CELL BIOLOGY

Human NK cells, which originate from the bone marrow, represent up to 15% of peripheral blood mononuclear cells. They are characterized by the expression of CD56 and by the absence of the T cell marker CD3. According to the surface expression density of CD56 and CD16, NK cells can be subdivided in two main subpopulations, namely the cytotoxic $CD56^{dim}CD16^{bright}$ and the immune regulatory $CD56^{bright}CD16^{dim}$ subsets (18). Although NK cells were originally considered as cells of innate immunity, they demonstrate qualities of the adaptive immunity such as immunological memory (19–22). In this regard, animal models and human studies indicate that NK cells are able to develop long-lasting antigen-specific memory (23–26). It has been demonstrated that memory-like NK cells display a less differentiated phenotype in $CD56^{dim}$ NK cells, which were $CD94^{+}NKG2A^{+}$ but $CD57^{-}KIR^{-}$ (27). The name "natural killer cell" originally came from their ability to kill tumor cells *in vitro* and *in vivo* without previous stimulation (22, 28–31). Their antitumor activity includes activity against acute lymphoblastic leukemia (32), acute myeloid leukemia (33), and neuroblastoma (34, 35). In addition to their antitumor activity, NK cells play an important role in the host response against various pathogens which includes viruses such as cytomegalovirus (CMV), Epstein–Barr virus (23, 36–38), or hepatitis B and C virus (37, 39, 40), and Gram-positive, Gram-negative, and intracellular bacteria, such as *Salmonella typhi*, *Escherichia coli* (41), or *Listeria monocytogenes* (42).

Natural killer cells eliminate their potential targets either by directly using cytotoxic molecules such as perforin or granzyme B, which are stored in granules, or by death receptor-mediated apoptosis (36). In addition, CD16 (FcγRIII) triggers antibody-dependent cell-mediated cytotoxicity on opsonized target cells (36). Education and differentiation are considered to be important mechanisms for both direct and antibody-dependent functionality of NK cells (43–45). Several models have been developed to explain the process of "education" (43, 45–49). In general, the expression of self-recognizing inhibitory receptors (SRIR) results in the development of NK cells toward fully functional mature form, which has been termed as "licensing" process (50). In contrast, the "disarming" model describes NK cells lacking SRIR that become anergic due to chronic activation (51). The more dynamic "rheostat model" has been used to describe that stronger inhibitory signaling through more SRIR interactions results in a greater functional responsiveness of NK cells (52, 53). Importantly, cytokine stimulation can prime SRIR-deficient NK cells to a functional state (50), and uneducated cells are also able to combat viral infections, as SRIR-deficient NK cells strongly respond toward murine CMV (54).

In addition to the direct cytotoxic abilities, NK cells have recently been classified closely to group 1 innate lymphoid cells, which are characterized by the production of IFN-γ, whereas type 2 cytokines are not produced (55). *Via* the release of chemokines and cytokines such as IFN-γ, tumor necrosis factor alpha (TNF-α), granulocyte-macrophage colony-stimulating factor (GM-CSF), or chemokine ligand 5 (CCL5) [regulated upon activation, normal T-cell expressed, and secreted (RANTES)], NK cells modulate the activity of various immune cells including neutrophils, DCs, and T cells (46, 56), which complements their direct anti-pathogen and antibody-mediated activities.

NK CELLS AND INVASIVE FUNGAL INFECTION: CLINICAL OBSERVATIONS

Although clinical data suggest the importance of NK cells in the risk and outcome of invasive fungal infection, the exact role of NK cells is difficult to determine as multiple cells are involved in the antifungal host response, and as these cells interact in a complex network with both positive and negative feedback mechanisms (7, 8). A recent study analyzed 51 patients undergoing allogeneic HSCT, among them 9 patients in whom proven or probable invasive aspergillosis occurred (10). The study evaluated both the quantitative and qualitative reconstitution of immune cells including polymorphonuclear cells, $CD4^+$ T cells, $CD8^+$ T cells, and NK cells, and the authors reported two important observations: first, transplant recipients suffering from invasive aspergillosis displayed insufficient NK cell recovery with cell counts remaining less than 200/µl as well as lower reactive oxygen species (ROS) production. Second, HSCT transplant recipients who were cured from invasive aspergillosis had significantly higher ROS production and higher NK cell counts as compared to those patients who had a poor outcome of the invasive fungal infection. As both cell count and ROS production were altered in each of the analyses, the importance of the NK cell count as single risk and single prognostic factor for invasive aspergillosis remains unresolved. Another study evaluated 396 patients undergoing solid organ transplantation (57). A total of 304 patients were kidney and 92 patients were liver transplant recipients, and median followed-up time was 504.5 days after transplantation. The analysis demonstrated that 1 month after transplantation, patients who did not develop invasive fungal disease at a later time point had significantly higher mean NK cell count as compared with those patients who developed fungal disease. In the non-transplant setting, larger clinical studies on the impact of NK cell-mediated immunity on fungal infections are lacking. Although it was observed that patients suffering from chronic mucocutaneous candidiasis (CMCC) have a decrease of both NK cell number and cytotoxic activity (58–60), the exact impact of NK cells in the pathogenesis of the infection or in the progression of the disease is hard to define, in particular as cell-mediated immunity is also impaired in patients with CMCC. Although it may very well be that the pathologic NK cell findings are a risk factor for CMCC, other possible explanations for the decreased NK cell count and NK cell activity include that the fungus had a negative impact on originally normal NK cells, or that the observation is an epiphenomenon only. Similarly, it was reported that a patient developed a *Trichophyton rubrum* infection during corticosteroid treatment for systemic lupus erythematosus (61). Although immunosuppressive therapy was stopped, the infection remained. Further evaluation demonstrated that both numbers and activity of NK cells were reduced. The authors speculated that the impairment of the NK cells was causing the infection, but again, one could also argue that the infection resulted in a decreased NK cell number and NK cell activity in this individual patient.

NK CELLS DAMAGE VARIOUS FUNGI *IN VITRO*

Multiple studies published over the last three decades demonstrate that both murine and human NK cells exhibit antifungal activity *in vitro* against various fungal pathogens, such as *Aspergillus fumigatus*, *Aspergillus niger*, *Candida albicans*, *Cryptococcus neoformans*, *Paracoccidioides brasiliensis*, *Rhizopus oryzae*, and other mucormycetes including *Lichthemia ramosa* or *Absidia corymbifera* (62–70) (**Figure 1**). NK cells damage the hyphal form of *A. fumigatus* and *R. oryzae*, but are not able to exhibit fungicidal activity toward conidia (62, 63, 65). In *C. albicans*, human NK cell are cytotoxic against germ tubes and additionally are able to phagocyte *C. albicans* yeasts (8 ± 0.5% of *C. albicans* yeasts were phagocytosed by NK cells within the first 2 h of interaction) (70). The lack of antifungal activity against conidia may be explained by the fact that conidia are often protected by capsules, by pigments such as melanin, or by hydrophobic layers, all of which may prevent recognition by various immune cells (71–74). For example, the rodlet/hydrophobin layer on dormant *A. fumigatus* conidia masks the recognition by the immune system and thus prevents an host immune response, whereas the genetical removal the rodlet/hydrophobin layer in dormant conidia of the *ΔrodA* mutant resulted in the induction of maturation and activation of human

DCs (71). Similarly, the lack of a capsule in the strain CAP67 of the yeast-like fungus *C. neoformans* leads to a higher expression of the cytotoxic molecule perforin by NK cells as compared to the encapsulated strain B3501 (75).

RECOGNITION OF FUNGI BY NK CELLS

Over the last years, there were major advances in the identification and characterization of receptors by which NK cells recognize fungal pathogens (**Figure 1**, **Table 1**). NK cells express unique activating receptors on their surface, which are called natural cytotoxicity receptors (NCR) 1–3 (NKp46, NKp44, and NKp30; CD335–CD337). Studies using blocking antibodies and siRNA to knockdown the NKp30 expression on the surface of the cell line YT demonstrated that NK cells are able to directly recognize *C. albicans* and *C. neoformans* by the NKp30 receptor, which further mediates killing of these fungi (68). However, polymorphonuclear neutrophils and granulocyte myeloid-derived suppressor cells may decrease the NKp30 expression on NK cells, which results in reduced cytotoxicity toward *A. fumigatus* and a

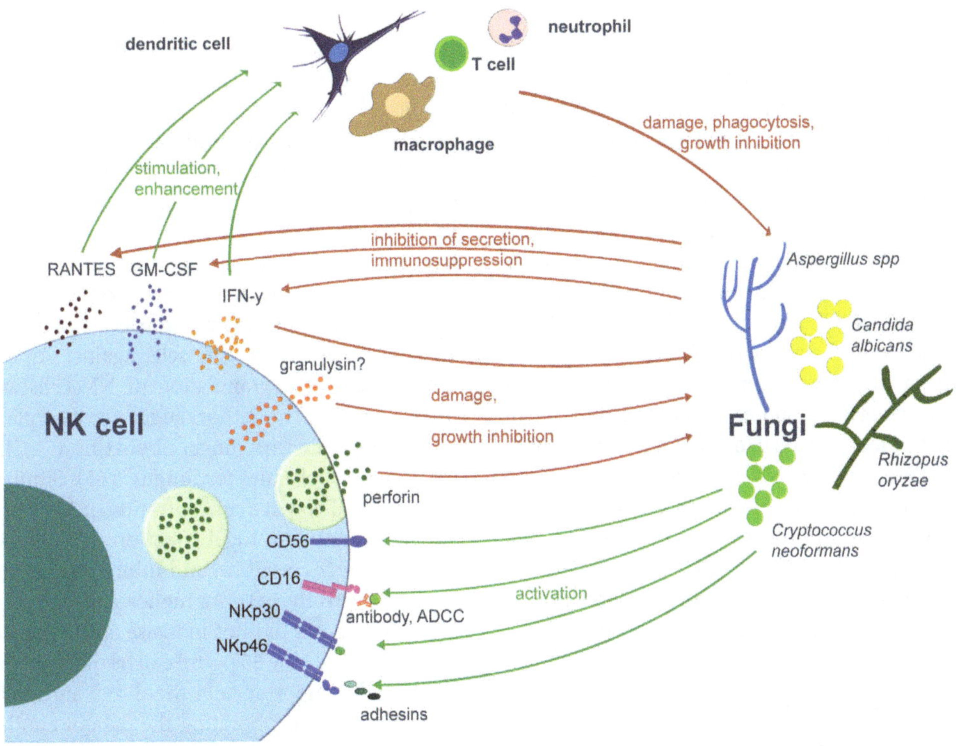

FIGURE 1 | Interplay of NK cells and fungal pathogens. Various fungal pathogens are able to activate NK cells. Once activated, NK cells directly damage fungi by cytotoxic molecules such as perforin or release cytokines, by which they modulate the antifungal host response *via* various immune cells. On the other hand, the fungus may compromise the host immune system. Green arrows indicate activation/stimulation, red arrows inhibition/damage. ADCC, antibody-dependent cell mediated cytotoxicity; IFN, interferon; GM-CSF, granulocyte-macrophage colony-stimulating factor; NK, natural killer.

TABLE 1 | Natural killer (NK) cell receptors in antifungal response.

Receptor	Origin	Ligand	Fungus	Remarks	Reference
NKp30	Human, YT cell line	Undefined pathogen-associated molecular pattern	*Candida albicans*, *Cryprococcus neoformans*	NKp30 required for YT cell cytotoxicity toward fungal pathogens *in vitro* siRNA knockdown of NKp30 results in decreased release of perforin Addition of anti-NKp30 antibody or inhibition of NKp30 via siRNA results in decreased antifungal activity	Li et al. (68)
NKp46 NCR1	Human Mouse	Fungal adhesins Epa1, Epa6, Epa7	*Candida glabrata*	Human NKp46 and mouse ortholog NCR1 bind *C. glabrata in vitro* Clearing of systemic *C. glabrata* infection *in vivo* depends on recognition of fungal adhesins by NCR1	Vitenshtein et al. (77)
CD56	Human	Unknown	*Aspergillus fumigatus*	Blocking of CD56 by inhibitory antibodies reduces fungal-mediated NK cell activation and inhibits amount of secreted cytokines *in vitro*	Ziegler et al. (80)
CD16	Mouse	Cryptococcal polysaccharide	*Cryptococcus neoformans*	Purified IgG fraction of rabbit anticryptococcal antibody augments growth inhibitory activity of murine splenic NK cells *in vitro*	Nabavi and Murphy (81)

decrease in IFN-γ secretion (76). Recently, the NKp46 receptor and its mouse ortolog NCR1 were identified to play an important role in the NK cell-mediated killing of *C. glabrata* (77). It was speculated whether NKp46/NCR1 may be a novel type of pattern recognition receptor, as these receptors not only recognize the *C. glabrata* adhesins Epa1, Epa6, and Epa7 but also bind viral adhesion receptors (77). The importance of the receptor is underlined by the observation that NCR1-deficient mice were unable to clear *C. glabrata* systemic infection (77). Because several fungi including *Aspergillus*, *Cryptococcus*, and *Coccidioides* express adhesins (78), further studies have to evaluate whether and to what extent these fungal adhesins are recognized by which of the NK cell receptors (79).

Recent studies suggested CD56 as pathogen recognition receptor, as it was demonstrated by flow cytometry that the fluorescence positivity of the surface receptor significantly decreased upon fungal contact (80). The authors could visualize the direct interaction of NK cells and *A. fumigatus via* CD56, which was reorganized and accumulated at this interaction site time dependently. Importantly, blocking of CD56 surface receptor reduced fungal-mediated NK cell activation and reduced cytokine secretion. Earlier studies have demonstrated that the low-affinity Fc-receptor CD16 [FcγRIIIa (CD16a) and FcγRIIIb (CD16b)] is also involved in the antifungal activity of NK cells, as NK cells inhibited the growth of *Cryptococci* more effectively in the presence of anti-cryptococcal IgG antibodies than in the presence of normal rabbit serum or medium (81). However, it is important to note that primary and pre-activated NK cells downregulate CD16 after contact with *C. albicans*, which has also been described for the cellular adhesin CD56 and immunoreceptor tyrosine-based activation motif-bearing receptors NKG2D (CD314) and NKp46 (CD335) (70). Taken together, we just begin to understand the complexity how NK cells are being activated by fungal pathogens.

DIRECT DAMAGE OF FUNGAL PATHOGENS BY NK CELLS

Various mechanisms are described by which NK cells directly kill tumor cells, which include the release of soluble cytotoxic molecules such as perforin or granzyme, or the induction of apoptosis by the Fas–FasL or the TNF pathway. Regarding fungal pathogens, several studies reported on the importance of lytic granules released by NK cells. For example, the use of monensin, which inhibits granule secretion, partially abrogated the growth inhibition of *C. neoformans* by human NK cells [reviewed in Ref. (79)]. It further became clear that mainly perforin and granulysin mediate the direct NK cell cytotoxicity toward fungal pathogens (67, 82). When pretreating human NK cells with concanamycin A (ConA), which induces accelerated perforin degradation *via* an increase of pH in the lytic granules, significantly less damage of *A. fumigatus* and *R. oryzae* hyphae can be observed as compared to the addition of untreated NK cells to the fungus (62, 63, 83). Other studies used purified perforin and reported on fungal damage of *A. fumigatus* hyphae (62), the inhibition of filamentation of *C. albicans* (84), and the inhibition of the metabolic activity of *C. albicans* and *R. oryzae* in a dose-dependent manner (63, 70). The fact that ConA did not totally abrogate NK cell-mediated fungal damage suggests that other molecules than perforin also participate in the antifungal activity of human NK cells, as reported for *A. fumigatus*, *C. albicans*, and *R. oryzae*. Interestingly, inhibition of perforin by ConA or by small interfering RNA decreased NK cell anti-cryptococcal activity, whereas inhibition of granulysin did not alter the antifungal effect (67). However, it has been shown that the defective anti-cryptococcal activity of NK cells from HIV-patients can be corrected by *ex vivo* treatment with interleukin (IL)-12 (68), as IL-12 restores the lower perforin expression in NK cells from HIV-infected patients as well as the defective granule polarization in response to *C. neoformans* (85). In tumor cells, perforin perforates the membrane of the target, which leads to an influx of water and a loss of intracellular molecules, resulting in cell lysis (86, 87). Similarly, granulysin disrupts the target cell membrane, which results in higher intracellular calcium and lower intracellular potassium concentrations, both of which ultimately activate caspases and programmed cell death (apoptosis) (88–92). However, it is important to note that the mechanisms of the antifungal effect of perforin and granulysin have not fully been elucidated to date.

There is an ongoing controversy on the direct antifungal effect of IFN-γ. One study reported on a direct IFN-γ-mediated antifungal activity of NK cells against *Aspergillus*, which was independent of degranulation of NK cells and their cytotoxic molecules (65). The authors suggested as explanation that "IFN-γ might cooperate with fungal ribotoxins, (…), transforming them into suicide molecules for fungus" (65). Similarly, it was demonstrated that IFN-γ at a concentration of 32 pg/ml exhibited a small but significant antifungal effect on *A. fumigatus*, *A. flavus*, and *Saccharomyces cerevisiae*, and inhibited the growth by 6, 11, and 17%, respectively (93). As higher concentrations of IFN-γ, e.g., 50 or 100 pg/ml, did not increase antifungal activity, and IFN-γ serum levels of 18 ± 30 pg/ml can be detected in healthy individuals (94), the importance of the direct antifungal effect *in vivo* is questionable. Corroborating the data of another report (70), no significant antifungal effects of IFN-γ were detected in *Candida* and *C. neoformans* (93). However, it is important to note that a combination of amphotericin B at a concentration of 1 μg/ml and IFN-γ at 32 pg/ml increased the efficacy of amphotericin B against *A. fumigatus*, which might be important for immunotherapeutic strategies.

Inducing apoptosis *via* the Fas–FasL or the TNF pathway is another mechanism by which NK cells are able to kill a target and has been described for various tumor cells as well as for pathogen infected cells (95, 96). Whereas data on apoptosis are missing for molds, apoptosis in yeast cells has been reported, but molecular mechanisms at the core of apoptotic execution is still unknown (97, 98). One recent study reported that blocking the death receptor ligands FasL and tumor necrosis factor-related apoptosis inducing ligand on the surface of human NK cells by antibodies did not have any impact on the antifungal activity (70). In addition, phagocytosis may be another mechanism of direct fungal damage by NK cells, which has been reported for *C. albicans* yeast (70). Notably, the IgG fraction of rabbit anti-cryptococcal serum enhanced the anti-cryptococcal activity of NK cells *via* their CD16 receptor (81).

MODULATION OF THE ANTIFUNGAL HOST RESPONSE BY NK CELLS

Upon stimulation, NK cells produce various cytokines, all of which modulate the host immunity against fungi. IFN-γ is one of the key molecules in the antifungal host response and is constitutively produced by NK cells (99). IFN-γ exhibits multiple effects on various immune cells. For example, IFN-γ is able to stimulate migration, adherence, phagocytosis, as well as oxidative killing by neutrophils and macrophages. Conditioned medium from co-incubation of NK cells and *C. albicans* enhanced polymorphonuclear neutrophil activation (70). In addition, data of a murine model demonstrated the pivotal role of IFN-γ-producing NK cells in inducing the phagocytic activity of splenic macrophages, thus mediating protection against systemic infection with *C. albicans* (100). As NK cells are the main source of IFN-γ in neutropenic mice suffering from aspergillosis, depletion of NK cells resulted in diminished IFN-γ levels in the lungs followed by an increased fungal load (101). Interestingly, the fungal load could be reduced by the transfer of wild-type IFN-γ producing NK cells, whereas this was not seen when transferring NK cells from IFN-γ-deficient mice. Because IFN-γ also enhances maturation of DCs and plays a pivotal role in the protective T_H1 cell response (11, 12, 102), the molecule was used as immunotherapy in invasive fungal disease. Whereas the administration of IFN-γ to mice with invasive aspergillosis was leading to reduced fungal burden and increased survival (103), available clinical data are inconclusive and do not allow a final conclusion on the usefulness of this strategy (11).

In addition to IFN-γ, NK cells produce soluble molecules such as GM-CSF and RANTES, both of which augment the host immune response *via* the stimulation of phagocytes and T cells, respectively (104–106).

INTERPLAY OF NK CELLS AND FUNGI

Fungi have developed strategies to counteract the complex and sophisticated antifungal immune response of the host. For example, *A. fumigatus* galactosaminogalactan induces apoptosis of polymorphonuclear neutrophils (107). Shedding of this molecule results in NK cell activation, which, in turn, leads to a Fas-dependent apoptosis-promoting signal in polymorphonuclear neutrophils (108). Galactosaminogalactan also induces IL-1 receptor antagonist, which leads to the suppression of IL-17 and IL-22 in peripheral blood mononuclear cells (109), and similar effects were observed with *Aspergillus* chitin (110). In addition, mycotoxins such as gliotoxin or aflatoxin (111) inhibit the phagocytic activity of macrophages, induce the apoptosis of monocytes, decrease the activation of nicotinamide adenine dinucleotide phosphate oxidase in neutrophils, and impair functional T cell responses (112–116), all of which hampers the host immune response toward the pathogen.

When NK cells are co-incubated with *A. fumigatus* or *R. oryzae*, lower levels of IFN-γ, GM-CSF, and RANTES are detected in the supernatant as compared to NK cells incubated alone (62, 63). Surprisingly, *A. fumigatus* increases the gene expression of IFN-γ in NK cells, but inhibits its release, thus leading to intracellular accumulation and decreased extracellular availability (117). Similarly, various mucormycetes affect the IFN-γ release by human NK cells (64). In contrast, earlier studies report that *C. neoformans* downregulates of the production of GM-CSF and TNF-α in unstimulated human NK cells, as assessed by gene expression and supernatant protein levels (118).

When looking at the fungal pathogen, it has been demonstrated that co-incubation of NK cells with *A. fumigatus* upregulated the expression of several stress-related fungal genes (117). This has been demonstrated for the heat shock protein *hsp90* or the ferric reductase *freB* (117). In *A. fumigatus*, Hsp90 plays an important role in the compensatory repair mechanisms of the cell wall in response to stress induced by antifungals, and Hsp90 has been described as a trigger for resistance to high concentrations of caspofungin, known as the paradoxical effect (119). FreB has recently been identified as an important enzyme in filamentous fungi which helps the fungus to adapt to iron starvation (120). Similarly, perforin-induced reduction of iron availability leads to the upregulation of the gene expression of *CSA2* in *C. albicans*, which is involved in the uptake of iron of human hemoglobin (84). Further characterization of specific interactions of the host immune system and fungal pathogens might identify novel targets for the antifungal armamentarium, e.g., the disruption of Hsp90 circuitry by Hsp90 inhibitors or anti-calcineurin drugs.

NK CELLS AND INVASIVE FUNGAL INFECTION: ANIMAL STUDIES

The few data of animal models clearly support the *in vitro* findings that NK cells play an important role in the antifungal host immune response. An early study in mice infected with *A. niger* demonstrated the association of the proliferation of NK cells and the inhibition of fungal growth (69). In addition, depletion of NK cells in mice inoculated with *C. neoformans* resulted in a considerably higher fungal load in the lungs as compared to untreated animals (121). In addition, antibody-mediated depletion of NK cells also decreased the phagocytosis of *C. albicans* by splenic macrophages as compared to controls (5.2 versus 21.5%) (100), and depletion of NK cells in mice *via* anti-asialo GM1 antibody resulted in enhanced susceptibility to *Histoplasma capsulatum* (122). Interestingly, in neutropenic mice, antibody-mediated depletion of NK cells also resulted in impaired clearance of the pathogen from the lungs and in a greater than twofold increase in mortality as compared to neutropenic mice with NK cells (123).

Importantly, the adoptive transfer of NK cells in mice lacking these cells can restore antifungal resistance. For example, in cyclophosphamide-pretreated mice suffering from cryptococcosis, the adoptive transfer of NK cell-enriched cell populations resulted in an enhanced clearance of the fungus as compared to controls receiving NK cell-depleted grafts (124, 125). As noted above, NK cell-derived IFN-γ plays an important role in the antifungal host response. NK cell depletion in neutropenic mice with invasive aspergillosis was leading to reduced lung IFN-γ levels and increased pulmonary fungal load, which was independent of T and B cell lymphocytes (101). However, the transfer of activated NK cells from wild-type, but not from IFN-γ-deficient mice resulted in better clearance of *A. fumigatus* from the lungs of both IFN-γ-deficient and wild-type recipients. Based on these findings, future studies have to assess in which clinical circumstances the adoptive transfer of NK cells to an immunocomoromised host suffering from an invasive fungal infection will be of benefit.

CONCLUSION AND PERSPECTIVES

There is increasing evidence that NK cells play an important role in the antifungal host response. *In vitro* data show that multiple fungal pathogens are able to activate NK cells, and further research will hopefully shed more light in the characterization of the complex interplay of NK cell receptors and fungal ligands. Once activated, NK cells directly damage the fungus by soluble cytotoxic molecules such as perforin, whereas the role of other mechanisms such as the induction of apoptosis *via* different pathways is still relatively unclear. In addition to the direct fungal damage, NK cells release multiple cytokines and IFNs by which they modulate the immune system, e.g., *via* neutrophils and T cells. As cure from an infectious complication not only depends on the successful activation of the immune system but also from a timely downregulation and resolution of the inflammatory process, further research needs to characterize the release of pro- and anti-inflammatory molecules. How and to what extent the fungus itself alters its gene expression profile in the presence of NK cells remains another research gap. In this regard, we have to learn how the fungus compromises the host immune system, which might offer new targets in our combat against the pathogen. In addition, animal studies will help to clarify the benefit and potential risks of using NK cells as adoptive preventive or therapeutic strategy, which may be a significant step toward decreasing morbidity and mortality of invasive fungal infection in the clinical setting.

AUTHOR CONTRIBUTIONS

All authors were involved in the concept of the manuscript, search and analysis of the references, and writing the manuscript; read and approved the final version of the manuscript.

REFERENCES

1. Zaoutis TE, Heydon K, Chu JH, Walsh TJ, Steinbach WJ. Epidemiology, outcomes, and costs of invasive aspergillosis in immunocompromised children in the United States, 2000. *Pediatrics* (2006) 117:e711–6. doi:10.1542/peds.2005-1161
2. Bitar D, Lortholary O, Le Strat Y, Nicolau J, Coignard B, Tattevin P, et al. Population-based analysis of invasive fungal infections, France, 2001–2010. *Emerg Infect Dis* (2014) 20:1149–55. doi:10.3201/eid2007.140087
3. McNeil MM, Nash SL, Hajjeh RA, Phelan MA, Conn LA, Plikaytis BD, et al. Trends in mortality due to invasive mycotic diseases in the United States, 1980-1997. *Clin Infect Dis* (2001) 33:641–7. doi:10.1086/322606
4. Kontoyiannis DP, Marr KA, Park BJ, Alexander BD, Anaissie EJ, Walsh TJ, et al. Prospective surveillance for invasive fungal infections in hematopoietic stem cell transplant recipients, 2001-2006: overview of the transplant-associated infection surveillance network (TRANSNET) database. *Clin Infect Dis* (2010) 50:1091–100. doi:10.1086/651263
5. Horn DL, Fishman JA, Steinbach WJ, Anaissie EJ, Marr KA, Olyaei AJ, et al. Presentation of the PATH Alliance® registry for prospective data collection and analysis of the epidemiology, therapy, and outcomes of invasive fungal infections. *Diagn Microbiol Infect Dis* (2007) 59:407–14. doi:10.1016/j.diagmicrobio.2007.06.008
6. Azie N, Neofytos D, Pfaller M, Meier-Kriesche HU, Quan SP, Horn D. The PATH (prospective antifungal therapy) Alliance® registry and invasive fungal infections: update 2012. *Diagn Microbiol Infect Dis* (2012) 73:293–300. doi:10.1016/j.diagmicrobio.2012.06.012
7. Lehrnbecher T, Koehl U, Wittekindt B, Bochennek K, Tramsen L, Klingebiel T, et al. Changes in host defence induced by malignancies and antineoplastic treatment: implication for immunotherapeutic strategies. *Lancet Oncol* (2008) 9:269–78. doi:10.1016/S1470-2045(08)70071-8
8. Lehrnbecher T, Foster C, Vázquez N, Mackall CL, Chanock SJ. Therapy-induced alterations in host defense in children receiving therapy for cancer. *J Pediatr Hematol Oncol* (1997) 19:399–417. doi:10.1097/00043426-199709000-00001
9. Bodey GP. Infectious complications of acute leukemia. *Med Times* (1966) 94:1076–85.
10. Stuehler C, Kuenzli E, Jaeger VK, Baettig V, Ferracin F, Rajacic Z, et al. Immune reconstitution after allogeneic hematopoietic stem cell transplantation and association with occurrence and outcome of invasive aspergillosis. *J Infect Dis* (2015) 212:959–67. doi:10.1093/infdis/jiv143
11. Lehrnbecher T, Kalkum M, Champer J, Tramsen L, Schmidt S, Klingebiel T. Immunotherapy in invasive fungal infection – focus on invasive aspergillosis. *Curr Pharm Des* (2013) 19:3689–712. doi:10.2174/1381612811319200010
12. Romani L. Immunity to fungal infections. *Nat Rev Immunol* (2004) 4:1–23. doi:10.1038/nri1255
13. Romani L. Immunity to fungal infections. *Nat Rev Immunol* (2011) 11:275–88. doi:10.1038/nri2939
14. Fisher BT, Robinson PD, Lehrnbecher T, Steinbach WJ, Zaoutis TE, Phillips B, et al. Risk factors for invasive fungal disease in pediatric cancer and hematopoietic stem cell transplantation: a systematic review. *J Pediatric Infect Dis Soc* (2017). doi:10.1093/jpids/pix030
15. Cunha C, Kurzai O, Löffler J, Aversa F, Romani L, Carvalho A. Neutrophil responses to aspergillosis: new roles for old players. *Mycopathologia* (2014) 178:387–93. doi:10.1007/s11046-014-9796-7
16. Borghi M, Renga G, Puccetti M, Oikonomou V, Palmieri M, Galosi C, et al. Antifungal Th immunity: growing up in family. *Front Immunol* (2014) 5:506. doi:10.3389/fimmu.2014.00506
17. Limon JJ, Skalski JH, Underhill DM. Commensal fungi in health and disease. *Cell Host Microbe* (2017) 22:156–65. doi:10.1016/j.chom.2017.07.002
18. Cooper MA, Fehniger TA, Caligiuri MA. The biology of human natural killer-cell subsets. *Trends Immunol* (2001) 22:633–40. doi:10.1016/S1471-4906(01)02060-9
19. Sun JC, Lopez-Verges S, Kim CC, DeRisi JL, Lanier LL. NK cells and immune "memory". *J Immunol* (2011) 186:1891–7. doi:10.4049/jimmunol.1003035
20. Narni-Mancinelli E, Vivier E, Kerdiles YM. The "T-cell-ness" of NK cells: unexpected similarities between NK cells and T cells. *Int Immunol* (2011) 23:427–31. doi:10.1093/intimm/dxr035
21. Kleinnijenhuis J, Quintin J, Preijers F, Joosten LAB, Jacobs C, Xavier RJ, et al. BCG-induced trained immunity in NK cells: role for non-specific protection to infection. *Clin Immunol* (2014) 155:213–9. doi:10.1016/j.clim.2014.10.005
22. Kiessling R, Klein E, Wigzell H. "Natural" killer cells in the mouse. I. Cytotoxic cells with specificity for mouse Moloney leukemia cells. Specificity and distribution according to genotype. *Eur J Immunol* (1975) 5:112–7. doi:10.1002/eji.1830050208
23. Lam VC, Lanier LL. NK cells in host responses to viral infections. *Curr Opin Immunol* (2017) 44:43–51. doi:10.1016/j.coi.2016.11.003
24. Arase H, Mocarski ES, Campbell AE, Hill AB, Lanier LL. Direct recognition of cytomegalovirus by activating and inhibitory NK cell receptors. *Science* (2002) 296:1323–6. doi:10.1126/science.1070884
25. Adams EJ, Juo ZS, Venook RT, Boulanger MJ, Arase H, Lanier LL, et al. Structural elucidation of the m157 mouse cytomegalovirus ligand for Ly49 natural killer cell receptors. *Proc Natl Acad Sci U S A* (2007) 104:10128–33. doi:10.1073/pnas.0703735104
26. Kielczewska A, Kim H-S, Lanier LL, Dimasi N, Vidal SM. Critical residues at the Ly49 natural killer receptor's homodimer interface determine functional

recognition of m157, a mouse cytomegalovirus MHC class I-like protein. *J Immunol* (2007) 178:369–77. doi:10.4049/jimmunol.178.1.369
27. Romee R, Schneider SE, Leong JW, Chase JM, Keppel CR, Sullivan RP, et al. Cytokine activation induces human memory-like NK cells. *Blood* (2012) 120:4751–60. doi:10.1182/blood-2012-04-419283
28. Malmberg K-J, Carlsten M, Björklund A, Sohlberg E, Bryceson YT, Ljunggren H-G. Natural killer cell-mediated immunosurveillance of human cancer. *Semin Immunol* (2017) 31:20–9. doi:10.1016/j.smim.2017.08.002
29. Herberman RR, Ortaldo JR, Bonnard GD. Augmentation by interferon of human natural and antibody-dependent cell-mediated cytotoxicity. *Nature* (1979) 277:221–3. doi:10.1038/277221a0
30. Ortaldo JR, Bonnard GD, Kind PD, Herberman RB. Cytotoxicity by cultured human lymphocytes: characteristics of effector cells and specificity of cytotoxicity. *J Immunol* (1979) 122:1489–94.
31. Biron CA, Welsh RM. Activation and role of natural killer cells in virus infections. *Med Microbiol Immunol* (1982) 170:155–72. doi:10.1007/BF02298196
32. Liu LL, Béziat V, Oei VYS, Pfefferle A, Schaffer M, Lehmann S, et al. Ex vivo expanded adaptive NK cells effectively kill primary acute lymphoblastic leukemia cells. *Cancer Immunol Res* (2017) 5:654–65. doi:10.1158/2326-6066.CIR-16-0296
33. Schlegel P, Ditthard K, Lang P, Mezger M, Michaelis S, Handgretinger R, et al. NKG2D signaling leads to NK cell mediated lysis of childhood AML. *J Immunol Res* (2015) 2015:473175. doi:10.1155/2015/473175
34. Castriconi R, Dondero A, Corrias MV, Lanino E, Pende D, Moretta L, et al. Natural killer cell-mediated killing of freshly isolated neuroblastoma cells: critical role of DNAX accessory molecule-1-poliovirus receptor interaction. *Cancer Res* (2004) 64:9180–4. doi:10.1158/0008-5472.CAN-04-2682
35. Kloess S, Huenecke S, Piechulek D, Esser R, Koch J, Brehm C, et al. IL-2-activated haploidentical NK cells restore NKG2D-mediated NK-cell cytotoxicity in neuroblastoma patients by scavenging of plasma MICA. *Eur J Immunol* (2010) 40:3255–67. doi:10.1002/eji.201040568
36. Vivier E, Tomasello E, Baratin M, Walzer T, Ugolini S. Functions of natural killer cells. *Nat Immunol* (2008) 9:503–10. doi:10.1038/ni1582
37. Béziat V, Dalgard O, Asselah T, Halfon P, Bedossa P, Boudifa A, et al. CMV drives clonal expansion of NKG2C+ NK cells expressing self-specific KIRs in chronic hepatitis patients. *Eur J Immunol* (2012) 42:447–57. doi:10.1002/eji.201141826
38. Saghafian-Hedengren S, Sohlberg E, Theorell J, Carvalho-Queiroz C, Nagy N, Persson J-O, et al. Epstein-Barr virus coinfection in children boosts cytomegalovirus-induced differentiation of natural killer cells. *J Virol* (2013) 87:13446–55. doi:10.1128/JVI.02382-13
39. Shabani Z, Bagheri M, Zare-Bidaki M, Hassanshahi G, Arababadi MK, Mohammadi Nejad M, et al. NK cells in hepatitis B virus infection: a potent target for immunotherapy. *Arch Virol* (2014) 159:1555–65. doi:10.1007/s00705-013-1965-3
40. Werner JM, Heller T, Gordon AM, Sheets A, Sherker AH, Kessler E, et al. Innate immune responses in hepatitis C virus-exposed healthcare workers who do not develop acute infection. *Hepatology* (2013) 58:1621–31. doi:10.1002/hep.26353
41. Garcia-Peñarrubia P, Koster FT, Kelley RO, McDowell TD, Bankhurst AD. Antibacterial activity of human natural killer cells. *J Exp Med* (1989) 169:99–113. doi:10.1084/jem.169.1.99
42. Wherry JC, Schreiber RD, Unanue ER. Regulation of gamma interferon production by natural killer cells in scid mice: roles of tumor necrosis factor and bacterial stimuli. *Infect Immun* (1991) 59:1709–15.
43. Anfossi N, André P, Guia S, Falk CS, Roetynck S, Stewart CA, et al. Human NK cell education by inhibitory receptors for MHC class I. *Immunity* (2006) 25:331–42. doi:10.1016/j.immuni.2006.06.013
44. Parsons MS, Zipperlen K, Gallant M, Grant M. Killer cell immunoglobulin-like receptor 3DL1 licenses CD16-mediated effector functions of natural killer cells. *J Leukoc Biol* (2010) 88:905–12. doi:10.1189/jlb.1009687
45. Horowitz A, Djaoud Z, Nemat-Gorgani N, Blokhuis J, Hilton HG, Béziat V, et al. Class I HLA haplotypes form two schools that educate NK cells in different ways. *Sci Immunol* (2016) 1:eaag1672. doi:10.1126/sciimmunol.aag1672
46. Campbell KS, Hasegawa J. NK cell biology: an update and future directions. *J Allergy Clin Immunol* (2013) 132:536–44. doi:10.1016/j.jaci.2013.07.006
47. Yawata M, Yawata N, Draghi M, Little A-M, Partheniou F, Parham P. Roles for HLA and KIR polymorphisms in natural killer cell repertoire selection and modulation of effector function. *J Exp Med* (2006) 203:633–45. doi:10.1084/jem.20051884
48. Yawata M, Yawata N, Draghi M, Partheniou F, Little A-M, Parham P. MHC class I-specific inhibitory receptors and their ligands structure diverse human NK-cell repertoires toward a balance of missing self-response. *Blood* (2008) 112:2369–80. doi:10.1182/blood-2008-03-143727
49. Horowitz A, Strauss-Albee DM, Leipold M, Kubo J, Nemat-Gorgani N, Dogan OC, et al. Genetic and environmental determinants of human NK cell diversity revealed by mass cytometry. *Sci Transl Med* (2013) 5:208ra145. doi:10.1126/scitranslmed.3006702
50. Kim S, Poursine-Laurent J, Truscott SM, Lybarger L, Song Y-J, Yang L, et al. Licensing of natural killer cells by host major histocompatibility complex class I molecules. *Nature* (2005) 436:709–13. doi:10.1038/nature03847
51. Fernandez NC, Treiner E, Vance RE, Jamieson AM, Lemieux S, Raulet DH. A subset of natural killer cells achieves self-tolerance without expressing inhibitory receptors specific for self-MHC molecules. *Blood* (2005) 105:4416–23. doi:10.1182/blood-2004-08-3156
52. Brodin P, Lakshmikanth T, Johansson S, Kärre K, Höglund P. The strength of inhibitory input during education quantitatively tunes the functional responsiveness of individual natural killer cells. *Blood* (2009) 113:2434–41. doi:10.1182/blood-2008-05-156836
53. Joncker NT, Fernandez NC, Treiner E, Vivier E, Raulet DH. NK cell responsiveness is tuned commensurate with the number of inhibitory receptors for self-MHC class I: the rheostat model. *J Immunol* (2009) 182:4572–80. doi:10.4049/jimmunol.0803900
54. Orr MT, Murphy WJ, Lanier LL. "Unlicensed" natural killer cells dominate the response to cytomegalovirus infection. *Nat Immunol* (2010) 11:321–7. doi:10.1038/ni.1849
55. Spits H, Artis D, Colonna M, Diefenbach A, Di Santo JP, Eberl G, et al. Innate lymphoid cells – a proposal for uniform nomenclature. *Nat Rev Immunol* (2013) 13:145–9. doi:10.1038/nri3365
56. Orange JS, Ballas ZK. Natural killer cells in human health and disease. *Clin Immunol* (2006) 118:1–10. doi:10.1016/j.clim.2005.10.011
57. Fernández-Ruiz M, López-Medrano F, San Juan R, Allende LM, Paz-Artal E, Aguado JM. Low natural killer cell counts and onset of invasive fungal disease after solid organ transplantation. *J Infect Dis* (2016) 213:873–4. doi:10.1093/infdis/jiv552
58. Palma-Carlos AG, Palma-Carlos ML. Chronic mucocutaneous candidiasis revisited. *Allerg Immunol (Paris)* (2001) 33:229–32.
59. Chiu S-J, Tsao C-H, Chen L-C, Kao C-C, Lue K-H, Huang J-L. Chronic mucocutaneous candidiasis in a 6-year-old boy. *J Microbiol Immunol Infect* (2004) 37:196–9.
60. De Moraes-Vasconcelos D, Orii NM, Romano CC, Iqueoka RY, Duarte AJS. Characterization of the cellular immune function of patients with chronic mucocutaneous candidiasis. *Clin Exp Immunol* (2001) 123:247–53. doi:10.1046/j.1365-2249.2001.01430.x
61. Akiba H, Motoki Y, Satoh M, Iwatsuki K, Kaneko F. Recalcitrant trichophytic granuloma associated with NK-cell deficiency in a SLE patient treated with corticosteroid. *Eur J Dermatol* (2001) 11:58–62.
62. Schmidt S, Tramsen L, Hanisch M, Latgé J-P, Huenecke S, Koehl U, et al. Human natural killer cells exhibit direct activity against *Aspergillus fumigatus* hyphae, but not against resting conidia. *J Infect Dis* (2011) 203:430–5. doi:10.1093/infdis/jiq062
63. Schmidt S, Tramsen L, Perkhofer S, Lass-Florl C, Hanisch M, Roger F, et al. *Rhizopus oryzae* hyphae are damaged by human natural killer (NK) cells, but suppress NK cell mediated immunity. *Immunobiology* (2013) 218:939–44. doi:10.1016/j.imbio.2012.10.013
64. Schmidt S, Schneider A, Demir A, Lass-Flörl C, Lehrnbecher T. Natural killer cell-mediated damage of clinical isolates of mucormycetes. *Mycoses* (2016) 59:34–8. doi:10.1111/myc.12431
65. Bouzani M, Ok M, McCormick A, Ebel F, Kurzai O, Morton CO, et al. Human NK cells display important antifungal activity against *Aspergillus fumigatus*, which is directly mediated by IFN-γ release. *J Immunol* (2011) 187:1369–76. doi:10.4049/jimmunol.1003593
66. Hidore MR, Nabavi N, Reynolds CW, Henkart PA, Murphy JW. Cytoplasmic components of natural killer cells limit the growth of *Cryptococcus neoformans*. *J Leukoc Biol* (1990) 48:15–26.

67. Ma LL, Wang CLC, Neely GG, Epelman S, Krensky AM, Mody CH. NK cells use perforin rather than granulysin for anticryptococcal activity. *J Immunol* (2004) 173:3357–65. doi:10.4049/jimmunol.173.5.3357
68. Li SS, Kyei SK, Timm-McCann M, Ogbomo H, Jones GJ, Shi M, et al. The NK receptor NKp30 mediates direct fungal recognition and killing and is diminished in NK cells from HIV-infected patients. *Cell Host Microbe* (2013) 14:387–97. doi:10.1016/j.chom.2013.09.007
69. Benedetto N, Sabatini P, Sellitto C, Romano Carratelli C. Interleukin-2 and increased natural killer activity in mice experimentally infected with *Aspergillus niger*. *Microbiologica* (1988) 11:339–45.
70. Voigt J, Hünniger K, Bouzani M, Jacobsen ID, Barz D, Hube B, et al. Human natural killer cells acting as phagocytes against *Candida albicans* and mounting an inflammatory response that modulates neutrophil antifungal activity. *J Infect Dis* (2014) 209:616–26. doi:10.1093/infdis/jit574
71. Aimanianda V, Bayry J, Bozza S, Kniemeyer O, Perruccio K, Elluru SR, et al. Surface hydrophobin prevents immune recognition of airborne fungal spores. *Nature* (2009) 460:1117–21. doi:10.1038/nature08264
72. Chai LYA, Netea MG, Sugui J, Vonk AG, van de Sande WWJ, Warris A, et al. *Aspergillus fumigatus* conidial melanin modulates host cytokine response. *Immunobiology* (2010) 215:915–20. doi:10.1016/j.imbio.2009.10.002
73. Kozel TR, Gotschlich EC. The capsule of *Cryptococcus neoformans* passively inhibits phagocytosis of the yeast by macrophages. *J Immunol* (1982) 129:1675–80.
74. Rappleye CA, Goldman WE. Fungal stealth technology. *Trends Immunol* (2008) 29:18–24. doi:10.1016/j.it.2007.10.001
75. Marr KJ, Jones GJ, Zheng C, Huston SM, Timm-McCann M, Islam A, et al. *Cryptococcus neoformans* directly stimulates perforin production and rearms NK cells for enhanced anticryptococcal microbicidal activity. *Infect Immun* (2009) 77:2436–46. doi:10.1128/IAI.01232-08
76. Mueller-Leisse J, Brueggemann S, Bouzani M, Schmitt A-L, Einsele H, Loeffler J. Polymorphonuclear neutrophils and granulocytic myeloid-derived suppressor cells inhibit natural killer cell activity toward *Aspergillus fumigatus*. *Med Mycol* (2015) 53:622–9. doi:10.1093/mmy/myv030
77. Vitenshtein A, Charpak-Amikam Y, Yamin R, Bauman Y, Isaacson B, Stein N, et al. NK cell recognition of *Candida glabrata* through binding of NKp46 and NCR1 to fungal ligands Epa1, Epa6, and Epa7. *Cell Host Microbe* (2016) 20:527–34. doi:10.1016/j.chom.2016.09.008
78. de Groot PWJ, Bader O, de Boer AD, Weig M, Chauhan N. Adhesins in human fungal pathogens: glue with plenty of stick. *Eukaryot Cell* (2013) 12:470–81. doi:10.1128/EC.00364-12
79. Ogbomo H, Mody CH. Granule-dependent natural killer cell cytotoxicity to fungal pathogens. *Front Immunol* (2017) 7:692. doi:10.3389/fimmu.2016.00692
80. Ziegler S, Weiss E, Schmitt A-L, Schlegel J, Burgert A, Terpitz U, et al. CD56 is a pathogen recognition receptor on human natural killer cells. *Sci Rep* (2017) 7:6138. doi:10.1038/s41598-017-06238-4
81. Nabavi N, Murphy JW. Antibody-dependent natural killer cell-mediated growth inhibition of *Cryptococcus neoformans*. *Infect Immun* (1986) 51:556–62.
82. Obata-Onai A, Hashimoto S, Onai N, Kurachi M, Nagai S, Shizuno K, et al. Comprehensive gene expression analysis of human NK cells and CD8(+) T lymphocytes. *Int Immunol* (2002) 14:1085–98. doi:10.1093/intimm/dxf086
83. Kataoka T, Shinohara N, Takayama H, Takaku K, Kondo S, Yonehara S, et al. Concanamycin A, a powerful tool for characterization and estimation of contribution of perforin- and Fas-based lytic pathways in cell-mediated cytotoxicity. *J Immunol* (1996) 156:3678–86.
84. Hellwig D, Voigt J, Bouzani M, Löffler J, Albrecht-Eckardt D, Weber M, et al. *Candida albicans* induces metabolic reprogramming in human NK cells and responds to perforin with a zinc depletion response. *Front Microbiol* (2016) 7:750. doi:10.3389/fmicb.2016.00750
85. Kyei SK, Ogbomo H, Li S, Timm-mccann M, Xiang RF, Huston SM. Mechanisms by which interleukin-12 corrects defective NK cell anticryptococcal activity in HIV-infected patients. *MBio* (2016) 7:e00878-16. doi:10.1128/mBio.00878-16
86. Duke RC, Persechini PM, Chang S, Liu C-C, Cohen JJ, Young JD. Purified perforin induces target cell lysis but not DNA fragmentation. *J Exp Med* (1989) 170:1451–6. doi:10.1084/jem.170.4.1451
87. Law RHP, Lukoyanova N, Voskoboinik I, Caradoc-Davies TT, Baran K, Dunstone MA, et al. The structural basis for membrane binding and pore formation by lymphocyte perforin. *Nature* (2010) 468:447–51. doi:10.1038/nature09518
88. Ernst WA, Thoma-Uszynski S, Teitelbaum R, Ko C, Hanson DA, Clayberger C, et al. Granulysin, a T cell product, kills bacteria by altering membrane permeability. *J Immunol* (2000) 165:7102–8. doi:10.4049/jimmunol.165.12.7102
89. Gamen S, Hanson DA, Kaspar A, Naval J, Krensky AM, Anel A. Granulysin-induced apoptosis. I. Involvement of at least two distinct pathways. *J Immunol* (1998) 161:1758–64.
90. Kaspar AA, Okada S, Kumar J, Poulain FR, Drouvalakis KA, Kelekar A, et al. A distinct pathway of cell-mediated apoptosis initiated by granulysin. *J Immunol* (2001) 167:350–6. doi:10.4049/jimmunol.167.1.350
91. Krensky AM, Clayberger C. Biology and clinical relevance of granulysin. *Tissue Antigens* (2009) 73:193–8. doi:10.1111/j.1399-0039.2008.01218.x
92. Okada S, Li Q, Whitin JC, Clayberger C, Krensky AM. Intracellular mediators of granulysin-induced cell death. *J Immunol* (2003) 171:2556–62. doi:10.4049/jimmunol.171.5.2556
93. El-Khoury M, Ligot R, Mahoney S, Stack CM, Perrone GG, Morton CO. The in vitro effects of interferon-gamma, alone or in combination with amphotericin B, tested against the pathogenic fungi *Candida albicans* and *Aspergillus fumigatus*. *BMC Res Notes* (2017) 10:364. doi:10.1186/s13104-017-2696-4
94. Katti MK. Assessment of serum IL-1, IL-2 and IFN-γ levels in untreated pulmonary tuberculosis patients: role in pathogenesis. *Arch Med Res* (2011) 42:199–201. doi:10.1016/j.arcmed.2011.04.012
95. Screpanti V, Wallin RPA, Grandien A, Ljunggren HG. Impact of FASL-induced apoptosis in the elimination of tumor cells by NK cells. *Mol Immunol* (2005) 42:495–9. doi:10.1016/j.molimm.2004.07.033
96. Guerra C, Johal K, Morris D, Moreno S, Alvarado O, Gray D, et al. Control of *Mycobacterium tuberculosis* growth by activated natural killer cells. *Clin Exp Immunol* (2012) 168:142–52. doi:10.1111/j.1365-2249.2011.04552.x
97. Madeo F, Herker E, Wissing S, Jungwirth H, Eisenberg T, Fröhlich KU. Apoptosis in yeast. *Curr Opin Microbiol* (2004) 7:655–60. doi:10.1016/j.mib.2004.10.012
98. Fröhlich KU, Fussi H, Ruckenstuhl C. Yeast apoptosis – from genes to pathways. *Semin Cancer Biol* (2007) 17:112–21. doi:10.1016/j.semcancer.2006.11.006
99. Mah AY, Cooper MA. Metabolic regulation of natural killer cell IFN-γ production. *Crit Rev Immunol* (2016) 36:131–47. doi:10.1615/CritRevImmunol.2016017387
100. Algarra I, Ortega E, Serrano MJ, Alvarez de Cienfuegos G, Gaforio JJ. Suppression of splenic macrophage *Candida albicans* phagocytosis following in vivo depletion of natural killer cells in immunocompetent BALB/c mice and T-cell-deficient nude mice. *FEMS Immunol Med Microbiol* (2002) 33:159–63. doi:10.1111/j.1574-695X.2002.tb00586.x
101. Park SJ, Hughes MA, Burdick M, Strieter RM, Mehrad B. Early NK cell-derived IFN-γ is essential to host defense in neutropenic invasive aspergillosis. *J Immunol* (2009) 182:4306–12. doi:10.4049/jimmunol.0803462
102. Boehm U, Klamp T, Groot M, Howard JC. Cellular responses to interferon-gamma. *Annu Rev Immunol* (1997) 15:749–95. doi:10.1146/annurev.immunol.15.1.749
103. Nagai H, Guo J, Choi H, Kurup V. Interferon-gamma and tumor necrosis factor-alpha protect mice from invasive aspergillosis. *J Infect Dis* (1995) 172:1554–60. doi:10.1093/infdis/172.6.1554
104. Homey B, Müller A, Zlotnik A. Chemokines: agents for the immunotherapy of cancer? *Nat Rev Immunol* (2002) 2:175–84. doi:10.1038/nri748
105. Richardson MD, Brownlie CE, Shankland GS. Enhanced phagocytosis and intracellular killing of *Candida albicans* by GM-CSF-activated human neutrophils. *J Med Vet Mycol* (1992) 30:433–41. doi:10.1080/02681219280000591
106. Roilides E, Holmes A, Blake C, Venzon D, Pizzo PA, Walsh TJ. Antifungal activity of elutriated human monocytes against *Aspergillus fumigatus* hyphae: enhancement by granulocyte-macrophage colony-stimulating factor and interferon-gamma. *J Infect Dis* (1994) 170:894–9. doi:10.1093/infdis/170.4.894
107. Fontaine T, Delangle A, Simenel C, Coddeville B, van Vliet SJ, van Kooyk Y, et al. Galactosaminogalactan, a new immunosuppressive polysaccharide of *Aspergillus fumigatus*. *PLoS Pathog* (2011) 7:e1002372. doi:10.1371/journal.ppat.1002372

108. Robinet P, Baychelier F, Fontaine T, Picard C, Debré P, Vieillard V, et al. A polysaccharide virulence factor of a human fungal pathogen induces neutrophil apoptosis *via* NK cells. *J Immunol* (2014) 192:5332–42. doi:10.4049/jimmunol.1303180
109. Gresnigt MS, Bozza S, Becker KL, Joosten LAB, Abdollahi-Roodsaz S, van der Berg WB, et al. A polysaccharide virulence factor from *Aspergillus fumigatus* elicits anti-inflammatory effects through induction of interleukin-1 receptor antagonist. *PLoS Pathog* (2014) 10:e1003936. doi:10.1371/journal.ppat.1003936
110. Becker KL, Aimanianda V, Wang X, Gresnigt MS, Ammerdorffer A, Jacobs CW, et al. *Aspergillus* cell wall chitin induces anti- and proinflammatory cytokines in human PBMCs via the Fc-γ receptor/Syk/PI3K pathway. *MBio* (2016) 7:e01823–15. doi:10.1128/mBio.01823-15
111. Abad A, Fernández-Molina JV, Bikandi J, Ramírez A, Margareto J, Sendino J, et al. What makes *Aspergillus fumigatus* a successful pathogen? Genes and molecules involved in invasive aspergillosis. *Rev Iberoam Micol* (2010) 27:155–82. doi:10.1016/j.riam.2010.10.003
112. Müllbacher A, Eichner RD. Immunosuppression in vitro by a metabolite of a human pathogenic fungus. *Proc Natl Acad Sci U S A* (1984) 81:3835–7. doi:10.1073/pnas.81.12.3835
113. Sutton P, Newcombe NR, Waring P, Mullbacher A. In vivo immunosuppressive activity of gliotoxin, a metabolite produced by human pathogenic fungi. *Infect Immun* (1994) 62:1192–8.
114. Stanzani M, Orciuolo E, Lewis R, Kontoyiannis DP, Martins SLR, St. John LS, et al. *Aspergillus fumigatus* suppresses the human cellular immune response via gliotoxin-mediated apoptosis of monocytes. *Blood* (2005) 105:2258–65. doi:10.1182/blood-2004-09-3421
115. Tsunawaki S, Yoshida LS, Nishida S, Kobayashi T. Fungal metabolite gliotoxin inhibits assembly of the human respiratory burst NADPH oxidase fungal metabolite gliotoxin inhibits assembly of the human respiratory burst NADPH oxidase. *Infect Immun* (2004) 72:3373–82. doi:10.1128/IAI.72.6.3373-3382.2004
116. Yamada A, Kataoka T, Nagai K. The fungal metabolite gliotoxin: immunosuppressive activity on CTL-mediated cytotoxicity. *Immunol Lett* (2000) 71:27–32. doi:10.1016/S0165-2478(99)00155-8
117. Schneider A, Blatzer M, Posch W, Schubert R, Lass-Flörl C, Schmidt S, et al. *Aspergillus fumigatus* responds to natural killer (NK) cells with upregulation of stress related genes and inhibits the immunoregulatory function of NK cells. *Oncotarget* (2016) 7:71062–71. doi:10.18632/oncotarget.12616
118. Murphy JW, Zhou A, Wong SC. Direct interactions of human natural killer cells with *Cryptococcus neoformans* inhibit granulocyte-macrophage colony-stimulating factor and tumor necrosis factor alpha production. *Infect Immun* (1997) 65:4564–71.
119. Lamoth F, Juvvadi PR, Steinbach WJ. Heat shock protein 90 (Hsp90): a novel antifungal target against *Aspergillus fumigatus*. *Crit Rev Microbiol* (2014) 42:1–12. doi:10.3109/1040841X.2014.947239
120. Blatzer M, Binder U, Haas H. The metalloreductase FreB is involved in adaptation of *Aspergillus fumigatus* to iron starvation. *Fungal Genet Biol* (2011) 48:1027–33. doi:10.1016/j.fgb.2011.07.009
121. Lipscomb MF, Alvarellos T, Toews GB, Tompkins R, Evans Z, Koo G, et al. Role of natural killer cells in resistance to *Cryptococcus neoformans* infections in mice. *Am J Pathol* (1987) 128:354–61.
122. Tewari RP, Von Behren LA. Immune responses in histoplasmosis, a prototype of respiratory mycoses. *Indian J Chest Dis Allied Sci* (2000) 42:265–9.
123. Morrison BE, Park SJ, Mooney JM, Mehrad B. Chemokine-mediated recruitment of NK cells is a critical host defense mechanism in invasive aspergillosis. *J Clin Invest* (2003) 112:1862–70. doi:10.1172/JCI18125
124. Hidore MR, Murphy JW. Natural cellular resistance of beige mice against *Cryptococcus neoformans*. *J Immunol* (1986) 137:3624–31.
125. Hidore MR, Murphy JW. Correlation of natural killer cell activity and clearance of *Cryptococcus neoformans* from mice after adoptive transfer of splenic nylon wool-nonadherent cells. *Infect Immun* (1986) 51:547–55.

8

Candida albicans Yeast, Pseudohyphal and Hyphal Morphogenesis Differentially Affects Immune Recognition

Liliane Mukaremera[1,2†], Keunsook K. Lee[1†], Hector M. Mora-Montes[3] and Neil A. R. Gow[1]*

[1]Aberdeen Fungal Group, Institute of Medical Sciences, Foresterhill, University of Aberdeen, Aberdeen, United Kingdom, [2]Department of Microbiology and Immunology, Medical School, University of Minnesota, Minneapolis, MN, United States, [3]Departamento de Biología, División de Ciencias Naturales y Exactas, Universidad de Guanajuato, Guanajuato, Mexico

***Correspondence:**
Neil A. R. Gow
n.gow@abdn.ac.uk

†These authors have contributed equally to this work.

Candida albicans is a human opportunist pathogen that can grow as yeast, pseudohyphae, or true hyphae *in vitro* and *in vivo*, depending on environmental conditions. Reversible cellular morphogenesis is an important virulence factor that facilitates invasion of host tissues, escape from phagocytes, and dissemination in the blood stream. The innate immune system is the first line of defense against *C. albicans* infections and is influenced by recognition of wall components that vary in composition in different morphological forms. However, the relationship between cellular morphogenesis and immune recognition of this fungus is not fully understood. We therefore studied various vegetative cell types of *C. albicans*, singly and in combination, to assess the consequences of cellular morphogenesis on selected immune cytokine outputs from human monocytes. Hyphae stimulated proportionally lower levels of certain cytokines from monocytes per unit of cell surface area than yeast cells, but did not suppress cytokine response when copresented with yeast cells. Pseudohyphal cells induced intermediate cytokine responses. Yeast monomorphic mutants had elevated cytokine responses under conditions that otherwise supported filamentous growth and mutants of yeast and hyphal cells that were defective in cell wall mannosylation or lacking certain hypha-specific cell wall proteins could variably unmask or deplete the surface of immunostimulatory ligands. These observations underline the critical importance of *C. albicans* morphology and morphology-associated changes in the cell wall composition that affect both immune recognition and pathogenesis.

Keywords: *Candida albicans*, cell wall, cytokine, immune recognition, morphogenesis

INTRODUCTION

Fungal pathogens are associated with a wide range of human diseases from superficial infections of the skin and mucosal surfaces to life-threatening systemic infections, depending on host health and immunocompetence. *Candida* species account collectively for as many as 400,000 cases of systemic fungal disease with associated mortality rates of up to 40% (1–4). Of these species, *Candida albicans* is the most common agent of disease and is characterized by its morphological plasticity. It is capable of vegetative growth *in vitro* and *in vivo* as ovoid budding yeast-like cells and as branching filamentous cells that exist as more or less elongated and constricted chains of yeast cells called pseudohyphae or parallel-sided hyphal cells (5–10). Other cell types, such as GUT, gray, and opaque cells, are a tristable system of specialized cells involved in colonization of specific body sites and in mating competence (10). We set out to characterize differences in the immune response by human peripheral blood mononuclear cells (PBMCs) to yeast cells, hyphae, and pseudohyphae as the three major morphological forms of *C. albicans*.

The innate immune system is the first line of defense against all invading organisms and plays a major role in resistance to infectious diseases in immunocompetent hosts (11). Phagocytes detect microbial pathogen-associated molecular patterns (PAMPs) *via* pattern-recognition receptors (PRRs), resulting in signaling-mediated transcription and secretion of inflammatory mediators, such as chemokines and cytokines that recruit neutrophils and other immune cells to the site of infection, resulting in localized killing of the pathogen and activation of the adaptive immune response (11–13).

C. albicans PAMPs that activate the inflammatory response are located in both the outer and inner layers of the intact cell wall (4, 11, 14–16). Mannans and glucans are the main elicitors of both cytokine production and phagocytosis and are recognized by a range of C-type lectins and toll-like receptors (TLRs) (4, 17–21). The *O*-linked mannans are sensed through the TLR4 receptor (17), β-mannan is recognized by galectin-3 (22–25), and α-linked *N*-mannans are recognized by the mannose receptor (MR), dectin-2, mincle, and DC-SIGN (21, 26). Opsonized β1,6-glucan acts as an immune agonist (27), and chitin is taken up by the MR and induces TLR9- and NOD2-dependent IL-10 production (4, 28).

Most immune recognition studies have focused on *C. albicans* yeast cells as the cell target; however, it is known that filamentous hyphal cells induce an altered immune response (4, 6, 8, 21, 29–32). The switch between yeast and hyphal growth is critical for virulence (6, 8, 33, 34), affecting numerous properties including the expression of morphology-dependent cell wall adhesins, invasins, proteases, and a raft of other phenotypic and biochemical properties, including the recently discovered candidalysin toxin (35). Mutants locked in either the yeast or hypha form are avirulent, suggesting that the ability to transit reversibly between these morphotypes potentiate the virulence of this fungus (7, 33, 35–40). Pseudohyphae are a distinct growth form that differs from both yeast cells and parallel-sided hyphae and are characterized by synchronously dividing elongated yeast cells (5, 7, 41, 42). Although pseudohyphal forms are generated by a wide range of *Candida* species, we know little about the immune response to pseudohyphal cells.

It is therefore important to understand the consequences of cellular morphogenesis of *C. albicans* on immune recognition and the activation of inflammation. Here, we demonstrate that *C. albicans* hyphae stimulated lower levels of cytokine production from human PBMCs than did yeast cells, but did not suppress the immune response of yeast cells in trans. Pseudohyphae elicited intermediate cytokine profiles between those of yeast and hyphae and again did not suppress yeast-induced cytokines. We also demonstrate that cell wall mannosylation and certain hypha-specific cell wall proteins affect morphology-dependent recognition by PBMCs.

MATERIALS AND METHODS

Strains, Media, and Culture Conditions Inducing Cellular Morphogenesis

Strains used in this work are listed in Table S1 in Supplementary Material. Cells were maintained and propagated at 30°C in either Sabouraud broth [1% (w/v) mycological peptone, 4% (w/v) glucose] or YPD broth [1% (w/v) yeast extract, 2% (w/v) mycological peptone, 2% (w/v) glucose]. The immune reposes to hyphae induced by multiple independent growth conditions were compared. Hyphae were generated using multiple independent methods: (i) 20% (v/v) fetal calf serum (FCS) or in RPMI 1640 supplemented with 2.5% (v/v) FCS, (ii) in YPD broth supplemented with 20% (v/v) FCS, (iii) in SC broth [0.68% (w/v) yeast nitrogen base without amino acids, 0.074% (w/v) amino acids buffered with 0.378% (w/v) PIPES] supplemented with 0.012% (w/v) fresh *N*-acetylglucosamine (GlcNAc), or (iv) in Lee's medium (43). Cultures were collected for use when greater 90–95% filamentation was obtained (typically after 3.5 h of incubation at 37°C). Hyphae were then washed twice in PBS and stored frozen at −20°C until used in cytokine induction experiments.

C. albicans pseudohyphae were produced using conditions published previously with modifications (41). Overnight cultures of *C. albicans* were collected by centrifugation, washed twice with 0.15 M NaCl, resuspended in 0.15 M NaCl, and incubated at room temperature for 24 h to induce starvation. After 24-h starvation, cells were inoculated into RPMI 1640 at a final concentration of 1×10^6 cells/ml and incubated at 25, 30, or 37°C with shaking for 6 h. Under these conditions, the vegetative morphology could be regulated by growth temperature alone, with yeast cells formed at 25°C, pseudohyphae at 30°C, and true hyphae at 37°C. Heat-killed (HK) cells were prepared after incubation at 56°C for 1 h, with killing verified by plating on YPD.

Samples of cells were fixed in 5% (v/v) formalin for morphological and microscopical analyses. All photomicrographs were taken on an Olympus BX50 outfitted with an Infinity 1 digital camera. Morphology indices, which are a measure of the extent of cellular elongation and hence discrimination of constricted pseudohyphae from parallel-sided hyphae, were determined as published (41). All measurements were made using the measurement tool in ImageJ 1.47v (http://imagej.nih.gov/ij), and MIs were calculated in Microsoft Excel.

Calculation of the Surface Area (SA) of Fungal Cells

The SA of all cells was based on microscopical measurements made from DIC images using a Zeiss Axioplan 2 microscope and captured by a Hamamatsu C4742-95 digital camera (Hamamatsu Photonics, Hamamatsu, Japan). All measurements created by ImageJ were exported in Microsoft Excel. The SA of yeast cells was calculated based on measurements of the radius calculated from the average of the largest and smallest cell diameters of yeast cells ($4\pi r^2$). Germ tube SA was taken as the SA of the mother yeast plus the SA of the daughter germ tube (true hypha). Hypha SA based on SA ($2\pi r^2 + 2\pi rl$) where the germ tube length (l) was measured from the base of the mother cell and the germ tube diameter was the average of the narrowest and widest diameter measurements made along each germ tube. At least 50 measurements, and 3–4 biological replicates, of SA of individual yeast and hyphal cells grown were made.

Cytokine Stimulation Assays

Blood samples were collected from healthy volunteers according to local guidelines and regulations, as approved by the College Ethics Review Board of the University of Aberdeen (CERB/2012/11/676). The PBMCs were used in this study and isolated using Ficoll-Paque™ PLUS (GE Healthcare) as previously described (44), with slight modifications. Unless otherwise indicated, 5×10^5 PBMCs in 100 μl were incubated in a round-bottom 96-well plate (Nunc) with 100 μl of fungal cells at 1×10^6 cells/ml. After incubation for 24 h at 37°C under 5% (v/v) CO_2, plates were centrifuged at 1,000 *g* for 10 min at room temperature, and supernatants were saved and kept at −20°C until use. For cytokine assays using mixed *C. albicans* cell types, PBMCs were first preincubated with 50 μl of cells of one morphology at 2×10^6 cells/ml for 1 h at 37°C under 5% (v/v) CO_2. Subsequently, 50 μl of a sample containing a second sample of yeast or hyphae cells at 2×10^6 cells/ml were added to PBMCs. Plates were then incubated for a further 24 h at 37°C, before supernatant collection and assay of induced cytokines. In experiments with PBMCs, the inoculum of hyphal cells was more or less aggregated. To assess the effect of cell aggregates on the cytokine stimulation, control experiments where hyphae were dispersed by ultrasonication before interaction with immune cells were performed, but theses did not show any significant differences with cultures of non-sonicated cells (data not shown). Therefore, steric blocking of monocyte access to fungal material did not explain the reduced response to hyphae that was observed.

TNFα, IL-1α, IL-1β, IL-6, and IL-10 concentrations were determined from coculture supernatants. For IL-1α quantification, stimulated PBMCs were disrupted by three sequential temperature shock cycles, and homogenates used for cytokine determination. All cytokine concentrations were determined using enzyme-linked immunosorbent assays (R&D Systems) according to the manufacturer's instructions.

Cell Wall Extraction and Analysis

C. albicans cells of different morphology were prepared as described above. Cells were collected by low-speed centrifugation and washed with ultrapure water, then broken using glass beads and a FastPrep machine (Qbiogene), homogenates were centrifuged at 13,000 *g* for 3 min, and pellets, containing the cell debris and walls, were washed five times with 1 M NaCl, resuspended in cell wall extraction buffer [50 mM Tris-HCl buffer pH 7.5, 2% (w/v) SDS, 0.3 M β-mercaptoethanol, and 1 mM EDTA], then boiled for 10 min, and washed three times with ultrapure water. Cell walls were freeze dried and stored at −20°C until used. The β-glucan, mannan, and chitin contents of cell wall preparations were determined by acid hydrolysis of the polymers and quantification of glucose, mannose, and glucosamine. Freeze-dried cell walls were hydrolyzed with 2 M trifluoroacetic acid as described previously (45), and acid hydrolyzates were analyzed by HPAEC-PAD (high-performance anion-exchange chromatography with pulsed amperometric detection) (46).

hPBMC Cell Damage Assay

Human PBMC damage was assessed by lactate dehydrogenase (LDH) released into the supernatant in the culture medium. After 24 h stimulation with *C. albicans* either heat-killed yeast (HKY) or HKH over a range of MOIs (*Candida* cells:hPBMCs) from 0.002:1 to 2:1. The LDH release was determined using the cytotoxicity detection kit (Roche Applied Science), according to the manufacturer's instructions. As a negative control for LDH release, 5×10^5 cells of hPBMCs were incubated with only the cell culture medium and incubated at 37°C with 5% CO_2 for 24 h. For the positive control maximum LDH release, 5×10^5 cells of hPBMCs was obtained by treatment with 2% Triton X-100 and incubated under the same conditions. The percentage of LDH release was calculated relative to the value for 100% cell death.

Statistical Analyses

The Mann–Whitney *U* test, *t*-test, or one-way ANOVA with a Dunnett's *post hoc* test in an appropriate parameter was used to analyze data. Results are presented as means ± SDs or SEMs and levels of significance determined at $p < 0.05$.

RESULTS

Differential Cytokine Induction by Yeast and Filamentous Cell Types

We used the cytokine response of human PBMCs as a read out to investigate the role of *C. albicans* morphogenesis on immune recognition. The cytokine profile of human PBMCs was compared when these immune cells were exposed to yeast cells and filamentous forms (true hyphae and pseudohyphae) of *C. albicans*. Yeast, pseudohyphal, and hyphal cells could all be induced *in vitro* using various culture conditions that preferentially stimulated a specific *C. albicans* cell morphology. Live and HK cells of different cell morphologies were also analyzed in our study. Across a wide range of conditions, heat killing increased the total amount of TNFα and other cytokines induced by yeast cells, and to a lesser extent, filamentous cells (**Figure 1**), suggesting that heat-treatment unmasks cytokine inducing PAMPs due to thermal disruption of components of the outer layer of the cell wall, thus exposing internal cytokine inductive cell layers to PRRs found on the surface of human PBMCs.

Under the conditions employed, more than 99% of yeast cells were obtained at 25°C and more than 94% of hyphae with at least two cell compartments were generated at 37°C (data not shown). Cell for cell, HK yeast cells induced significantly more TNFα than hyphal cells (**Figure 1A**). Germ tubes/hyphae induced less TNFα despite the presence of the parent yeast cell, implying that hypha formation may suppress TNFα production that would be normally associated with the cell surface of HK yeast cells (**Figures 1A–C** and **3**).

TNFα production induced by *C. albicans* was dose dependent (**Figure 1B**). Live yeast cells stimulated lower cytokine production compared to HK yeast cells—a difference that was less apparent when comparing live and HK true hyphal cells (**Figure 1B**). Both live and HK hyphae stimulated poor TNFα production compared to that of HK yeast cells (**Figures 1B,C**). In addition, LDH activity

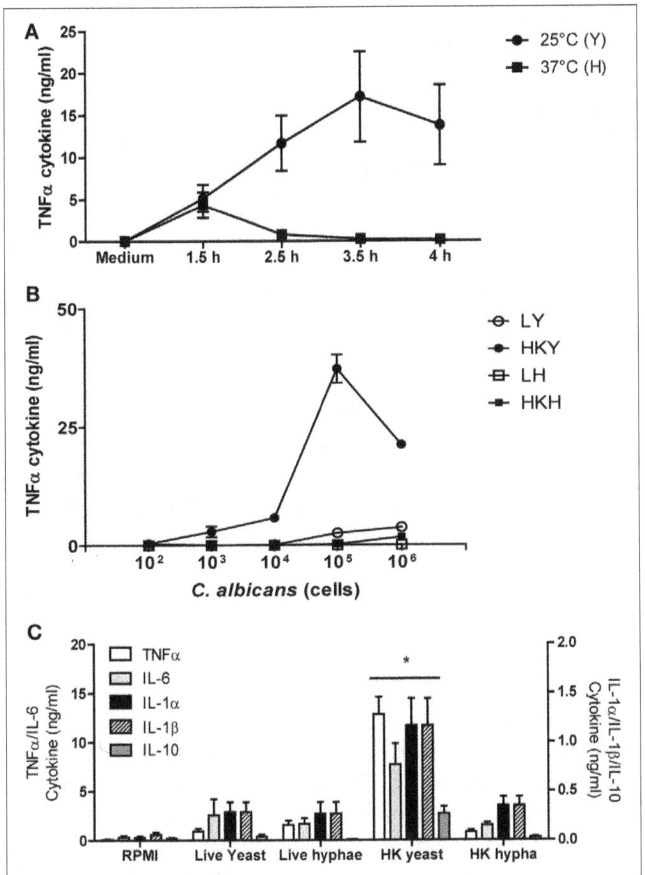

FIGURE 1 | TNFα stimulation with *Candida albicans* yeast and hyphal cells by human peripheral blood mononuclear cells (PBMCs). **(A)** Cytokine production by human PBMCs stimulated with yeasts cells (Y) of *C. albicans* NGY152 grown at 25°C (closed circles) or hyphae (H) grown at 37°C (closed squares) in RPMI 1640 + 2.5% fetal calf serum (FCS). Error bars = SEM ($n = 3$). **(B)** Dose-dependent stimulation of TNFα production by human PBMCs when stimulated with different forms of *C. albicans* NGY152 grown in RPMI 1640 + 2.5% FCS. Heat-killed yeasts (HKY), closed circles; live yeasts (LY), open circles; HK hyphae (HKH), closed squares; live hyphae (LH), open squares. Error bars = SEM ($n = 6$). In these experiments, a total of 5×10^5 PBMCs were used in each treatment and so the MOI varied from 0.0002:1 to 2:1. **(C)** Cytokine production by human PBMCs stimulated with the different morphological forms of *C. albicans* NGY152. In each treatment, an inoculum of 1×10^6 cells/ml was used. Results are means ± SEM ($n = 6$; $^*p < 0.05$).

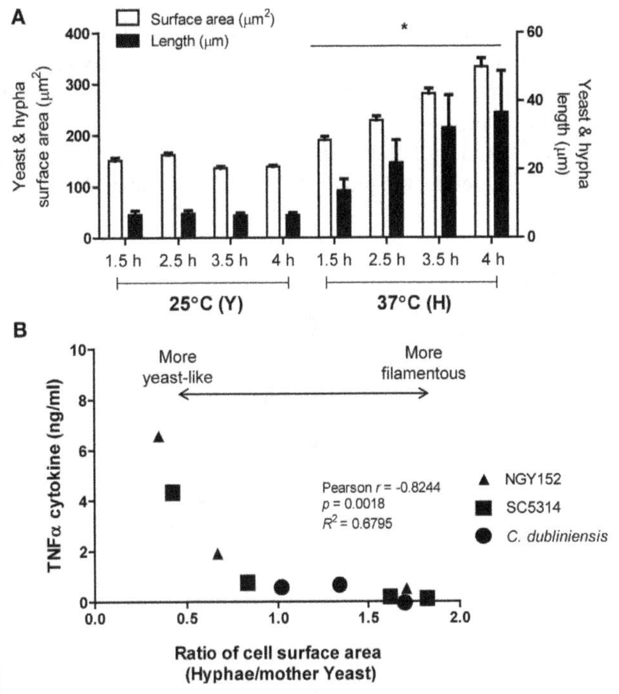

FIGURE 2 | Cell surface area (SA) of hyphal forming cells negatively correlated with TNFα stimulation. **(A)** Cell SA and cell size of *Candida albicans* SC5314 yeast (Y) or hyphae (H) grown at either 25 or 37°C for 1.5, 2.5, 3.5, and 4 h ($^*p < 0.05$). Error bars are SEM ($n > 50$ individual cells). **(B)** Relationship between TNFα production and extent of cell elongation expressed as the ratio of the hyphal cell area and the mother yeast cell area for *C. albicans* SC5314 and NGY152, and *Candida dubliniensis* CD36.

released into the supernatant was measured after 24 h stimulation with *C. albicans* HKY or HKH. There was no significant difference between *C. albicans* stimulated and non-stimulated hPBMCs (Figure S1 in Supplementary Material). Therefore, although TNFα production by hPBMCs incubated with 1×10^6 cells of HKY was significantly reduced, this was not due a loss of viability of hPBMCs. Similar results were obtained for a range of other cytokines, including IL-1α, IL-1β, IL-6, and IL-10 (**Figure 1C**).

We next investigated how hypha cell SA correlated with TNFα production by human PBMCs. Cell SA and cell size (diameter or length) of *C. albicans* yeast and hyphae were calculated assuming yeast cells were elliptical spheres, and germ tubes were parallel-sided cylinders. The size and SA of yeast plus associated germ tubes cells grown at 25 and 37°C are shown in **Figure 2A**. SA and length of hyphae increased by time. Under these conditions (at 3.5 h) of growth, yeasts had a mean diameter of 6.6 ± 0.1 μm (mean ± SEM) and mean SA of 136 ± 3.1 μm², respectively (**Figure 2A**). Hyphae had approximately twofold increased SA and were fivefold longer than the yeast cell diameter at the time cells were harvested. These values are comparable with those in previous reports (47). The average growth rate of hyphae grown in RPMI1640 plus 2.5% serum was 9.0 ± 1.1 μm/h. For *C. albicans* strains SC5314, NGY152, and the hypha-forming species *Candida dubliniensis* (strain CD36), there was a negative correlation between hypha to yeast cell surface ratio and TNFα production by human PBMCs (**Figure 2B**). Longer hyphae induced progressively less TNFα production per unit of cell surface (data not shown). We conclude that hyphae induce less TNFα than yeast cells and that the hypha surface may in some way suppress TNFα production by the cell wall of the attached parent yeast cell or that the yeast cell wall may be modified during the process of germ tube formation, so that it becomes less inductive of cytokine formation.

Hypha Formation and Cytokine Induction by Human PBMCs

In order to confirm whether this observation was indeed related to cell morphology rather than the growth conditions used to generate yeast and hyphae, we compared the immune response of hyphae generated in different growth media. Live and HK hyphae generated in either YPD medium supplement with FCS, Lee's medium, minimal medium (SC) added with GlcNAc, or in dilute FCS, were universally poorer inducers of TNFα, IL-1α, IL-1β, IL-6, and IL-10 (Table S1 in Supplementary Material) than yeast cells. Therefore, the reduced ability of *C. albicans* hyphae to stimulate cytokine production was independent of the hyphal-inducing growth conditions used.

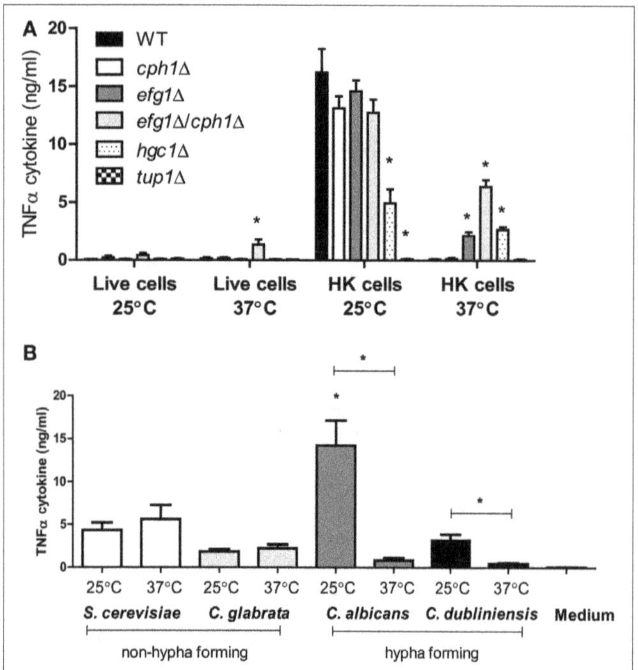

FIGURE 3 | TNFα production by human peripheral blood mononuclear cells stimulated with morphological mutants of *Candida albicans* mutants or other yeast species. (A) *C. albicans* NGY152 (WT), JKC19 (*cph1*Δ), HLC52 (*efg1*Δ), HLC54 (*cph1*Δ/*efg1*Δ), WYZ12.2 (*hgc1*Δ), and Bca2-10 (*tup1*Δ). Results are means ± SEM ($n = 6$; $^*p < 0.05$). **(B)** TNFα stimulation by non-hypha-forming species *Saccharomyces cerevisiae* (S288C) and *Candida glabrata* (ATCC 2001) compared to hypha-forming species *C. albicans* (NGY152) and *Candida dubliniensis* (CD36) ($^*p < 0.05$). Error bars = SEM ($n = 9$).

Next, we investigated the TNFα simulation by yeast cells of *Candida glabrata* and *Saccharomyces cerevisiae* (48), which, unlike *C. albicans* and *C. dubliniensis*, are not able to form hyphae or pseudohyphae. Yeast cells of *S. cerevisiae*, *C. glabrata*, and *C. dubliniensis* stimulated comparable levels of TNFα cytokine when grown at 25 and 37°C (**Figure 3B**). *C. dubliniensis* yeast cells induced less TNFα than *C. albicans*, when grown at 25°C. However, as with *C. albicans*, *C. dubliniensis* yeast grown at 25°C induced more cytokine than hyphae grown at 37°C. Therefore, the hyphae of both *C. albicans* and *C. dubliniensis* stimulated less TNFα than the respective yeast form.

We then assessed the ability of various mutants that regulate morphogenesis to stimulate cytokine production. The *cph1*Δ mutant was still able to form hyphae under the experimental conditions used (93% hypha production), and these cells did not stimulate a high level of TNFα by human PBMCs (**Figure 3A**). In comparison, the *efg1*Δ mutant mainly produced pseudohyphae (more than 90%) and stimulated only about 15% of TNFα of the control HK wild-type yeast cells. The *cph1*Δ/*efg1*Δ double mutant was unable to form hyphae at 37°C and stimulated significantly higher amounts of TNFα at 37°C than the hyphal wild-type parent (**Figure 3A**). Another yeast-locked *hgc1*Δ mutant also induced higher levels of TNFα at 37°C, although surprisingly this was also reduced at 25°C, indicating that Hgc1 influences TNFα stimulation in human PBMCs for both yeast and hyphae. By contrast, the pseudohypha-locked *tup1*Δ mutant stimulated a poor cytokine production at both 25 and 37°C (**Figure 3A**). Similar results for TNFα were observed for IL-1α, IL-1β, IL-6, and IL-10 (data not shown).

Next, we investigated the apparent ability of the germ tube to inhibit the ability of the mother yeast cells to stimulate TNFα cytokine production. PBMCs were pretreated with live or HK yeast or hyphae for 1 h, then a second stimulus of the same or another morphotype was added. PBMCs preincubated with HK yeast cells and then stimulated with either live or HK hyphae were not compromised in their ability to produce TNFα (**Figure 4**). Reciprocally when HK hyphae were preincubated with PBMCs

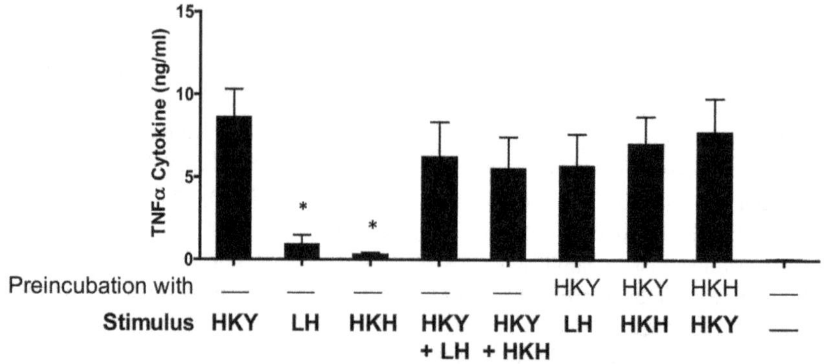

FIGURE 4 | Stimulation of cytokine production by human peripheral blood mononuclear cells (PBMCs) interacting with *Candida albicans* yeast cells and hyphae. Human PBMCs in RPMI 1640 were preincubated 1 h with either *C. albicans* NGY152 yeast cells or hyphae and then stimulated with a second cell type for 24 h. HKY, heat-killed yeast; LH, live hyphae; HKH, heat-killed hyphae ($^*p < 0.05$; $n = 12$).

and then stimulated with HK yeast cells, there was a no significant reduction in the cytokine response (**Figure 4**). When yeast cells and hyphae were mixed together in a ratio 1:1, there was a strong cytokine production comparable to that elicited with HK yeast cells alone. Therefore, germ tubes with an attached parent yeast cell did not induce a response that would normally be associated with free yeast cells; however, hyphae did not block cytokine stimulation by yeast cells presented in trans.

The possibility that *C. albicans* reduced cytokine production by hyphae was due to blocking receptors on immune cells was tested by coincubating hyphal cells with various TLR ligands including Pam_3CSk_4, LPS, zymosan, flagellin, and curdlan. However, *C. albicans* hyphae did not block nor reduce TNFα, IL-1β, or IL-1α stimulated by these TLRs ligands used (Figure S2 in Supplementary Material).

Cell Wall Composition and the Immune Response

The fungal cell wall contains most of the PAMPs recognized by the innate immune cells (4, 11). Thus, we next assessed the ability of yeast and hyphal cells with specific cell wall defects to stimulate cytokine production by human PBMCs. A *chs3Δ* null mutant with a low chitin content at the cell wall (49), and a *mnn4Δ* mutant (50) lacking cell wall mannosylphosphate, were unaffected in the PBMC-induced cytokine production, compared to wild-type control cells (**Figure 5A**). A *pmr1Δ* mutant (51), which is deficient in yeast and hyphal cell wall *N*- and *O*-linked mannan, induced a reduced cytokine response by HK yeast cells, but an increased cytokines response from live and HK hyphae. This suggests that for yeast cells the lack of mannan reduced the overall immune response, while in hyphae the major effect of mannan depletion was to reveal subsurface immunostimulatory ligands such as β-glucan. In the *O*-mannosylation *mnt1/mnt2Δ* mutant (52), and the core *N*-mannan *mns1Δ* mutant (45) the secretion of most cytokines was enhanced or not affected in yeast or hyphal cells. IL-1α secretion from monocytes was enhanced to the greatest extend in the *pmr1Δ*, *mnt1/mnt2Δ*, and *mns1Δ* mutants in both yeast and hyphal cells (**Figure 5B**).

We compared the cytokine levels produced by a number of mutants that lacked hypha-associated cell wall proteins including *als3Δ* (53), *hwp1Δ* (54), *hyr1Δ* (55), and *ece1Δ* (56) with those stimulated with wild-type control cells. Only the *hwp1Δ* HK mutant hyphae stimulated a higher cytokine production than wild-type control cells (**Figure 5C**). Unexpectedly, despite the hypha-specific expression pattern for *HYR1* (55), the *hyr1Δ* mutant yeast cells stimulated a slightly reduced cytokine response from human PBMCs compared to wild-type control cells (**Figure 5C**). The *hwp1Δ* mutant showed no significant differences in mannan, glucan, and chitin content of the cell wall, when compared to wild-type control cells in both morphologies (**Table 1**), suggesting that this proteins may act in masking cytokine stimulating PAMPs in the cell wall. By contrast, yeast and hyphal cells of the *mns1Δ* and *pmr1Δ* mutants displayed a significant reduction in cell wall mannan and increased levels of glucan (**Table 1**). Therefore, cell wall mannosylation and the presence of Hwp1 were important for the reduced ability of hyphae of *C. albicans* to induce cytokines by human PBMCs.

We also tested the effect of deletion of the yeast-specific gene *PGA29* on cytokine production by human PBMCs and noted that this HK mutant induced less TNFα under conditions of yeast growth (Figure S3 in Supplementary Material). The reconstituted heterozygous *pga29/PGA29* mutant restored the TNFα induction to normal levels. Therefore, morphology-specific cell wall proteins of both yeast and hyphae influenced immune recognition.

C. albicans Pseudohyphae Stimulate Intermediate Cytokine Levels from Human PBMCs

We then examined the ability of pseudohyphae to induce cytokine production. We deployed a method in which changes in temperature alone could generate yeast cells, pseudohyphae, or hyphae (41, 57). When *C. albicans* NGY152 was grown in RPMI 1640 medium at a neutral pH and at 30°C for 6 h (**Figure 6A**), it reproducibly resulted in a largely pseudohyphal population (~90%). For this strain, growth at 25°C yielded yeast cells (MI = 0.65 ± 0.06, mean ± SEM), 30°C yielded pseudohyphae (MI = 2.34 ± 0.19), and 37°C yielded hyphal forms (MI = 8.65 ± 0.73) (**Figure 6B**).

Next, we investigated cytokine production of human PBMCs stimulated with pseudohyphae in comparison to yeast and hyphae. In a range of experiments pseudohyphal cell populations generated reproducibly intermediate levels of TNFα and other cytokines from live and HK cells, although the differences were not always significant at $p < 0.05$ and the level of significance varied depending on whether the average MI of a given population of pseudohyphae was sufficiently distinct from that of populations of yeast cells or hyphae (**Figures 6A–D**). There was a statistically significant correlation between the level of TNFα and IL-1β cytokine from PBMCs and the MI of *C. alb*icans cells inducing these cytokines (**Figure 6E**).

DISCUSSION

Multiple independent studies have proposed a positive correlation between the formation of *C. albicans* hyphae and an enhanced capacity for tissue invasion, damage, and virulence (6, 33, 39). However, the significance of *C. albicans* morphogenesis on the innate immune response has not been fully characterized. Here, the interaction of yeasts, pseudohyphae, and hyphae of this fungus with cells of the human innate immune system was investigated using cytokine production by human PBMCs as an immunoassay readout. We demonstrate that yeast cells generated more inflammatory cytokines from PBMCs than hyphae, and that pseudohyphae generated intermediate cytokine levels. These differences were observed in independent strains for cells generated in different growth media. Heat killing of cells has been used frequently in immunological studies of *C. albicans* to prevent cells undergoing filamentation in response to serum components of cell culture media when exposing *Candida* to immune cells during cytokine induction assays (58, 59). HK cells had enhanced immune responses, which has been interpreted as being due to heat-induced permeabilization of the cell wall and subsequent exposure of the underlying β1,3-glucan layer, which is strongly immunogenic (18). Our data support this hypothesis and suggest that HK cells generate a greater cytokine signal because more

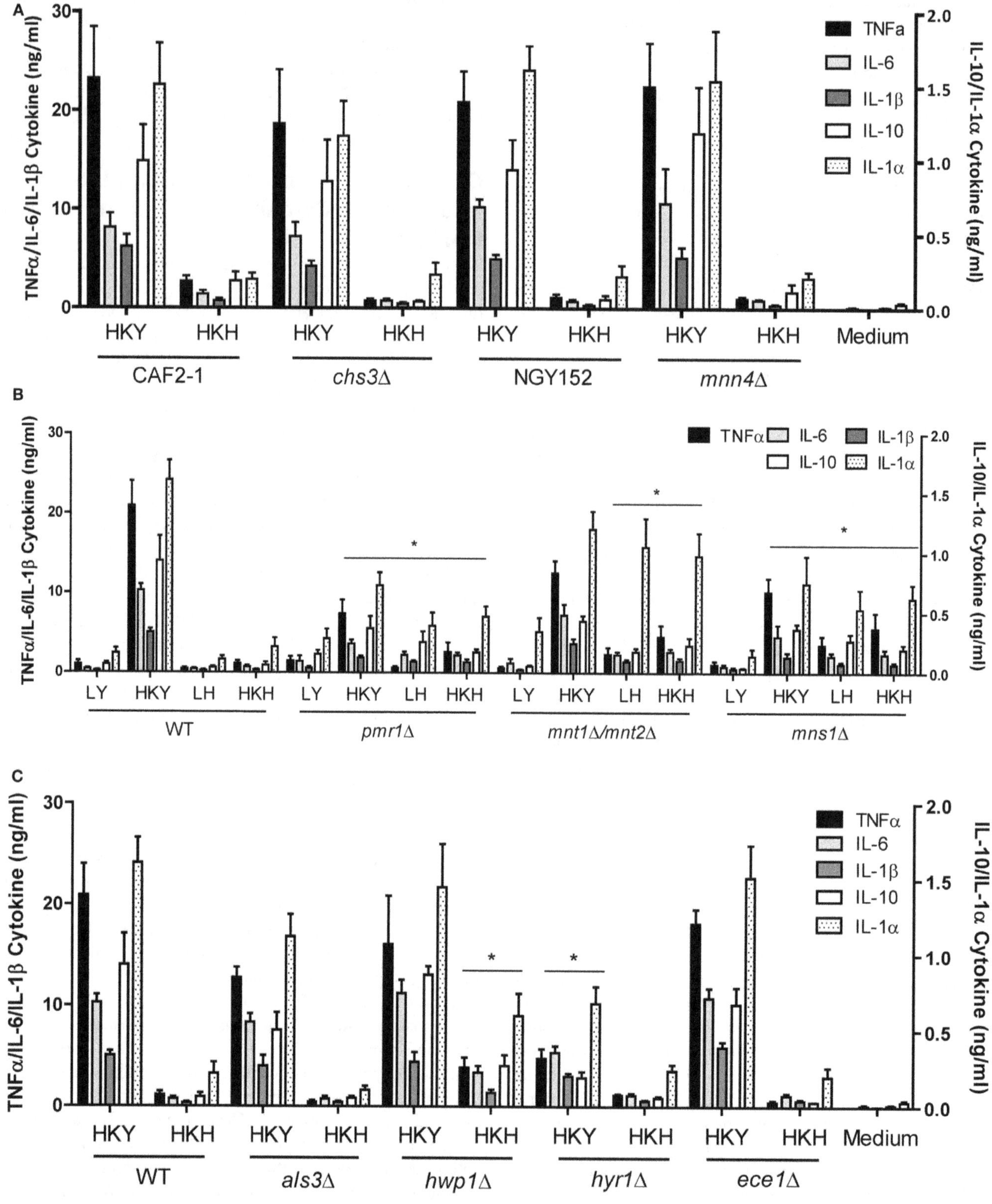

FIGURE 5 | Cytokine production stimulated by cell wall mutants of yeast and hyphal cells. (A) Cytokine production stimulated by human PBMCs with LY—live yeast; HKY—heat-killed yeast; LH—live hyphae; HKH—heat-killed hyphae; *Candida albicans mnn4*Δ and *chs3*Δ and control strains, NGY152 and CAF2-1. **(B)** Cytokine stimulation with mannosylation defective mutants, *pmr1*Δ, *mnt1*Δ/*mnt2*Δ, and *mns1*Δ. **(C)** *als3*Δ, *hwp1*Δ, *hyr1*Δ, and *ece1*Δ. Results presented as mean ± SEM (n = 6), and the asterisks indicate comparison of the wild-type values and the mutant strains (*$p < 0.05$).

TABLE 1 | Cell wall composition of *Candida albicans* strains.

Strain	Glucosamine	Glucose	Mannose
Yeast morphology			
WT	1.01 ± 0.4	58.31 ± 2.25	40.68 ± 2.19
hwp1Δ	0.77 ± 0.46	52.99 ± 0.77*	46.24 ± 0.34*
mns1Δ	0.91 ± 1.18	88.71 ± 2.34*	10.38 ± 0.96*
pmr1Δ	1.50 ± 2.05	99.55 ± 3.63*	0.50 ± 1.33*
Hypha morphology			
WT	4.77 ± 0.32#	87.18 ± 1.54#	8.06 ± 0.99#
hwp1Δ	5.63 ± 0.93#	83.68 ± 2.57#	10.68 ± 1.75#
mns1Δ	6.10 ± 1.34#	87.61 ± 1.59	6.29 ± 0.18#
pmr1Δ	1.48 ± 0.74*	97.72 ± 2.01*	0.80 ± 0.68*,#

*Means ± SD (n = 3) *p < 0.05 when comparing the mutant strain with the wild-type control cells.*
#p < 0.05 when comparing hyphae with yeast cells.

PAMPs can engage collaboratively with PRRs, thus resulting in coreceptor amplification of the cytokine response (18, 60–62).

Although the hyphae used in these experiments also had a parental yeast cell, the combined cytokine signal due to the hypha plus parent yeast cell was significantly less than that expected from the yeast cell alone. This may suggest that either the yeast cell surface of germ tube matures to become different from that of a free yeast cell or that an unknown mechanism operates in germ tubes that are able to block cytokine induction due to the mother yeast cell. However, if a blocking signal is present, it does not operate in "trans" since hyphae added after free yeast cells were used to stimulate PBMCs did not interfere with the ensuing yeast cell stimulated cytokine response. Interestingly, hyphae of *C. dubliniensis* also stimulated less cytokine from PBMCs than yeast cells. The genomes of *C. albicans* and *C. dubliniensis* are 95% identical, and the cell walls are also thought to be of similar composition, although there are notable differences in the cell wall proteome (63). These closely related *Candida* species therefore show both common aspects and some differences in the nature of the immune response to yeast and hyphal cells.

Different immune cell types respond differently to *C. albicans* yeast and hyphae. For example, *C. albicans* hyphae induce higher levels of TNFα than yeast cells in macrophages (64, 65), while yeast and hyphae stimulate comparable levels of IL-8 cytokine by human neutrophils (47). It was shown that *C. albicans* induced different cytokine responses from oral and vaginal epithelial cells, and that hyphae induced higher cytokine levels than yeast cells in both epithelial cell types (32, 66). However, our findings reinforce previous studies where *C. albicans* filaments (hyphae and pseudohyphae) were reported to stimulate the production of less IL-12, IFN-γ, IL-1β, and IL-12p70 by human PBMCs and murine splenic lymphocytes than *C. albicans* yeast cells (30, 58, 67–69). It was also previously reported that TLR4-mediated pro-inflammatory signals were diminished during the germination of *C. albicans* yeast cells into hyphae (30). Supporting this, we show that *C. albicans* cells grown at 37°C have a progressively reduced TNFα cytokine response. In addition, it was reported that *C. albicans* hyphal cell walls also stimulated less chemokines than yeast cell walls (68), and it was suggested that this may be due to surface expression of β1,6-glucan being lower on hyphae compared to yeast cells. The cell SA of each individual hyphal compartment is larger than that of a yeast cell, and hyphae have no bud scars where inner wall layers are exposed (29). Therefore, it is possible that the density of certain immune agonists is less concentrated on the hyphal surface than on yeast cells. Also, progressive elongation of hyphae *in vivo* has been shown to result in increasing exposures of β1,3-glucan (70). Hence, cellular morphogenesis leading to filamentous growth of *C. albicans* leads to important progressive modifications of cell wall composition and architecture that has profound and differing effects on the immune response.

Cell wall polysaccharide analysis showed that yeast cell walls contained significantly higher amounts of mannan but lower amounts chitin and glucan compared to that of hyphal cell walls (**Table 1**). The reduction of mannan and increase in chitin content of hyphal cell walls might also be related to the lower cytokine responses to *C. albicans* hyphae (28, 45, 71, 72). Our results underline the importance of *N*- and *O*-linked mannans in the recognition of *C. albicans* hyphae by human PBMCs (**Figure 5**) since *N*- and *O*-mannan mutants (45, 52), but not chitin and phosphomannan mutants, stimulated the production of higher levels of cytokines that wild-type hyphae.

Although the primary polysaccharides in the cell wall are likely to have a major influence on immune recognition, it was noted that a HK *hwp1Δ* cell wall protein deletion mutant induced an increased cytokine signal, despite having no measurable alteration in hyphal mannan or glucan content. Similarly, a mutant lacking *MNS1* grown under hyphal-inducing conditions showed insignificant changes in cell wall components, but substantial reduction in cytokine production. However, the *mns1* yeast cells had 34% increased glucan as a compensation of 70% reduction in mannan, and a reduced cytokine profile. Therefore, there was no direct or universal correlation between cytokine induction and gross cell wall polysaccharide composition.

Our observations suggest that surface proteins, polysaccharides, and virulence factors are regulated or modified during filamentous growth resulting in changes in the immune response. Such changes in the incorporation of surface cell wall proteins on cells of different morphology could mask or unmask PAMPs, thereby blocking or promoting PRR engagement.

The presence of *C. albicans* hyphae could potentially compete with yeast cells for the ability to bind PRRs and stimulate immune cells. This would be important if specific yeast cell wall proteins are important for immune recognition and activation. We observed that a *pga29* mutant grown in the yeast form stimulated less TNFα from human PBMCs. This cell wall protein Pga29 has homologs in several pathogenic *Candida* spp. and is abundant in yeast cell walls in *C. albicans* but not in hyphae (73). Deletion of *PGA29* resulted in decreased glucan–mannan in the cell wall, and reduction of TNFα, IL-6, and IL-8 stimulated by oral reconstituted human epithelial cells (74). Therefore, both yeast and hypha-specific cell wall proteins may directly modulate immune responses.

It is also possible that *C. albicans* hyphal cells may produce secreted molecules that suppress immune recognition. Quorum-sensing molecules, such as farnesol, tyrosol, phenylethanol, and tryptophol, produced by *C. albicans*, play a key role in morphogenesis (75–77), and tyrosol acts negatively on cytokine production stimulated by RAW 264.7 macrophages induced

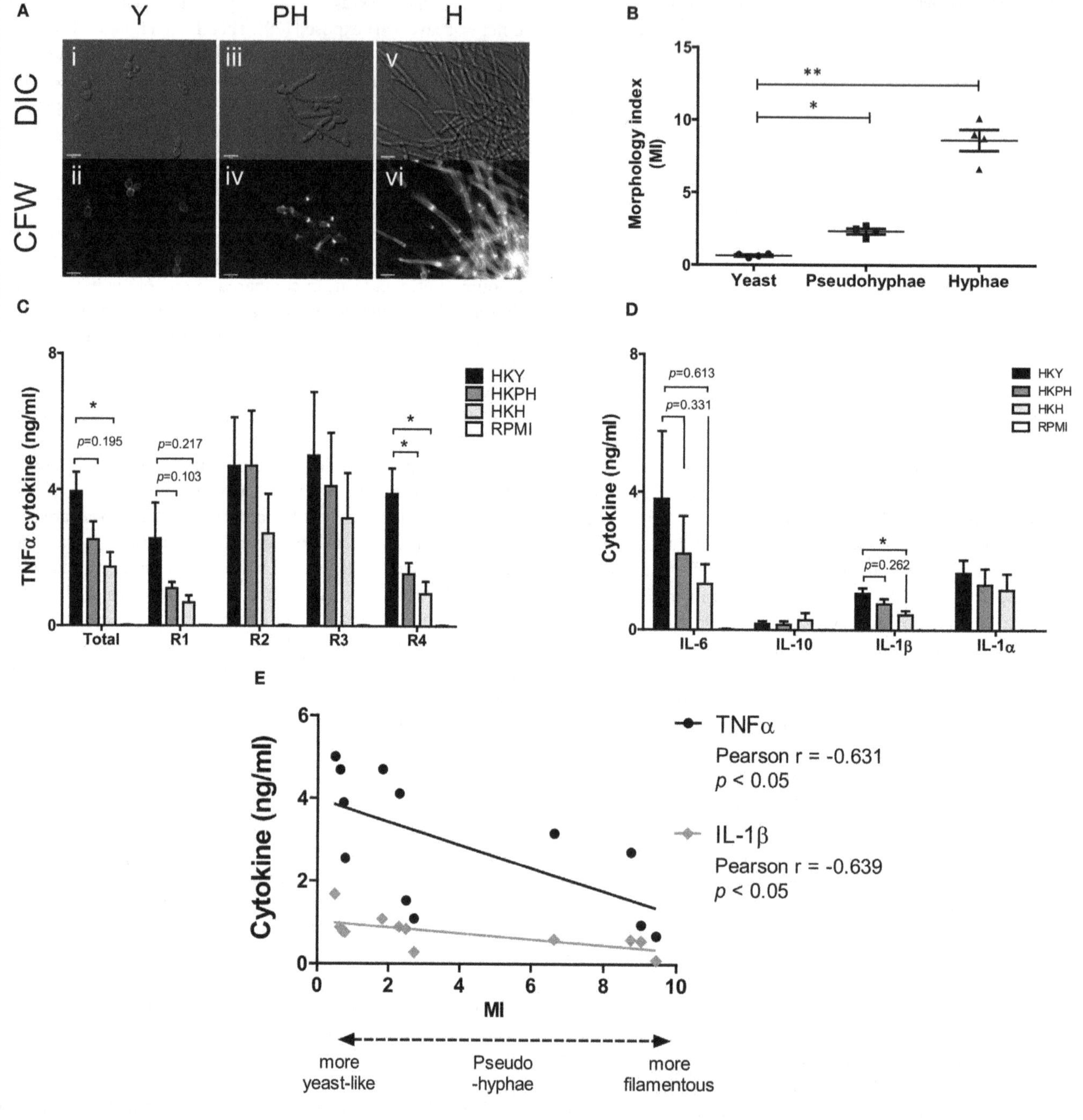

FIGURE 6 | Cytokine production by hPBMCs stimulated by different *Candida albicans* morphological forms. **(A)** Yeasts (i–ii), pseudohyphae (iii–iv), or hyphae (v–vi) of *C. albicans* NGY152 were grown in RPMI 1640 (pH 7) for 6 h at 25, 30, and 37°C, respectively, fixed, and stained with 25 μg/ml CFW to visualize the cell wall. Scale bars = 10 μm. **(B)** Morphological index (MI) of yeast, pseudohyphal, and hyphal cells was measured. Error bars are SEMs (averages from 50 cell measurements and 4 biological replicates) (*$p < 0.05$; **$p < 0.01$). **(C)** TNFα cytokine production elicited by human peripheral blood mononuclear cells (PBMCs) with HK NGY152 of yeast (Y), pseudohypha (PH), and hypha (H) cells. Each replicate (R1–R4) were averaged as total values. Data are means ± SEM ($n > 6$; *$p < 0.05$). **(D)** IL-6, IL-1β, IL-1α, and IL-10 cytokine production elicited by human PBMCs with HK of yeast (Y), pseudohypha (PH), and hypha (H) cells. Data are means ± SEM ($n > 6$; *$p < 0.05$). **(E)** Correlation between TNFα or IL-1β cytokine and MI. Results are Person *R* values ($n = 4$ biological replica).

by lipopolysaccharide (78). However, we showed that neither live nor HK hyphae could suppress yeast cell-induced cytokine production in trans; therefore, soluble factors were not suggested as playing a significant role in our experiments.

Our observations and those of previous studies (30, 58, 68, 69) demonstrate that *C. albicans* hyphae stimulated lower cytokine production by PBMCs than *C. albicans* yeast cells, thus indicating that *C. albicans* hyphae may help to evade or alter the host immune response. However, it is clear that *C. albicans* hyphae induced strong cytokine responses and caused more damage to epithelial cells, while yeast cells did not trigger cytokine responses (66, 79, 80). Also, *C. albicans* hyphae induce stronger cytokine responses that yeast cells from macrophages (64, 65). The common denominator of these various reports is that cellular morphogenesis plays an important role in determining the immune response to *C. albicans*, but the nature of this response is both host cell type specific and pathogen morphotype dependent. These data underline the perspective that *C. albicans* presents a moving target to the cells of the innate immune response.

AUTHOR CONTRIBUTIONS

LM and KL performed experiments. NG, HM-M, LM, and KL conceived and designed experiments and analyzed the data. NG and HM-M supervised the project. LM, KL, and NG contributed to writing of the manuscript. All the authors reviewed the manuscript.

ACKNOWLEDGMENTS

The authors thank Amy Whittington for preliminary experiments on *in vitro* induction of pseudohyphae and Mihai Netea for discussions. The authors also thank Michael Weig for the pga29 strains.

FUNDING

NG and AW were supported by the Wellcome Trust (086827, 075470, 097377, 101873, and 200208); the European Union ALLFUN (FP7/2007 2013, HEALTH-2010-260338), and the MRC Centre for Medical Mycology for funding (N006364/1). LM was supported by a SORSAS (Scottish Overseas Research Students Award Scheme) from the University of Aberdeen and Funding from the Rwandan Government.

SUPPLEMENTARY MATERIAL

FIGURE S1 | Cell damage assay of hPBMC stimulated with *Candida albicans*. Lactate dehydrogenase activity released from 5×10^5 hPBMCs into the culture medium was determined after 24 h stimulated with either *C. albicans* heat-killed yeast or HKH at the different number of cells from 1×10^2 to 1×10^6 cells. The result represented as a percentage relative to 100% cell death of hPBMCs when killed with 2% Triton-X-100. Error bars = SEM (n = 4).

FIGURE S2 | Cytokine production by hPBMCs stimulated by different *Candida albicans* coincubated with toll-like receptors (TLRs) ligands. Human peripheral blood mononuclear cells were stimulated using a mixture of *C. albicans* cells and TLRs ligands. Cells were either live (L) or heat-killed (HK), and yeast (Y) or hyphae (H). TLRs ligands used were flagellin (for TLR5), LPS (for TLR4), Pam_3CSK_4 (for TLR2/TLR1), zymosan, and curdlan (for Dectin-1). The cytokines measured were TNF-α **(A)**, IL-6 **(B)**, IL-1β **(C)**, IL-1α **(D)**, and IL-10 **(E)**. IL-10 was barely detectable and could not be evaluated. Data are means ± SEM ($n > 3$; $^*p < 0.05$). ND, not detectable.

FIGURE S3 | TNFα cytokine production by hPBMCs incubated with *Candida albicans* lacking *PGA29*. *C. albicans* cells lacking *PGA29* was grown in RPMI 1640 + 2.5% fetal calf serum at 25 or 37°C for 3.5 h. Cells were collected and heat killed. The mutant was incubated with hPBMCs for 24 h. Then, TNFα cytokine production was determined (see Methods and Materials). Data are means ± SEM (n > 9; $^*p < 0.05$; $^{***}p < 0.001$).

TABLE S1 | *C. albicans* and other fungal strains used in this study.

REFERENCES

1. Gudlaugsson O, Gillespie S, Lee K, Vande Berg J, Hu J, Messer S, et al. Attributable mortality of nosocomial candidemia, revisited. *Clin Infect Dis* (2003) 37:1172–7. doi:10.1086/378745
2. Pappas PG, Rex JH, Lee J, Hamill RJ, Larsen RA, Powderly W, et al. A prospective observational study of candidemia: epidemiology, therapy, and influences on mortality in hospitalized adult and pediatric patients. *Clin Infect Dis* (2003) 37:634–43. doi:10.1086/376906
3. Kullberg BJ, Arendrup MC. Invasive candidiasis. *N Engl J Med* (2015) 373:1445–56. doi:10.1056/NEJMra1315399
4. Erwig LP, Gow NAR. Interactions of fungal pathogens with phagocytes. *Nat Rev Microbiol* (2016) 14:163–76. doi:10.1038/nrmicro.2015.21
5. Sudbery PE, Gow NAR, Berman J. The distinct morphogenic states of *Candida albicans*. *Trends Microbiol* (2004) 12:317–24. doi:10.1016/j.tim.2004.05.008
6. Gow NAR, van de Veerdonk FL, Brown AJP, Netea MG. *Candida albicans* morphogenesis and host defence: discriminating invasion from colonization. *Nat Rev Microbiol* (2011) 10:112–22. doi:10.1038/nrmicro2711
7. Sudbery PE. Growth of *Candida albicans* hyphae. *Nat Rev Microbiol* (2011) 9:737–48. doi:10.1038/nrmicro2636
8. Gow NAR, Hube B. Importance of the *Candida albicans* cell wall during commensalism and infection. *Curr Opin Microbiol* (2012) 15:406–12. doi:10.1016/j.mib.2012.04.005
9. Kullberg BJ, Arendrup MC. Invasive candidiasis. *N Engl J Med* (2016) 374:793–5. doi:10.1056/NEJMc1514201
10. Sellam A, Whiteway M. Recent advances on *Candida albicans* biology and virulence. *F1000Res* (2016) 5:2582. doi:10.12688/f1000research.9617.1
11. Netea MG, Brown GD, Kullberg BJ, Gow NAR. An integrated model of the recognition of *Candida albicans* by the innate immune system. *Nat Rev Microbiol* (2008) 6:67–78. doi:10.1038/nrmicro1815
12. Hoebe K, Janssen E, Beutler B. The interface between innate and adaptive immunity. *Nat Immunol* (2004) 5:971–4. doi:10.1038/ni1004-971
13. Medzhitov R. Recognition of microorganisms and activation of the immune response. *Nature* (2007) 449:819–26. doi:10.1038/nature06246
14. Cheng SC, Joosten LA, Kullberg BJ, Netea MG. Interplay between *Candida albicans* and the mammalian innate host defense. *Infect Immun* (2012) 80:1304–13. doi:10.1128/IAI.06146-11
15. Netea MG, Joosten LA, van der Meer JW, Kullberg BJ, van de Veerdonk FL. Immune defence against *Candida* fungal infections. *Nat Rev Immunol* (2015) 15:630–42. doi:10.1038/nri3897
16. Gow NAR, Netea MG. Medical mycology and fungal immunology: new research perspectives addressing a major world health challenge. *Philos Trans R Soc Lond B Biol Sci* (2016) 371. doi:10.1098/rstb.2015.0462
17. Netea MG, Gow NAR, Munro CA, Bates S, Collins C, Ferwerda G, et al. Immune sensing of *Candida albicans* requires cooperative recognition of mannans and glucans by lectin and toll-like receptors. *J Clin Invest* (2006) 116:1642–50. doi:10.1172/JCI27114
18. Gow NAR, Netea MG, Munro CA, Ferwerda G, Bates S, Mora-Montes HM, et al. Immune recognition of *Candida albicans* beta-glucan by dectin-1. *J Infect Dis* (2007) 196:1565–71. doi:10.1086/523110

19. Cambi A, Netea MG, Mora-Montes HM, Gow NAR, Hato SV, Lowman DW, et al. Dendritic cell interaction with *Candida albicans* critically depends on *N*-linked mannan. *J Biol Chem* (2008) 283:20590–9. doi:10.1074/jbc.M709334200
20. Heinsbroek SEM, Taylor PR, Martinez FO, Martinez-Pomares L, Brown GD, Gordon S. Stage-specific sampling by pattern recognition receptors during *Candida albicans* phagocytosis. *PLoS Pathog* (2008) 4:e1000218. doi:10.1371/journal.ppat.1000218
21. McKenzie CGJ, Koser U, Lewis LE, Bain JM, Mora-Montes HM, Barker RN, et al. Contribution of *Candida albicans* cell wall components to recognition by and escape from murine macrophages. *Infect Immun* (2010) 78:1650–8. doi:10.1128/IAI.00001-10
22. Jouault T, El Abed-El Behi M, Martínez-Esparza M, Breuilh L, Trinel PA, Chamaillard M, et al. Specific recognition of *Candida albicans* by macrophages requires galectin-3 to discriminate *Saccharomyces cerevisiae* and needs association with TLR2 for signaling. *J Immunol* (2006) 177:4679–87. doi:10.4049/jimmunol.177.7.4679
23. Kohatsu L, Hsu DK, Jegalian AG, Liu FT, Baum LG. Galectin-3 induces death of *Candida* species expressing specific beta-1,2-linked mannans. *J Immunol* (2006) 177:4718–26. doi:10.4049/jimmunol.177.7.4718
24. Linden JR, De Paepe ME, Laforce-Nesbitt SS, Bliss JM. Galectin-3 plays an important role in protection against disseminated candidiasis. *Med Mycol* (2013) 51:641–51. doi:10.3109/13693786.2013.770607
25. Courjol F, Jouault T, Mille C, Hall R, Maes E, Sendid B, et al. Beta-1,2-mannosyltransferases 1 and 3 participate in yeast and hyphae *O*- and *N*-linked mannosylation and alter *Candida albicans* fitness during infection. *Open Forum Infect Dis* (2015) 2:ofv116. doi:10.1093/ofid/ofv116
26. Harris M, Mora-Montes HM, Gow NAR, Coote PJ. Loss of mannosylphosphate from *Candida albicans* cell wall proteins results in enhanced resistance to the inhibitory effect of a cationic antimicrobial peptide via reduced peptide binding to the cell surface. *Microbiology* (2009) 155:1058–70. doi:10.1099/mic.0.026120-0
27. Rubin-Bejerano I, Abeijon C, Magnelli P, Grisafi P, Fink GR. Phagocytosis by human neutrophils is stimulated by a unique fungal cell wall component. *Cell Host Microbe* (2007) 2:55–67. doi:10.1016/j.chom.2007.06.002
28. Wagener J, Malireddi RKS, Lenardon MD, Köberle M, Vautier S, MacCallum DM, et al. Fungal chitin dampens inflammation through IL-10 induction mediated by NOD2 and TLR9 activation. *PLoS Pathog* (2014) 10. doi:10.1371/journal.ppat.1004050
29. Gantner BN, Simmons RM, Underhill DM. Dectin-1 mediates macrophage recognition of *Candida albicans* yeast but not filaments. *EMBO J* (2005) 24:1277–86. doi:10.1038/sj.emboj.7600594
30. Van Der Graaf CAA, Netea MG, Verschueren I, Van Der Meer JWM, Kullberg BJ. Differential cytokine production and toll-like receptor signaling pathways by *Candida albicans* blastoconidia and hyphae. *Infect Immun* (2005) 73:7458–64. doi:10.1128/IAI.73.11.7458-7464.2005
31. Cheng SC, van de Veerdonk FL, Lenardon M, Stoffels M, Plantinga T, Smeekens S, et al. The dectin-1/inflammasome pathway is responsible for the induction of protective T-helper 17 responses that discriminate between yeasts and hyphae of *Candida albicans*. *J Leukoc Biol* (2011) 90:357–66. doi:10.1189/jlb.1210702
32. Moyes DL, Murciano C, Runglall M, Islam A, Thavaraj S, Naglik JR. *Candida albicans* yeast and hyphae are discriminated by MAPK signaling in vaginal epithelial cells. *PLoS One* (2011) 6:e26580. doi:10.1371/journal.pone.0026580
33. Lo HJ, Köhler JR, Didomenico B, Loebenberg D, Cacciapuoti A, Fink GR. Nonfilamentous *C. albicans* mutants are avirulent. *Cell* (1997) 90:939–49. doi:10.1016/S0092-8674(00)80358-X
34. Gow NAR, Brown AJP, Odds FC. Fungal morphogenesis and host invasion. *Curr Opin Microbiol* (2002) 5:366–71. doi:10.1016/S1369-5274(02)00338-7
35. Moyes DL, Wilson D, Richardson JP, Mogavero S, Tang SX, Wernecke J, et al. Candidalysin is a fungal peptide toxin critical for mucosal infection. *Nature* (2016) 532:64–8. doi:10.1038/nature17625
36. Ghannoum MA, Spellberg B, Saporito-Irwin SM, Fonzi WA. Reduced virulence of *Candida albicans PHR1* mutants. *Infect Immun* (1995) 63:4528–30.
37. Calera JA, Zhao XJ, Calderone R. Defective hyphal development and avirulence caused by a deletion of the *SSK1* response regulator gene in *Candida albicans*. *Infect Immun* (2000) 68:518–25. doi:10.1128/IAI.68.2.518-525.2000
38. Murad AMA, Leng P, Straffon M, Wishart J, Macaskill S, MacCallum D, et al. NRG1 represses yeast-hypha morphogenesis and hypha-specific gene expression in *Candida albicans*. *EMBO J* (2001) 20:4742–52. doi:10.1093/emboj/20.17.4742
39. Saville SP, Lazzell AL, Monteagudo C, Lopez-Ribot JL. Engineered control of cell morphology in vivo reveals distinct roles for yeast and filamentous forms of *Candida albicans* during infection. *Eukaryot Cell* (2003) 2:1053–60. doi:10.1128/EC.2.5.1053-1060.2003
40. Zheng X, Wang Y, Wang Y. Hgc1, a novel hypha-specific G1 cyclin-related protein regulates *Candida albicans* hyphal morphogenesis. *EMBO J* (2004) 23:1845–56. doi:10.1038/sj.emboj.7600195
41. Merson-Davies LA, Odds FC. A morphology index for characterization of cell shape in *Candida albicans*. *J Gen Microbiol* (1989) 135:3143–52.
42. Berman J, Gow NAR. Chapter 3. Cell cycle of fungal pathogens. In: San-Blas G, Calderone RA, editors. *Pathogenic Fungi: Structural Biology and Taxonomy*. Norfolk, UK: Caster Academic Press (2004). p. 101–25.
43. Lee KL, Buckley HR, Campbell CC. An amino acid liquid synthetic medium for the development of mycelial and yeast forms of *Candida albicans*. *Sabouraudia* (1975) 13:148–53. doi:10.1080/00362177585190271
44. Endres S, Ghorbani R, Lonnemann G, van der Meer JWM, Dinarello CA. Measurement of immunoreactive interleukin-1ß from human mononuclear cells: optimization of recovery, intrasubject consistency, and comparison with interleukin-1a and tumor necrosis factor. *Clin Immunol Immunopathol* (1988) 49:424–38. doi:10.1016/0090-1229(88)90130-4
45. Mora-Montes HM, Bates S, Netea MG, Diaz-Jimenez DF, Lopez-Romero E, Zinker S, et al. Endoplasmic reticulum alpha-glycosidases of *Candida albicans* are required for N glycosylation, cell wall integrity, and normal host-fungus interaction. *Eukaryot Cell* (2007) 6:2184–93. doi:10.1128/EC.00350-07
46. Plaine A, Walker L, Da Costa G, Mora-Montes HM, McKinnon A, Gow NA, et al. Functional analysis of *Candida albicans* GPI-anchored proteins: roles in cell wall integrity and caspofungin sensitivity. *Fungal Genet Biol* (2008) 45:1404–14. doi:10.1016/j.fgb.2008.08.003
47. Hosseinzadeh A, Urban CF. Novel insight into neutrophil immune responses by dry mass determination of *Candida albicans* morphotypes. *PLoS One* (2013) 8:e77993. doi:10.1371/journal.pone.0077993
48. Fidel PL Jr, Vazquez JA, Sobel JD. *Candida glabrata*: review of epidemiology, pathogenesis, and clinical disease with comparison to *C. albicans*. *Clin Microbiol Rev* (1999) 12:80–96.
49. Bulawa CE, Miller DW, Henry LK, Becker JM. Attenuated virulence of chitin-deficient mutants of *Candida albicans*. *Proc Natl Acad Sci U S A* (1995) 92:10570–4. doi:10.1073/pnas.92.23.10570
50. Hobson RP, Munro CA, Bates S, MacCallum DM, Cutler JE, Heinsbroek SE, et al. Loss of cell wall mannosylphosphate in *Candida albicans* does not influence macrophage recognition. *J Biol Chem* (2004) 279:39628–35. doi:10.1074/jbc.M405003200
51. Bates S, MacCallum DM, Bertram G, Munro CA, Hughes HB, Buurman ET, et al. *Candida albicans* Pmr1p, a secretory pathway P-type Ca^{2+}/Mn^{2+}-ATPase, is required for glycosylation and virulence. *J Biol Chem* (2005) 280:23408–15. doi:10.1074/jbc.M502162200
52. Munro CA, Bates S, Buurman ET, Hughes HB, Maccallum DM, Bertram G, et al. Mnt1p and Mnt2p of *Candida albicans* are partially redundant alpha-1,2-mannosyltransferases that participate in *O*-linked mannosylation and are required for adhesion and virulence. *J Biol Chem* (2005) 280:1051–60. doi:10.1074/jbc.M411413200
53. Zhao X, Oh SH, Cheng G, Green CB, Nuessen JA, Yeater K, et al. *ALS3* and *ALS8* represent a single locus that encodes a *Candida albicans* adhesin; functional comparisons between Als3p and Als1p. *Microbiology* (2004) 150:2415–28. doi:10.1099/mic.0.26943-0
54. Sundstrom P, Balish E, Allen CM. Essential role of the *Candida albicans* transglutaminase substrate, hyphal wall protein 1, in lethal oroesophageal candidiasis in immunodeficient mice. *J Infect Dis* (2002) 185:521–30. doi:10.1086/338836
55. Bailey DA, Feldmann PJF, Bovey M, Gow NAR, Brown AJP. The *Candida albicans HYR1* gene, which is activated in response to hyphal development,

belongs to a gene family encoding yeast cell wall proteins. *J Bacteriol* (1996) 178:5353–60. doi:10.1128/jb.178.18.5353-5360.1996
56. Birse CE, Irwin MY, Fonzi WA, Sypherd PS. Cloning and characterization of *ECE1*, a gene expressed in association with cell elongation of the dimorphic pathogen *Candida albicans*. *Infect Immun* (1993) 61:3648–55.
57. Hornby JM, Dumitru R, Nickerson KW. High phosphate (up to 600 mM) induces pseudohyphal development in five wild type *Candida albicans*. *J Microbiol Methods* (2004) 56:119–24. doi:10.1016/j.mimet.2003.09.021
58. Chiani P, Bromuro C, Torosantucci A. Defective induction of interleukin-12 in human monocytes by germ-tube forms of *Candida albicans*. *Infect Immun* (2000) 68:5628–34. doi:10.1128/IAI.68.10.5628-5634.2000
59. Beaussart A, Alsteens D, El-Kirat-Chatel S, Lipke PN, Kucharíková S, Van Dijck P, et al. Single-molecule imaging and functional analysis of Als adhesins and mannans during *Candida albicans* morphogenesis. *ACS Nano* (2012) 6:10950–64. doi:10.1021/nn304505s
60. Brown GD, Herre J, Williams DL, Willment JA, Marshall ASJ, Gordon S. Dectin-1 mediates the biological effects of ß-glucans. *J Exp Med* (2003) 197:1119–24. doi:10.1084/jem.20021890
61. Gantner BN, Simmons RM, Canavera SJ, Akira S, Underhill DM. Collaborative induction of inflammatory responses by dectin-1 and toll-like receptor 2. *J Exp Med* (2003) 197:1107–17. doi:10.1084/jem.20021787
62. Dennehy KM, Willment JA, Williams DL, Brown GD. Reciprocal regulation of IL-23 and IL-12 following co-activation of Dectin-1 and TLR signaling pathways. *Eur J Immunol* (2009) 39:1379–86. doi:10.1002/eji.200838543
63. Jackson AP, Gamble JA, Yeomans T, Moran GP, Saunders D, Harris D, et al. Comparative genomics of the fungal pathogens *Candida dubliniensis* and *Candida albicans*. *Genome Res* (2009) 19:2231–44. doi:10.1101/gr.097501.109
64. Blasi E, Pitzurra L, Puliti M, Bartoli A, Bistoni F. *Candida albicans* hyphal form enhances tumor necrosis factor mRNA levels and protein secretion in murine ANA-1 macrophages. *Cell Immunol* (1992) 142:137–44. doi:10.1016/0008-8749(92)90275-T
65. Matuschak GM, Lechner AJ. The yeast to hyphal transition following hematogenous candidiasis induces shock and organ injury independent of circulating tumor necrosis factor-alpha. *Crit Care Med* (1997) 25:111–20. doi:10.1097/00003246-199701000-00022
66. Moyes DL, Runglall M, Murciano C, Shen C, Nayar D, Thavaraj S, et al. A biphasic innate immune MAPK response discriminates between the yeast and hyphal forms of *Candida albicans* in epithelial cells. *Cell Host Microbe* (2010) 8:225–35. doi:10.1016/j.chom.2010.08.002
67. d'Ostiani CF, Del Sero G, Bacci A, Montagnoli C, Spreca A, Mencacci A, et al. Dendritic cells discriminate between yeasts and hyphae of the fungus *Candida albicans*. Implications for initiation of T helper cell immunity in vitro and in vivo. *J Exp Med* (2000) 191:1661–74. doi:10.1084/jem.191.10.1661
68. Torosantucci A, Chiani P, Cassone A. Differential chemokine response of human monocytes to yeast and hyphal forms of *Candida albicans* and its relation to the ß-1,6 glucan of the fungal cell wall. *J Leukoc Biol* (2000) 68(6):923–32.
69. Van De Veerdonk FL, Joosten LAB, Devesa I, Héctor MM, Kanneganti T, Dinarello CA, et al. Bypassing pathogen-induced inflammasome activation for the regulation of interleukin-1ß production by the fungal pathogen *Candida albicans*. *J Infect Dis* (2009) 199:1087–96. doi:10.1086/597274
70. Wheeler RT, Kombe D, Agarwala SD, Fink GR. Dynamic, morphotype-specific *Candida albicans* β-glucan exposure during infection and drug treatment. *PLoS Pathog* (2008) 4:e1000227. doi:10.1371/journal.ppat.1000227
71. Bates S, De La Rosa JM, MacCallum DM, Brown AJP, Gow NAR, Odds FC. *Candida albicans* Iff11, a secreted protein required for cell wall structure and virulence. *Infect Immun* (2007) 75:2922–8. doi:10.1128/IAI.00102-07
72. Mora-MontesHM,NeteaMG,FerwerdaG,LenardonMD,BrownGD,MisuraAS, et al. Recognition and blocking of innate immunity cells by *Candida albicans* chitin. *Infect Immun* (2011) 79:1961–70. doi:10.1128/IAI.01282-10
73. De Boer AD, De Groot PWJ, Weindl G, Schaller M, Riedel D, Diez-Orejas R, et al. The *Candida albicans* cell wall protein Rhd3/Pga29 is abundant in the yeast form and contributes to virulence. *Yeast* (2010) 27:611–24. doi:10.1002/yea.1790
74. Vavala E, Mignogna G, Spano F, Stringaro A, Colone M, Sanguinetti M, et al. The cell wall protein Rhd3/Pga29 is over-expressed in *Candida albicans* upon micafungin treatment. *J Chemother* (2013) 25:332–40. doi:10.1179/1973947813Y.0000000091
75. HornbyJM, JensenEC, LisecAD, TastoJJ, JahnkeB, ShoemakerR, etal. Quorum sensing in the dimorphic fungus *Candida albicans* is mediated by farnesol. *Appl Environ Microbiol* (2001) 67:2982–92. doi:10.1128/AEM.67.7.2982-2992.2001
76. Chen H, Fujita M, Feng Q, Clardy J, Fink GR. Tyrosol is a quorum-sensing molecule in *Candida albicans*. *Proc Natl Acad Sci U S A* (2004) 101:5048–52. doi:10.1073/pnas.0401416101
77. Chen H, Fink GR. Feedback control of morphogenesis in fungi by aromatic alcohols. *Genes Dev* (2006) 20:1150–61. doi:10.1101/gad.1411806
78. Lu J, Huang G, Wang Z, Zhuang S, Xu L, Song B, et al. Tyrosol exhibits negative regulatory effects on LPS response and endotoxemia. *Food Chem Toxicol* (2013) 62:172–8. doi:10.1016/j.fct.2013.08.031
79. Dalle F, Wächtler B, L'Ollivier C, Holland G, Bannert N, Wilson D, et al. Cellular interactions of *Candida albicans* with human oral epithelial cells and enterocytes. *Cell Microbiol* (2010) 12:248–71. doi:10.1111/j.1462-5822.2009.01394.x
80. Moyes DL, Murciano C, Runglall M, Kohli A, Islam A, Naglik JR. Activation of MAPK/c-Fos induced responses in oral epithelial cells is specific to *Candida albicans* and *Candida dubliniensis* hyphae. *Med Microbiol Immunol* (2012) 201:93–101. doi:10.1007/s00430-011-0209-y

9

Protein Deiminase 4 and CR3 Regulate *Aspergillus fumigatus* and β-Glucan-Induced Neutrophil Extracellular Trap Formation, but Hyphal Killing is Dependent Only on CR3

*Heather L. Clark[1,2,3], Serena Abbondante[2,3], Martin S. Minns[2,3], Elyse N. Greenberg[2,3], Yan Sun[1] and Eric Pearlman[2,3]**

[1] *Department of Ophthalmology and Visual Sciences, Case Western Reserve University, Cleveland, OH, United States,* [2] *Department of Ophthalmology, University of California Irvine, Irvine, CA, United States,* [3] *Department of Physiology and Biophysics, University of California Irvine, Irvine, CA, United States*

Correspondence:
Eric Pearlman
eric.pearlman@uci.edu

Neutrophil extracellular trap (NET) formation requires chromatin decondensation before nuclear swelling and eventual extracellular release of DNA, which occurs together with nuclear and cytoplasmic antimicrobial proteins. A key mediator of chromatin decondensation is protein deiminase 4 (PAD4), which catalyzes histone citrullination. In the current study, we examined the role of PAD4 and NETosis following activation of neutrophils by *A. fumigatus* hyphal extract or cell wall β-glucan (curdlan) and found that both induced NET release by human and murine neutrophils. Also, using blocking antibodies to CR3 and Dectin-1 together with CR3-deficient CD18$^{-/-}$ and Dectin-1$^{-/-}$ murine neutrophils, we found that the β-glucan receptor CR3, but not Dectin-1, was required for NET formation. NETosis was also dependent on NADPH oxidase production of reactive oxygen species (ROS). Using an antibody to citrullinated histone 3 (H3Cit) as an indicator of PAD4 activity, we show that β-glucan stimulated NETosis occurs in neutrophils from C57BL/6, but not PAD4$^{-/-}$ mice. Similarly, a small molecule PAD4 inhibitor (GSK484) blocked NET formation by human neutrophils. Despite these observations, the ability of PAD4$^{-/-}$ neutrophils to release calprotectin and kill *A. fumigatus* hyphae was not significantly different from C57BL/6 neutrophils, whereas CD18$^{-/-}$ neutrophils exhibited an impaired ability to perform both functions. We also detected H3Cit in *A. fumigatus* infected C57BL/6, but not PAD4$^{-/-}$ corneas; however, we found no difference between C57BL/6 and PAD4$^{-/-}$ mice in either corneal disease or hyphal killing. Taken together, these findings lead us to conclude that although PAD4 together with CR3-mediated ROS production is required for NET formation in response to *A. fumigatus*, PAD4-dependent NETosis is not required for *A. fumigatus* killing either *in vitro* or during infection.

Keywords: ***Aspergillus*****, neutrophil extracellular trap, protein deiminase 4, CR3, keratitis**

INTRODUCTION

Neutrophil extracellular trap (NET) formation is a coordinated form of neutrophil cell death, first described by Zychlinsky and colleagues in which genomic DNA is released from neutrophils and traps and mediates killing of pathogenic bacteria, fungi, and parasites (1–3). The molecular events in this process involve protein kinase C, Raf, Mek, and Erk activation, which leads to activation of NADPH oxidase, production of reactive oxygen species (ROS), and mobilization of neutrophil elastase (NE) into the nucleus, where it functions to degrade histones, resulting in chromatin decondensation (1). NETosis also requires activation of protein deiminase 4 (PAD4) in the nucleus, which converts positively charged arginine residues to neutral citrulline. Histone citrullination also mediates chromatin decondensation and nuclear swelling (4–8).

We reported that neutrophils play a critical role in fungal killing and in corneal infections with the pathogenic molds *Aspergillus* and *Fusarium*, which are major causes of blindness and visual impairment worldwide (9, 10). We demonstrated an essential role for neutrophil NADPH oxidase and for the antimicrobial peptide calprotectin (CP) in fungal killing *in vitro* and in murine models of fungal keratitis (11, 12).

In the current study, we examined the role of PAD4 in NET formation in response to *Aspergillus fumigatus* or cell wall β-glucan and show that although PAD4 is required for NET formation *in vitro* and during corneal infection, it is not required for hyphal killing *in vitro* or during infection. Instead, we demonstrate that CR3 (CD11b/CD18), which also binds β-glucan, is required for production of reactive oxygen, hyphal killing, and CP release. We conclude that although NETs are generated by *A. fumigatus* hyphae, they are not required for hyphal killing *in vitro* or during corneal infection.

RESULTS

A. fumigatus and β-Glucan Induce Neutrophil Extracellular Traps From Human and Mouse Neutrophils

Although NETs have a distinctive appearance in fixed cells, NETs in live cell cultures are more diffuse (7), which we also found after incubating human peripheral blood neutrophils with *A. fumigatus* hyphal extract (AspHE), particulate β-glucan (curdlan), or phorbol myristic acid (PMA) when incubated with the cell-impermeable DNA stain SYTOX Green (**Figure 1A**).

Quantification of SYTOX Green showed that extracellular DNA increased over time (**Figure 1B**). Total DNA released over 20 h (area under the curve of **Figure 1B**) showed that all three stimuli induced a significant increase in DNA release from human peripheral blood neutrophils compared with media alone (**Figure 1C**). Similarly, mouse bone marrow neutrophils released DNA in response to AspHE and curdlan (**Figures 1D,E**), although PMA did not stimulate murine bone marrow neutrophils (not shown).

β-Glucan-Induced NETosis Requires Production of ROS

Reactive oxygen species is required for NETosis in human neutrophils following stimulation with PMA, although ROS-independent NET formation has also been reported (13–15). To examine if ROS has a role in NET formation in response to *A. fumigatus*, human neutrophils were incubated with PMA, curdlan, or AspHE in the presence of the NADPH oxidase inhibitor diphenyl iodonium (DPI). We found that DPI inhibited DNA release in response to all stimuli (**Figures 2A,B**), indicating a requirement for NADPH oxidase-generated ROS in NET formation in response to fungal cell wall components.

CR3 Mediates NET Formation and ROS Production in Response to β-Glucan

C-type lectin receptors, including Dectin-1, Dectin-2, and Dectin-3 (also called macrophage c-type lectin) on murine macrophages recognize fungal cell wall components, including β-glucan and α-mannose (16). Neutrophils constitutively express the C-type lectin Dectin-1 and the β2-integrin CR3 (Mac-1, CD11b/CD18), which in addition to the complement binding I-domain, has a lectin binding domain that recognizes β-glucan (17). The lectin binding domain mediates ROS production in response to *Candida* and *Aspergillus* (11, 13), although maximal production of ROS and NETs depends on activation of both domains of this unique receptor in the presence of complement (15).

To determine the relative contribution of CR3 and Dectin-1 in ROS production and NET formation, human peripheral blood neutrophils were incubated with particulate β-glucan (curdlan) together with antibodies to either Dectin-1 or CR3. We found significantly reduced extracellular DNA in the presence of anti-CR3 (**Figure 3A**), whereas anti-Dectin-1 resulted in increased DNA release (**Figure 3B**), which is consistent with an earlier report on NETosis induced by *Candida* hyphae compared with yeast (18). As ROS is required for NET formation, we also examined the role of CR3 and Dectin-1 in ROS production, and found that curdlan-induced ROS production was inhibited by anti-CR3, but not anti-Dectin-1 (**Figure 3C**).

These findings were reproduced in bone marrow neutrophils from Dectin-$1^{-/-}$ and from $CD18^{-/-}$ mice, where NETosis was dependent on CD18 expression, and there was no effect of Dectin-1 deletion on β-glucan-induced NET formation or ROS production (**Figures 3D,E**). We therefore conclude that CR3 rather than Dectin-1 is the predominant β-glucan receptor required for ROS production and NET release in human and murine neutrophils.

PAD4 Is Required for NET Formation Induced by β-Glucan

Conversion of arginines to neutral citrullines is mediated by the protein deimidase family of enzymes (19); however, only PAD4 is present in the nucleus, where it mediates citrullination of histones and subsequent chromatin decondensation.

To examine if PAD4 has a role in NET formation in response to fungal cell wall components, we visualized NET formation

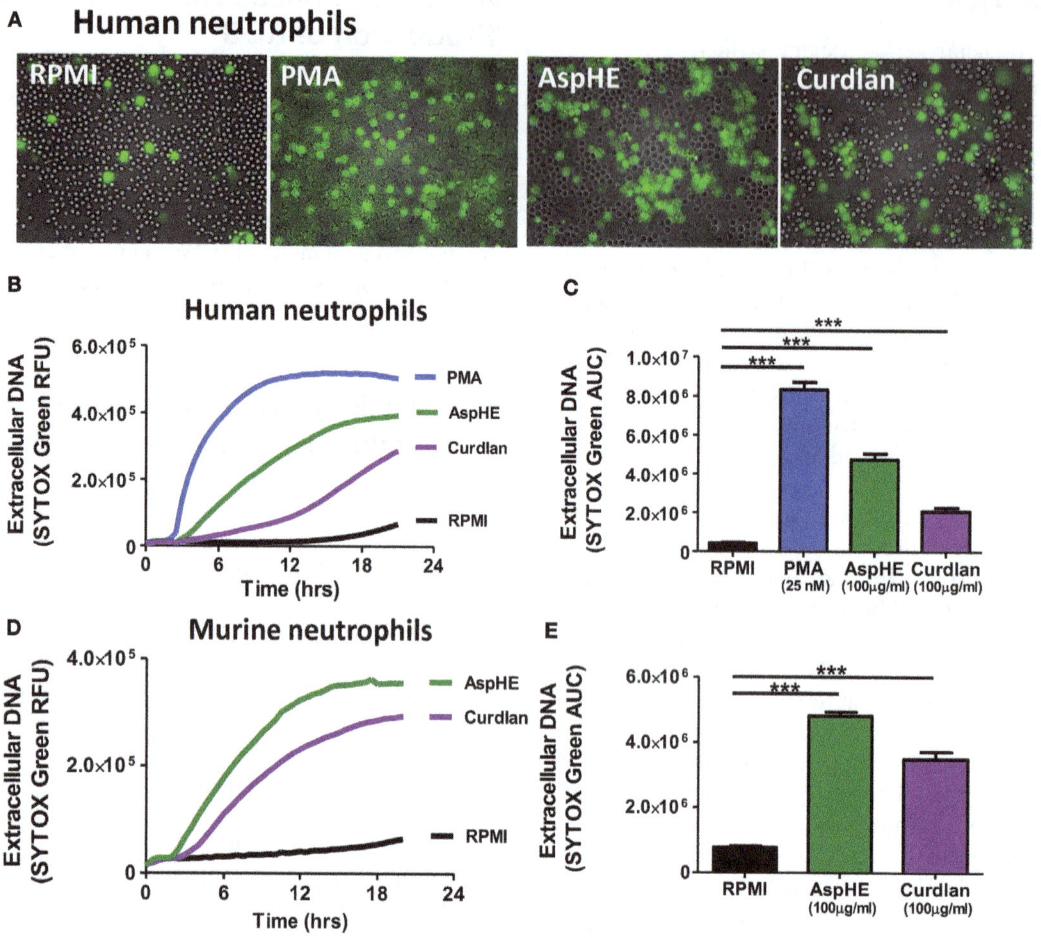

FIGURE 1 | *Aspergillus fumigatus* and β-glucan induce neutrophil extracellular trap formation in human and murine neutrophils. **(A)** Representative images showing DNA release by SYTOX Green staining in human peripheral blood neutrophils 20 h after stimulation with 25 nM phorbol myristic acid (PMA), 100 µg/ml *A. fumigatus* hyphal extract (AspHE), or 100 µg/ml particulate β-glucan (curdlan); original magnification is 200×. **(B)** DNA release overtime shown as relative fluorescent units (RFU) measured by SYTOX Green; **(C)** total extracellular DNA after 20 h calculated as area under the curve (AUC). **(D,E)** Extracellular DNA from mouse peritoneal neutrophils incubated with AspHE or curdlan and quantified by SYTOX Green RFU and AUC. Asterisks (***) indicate $p < 0.001$ based on one way ANOVA with Tukey post hoc analysis. Experiments were repeated five times with similar results.

in β-glucan stimulated neutrophils from C57BL/6 and PAD4$^{-/-}$ mice using antibodies to citrullinated histone H3 (H3Cit). We found that in response to curdlan, neutrophils from C57BL/6 mice generated characteristic NET structures that were also H3Cit^{+} (**Figures 4A–E**). In contrast, stimulated PAD4$^{-/-}$ neutrophils retain their lobular nuclei and were negative for H3Cit (**Figures 4C,F**). An early stage of NETosis is NE translocation to the nucleus (4), which is clearly detected in C57BL/6 neutrophils; however, elastase remained in the cytoplasm of PAD4$^{-/-}$ neutrophils (**Figures 4C,F**).

Protein deiminase 4-dependent NET formation by murine and human neutrophils was quantified by SYTOX green. Consistent with representative images, PAD4$^{-/-}$ neutrophils released significantly less DNA than C57BL/6 neutrophils following incubation with curdlan (**Figure 5A**). To investigate if there is a role for PAD4 in NET formation by human neutrophils, we used small molecule PAD4 inhibitors that inhibit NET formation *in vitro* (19). Curdlan-stimulated human neutrophils were incubated with the PAD4 inhibitor GSK484 or with the negative control compound GSK106. As shown in **Figures 5B,C**, DNA release in response to *Aspergillus* was significantly reduced in the presence of GSK484, whereas the negative control GSK106 did not inhibit DNA release.

Together, these findings clearly demonstrate that PAD4 citrullination is required for NET formation by murine and human neutrophils.

CR3 but Not PAD4 Is Required for Calprotectin Release *In Vitro*

The antimicrobial peptide calprotectin (CP; S100A8/A9) is a major component of NETs in response to *Candida albicans* and is required for NET-mediated killing (3). CP was found to be an essential NET component in controlling *A. fumigatus* following gene therapy for chronic granulomatous disease (20), and we

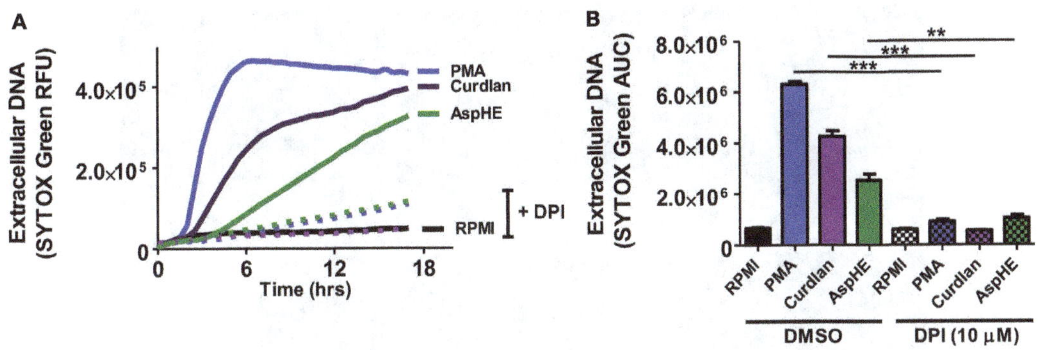

FIGURE 2 | Neutrophil extracellular trap (NET) formation is dependent on reactive oxygen species (ROS). Human neutrophils were stimulated 20 h with phorbol myristic acid (PMA), AspHE, or curdlan in the presence of the ROS inhibitor diphenyl iodonium (DPI) (10 μM). NET formation was quantified by SYTOX Green over time **(A)**, and total SYTOX over 18 h is shown as area under the curve (AUC) **(B)**. ANOVA with Tukey post hoc analysis showed ***$p < 0.001$ and **$p < 0.01$. Experiments were repeated four times with similar results.

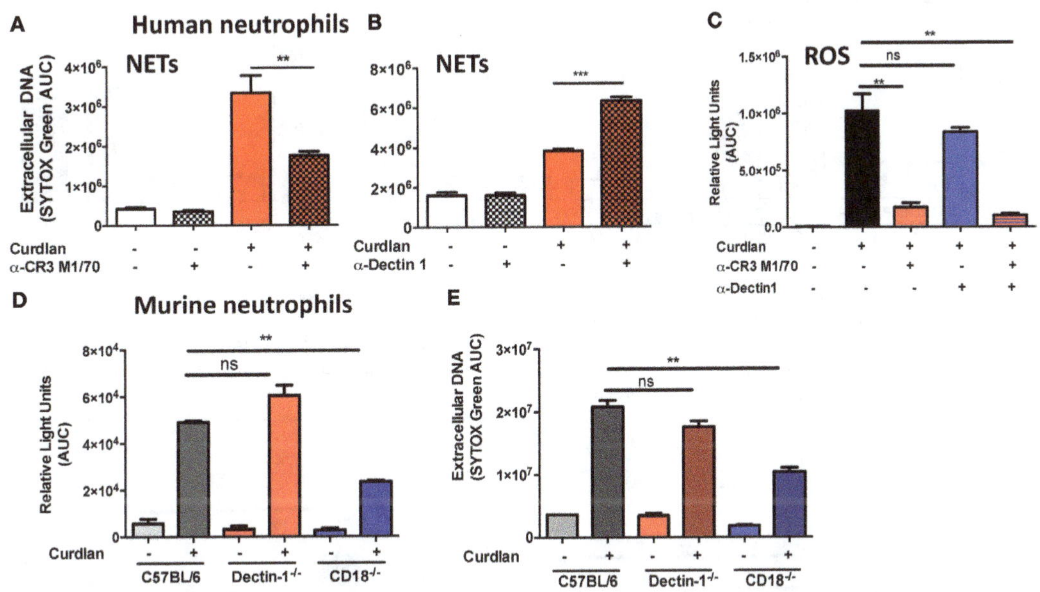

FIGURE 3 | Distinct roles for CR3 and Dectin-1 in β-glucan-induced reactive oxygen species (ROS) production and neutrophil extracellular trap (NET) formation. **(A–C)** Human neutrophils; **(D,E)** murine neutrophils. Neutrophils were incubated with β-glucan (curdlan) in the presence of the anti-CR3 blocking antibody M1/70 (30 μg/ml) **(A)** or with the anti-Dectin-1 blocking antibody 22H8 (Invivogen, 20 μg/ml) **(B)**. **(A,B)** DNA release was quantified by SYTOX Green and expressed as area under the curve. **(C)** ROS production measured by luminol. **(D,E)** DNA release and ROS production by mouse bone marrow neutrophils from C57BL/6, Dectin-1$^{-/-}$, and CD18$^{-/-}$ mice stimulated with curdlan. *p* Values are biological replicates of at least three repeat experiments and were calculated using ANOVA with Tukey post hoc analysis (***$p < 0.001$, **$p < 0.01$, and *$p < 0.05$).

reported that CP inhibits *A. fumigatus* hyphal growth by sequestering zinc *in vitro* and in *Aspergillus* keratitis (12).

To determine if CP is associated with NETs, we examined CP release in CR3 (CD18$^{-/-}$) and PAD4$^{-/-}$ neutrophils following stimulation with curdlan. Bone marrow neutrophils from C57BL/6, CD18$^{-/-}$, and PAD4$^{-/-}$ mice were incubated with curdlan 2h (prior to NET formation) or for 16 (after NET formation), and the CP subunit S100A8 was measured in cell-free supernatants by ELISA.

Whereas there was no significant difference in S100A8 between C57BL/6 and PAD4$^{-/-}$ neutrophils released in response to curdlan at either time point, CD18$^{-/-}$ neutrophils produced significantly less S100A8 at both time points (**Figure 6**). There was no difference in production of S100A8 in response to total hyphal extracts (Figure S1 in Supplementary Material).

These data indicate that CP is released from neutrophils in the absence of PAD4-dependent NET formation, and that release in response to curdlan requires CR3 activation.

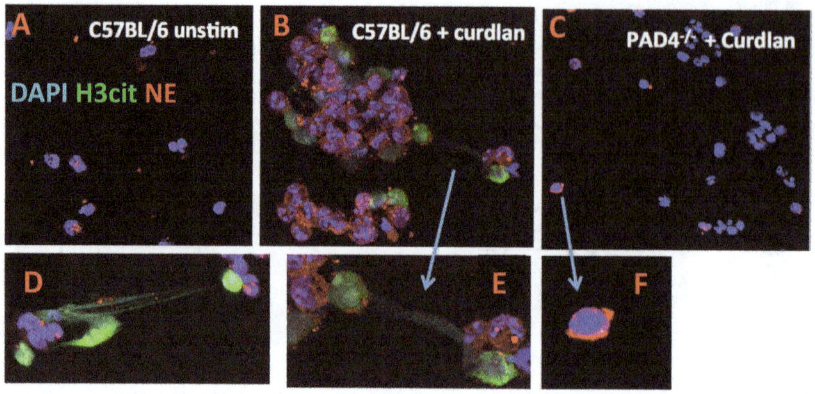

FIGURE 4 | β-Glucan-induced neutrophil extracellular trap formation. Curdlan-stimulated bone marrow neutrophils from C57BL/6 and PAD4$^{-/-}$ mice. Neutrophils were immunostained with antibodies to citrullinated histone 3 (H3Cit), neutrophil elastase (NE), and DAPI nuclear stain **(A–C)** 200×; **(D–F)** 400×.

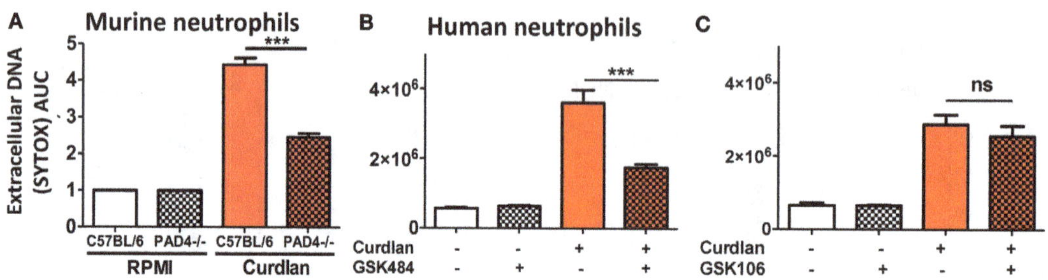

FIGURE 5 | Protein deiminase 4 (PAD4)-dependent neutrophil extracellular trap formation. **(A)** Bone marrow neutrophils from C57BL/6 and PAD4$^{-/-}$ mice were incubated 20 h with particulate β-glucan (curdlan) in RPMI, and DNA release was quantified by SYTOX Green. Values were normalized to unstimulated neutrophils (RPMI). **(B,C)** Human peripheral blood neutrophils incubated with curdlan and 10 μM specific PAD4 inhibitor GSK484 **(B)** or with the related, non-inhibitory compound GSK106 **(C)**. *p* Values are biological replicates of at least three repeat experiments and were calculated using ANOVA with Tukey post hoc analysis (***$p < 0.01$; **$p < 0.05$; ns, not significant). Experiments were repeated twice with similar results.

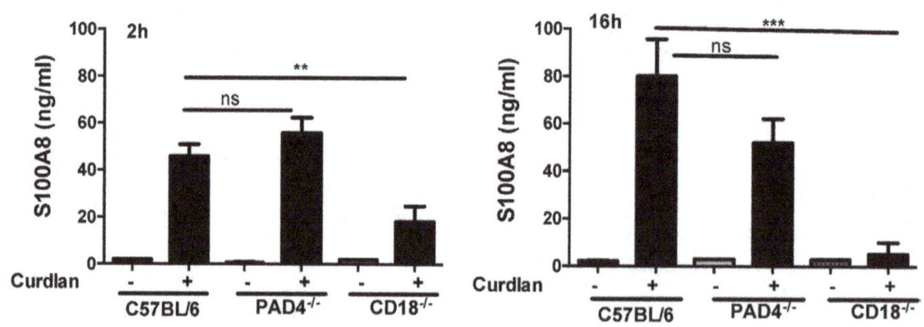

FIGURE 6 | CD18-dependent calprotectin (CP) (S100A8/A9) production. Bone marrow neutrophils from C57BL/6, PAD4$^{-/-}$, and CD18$^{-/-}$ mice were incubated 2 or 16 h with curdlan, and CP/S100A8 was quantified by ELISA. *p* Values are biological replicates of three repeat experiments and were calculated using ANOVA using a Tukey post hoc analysis (***$p < 0.001$; **$p < 0.01$; ns, not significant). S100A8 production to AspHE was similar in all groups (Figure S1 in Supplementary Material).

CR3, but Not PAD4, Is Required for Neutrophil Inhibition of *A. fumigatus* Hyphal Growth

To determine whether NETs regulate fungal growth *in vitro*, 2×10^5 human neutrophils were incubated with *A. fumigatus* hyphae in the presence of the anti-CR3 blocking antibody M1/70. Also, *A. fumigatus* hyphae were incubated with neutrophils from C57BL/6 and PAD4$^{-/-}$ mice. *A. fumigatus* hyphal growth over 18 h was quantified using calcofluor white, which binds cell wall chitin, and percent fungal mass was quantified based on hyphal growth in media alone (100%).

Human neutrophils significantly inhibited fungal growth compared with hyphae grown in media alone; however, this was reversed in the presence of blocking antibody to CR3 (**Figure 7A**). Similarly, hyphal growth was impaired when incubated with 2×10^5 C57BL/6 or PAD4$^{-/-}$ neutrophils, but not with neutrophils from CD18$^{-/-}$ mice (**Figure 7B**).

Together, these data demonstrate that CR3 signaling is required for fungal growth inhibition and/or killing by neutrophils *in vitro*, whereas there is no apparent role for PAD4.

PAD4 Is Not Required for *A. fumigatus* Killing, Corneal Disease, or Neutrophil Recruitment to Infected Corneas

Fungal keratitis is characterized by an early and profound infiltration of neutrophils to the corneal stroma in patients (21), and in murine models where these cells are required for hyphal killing and which mediate corneal opacification (9, 10).

To determine if PAD4 is required for NET formation in the cornea, and if NETs have a role in fungal killing at this site, corneas of C57BL/6 and PAD4$^{-/-}$ mice were infected with 1×10^5 RFP expressing *A. fumigatus* conidia (Af293), and after 48 h, corneal sections were examined for neutrophil infiltration and NET formation (H3Cit$^+$). H3Cit staining was evident in corneas of *A. fumigatus* infected C57BL/6, but not PAD4$^{-/-}$ mice (**Figure 8A**). Also, quantification of multiple sections showed a significant difference in H3Cit, but no significant difference in total Ly6G$^+$ cells between C57BL/6 and PAD4$^{-/-}$ mice (Figure S2 in Supplementary Material).

Total cells in infected corneas were examined by flow cytometry following collagenase digestion. As shown in **Figure 8B**, epithelial cells were identified as CD45$^-$, EpCam$^+$, which comprised <5% total cells, whereas >75% of total cells were CD45$^+$. Neutrophils were identified in the CD45$^+$ population as Ly6G/CD11b$^+$, with the remaining CD45$^+$ cells being Ly6C/CD11b$^+$ monocytes. Neutrophils comprised 40–60% total cells in infected corneas; however, there was no difference in the percentage of neutrophils between infected C57BL/6 and PAD4$^{-/-}$ corneas (**Figure 8C**; Figure S2 in Supplementary Material).

There were also no significant differences between infected C57BL/6 and PAD4$^{-/-}$ mice in the severity of corneal opacification, RFP-Af293 hyphal mass or CFU (**Figures 8D,E**). We also found no significant difference in CFU between C57BL/6 and PAD4$^{-/-}$ mice following infection with an *A. fumigatus* keratitis clinical isolate (Af BP) (**Figures 8F,G**). Collectively, these findings show that although PAD4-dependent NET formation is detected in infected corneas, they do not have an essential role in regulating fungal corneal infections.

DISCUSSION

A proposed sequence of events for NET formation by Zychlinsky and colleagues envisions an initial activation of neutrophils, assembly of the NADPH oxidase complex and production of ROS, resulting in bacterial entrapment and killing (1, 22). Human and mouse neutrophils with mutations or deletions in NADPH oxidase proteins cannot undergo NETosis *in vitro* or in a murine model of pulmonary aspergillosis (14). Elastase translocation to the nucleus is also required, and NETs are not detected following inhibition of elastase activity or in elastase deficient neutrophils (4).

Neutrophil extracellular traps have also been detected *in vivo* using two-photon microscopy, including in a murine model of pulmonary aspergillosis that shows hyphae in close association with neutrophils and extracellular DNA (23). These and other elegant studies leave little doubt that NETs are generated in response to bacteria, fungi and parasites. The controversy comes in to play in determining the role of NETs in killing pathogenic fungi. In the same pulmonary aspergillosis study, NETs did not kill *A. fumigatus*, although the authors suggest that NETs may have a role in inhibiting hyphal growth (23).

Human neutrophils from healthy, but not patients with chronic granulomatous disease (CGD) form NETs in response to *A. fumigatus* hyphae; however, DNAse treatment had no effect on hyphal killing in these patients, arguing against a role for NETs (24). Conversely, DNAse treatment inhibited the ability of human neutrophils to kill *A. fumigatus* germ tubes and hyphae (25, 26), thereby implicating a protective role for NETs in *A. fumigatus* infection.

In agreement with our current observations, the CGD study also showed that *A. fumigatus* conidia are recognized by CR3

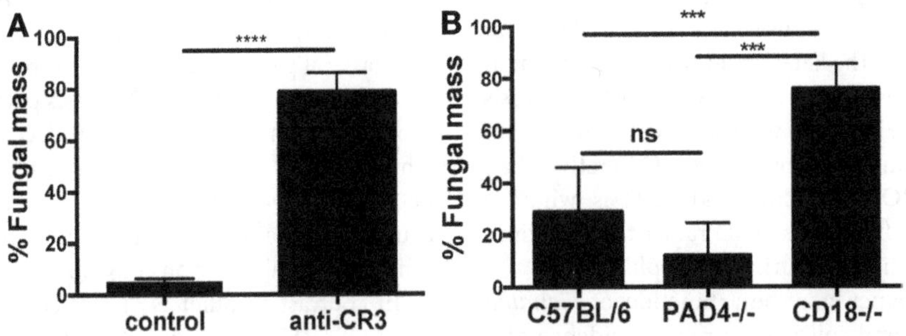

FIGURE 7 | CR3, but not protein deiminase 4 (PAD4), is required for neutrophil inhibition of *Aspergillus fumigatus* hyphal growth. **(A,B)** *A. fumigatus* hyphae incubated 18 h with human neutrophils in RPMI alone or with anti-CR3 M1/70 (20 µg/ml) **(A)**. Fungal mass was quantified by calcofluor white fluorescent chitin stain and presented as percent of total hyphae in the absence of neutrophils. **(B)** Percent fungal mass in bone marrow neutrophils from C57BL/6, CD18$^{-/-}$, or PAD4$^{-/-}$ mice following 18 h incubation with *A. fumigatus* hyphae. *p* Values are biological replicates of three repeat experiments and were calculated using Student's *t*-test **(A)** or ANOVA with a Tukey post hoc analysis **(B)** (****$p < 0.0001$; ***$p < 0.001$; ns, not significant).

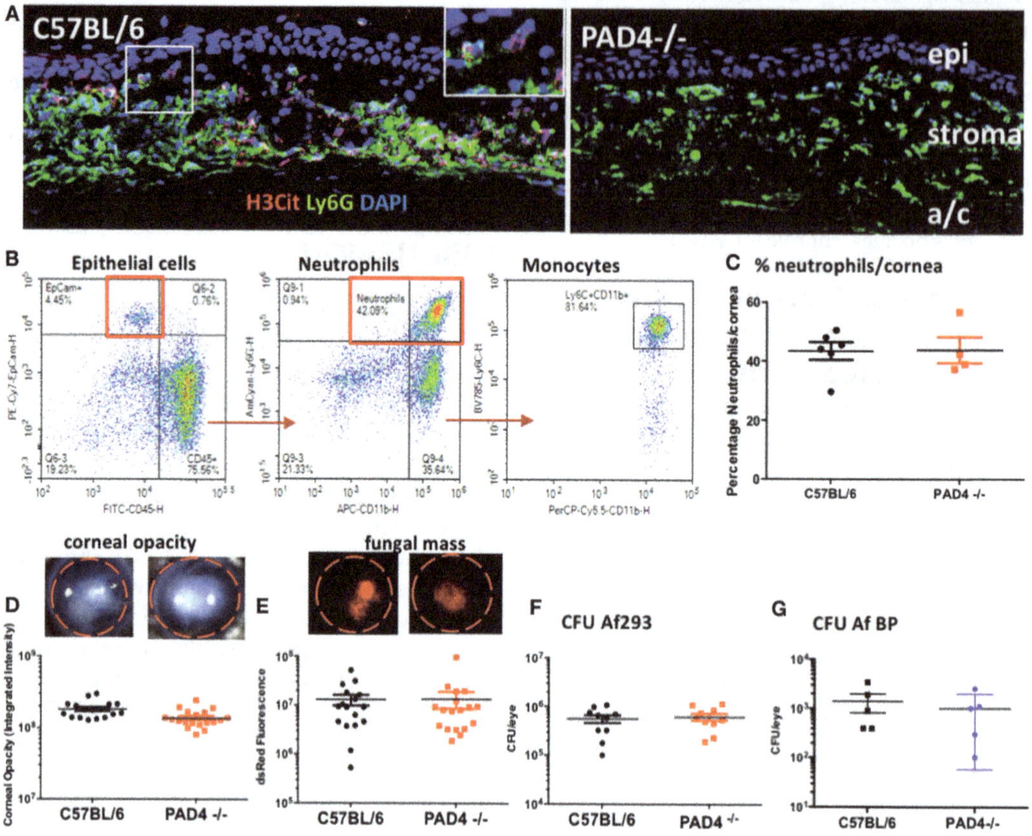

FIGURE 8 | *Aspergillus fumigatus* corneal infection in PAD4$^{-/-}$ mice. Corneas of C57BL/6 and PAD4$^{-/-}$ mice were infected with dsRed expressing *A. fumigatus*. **(A)** Corneal sections immunostained with antibodies to Ly6G and citrullinated histone 3 (H3Cit) and counterstained with DAPI nuclear stain. Epi, stroma = corneal epithelium and corneal stroma. Highlighted area shows H3Cit staining in neutrophils. Original magnification is 400x. **(B)** Representative flow cytometry scatter plots showing total cells from infected C57BL/6 corneas that include CD45$^-$ epithelial cells, CD45$^+$Ly6G$^+$ neutrophils, and Ly6C high monocytes. **(C)** Percent neutrophils in infected corneas from C57BL/6 and PAD4$^{-/-}$ mice [percent Ly6G$^+$ neutrophils in infected corneas (representative scatter plots from C57BL/6 and PAD4$^{-/-}$ mice are shown in Figure S2 in Supplementary Material)]. **(D,E)** Representative corneas showing opacification and RFP expressing *A. fumigatus* hyphae. **(F,G)** Quantification of corneal opacity, dsRed as a measure of fungal mass, and CFU. Each data point represents an individual cornea. $p > 0.05$ using Student's *t*-test analyses for panels **(C–G)**, indicating that there are no statistically significant differences between C57BL/6 and PAD4$^{-/-}$ mice for any of these parameters. These data are representative of five repeat experiments.

rather than Dectin-1 on human neutrophils and mediates non-oxidative killing (24). This observation is supported by a report showing that Dectin-1 negatively regulates hyphae-induced NET formation by human neutrophils (18), and by an earlier study showing that human neutrophils use CR3 to form NETs in response to *C. albicans* (27). The latter study also reported that in murine neutrophils, Dectin-1 rather than CR3 mediates NETosis induced by *C. albicans*. However, we used neutrophils from Dectin-1$^{-/-}$ and CD18$^{-/-}$ mice to show that it is CR3 rather than Dectin-1 that mediates ROS production and NETosis, which is consistent with our earlier finding that CR3 rather than Dectin-1 that mediates ROS production by murine neutrophils (11).

Although this discrepancy may be a function of *Candida* vs. *Aspergillus*, Reichner and colleagues provide evidence of a second NETosis pathway in the presence of extracellular matrix components such as fibronectin (13, 15). Whereas the classical pathway of NETosis described by Zychlinsky requires chromatin decondensation mediated by elastase translocation to the nucleus that is ROS dependent and occurs over a period of hours (1, 22), Reichner describes a rapid process (<30 min) of NET formation induced by *Candida* hyphae, which is independent of ROS formation (15).

As our studies show elastase in the nucleus, that ROS is required for NET formation, and that this process occurs over a number of hours, we conclude that NETosis progresses through the classical pathway. However, it is possible that in the presence of extracellular matrix, the NETosis pathway regulated by matrix proteins may also be activated; indeed, this may in part explain why we found no role for PAD4 in infected corneas even while detecting PAD4-dependent H3Cit. Activation of both pathways could also explain discrepancies in the role of PAD4 described in other microbial infections (28–30).

In contrast to other NET-related mediators such as elastase and ROS, PAD4 specifically regulates histone citrullination and is unique among the protein deiminase family in being localized to the nucleus (31, 32). Therefore, the only phenotype of PAD4$^{-/-}$ neutrophils should be an inability to form NETs so we focused on the role of PAD4 in neutrophil responses to *A. fumigatus*. Furthermore, although PAD4-dependent NETosis has been reported in mouse models of bacterial and parasitic infections, and in autoimmunity (4, 33), there are no reports on the role of PAD4 in fungal infections.

In this study, we visualized citrullinated histone H3 associated with NETs following β-glucan stimulation of C57BL/6, but not PAD4$^{-/-}$ neutrophils, and NETosis measured by SYTOX was also dependent on PAD4. Given that β-glucan is a major cell wall surface component of molds and yeast following germination, these findings indicate that most pathogenic fungi would stimulate NET formation. However, PAD4$^{-/-}$ neutrophils did not exhibit impaired CP release or have any role in hyphal killing *in vitro*; furthermore, although H3Cit was detected in *A. fumigatus* infected corneas, we found no difference in hyphal growth or corneal opacification between C57BL/6 and PAD4$^{-/-}$ mice. Therefore, at least under these experimental conditions, PAD4-dependent NET formation is not required to control hyphal growth or fungal infection.

Following corneal infection with *A. fumigatus*, we found only localized H3Cit staining compared with the large neutrophil infiltrate, so it is possible that the absence of a phenotype is a consequence of relatively few NETs being formed; however, it is more likely that even though antimicrobial peptides are associated with NETs, NETosis is not required for CP release, iron sequestration or ROS production, all of which are important in controlling hyphal growth *in vitro* and in infection models (11, 12, 34). These findings are consistent with other studies in which PAD4-dependent NETs were not required to control bacterial CFU in a cecal ligation model of peritonitis (30) or for controlling influenza (29), although PAD4$^{-/-}$ mice showed an impaired ability to control *Shigella flexneri* infection (4). Both ROS and PAD4 independent NETosis have been described for *Leishmania amazonensis* promastigotes (33).

Instead of PAD4, we found that CR3 was required for ROS production in response to curdlan and *A. fumigatus*, release of CP, and *A. fumigatus* hyphal killing. Although CR3 was also required for NET formation, these findings do not implicate NETs in fungal killing as production of ROS and CP may be independent of NETosis. Indeed, PAD4$^{-/-}$ neutrophils released comparable levels of CP as C57BL/6 neutrophils within 2 h, which is earlier than we can detect NET formation, and indicates that CP release is NETosis independent.

Taken together, CR3 appears to be the β-glucan receptor that leads to PAD4 activation and NETosis on human and murine neutrophils, which is dependent on ROS; however, although NETs contain antimicrobial peptides, we conclude that NET formation is not required for CP release or to regulate *A. fumigatus* hyphal growth *in vitro* or in the fungal keratitis model. Furthermore, because CD18 (LFA1) binding to ICAM-1 on capillary endothelial cells is required for neutrophil attachment and extravasation, CD18$^{-/-}$ neutrophils are not recruited to infected tissues; therefore, we were unable to examine CR3 recognition of *Aspergillus* in infected corneas.

Although the role of NETs in microbial killing appears to be controversial, NETs have also been implicated in tissue damage during infection and in autoimmune disease including rheumatoid arthritis, lupus, vasculitis, acute respiratory distress syndrome, and sepsis. This is due in part to release of histones that are abundant in NETs and which have direct cytotoxic activity (35). One example is intravenous injection of methicillin resistant *Staphylococcus aureus*, which resulted in PAD4-dependent NET formation in the liver and resulting hepatic injury (36). By contrast, we found that corneal opacity as a measure of tissue damage in fungal keratitis was not reduced in *A. fumigatus* infected PAD4$^{-/-}$ mice, indicating that NETs do not appear to regulate blinding corneal disease related to fungal infection. NETs have been reported in *Pseudomonas aeruginosa* keratitis, although ExoS-expressing strains are more susceptible than ExoU to NET-mediated bacterial killing (37).

A recent review of NETs proposes a clear distinction between ROS and elastase-dependent NETs, which have antimicrobial activity, and a second ROS independent, PAD4-mediated mechanism of DNA release termed leukotoxic hypercitrullination, which is triggered by elevated intracellular calcium (which activates PAD4) and is associated with autoimmunity (38). Our findings reveal β-glucan-induced NET formation that is both ROS and PAD4 dependent and is associated with intranuclear elastase, thereby suggesting this dichotomy is not so clear. The same review also notes that the main purpose of PAD4-mediated histone citrullination is to alter the chromatin and regulate gene transcription, whereas elastase digestion of chromatin is also required for NETosis. Our observations that release of extracellular DNA can be blocked by inhibiting PAD4 or ROS production makes it unlikely that we are seeing two distinct pathways.

In conclusion, this study demonstrates an essential role for CR3, ROS, and PAD4 in NET formation in response to *Aspergillus* and to β-glucan but shows that PAD4-dependent NETosis is not required for either hyphal killing or for tissue damage in the cornea.

MATERIALS AND METHODS

Ethics Statement

Human peripheral blood was collected from healthy donors between ages of 18 and 65 years in accordance with the Declaration of Helsinki guidelines and with the approval of the Institutional Review Board of the University of California (Irvine, CA, USA). Informed consent was obtained in writing from each volunteer.

All animals were treated in accordance with the guidelines provided in the Association for Research in Vision and Ophthalmology ARVO statement for the Use of Animals in Ophthalmic and Vision Research. All animal studies were conducted following approval of the Institutional Animal Care and Use Committee of Case Western Reserve University and the University of California, Irvine.

Human Peripheral Blood Neutrophils

Whole blood RBCs were separated in 3% dextran (Sigma-Aldrich, St. Louis, MO, USA) PBS, and neutrophils were purified from remaining cells by overlay on a Ficoll (GE Healthcare) density gradient and centrifugation at 500 × *g* for 25 min. Remaining RBCs were lysed, and neutrophils were resuspended in RPMI 1640 medium. Purity (~90%) was assessed by flow cytometry using antihuman D16 and CD66b Abs (eBioscience, San Diego, CA, USA).

Source of Mice

$CD18^{-/-}$ mice were originally provided by Claire Doerschuk (University of North Carolina, Chapel Hill, NC, USA). Age- and sex-matched C57BL/6 mice were purchased from Jackson Laboratories (Bar Harbor, ME, USA). $PAD4^{-/-}$ mice were originally provided by Dr. Kerri Mowen at Scripps Research Institute. All animal experiments were conducted with sex- and age-matched mice, and animal studies were compliant with all applicable provisions established by the Animal Welfare Act and the Public Health Services Policy on the Humane Care and Use of Laboratory Animals.

A. fumigatus Strains and Culture

The strain used in these studies was a keratitis clinical isolate obtained from the Bascom-Palmer Eye Institute, *A. fumigatus* BP, whereas the strain used for corneal infection experiments was the Af293-expressing red fluorescent protein used in our prior studies (12). Fungi were cultured on Sabouraud dextrose agar at 37°C for 3–5 days for sporulation, and conidia were isolated by disruption in PBS and filtration through sterile cotton gauze. For hyphal killing experiments, conidia were grown in Sabouraud dextrose broth (SDB), at 3,000 conidia/well of 96-well plate until germination (6 h), washed in sterile PBS and co-incubated with neutrophils. For AspHE preparation, conidia were grown in 500 ml SDB at 37°C for 5 days. SDB was removed from the fungi by vacuum filtration, and fungal mass was homogenized in a mortar and pestle under liquid nitrogen. Fungal homogenate was resuspended in RPMI 1640 without phenol red and filtered through a 70 μM cell strainer. Protein content was measured by BCA assay (ThermoFisher), and AspHE stocks were stored at −20°C.

Neutrophil Isolation

Human neutrophils were isolated from the blood of healthy donors age 18–50. All human studies were approved by the University of California, Irvine institutional review board. Whole blood was mixed 1:1 with 3% dextran-PBS for 20 min to sediment red blood cells. The upper layer was overlaid on Ficoll Hypaque (GE Healthcare) and centrifuged at 500 × *g* for 25 min. The pellet containing granulocytes and RBCs was treated with 1× RBC Lysis Buffer (eBioscience) and spun at 300 × *g* for 5 min to obtain a granulocyte pellet. Cells were resuspended in RPMI 1640 and counted. Typical purity was >95%. Total bone marrow was isolated from the tibias, and femurs of mice and neutrophils were purified using the EasySep mouse neutrophil enrichment kit (Stemcell), routinely yielding >90% neutrophil population.

SYTOX Green Assay for Extracellular DNA

Neutrophils were resuspended in RPMI 1640, no phenol red (Life Technologies) plus 10% FBS. Murine GM-CSF (20 ng/ml, R&D Systems) and 200 μM $CaCl_2$ were added to media for overnight mouse neutrophil experiments. In some assays, neutrophils were incubated at 37°C with inhibitors or blocking antibodies for 30 min before stimulation. Diphenyliodonium (DPI, Sigma-Aldrich) and a 10 mM stock solution in DMSO were prepared. The PAD4 inhibitors GSK484 and GSK106 described in Ref. (19) were purchased from Cayman chemical, and 40 mM of stock solutions was prepared in DMSO. Blocking antibody for CR3, LEAF purified antihuman/mouse CD11b, M1/70 was purchased from BioLegend. Anti-Dectin-1 22H8 blocking antibody was purchased from Invivogen. 2×10^5 cells/well for human or 1×10^5 cells/well for mice were added to black 96-well plates with optical bottoms (Corning) ± RPMI only, PMA (25 nM), particulate β-glucan (curdlan) (100 μg/ml) or AspHE (100 μg/ml) and 1 μM SYTOX Green nucleic acid stain (Life Technologies). Plates were incubated at 37°C, 5% CO_2 in a Biotek Cytation 5 imaging plate reader, and fluorescence was measured every 30 min at 504/523 nm for up to 24 h. Plates were imaged at 40–200× using brightfield or GFP filters.

Quantification of Reactive Oxygen

Neutrophils were resuspended in RPMI 1640 without phenol red (Life Technologies). In some assays neutrophils were incubated at 37°C with inhibitors or blocking antibodies for 30 min before stimulation. 2×10^5 cells/well were added to black 96-well plates with optical bottoms (Corning) ± RPMI only or curdlan (100 μg/ml) plus 500 μM luminol (Sigma-Aldrich) in the absence of serum, and luminescence was measured every 2 min for 2 h on a Biotek Cytation 5.

Immunocytochemistry and Fluorescence Imaging

Neutrophils were resuspended in RPMI 1640, no phenol red, 2% FBS at 2×10^6 cells/ml. In some assays, neutrophils were incubated at 37°C with cytokines, inhibitors or blocking antibodies for 30 min before stimulation. Cells were plated on glass bottom 8-well chamber slides (Ibidi) or poly-L-lysine coated glass coverslips (Neuvitro) ± RPMI only or curdlan (100 μg/ml) for up to 24 h. Media were removed, and cells were fixed for 30 min in 4% formaldehyde in PBS. Cells were permeabilized in 0.1% Triton-X100 in PBS for 15 min and washed in PBS. Cells were stained for H3Cit (Abcam 5103) 1:100 and NE (SCBT) at 1:50 overnight at 4°C. Slides were washed in PBST, and donkey anti-rabbit Alexafluor 488 or donkey anti-goat Alexafluor 568 (Life Technologies) was added for 1 h at RT. Slides were washed in PBST, and 100 μl of PBS-DAPI was added to slides. Slides were imaged at 200× on a Biotek Cytation 5 using GFP, RFP and DAPI filters and on a Leica confocal at 600×.

S100A8 ELISA

Mouse neutrophils were incubated in RPMI 1640 + 10% FBS+20 ng/ml GM-CSF (R&D Systems) ± curdlan (100 μg/ml) or AspHE (100 μg/ml) at 1×10^5 cells/well in 96-well plates as described (12). Plates were incubated at 37°C for 2 or 16 h, centrifuged at 300 × *g* for 3 min, and cell-free supernatants were collected. S100A8 was measured by ELISA (R&D Systems) according to the manufacturer's directions.

Fungal Growth Inhibition Assay

These assays were performed as described recently (12). Briefly, *A. fumigatus* conidia were grown to a hyphal stage in 96-well plates and incubated 18 h at 37°C with 2×10^5 neutrophils/well. Following incubation, the supernatant was removed, and wells were stained with 50 μl Calcofluor white chitin stain (Sigma-Aldrich) for 10 min. Wells were washed three times in ddH_2O, and fluorescence was read on a Biotek Cytation 5 at 360/440 nM.

A. fumigatus Corneal Infection

Mice were anesthetized, the corneal epithelium was penetrated with a 30 G needle, and 2 μl containing 50,000 conidia (dsRed Af293) were injected into the corneal stroma using a 33 G Hamilton syringe as described (12).

After 48 h, mice were euthanized, and corneas were imaged by brightfield to detect corneal opacity, and by fluorescence to detect dsRed hyphae. Images were analyzed, and corneal opacity and dsRed were quantified using Metamorph with the parameters described by us in detail (11, 34). Whole eyes were homogenized using a Retsch Mixer Mill bead homogenizer (QIAGEN Sciences, Germantown, MD, USA), and colony forming units were counted manually.

Flow Cytometry

Corneas were carefully dissected to remove adherent iris material and digested 1 h in collagenase type 1 (80u/cornea; Sigma-Aldrich, cat no 234153). Total cells were collected and incubated with Fc block anti-mouse CD16/CD32 (clone 93, 16-0161-86; eBioscience), followed by anti-mouse neutrophil antibody (Ly6G, NIMP-R14-PE, ab125259; Abcam, Cambridge, MA, USA), and anti-CD11b-APC FAB1124A (R&D Systems, Minneapolis, MN, USA). We also used CD45-FITC (30-F11), Ly6C APC-Cy7 (HK1.4), and Ep-CAM-PECy7 (G8.8), all from BioLegend. Total cells were examined in an ACEA Novocyte™ flow cytometer and analyzed following appropriate compensation.

Immunofluorescence Staining of Mouse Corneas

Whole corneas were excised and immediately embedded in optimal cutting temperature (Thermo Fisher Scientific). Frozen sections (10 μm) were mounted on Superfrost™ Plus™ slides and stored at −80°C. Before staining, the slices were placed on a 37°C hot plate for 10 min followed by submersion in acetone for 10 min at −20°C. The slides were washed in PBS twice, permeabilized 5 min in 0.1% Triton-X/PBS, and incubated at room temperature for 1 h in blocking buffer containing 2% BSA and 0.1% Tween 20 with 1:200 Fc block (Anti-CD16/32; Tonbo Biosciences), and 10% donkey serum (Vector Labs).

Corneal sections (5 μm) were then stained at room temperature for 2 h with Ly6G antibody NIMPR14 at 40 μg/ml (Abcam) and 1:50 Rabbit polyclonal antibody to histone H3 (citrulline R2 + R8 + R17) (Abcam). Slides were rinsed three times in PBS, and then secondary antibodies, donkey anti-rabbit Alexa Fluor 555 or goat anti-rat Alexa Fluor 488, were applied at 1:1,000 (Invitrogen) for 1 h at room temperature. Slides were rinsed and mounted in Fluoromount with DAPI (Thermo Fisher Scientific). All images were acquired within 24 h.

Statistical Analysis

Experimental data from *in vitro* and *in vivo* studies were analyzed for significance from at least three independent experiments. Statistical significance for multiple parameters was determined using one-way ANOVA with Tukey *post hoc* analyses, or using Student's *t*-test when only two parameters were compared.

All statistical analyses were performed with GraphPad Prism software, v6.0c (La Jolla, CA, USA). A p value < 0.05 was considered significant as indicated in the figure legends ($^{*}p \leq 0.05$, $^{**}p \leq 0.01$, and $^{***}p \leq 0.001$).

AUTHOR CONTRIBUTIONS

HC, SA, MM, YS, and EG: experimental design, performance, and data analysis. HC and EP: manuscript preparation.

ACKNOWLEDGMENTS

We thank Laura Mendez-Luque and Michaela Marshall for excellent technical assistance. This work was supported by National Eye Institute Grant R01 EY18612 (to EP), the National Eye Institute National Research Service Award F30EY025548 (to HC), MSTP Grant T32 GM007250 (HC), and the Visual Sciences Research Center Core Grant P30EY011373. Studies were also supported by a grant from the Research to Prevent Blindness Foundation.

REFERENCES

1. Brinkmann V, Reichard U, Goosmann C, Fauler B, Uhlemann Y, Weiss DS, et al. Neutrophil extracellular traps kill bacteria. *Science* (2004) 303(5663): 1532–5. doi:10.1126/science.1092385
2. Guimaraes-Costa AB, Nascimento MT, Froment GS, Soares RP, Morgado FN, Conceicao-Silva F, et al. *Leishmania amazonensis* promastigotes induce and are killed by neutrophil extracellular traps. *Proc Natl Acad Sci U S A* (2009) 106(16):6748–53. doi:10.1073/pnas.0900226106
3. Urban CF, Ermert D, Schmid M, Abu-Abed U, Goosmann C, Nacken W, et al. Neutrophil extracellular traps contain calprotectin, a cytosolic protein complex involved in host defense against *Candida albicans*. *PLoS Pathog* (2009) 5(10):e1000639. doi:10.1371/journal.ppat.1000639
4. Papayannopoulos V, Metzler KD, Hakkim A, Zychlinsky A. Neutrophil elastase and myeloperoxidase regulate the formation of neutrophil extracellular traps. *J Cell Biol* (2010) 191(3):677–91. doi:10.1083/jcb.201006052
5. Hakkim A, Fuchs TA, Martinez NE, Hess S, Prinz H, Zychlinsky A, et al. Activation of the Raf-MEK-ERK pathway is required for neutrophil extracellular trap formation. *Nat Chem Biol* (2011) 7(2):75–7. doi:10.1038/nchembio.496
6. Remijsen Q, Vanden Berghe T, Wirawan E, Asselbergh B, Parthoens E, De Rycke R, et al. Neutrophil extracellular trap cell death requires both autophagy and superoxide generation. *Cell Res* (2011) 21(2):290–304. doi:10.1038/cr.2010.150
7. Neeli I, Radic M. Opposition between PKC isoforms regulates histone deimination and neutrophil extracellular chromatin release. *Front Immunol* (2013) 4:38. doi:10.3389/fimmu.2013.00038
8. Kenno S, Perito S, Mosci P, Vecchiarelli A, Monari C. Autophagy and reactive oxygen species are involved in neutrophil extracellular traps release induced by *C. albicans* morphotypes. *Front Microbiol* (2016) 7:879. doi:10.3389/fmicb.2016.00879
9. Tarabishy AB, Aldabagh B, Sun Y, Imamura Y, Mukherjee PK, Lass JH, et al. MyD88 regulation of *Fusarium keratitis* is dependent on TLR4 and IL-1R1 but not TLR2. *J Immunol* (2008) 181(1):593–600. doi:10.4049/jimmunol.181.1.593
10. Leal SM Jr., Cowden S, Hsia YC, Ghannoum MA, Momany M, Pearlman E. Distinct roles for Dectin-1 and TLR4 in the pathogenesis of *Aspergillus fumigatus* keratitis. *PLoS Pathog* (2010) 6:e1000976. doi:10.1371/journal.ppat.1000976
11. Leal SM Jr., Vareechon C, Cowden S, Cobb BA, Latge JP, Momany M, et al. Fungal antioxidant pathways promote survival against neutrophils during infection. *J Clin Invest* (2012) 122(7):2482–98. doi:10.1172/JCI63239
12. Clark HL, Jhingran A, Sun Y, Vareechon C, de Jesus Carrion S, Skaar EP, et al. Zinc and manganese chelation by neutrophil S100A8/A9 (calprotectin) limits extracellular *Aspergillus fumigatus* hyphal growth and corneal infection. *J Immunol* (2016) 196(1):336–44. doi:10.4049/jimmunol.1502037

13. Byrd AS, O'Brien XM, Johnson CM, Lavigne LM, Reichner JS. An extracellular matrix-based mechanism of rapid neutrophil extracellular trap formation in response to *Candida albicans*. *J Immunol* (2013) 190(8): 4136–48. doi:10.4049/jimmunol.1202671
14. Rohm M, Grimm MJ, D'Auria AC, Almyroudis NG, Segal BH, Urban CF. NADPH oxidase promotes neutrophil extracellular trap formation in pulmonary aspergillosis. *Infect Immun* (2014) 82(5):1766–77. doi:10.1128/IAI.00096-14
15. O'Brien XM, Reichner JS. Neutrophil integrins and matrix ligands and NET release. *Front Immunol* (2016) 7:363. doi:10.3389/fimmu.2016.00363
16. Underhill DM, Pearlman E. Immune interactions with pathogenic and commensal fungi: a two-way street. *Immunity* (2015) 43(5):845–58. doi:10.1016/j.immuni.2015.10.023
17. Thornton BP, Vetvicka V, Pitman M, Goldman RC, Ross GD. Analysis of the sugar specificity and molecular location of the beta-glucan-binding lectin site of complement receptor type 3 (CD11b/CD18). *J Immunol* (1996) 156(3):1235–46.
18. Branzk N, Lubojemska A, Hardison SE, Wang Q, Gutierrez MG, Brown GD, et al. Neutrophils sense microbe size and selectively release neutrophil extracellular traps in response to large pathogens. *Nat Immunol* (2014) 15(11): 1017–25. doi:10.1038/ni.2987
19. Lewis HD, Liddle J, Coote JE, Atkinson SJ, Barker MD, Bax BD, et al. Inhibition of PAD4 activity is sufficient to disrupt mouse and human NET formation. *Nat Chem Biol* (2015) 11(3):189–91. doi:10.1038/nchembio.1735
20. Bianchi M, Niemiec MJ, Siler U, Urban CF, Reichenbach J. Restoration of anti-*Aspergillus* defense by neutrophil extracellular traps in human chronic granulomatous disease after gene therapy is calprotectin-dependent. *J Allergy Clin Immunol* (2011) 127(5):1243–52.e7. doi:10.1016/j.jaci.2011.01.021
21. Karthikeyan RS, Priya JL, Leal SM Jr., Toska J, Rietsch A, Prajna V, et al. Host response and bacterial virulence factor expression in *Pseudomonas aeruginosa* and *Streptococcus pneumoniae* corneal ulcers. *PLoS One* (2013) 8(6):e64867. doi:10.1371/journal.pone.0064867
22. Fuchs TA, Abed U, Goosmann C, Hurwitz R, Schulze I, Wahn V, et al. Novel cell death program leads to neutrophil extracellular traps. *J Cell Biol* (2007) 176(2):231–41. doi:10.1083/jcb.200606027
23. Bruns S, Kniemeyer O, Hasenberg M, Aimanianda V, Nietzsche S, Thywissen A, et al. Production of extracellular traps against *Aspergillus fumigatus* in vitro and in infected lung tissue is dependent on invading neutrophils and influenced by hydrophobin RodA. *PLoS Pathog* (2010) 6(4):e1000873. doi:10.1371/journal.ppat.1000873
24. Gazendam RP, van Hamme JL, Tool AT, Hoogenboezem M, van den Berg JM, Prins JM, et al. Human neutrophils use different mechanisms to kill *Aspergillus fumigatus* conidia and hyphae: evidence from phagocyte defects. *J Immunol* (2016) 196(3):1272–83. doi:10.4049/jimmunol.1501811
25. McCormick A, Heesemann L, Wagener J, Marcos V, Hartl D, Loeffler J, et al. NETs formed by human neutrophils inhibit growth of the pathogenic mold *Aspergillus fumigatus*. *Microbes Infect* (2010) 12(12–13):928–36. doi:10.1016/j.micinf.2010.06.009
26. Lee MJ, Liu H, Barker BM, Snarr BD, Gravelat FN, Al Abdallah Q, et al. The fungal exopolysaccharide galactosaminogalactan mediates virulence by enhancing resistance to neutrophil extracellular traps. *PLoS Pathog* (2015) 11(10):e1005187. doi:10.1371/journal.ppat.1005187
27. Marcos V, Nussbaum C, Vitkov L, Hector A, Wiedenbauer EM, Roos D, et al. Delayed but functional neutrophil extracellular trap formation in neonates. *Blood* (2009) 114(23):4908–4911; author reply 4911–4902. doi:10.1182/blood-2009-09-242388
28. Li P, Li M, Lindberg MR, Kennett MJ, Xiong N, Wang Y. PAD4 is essential for antibacterial innate immunity mediated by neutrophil extracellular traps. *J Exp Med* (2010) 207(9):1853–62. doi:10.1084/jem.20100239
29. Hemmers S, Teijaro JR, Arandjelovic S, Mowen KA. PAD4-mediated neutrophil extracellular trap formation is not required for immunity against influenza infection. *PLoS One* (2011) 6(7):e22043. doi:10.1371/journal.pone.0022043
30. Martinod K, Fuchs TA, Zitomersky NL, Wong SL, Demers M, Gallant M, et al. PAD4-deficiency does not affect bacteremia in polymicrobial sepsis and ameliorates endotoxemic shock. *Blood* (2015) 125(12):1948–56. doi:10.1182/blood-2014-07-587709
31. Nakashima K, Hagiwara T, Yamada M. Nuclear localization of peptidylarginine deiminase V and histone deimination in granulocytes. *J Biol Chem* (2002) 277(51):49562–8. doi:10.1074/jbc.M208795200
32. Wang Y, Li M, Stadler S, Correll S, Li P, Wang D, et al. Histone hypercitrullination mediates chromatin decondensation and neutrophil extracellular trap formation. *J Cell Biol* (2009) 184(2):205–13. doi:10.1083/jcb.200806072
33. Rochael NC, Guimaraes-Costa AB, Nascimento MT, DeSouza-Vieira TS, Oliveira MP, Garcia e Souza LF. Classical ROS-dependent and early/rapid ROS-independent release of neutrophil extracellular traps triggered by *Leishmania* parasites. *Sci Rep* (2015) 5:18302. doi:10.1038/srep18302
34. Leal SM Jr, Roy S, Vareechon C, Carrion S, Clark H, Lopez-Berges MS, et al. Targeting iron acquisition blocks infection with the fungal pathogens *Aspergillus fumigatus* and *Fusarium oxysporum*. *PLoS Pathog* (2013) 9(7): e1003436. doi:10.1371/journal.ppat.1003436
35. Saffarzadeh M, Juenemann C, Queisser MA, Lochnit G, Barreto G, Galuska SP, et al. Neutrophil extracellular traps directly induce epithelial and endothelial cell death: a predominant role of histones. *PLoS One* (2012) 7(2):e32366. doi:10.1371/journal.pone.0032366
36. Kolaczkowska E, Jenne CN, Surewaard BG, Thanabalasuriar A, Lee WY, Sanz MJ, et al. Molecular mechanisms of NET formation and degradation revealed by intravital imaging in the liver vasculature. *Nat Commun* (2015) 6: 6673. doi:10.1038/ncomms7673
37. Shan Q, Dwyer M, Rahman S, Gadjeva M. Distinct susceptibilities of corneal *Pseudomonas aeruginosa* clinical isolates to neutrophil extracellular trap-mediated immunity. *Infect Immun* (2014) 82(10):4135–43. doi:10.1128/IAI.02169-14
38. Konig MF, Andrade F. A critical reappraisal of neutrophil extracellular traps and NETosis mimics based on differential requirements for protein citrullination. *Front Immunol* (2016) 7:461. doi:10.3389/fimmu.2016.00461

10

Innate Immunity Induced by the Major Allergen Alt a 1 from the Fungus *Alternaria* is Dependent Upon Toll-Like Receptors 2/4 in Human Lung Epithelial Cells

Tristan Hayes[1,2†], Amanda Rumore[3†], Brad Howard[1], Xin He[1], Mengyao Luo[1], Sabina Wuenschmann[4], Martin Chapman[4], Shiv Kale[5], Liwu Li[1], Hirohito Kita[6] and Christopher B. Lawrence[1*]*

[1] *Department of Biological Sciences, Virginia Tech, Blacksburg, VA, United States,* [2] *Department of Pediatrics, School of Medicine, Indiana University Bloomington, Indianapolis, IN, United States,* [3] *Department of Biology, Randolph College, Lynchburg, VA, United States,* [4] *Indoor Biotechnologies, Charlottesville, VA, United States,* [5] *Biocomplexity Institute, Virginia Tech, Blacksburg, VA, United States,* [6] *Division of Allergic Diseases, Internal Medicine, Mayo Clinic, Rochester, MN, United States*

***Correspondence:**
Hirohito Kita
kita.hirohito@mayo.edu;
Christopher B. Lawrence
cblawren@vt.edu

†These authors have contributed equally to this work.

Allergens are molecules that elicit a hypersensitive inflammatory response in sensitized individuals and are derived from a variety of sources. Alt a 1 is the most clinically important secreted allergen of the ubiquitous fungus, *Alternaria*. It has been shown to be a major allergen causing IgE-mediated allergic response in the vast majority of *Alternaria*-sensitized individuals. However, no studies have been conducted in regards to the innate immune eliciting activities of this clinically relevant protein. In this study, recombinant Alt a 1 was produced, purified, labeled, and incubated with BEAS-2B, NHBE, and DHBE human lung epithelial cells. Alt a 1 elicited strong induction of IL-8, MCP-1, and Gro-a/b/g. Using gene-specific siRNAs, blocking antibodies, and chemical inhibitors such as LPS-RS, it was determined that Alt a 1-induced immune responses were dependent upon toll-like receptors (TLRs) 2 and 4, and the adaptor proteins MYD88 and TIRAP. Studies utilizing human embryonic kidney cells engineered to express single receptors on the cell surface such as TLRs, further confirmed that Alt a 1-induced innate immunity is dependent upon TLR4 and to a lesser extent TLR2.

Keywords: *Alternaria*, allergen, innate immunity, toll-like receptors, mold, fungus–host interaction

INTRODUCTION

Besides being a common cause of allergic rhinitis, sensitivity to the airborne fungus *Alternaria alternata* is believed to be a common cause of allergic/atopic asthma. Epidemiological studies from locations worldwide indicate that *Alternaria* sensitivity is closely linked with the development of asthma and up to 70% of mold-allergic patients have skin prick test (SPT) reactivity to *Alternaria* (1–3). *Alternaria* sensitivity has been shown to not only be a risk factor for asthma but can also directly lead to the development of severe and potentially fatal asthma often more than any other fungus (1–5). In addition, *Alternaria* sensitization has been determined to be one of the most important factors in the onset of childhood asthma in the southwest desert regions of the US and other arid regions in the world (2, 6, 7). *Alternaria* spores are ubiquitous, routinely found in atmospheric surveys in the US and in other countries and are the most frequently encountered fungal spore type (8). Airborne spore counts are often 1,000-fold greater than pollen counts, and exposures are often longer in duration. Indeed, it has long been speculated that this type of exposure may be partially responsible for both the chronic nature and severity of asthma in *Alternaria*-sensitized individuals (9). Indeed, in a survey by the National Institute of Environmental Health & Safety of 831 homes, containing 2,456 individuals, it was found that the prevalence of current symptomatic asthma correlated with increasing indoor *Alternaria* concentrations (3). Higher levels of *Alternaria* antigens in the environment significantly increased odds of having had asthma symptoms during the preceding year, more so than other examined antigens.

Although some research has been performed on the physiological and molecular identification of *Alternaria* allergens, approximately three major and five minor allergenic proteins have been described to date (10, 11). In general, the biological role of these allergens and other fungal products in the development of allergy and asthma is poorly understood. There is clearly a need to elucidate the role of *Alternaria* immunoreactive proteins and other molecules in the development of asthma from mechanistic perspectives.

Many of the known *Alternaria* allergens are intracellular proteins with clinically relevant homologs being reported in other fungi with known functions such as enolase, ribosomal proteins, nuclear transport factor, and aldehyde dehydrogenase to name a few (11–13). Alt a 1, the major allergen produced by *Alternaria* spp. namely *A. alternata*, is a relatively small (157 amino acids) secreted protein with no clear function in fungal metabolism or ecology (14, 15). Its protein sequence and β-barrel structure is unique among fungal allergens with no known cross reactivity to other allergens (16–20). Diagnosis of *A. alternata* sensitization is often hampered by the variability and complexity of fungal extracts, and thus simplification of the diagnostic procedures with purified allergens has been investigated. Currently, in some allergy clinics in the US, pure Alt a 1 protein is often used to assess sensitization in SPTs in lieu of total fungal extract because it produces the same reaction as total antigen extracts in the majority (80–90%) of human subjects (21–23). Furthermore, Alt a 1, either in its natural or recombinant form, is sufficient for a reliable diagnosis of *A. alternata* sensitization and induces skin prick reactivity comparable with that produced by commercially available *A. alternata* extract (21–23).

In this study, we investigated and report for the first time the innate immunostimulatory activities of Alt a 1 in human bronchial epithelial cells. We found Alt a 1 has potent cytokine and chemokine inducing activity. Moreover, this activity was found to be dependent upon toll-like receptors (TLR2 and TLR4) and associated signaling pathways. This study is the very first in regards to defining the potential role of a single purified *Alternaria* product or protein in innate immunity. Results of these studies are discussed.

MATERIALS AND METHODS

Vector Construction and Transformation of *Pichia pastoris*

An Alt a 1 cDNA harboring vector (pGAPZ, Thermo Fisher Scientific, Waltham, MA, USA) for expression in *P. pastoris* was provided as a generous gift from Dr. Martin Chapman (Indoor Biotechnologies, Charlottesville, VA, USA). Briefly, the pGAPZ-Alt a 1 vector contained a 6× poly-histidine tag for purification *via* immobilized metal ion affinity chromatography (IMAC) and allowed for zeocin to be used for selection. The pGAPZ-Alt a 1 plasmid was transformed into *P. pastoris* GS115 (Thermo Fisher Scientific, Waltham, MA, USA) *via* heat shock and plated on media containing zeocin according to the manufacturer's protocols (Thermo Fisher Scientific, Waltham, MA, USA). Next, as per the manufacturer's protocols, zeocin-resistant *P. pastoris* colonies were then screened for the presence of Alt a 1 using colony-based PCR using forward primer 5′-gtctggaagatctccgagttttacggacgcaag-3′ and the reverse primer 5′-cttgcgtccgtaaaactcggagatcttccagac-3′. Positive colonies were selected and used for downstream expression and production of rAlt a 1 in *P. pastoris* GS115.

Protein Expression and Purification

The rAlt a 1 protein was expressed in *P. pastoris* GS115 according to the manufacturer's instructions (Thermo Fisher Scientific, Waltham, MA, USA) and purification followed a typical IMAC protocol (Qiagen Inc., Valencia, CA, USA). Briefly, yeast was grown in 500 mL yeast extract peptone dextrose broth at 22°C while shaking at 180 RPM. After 60 h, the culture media was separated into cells and supernatant by centrifuge at 5,000 × *g* for 10 min. The supernatant was then buffer exchanged with 2 L of lysis buffer (50 mM NaH_2PO_4, 500 mM NaCl, 30 mM Imidazole, pH 8.0). After concentrating to 25 mL, supernatant was then applied to NiNTA resin (Qiagen Inc., Valencia, CA, USA) that had been washed and equilibrated in lysis buffer per manufacturer's protocols. Four column volumes of lysis buffer were flowed through the column. Next, 5 mL elution buffer (50 mM NaH_2PO_4, 500 mM NaCl, 50 mM imidazole, pH 8.0) was applied to the column. Elution buffer with increasing imidazole concentrations (100, 150, and 200 mM, respectively) was then applied. rAlt a 1 protein eluted at 200 mM imidazole concentration.

Purity was assessed *via* 15% SDS-polyacrylamide gel electrophoresis. As expected, the rAlt a 1 protein appeared to be a heterodimer consisting of 14.4 and 17 kDa bands under denaturing conditions. Amicon Ultra Centrifugal Filters MWCO 10 kDA (Sigma-Aldrich, St. Louis, MO, USA) were used to concentrate proteins, and proteins were buffer exchanged with endotoxin-free PBS, pH 7.4 (Thermo Fisher Scientific, Waltham, MA, USA) for downstream endotoxin removal and applications. Approximately 20 mg/L of rAlt a 1 was typically obtained following purification.

Endotoxin Removal and Quantification of rAlt a 1

Even though protein was produced in yeast, potential endotoxin contamination was removed from purified Alt a 1 using endotoxin removal columns (Detoxi-Gel endotoxin removing columns, Thermo Fisher Scientific, Waltham, MA, USA). Briefly, resin was equilibrated in 1% sodium deoxycholate followed by five volume washes of PBS. 1 mL of protein was loaded onto the column and incubated for 1 h. Protein was eluted by addition of endotoxin-free PBS, pH7.4 (Thermo Fisher Scientific, Waltham, MA, USA).

Quantification of endotoxin levels was performed using an enzyme-linked immunosorbent assay (ELISA) Kit (Biomatik,

ON, Canada). Briefly, 50 µL of protein was assessed following the manufacturer's protocol. Samples were run in duplicate in 96-well plate format and were read on a Versa MAX ELISA Microplate Reader (Molecular Devices, Sunnyvale, CA, USA) at room temperature. Measurements at OD_{450} were corrected against values obtained at OD_{570} following the manufacturer's suggestions. A standard curve was generated for each reading and generated using R software. Endotoxin/LPS concentration was determined using the standard curve and tabulated in ng/mL of LPS. Experiments were performed at least five times/protein preparation. In all experiments, purified rAlt a 1 contained below the detectable limit of endotoxin (<0.01 ng/mL). After testing for homogeneity of variances, Tukey's HSD was performed and adjusted (if applicable).

Membrane-Based Cytokine Arrays

Human cell culture supernatants were assayed for general secretion of different cytokines and chemokines using the RayBio C-Series Human Cytokine Antibody Array C1 per manufacturer's protocols (RayBiotech, Norcross, GA, USA). BEAS-2B cells were grown in DMEM + 1% Pen/Strep/10% FBS. NHBE/DHBE were grown in BEGM media per the manufacturer's protocols (Lonza, Walkersville, MD, USA). Cells were incubated at 37°C/5% CO_2. Approximately 4×10^6 BEAS-2B (ATCC CRL 9609, Manassas, VA, USA) or 4×10^6 NHBE/DHBE (Lonza, Walkersville, MD, USA) cells were starved for 4 h prior to the addition of 50 µg rAlt a 1 and incubated for 24 h. Supernatants were collected and used in downstream experiments per the manufacturer's protocols (RayBiotech, Norcross, GA, USA). Briefly, membranes were blocked with the blocking buffer and then washed. The membranes were then treated with the samples for 2 h at RT shaking at 90 RPM. After an additional wash, the biotinylated antibody cocktail was used to cover the membranes. After a 2-h incubation at RT with shaking at 90 RPM another wash step was conducted. Afterward, the membranes were covered with horseradish peroxidase streptavidin concentrate and incubated for 2 h at RT with shaking at 90 RPM. The membranes were then washed and signals were detected using chemiluminescence. Briefly, membranes were washed with two detection buffers provided by RayBiotech (Norcross, GA, USA) and exposed continuously from 5 to 600 s with images taken at multiple intervals in between using BioRad Chemi Doc CRS+ System with Image Lab Software (BioRad, Berkeley, CA, USA). Images were then exported with no correction or image modification.

Enzyme-Linked Immunosorbent Assays

Enzyme-linked immunosorbent assays were performed using Human IL-8, MCP-1, and GRO (a/b/g) ELISA MAX (BioLegend, San Diego, CA, USA) kits. Supernatants from cells treated with rAlt a 1 were examined following the manufacturer's protocol. Samples were run in duplicate in 96-well plate format and were read on a Versa MAX ELISA Microplate Reader (Molecular Devices, Sunnyvale, CA, USA) at room temperature. Measurements at OD_{450} were corrected against values obtained at OD_{570} following the manufacturer's suggestions. A standard curve was generated for each reading and generated using R software. Cytokine/chemokine concentrations were determined using the standard curve and tabulated in pg/mL. Experiments were performed at least five times. After testing for homogeneity of variances, Tukey's HSD was performed and adjusted (if applicable).

Human Embryonic Kidney (HEK) 293 Cells Engineered to Express TLRs and Measurement of NF-κB Activity

Human embryonic kidney 293-Blue hTLR4 cells expressing TLR4, MD2/CD14 co-receptor genes and a secreted embryonic alkaline phosphatase (SEAP) reporter gene under control of an IL-12 promoter and HEK-Blue Null 2 cells lacking TLR4 receptor but expressing the IL-12 promoter and SEAP reporter gene (Invivogen, San Diego, CA, USA) were seeded in a 96-well plate. The final volume of culture media was 200 µL DMEM + 1% Pen/Strep/10% FBS. After 16 h at 37°C/5% CO_2, the media was removed from the cells. Cells were then starved for 2 h in 200 µL DMEM + 1% Pen/Strep. Cells were pretreated with 5 ng/mL ultrapure LPS-RS (Invivogen, San Diego, CA, USA), 10 µg/mL anti-hTLR4-IgG or 10 µg/mL mouse IgG 1 control antibody (antibodies from Invivogen, San Diego, CA, USA) for 1 h. Then cells were treated with 1 µg rAlt a 1. Cells were then incubated at 37°C/5% CO_2 for 24 h. Afterward 20 µL of the cell supernatant was added to 180 µL QUANTI-Blue reagent (Invivogen, San Diego, CA, USA). After incubation for 3 h at 37°C, the plate was read at 655 nM (VersaMax ELISA microplate reader) at RT. After testing for homogeneity of variances, Tukey's HSD was performed and adjusted (if applicable).

Human embryonic kidney 293-Blue hTLR2 cells expressing TLR2 and CD14 co-receptor genes and an SEAP reporter gene under control of the interferon $(IFN)_\beta$ minimal promoter were seeded in a 96-well plate, final volume was 200 µL DMEM + 1% Pen/Strep/10% FBS. After 16 h at 37°C/5% CO_2, the media was removed from the cells. Cells were then starved for 2 h in 200 µL DMEM + 1% Pen/Strep. Cells were pretreated with 10 µg/mL human IgA2-control, 10 µg/mL anti-hCD14-IgA, and 1 µg/mL Mab-hMD2 (all from Invivogen, San Diego, CA, USA), for 2 h. Then cells were treated with 1 µg rAlt a 1. Cells were then incubated at 37°C/5% CO_2, for 24 h. Afterward 20 µL of the cell supernatant was added to 180 µL QUANTI-Blue reagent (Invivogen, San Diego, CA, USA). After incubation for 3 h at 37°C, the plate was read at 655 nM (VersaMax ELISA microplate reader) at RT. After testing for homogeneity of variances, Tukey's HSD was performed and adjusted (if applicable).

Human embryonic kidney 293-Blue hTLR5 cells expressing TLR5 gene and an SEAP reporter gene under control of an AP-1 promoter were seeded on a 96-well plate. Cells were treated with 100 ng/mL of FLA-ST Ultrapure (Invivogen, San Diego, CA, USA) or 1 µg rAlt a 1. This purified flagellin from *Salmonella typhimurium* is detected by TLR5 resulting in MyD88-mediated NF-κB activation. Cells were incubated overnight at 37°C/5% CO_2. After incubation, 20 µL of the cell supernatant was added to 180 µL QUANTI-Blue reagent (Invivogen). After incubation for 3 h at 37°C, the plate was read at 655 nM (VersaMax ELISA microplate reader) at RT. After testing for homogeneity of variances, Tukey's HSD was performed and adjusted (if applicable).

Blocking Antibodies in BEAS-2B Cells

2.5 × 10^5 BEAS-2B cells were plated in 1 mL DMEM + 1% Pen/Strep/10% FBS. After 24 h, 10 μg/mL of either anti-hTLR2-IgA, 10 μg/mL anti-hTLR4-IgG, 10 μg/mL human IgA2-control, or 10 μg/mL mouse-IgG1-control (all from Invivogen, San Diego, CA, USA) was added. After 2 h, 100 μg rAlt a 1 was added. Cells were then incubated for 24 h at 37°C/5% CO_2. Supernatants were then collected and assayed for cytokines *via* ELISA as described previously.

Gene Knockdown Using siRNAs in BEAS-2B Cells

3.0 × 10^5 BEAS-2B cells were seeded and cultured to 70% confluency in 24-well plates containing DMEM with 10% FBS. The cells were then transfected with 10 nM of either scrambled control, TLR2, TLR4, TIRAP, or MyD88 siRNAs (Santa Cruz Biotechnology, Santa Cruz, CA, USA) in serum-free Opti-MEM medium (Invitrogen, Carlsbad, CA, USA) using Lipofectamine RNA iMAX Reagent (Invitrogen, Carlsbad, CA, USA) according to the manufacturer's protocols. After 24 h, cells were treated with either 50 μg rAlt a 1 or where appropriate, 5 ng/mL of LPS (Sigma-Aldrich, St. Louis, MO, USA). To determine efficacy of gene silencing, western blot analysis was performed 24 h after transfection.

Statistical Analysis

Data are expressed as means and SDs. Data were tested for homogeneity of variances and appropriated analysis of variances tests were performed and adjusted accordingly. Downstream analysis of all numerical data utilized R software and packages. Packages used for analyzing data included Coin, Car, Drc, Multcomp, and Sandwich (24–28).

RESULTS

Alt a 1 Induces Innate Immune Responses in BEAS-2B Bronchial Epithelial Cells

To initially characterize the innate immune response induced by rAlt a 1 in bronchial epithelial cells *in vitro*, we used human cytokine/chemokine arrays harboring antibodies corresponding to 23 target molecules. Our results indicated that Alt a 1 induced the secretion of several cytokines and chemokines in BEAS-2B human bronchial epithelial airway cells—primarily MCP-1 (CCL2), IL-8, and GRO-a/b/g (CXCL1/2/3) (**Figure 1**). Similar results were obtained in experiments using NHBE and DHBE cells (data not shown). There were no marked differences between responses in BEAS-2B, NHBE, and DHBE cells. There was some indication that IL-15 may also be inducible by Alt a 1 in our array studies but was not explored further.

After finding that rAlt a 1 induces the secretion of several innate immune cytokines and chemokines *via* array blots, determining if there was a time-dependent secretion of IL-8 in BEAS-2B cells was conducted *via* ELISA assay (**Figure 2**). The goal of this experiment was to characterize the temporal aspects of IL-8 secretion and to determine if 24 h post treatment was optimal for supernatant collection. Human cells were incubated with Alt a 1 for time periods ranging from 15 min to 24 h. Significant increases of IL-8 secretion occurred after cells were incubated with Alt a 1 for 12 h. However, 24 h was the time point at which IL-8 secretion was the highest (**Figure 2A**). We also determined if Alt a 1 induces IL-8 in a dose-dependent manner and found this to be the case (**Figure 2B**). We found very strong induction of IL-8 with as little as 10 μg of rAlt a 1 with a maximum induction using 150 μg of protein. This indicates Alt a 1 is quite potent at inducing IL-8 in BEAS-2B cells even at lower concentrations.

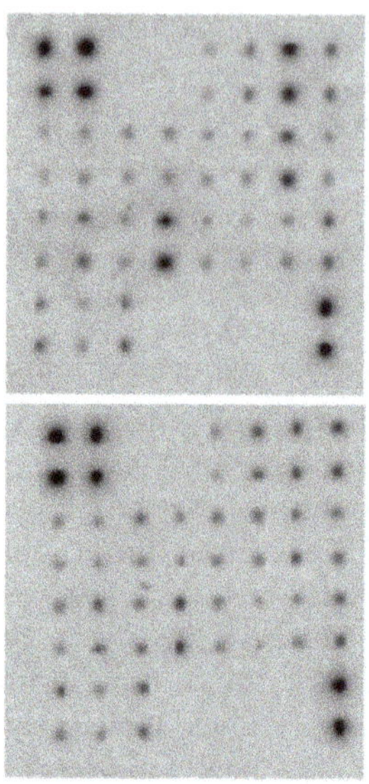

Alt a 1							
POS	POS	NEG	NEG	GCSF	GM-CSF	**GRO a/b/g**	GRO alpha
POS	POS	NEG	NEG	GCSF	GM-CSF	**GRO a/b/g**	GRO alpha
IL-1 alpha	IL-2	IL-3	IL-5	IL-6	IL-7	**IL-8**	IL-10
IL-1 alpha	IL-2	IL-3	IL-5	IL-6	IL-7	**IL-8**	IL-10
IL-13	IL-15	IFN-gamma	**MCP-1**	MCP-2	MCP-3	MIG	RANTES
IL-13	IL-15	IFN-gamma	**MCP-1**	MCP-2	MCP-3	MIG	RANTES
TGF-beta 1	TNF alpha	TNF beta	BLANK	BLANK	BLANK	BLANK	POS
TGF-beta 1	TNF alpha	TNF beta	BLANK	BLANK	BLANK	BLANK	POS

PBS Treated Cells							
POS	POS	NEG	NEG	GCSF	GM-CSF	GRO a/b/g	GRO alpha
POS	POS	NEG	NEG	GCSF	GM-CSF	GRO a/b/g	GRO alpha
IL-1 alpha	IL-2	IL-3	IL-5	IL-6	IL-7	IL-8	IL-10
IL-1 alpha	IL-2	IL-3	IL-5	IL-6	IL-7	IL-8	IL-10
IL-13	IL-15	IFN-gamma	MCP-1	MCP-2	MCP-3	MIG	RANTES
IL-13	IL-15	IFN-gamma	MCP-1	MCP-2	MCP-3	MIG	RANTES
TGF-beta 1	TNF alpha	TNF beta	BLANK	BLANK	BLANK	BLANK	POS
TGF-beta 1	TNF alpha	TNF beta	BLANK	BLANK	BLANK	BLANK	POS

FIGURE 1 | Cytokine profiling of rAlt a 1 treated BEAS-2B cells. 5.0 × 10^5 BEAS-2B cells were treated with 50 μg rAlt a 1 or 50 μL of endotoxin-free, sterile PBS (negative control). Cytokine array blots (*top left*) and corresponding maps of targets (*top right*) derived from cells treated with rAlt a 1, cytokine array blot (*bottom left*) and corresponding map of targets derived from cells treated with PBS (*bottom right*). Comparisons were made between the two blots and cytokines and chemokines highlighted in blue are those that were found to be qualitatively stronger in cells treated with rAlt a 1.

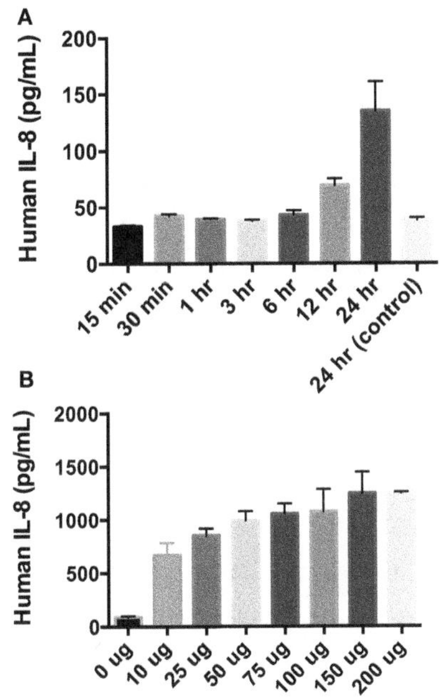

FIGURE 2 | Temporal and dose dependency of Alt a 1 induced IL-8 in BEAS-2B cells. **(A)** 2.0 × 10^5 BEAS-2B cells were grown in RPMI + FBS + 1% Pen Strep. Cells were starved for 6 h prior to induction with rAlt a 1 or endotoxin-free sterile PBS. The starve media consisted of RPMI + 1% Pen Strep without FBS. Cells were treated with 50 µg rAlt a 1 for the specified time. Supernatants were collected and assayed *via* BIOLEGEND IL-8 ELISAMAX. After testing for homogeneity of variances, Tukey's HSD was performed and adjusted ($^*p < 0.001$). Data are represented as mean (SD). Comparisons were made between rAlt a 1 treated and untreated cells (PBS-treated 24 h control). **(B)** 5 × 10^5 BEAS-2B cells were grown in RPMI + FBS + 1% Pen Strep. They were then starved for 6 h. The starve media was RPMI + 1% Pen Strep. Cells were treated with rAlt a 1 or PBS (0 µg) for 24 h. Media was collected and assayed *via* BIOLEGEND IL-8 ELISAMAX. Data are represented as mean (SD). Comparisons were made between Alt a 1-treated and control PBS-treated cells ($^*p < 0.001$).

Additional ELISA assays were next used instead to quantify and confirm the levels of secreted cytokines/chemokines, MCP-1 (CCL2), IL-8, and GRO-a/b/g (CXCL1/2/3). Human BEAS-2B cells were treated with rAlt a 1 for 24 h (**Figure 3**). The ELISA results confirmed the cytokine array blots and showed that levels of human IL-8, MCP-1, and GRO-a/b/g were significantly increased in rAlt a 1 treated cells.

Gene Knockdown Approaches Using siRNAs Indicate Alt a 1 Induction of Innate Immune Responses Is Dependent Upon TLR Signaling in BEAS-2B Cells

To determine the potential role of known pattern recognition receptors (PRRs) such as TLRs and associated signaling pathways in Alt a 1-induced innate immune responses in bronchial epithelial cells (BEAS-2B), a gene knockdown approach using siRNAs was used initially. A suite of gene-specific siRNAs (MyD88, PI-3-K, TIRAP, TLR2, TLR3, TLR4) or scrambled control siRNA (scRNA) were transfected into BEAS-2B cells, then treated with rAlt a 1 for 24 h. We confirmed knockdown of target genes using quantitative reverse transcription PCR. We typically obtained >70% gene-specific knockdown efficiency (data not shown). Supernatants were then collected and assayed for IL-8 levels. These cells showed no consistent reduction in IL-8 secretion when PI-3-K and TLR3 were knocked down (data not shown). In repeated experiments, Alt a 1-treated cells showed decreased IL-8 secretion following incubation with siRNAs corresponding to MyD88, TIRAP, TLR2, and TLR4, compared to scRNA controls (**Figure 4**). We found that silencing of TLR4 resulted in complete abolishment of Alt a 1 induced IL-8 when compared to scRNA control treated cells. In comparison to silencing of TLR4, the effect of silencing TLR2 was statistically significant but was not as robust in these experiments. Interestingly, akin to our results with TLR4-specific siRNAs, we found that silencing of TIRAP or MyD88 resulted in virtually complete abolishment of Alt a 1 induced IL-8 when compared to scRNA control treated cells indicating the importance of these adaptor proteins downstream of TLR-receptors. Collectively, this data indicated that Alt a 1-induced innate immune responses are dependent upon these receptors and downstream adaptors in BEAS-2B cells (**Figure 4**).

Blocking Antibody and Antagonist Approaches Demonstrate Alt a 1 Induction of Innate Immune Responses Is Dependent Upon TLR Signaling in BEAS-2B Cells

We confirmed the results of our siRNA gene knockdown experiments using TLR2 and TLR4 blocking antibodies. In preliminary experiments using TLR4 blocking antibodies, results indicated that TLR4 is important for Alt a 1 induction of MCP-1 (CCL2), IL-8, and GRO-a/b/g (CXCL1/2/3) in BEAS-2B cells (data not shown).

Next we incorporated control antibodies (non-blocking), and TLR4 and TLR2 specific blocking antibodies (**Figure 5**). Blocking TLR4 resulted in a much more pronounced reduction in Alt a 1-induced IL-8 compared to blocking TLR2. We also examined if combining TLR2 and TLR4 blocking antibodies would have an additive effect in regards to dampening Alt a 1 induced IL-8 and found this to be the case. Pretreating cells with both TLR2 and TLR4 blocking antibodies completely abolished Alt a 1-induced IL-8 but was not statistically significant when compared to blocking TLR4 alone and may warrant further investigation. Collectively, these results suggested that Alt a 1-induced IL-8 in BEAS-2B cells is primarily dependent upon TLR4 with a minor contribution from TLR2.

Engineered HEK 293 Cells Demonstrate Alt a 1-Induced NF-κB Signaling Is TLR 2 and 4 Dependent

To further examine the importance of TLR4 in the initiation of the innate immune response to Alt a 1, we used HEK 293 cells engineered to express specific cell surface receptors such as TLR2, TLR4, or TLR5. These cells are also engineered with a reporter system whereby an NF-κB-dependent gene promoter is fused to a

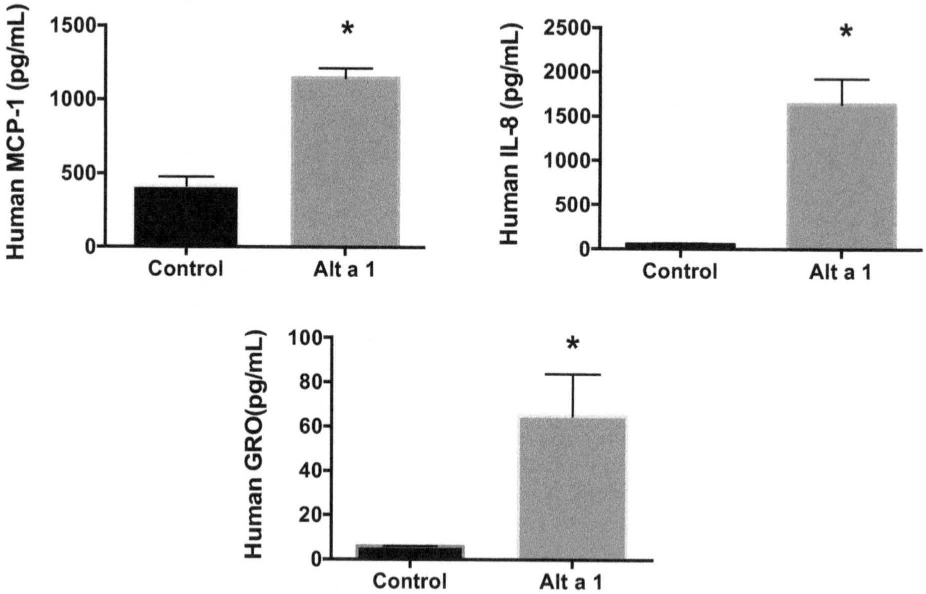

FIGURE 3 | Induction of cytokines and chemokines in BEAS-2B cells treated with Alt a 1. 5.0 × 10^5 human BEAS-2B cells were treated with 50 µg rAlt a 1 for 24 h. Supernatant was collected and cytokine/chemokine levels were determined using BIOLEGEND ELISAMAX [MCP-1 (CCL2), IL-8, and GRO-a/b/g (CXCL1/2/3)]. Data are represented as mean (SD). After testing for homogeneity of variances, Tukey's HSD was performed and adjusted (*$p < 0.001$).

gene encoding a secreted form of alkaline phosphatase (SEAP). In initial experiments, HEK-Blue hTLR4 cells were used to determine if Alt a 1 could activate NF-κB signaling *via* TLR4 (**Figure 6**). We first optimized the systems using cells treated with a TLR4-specific agonist LPS (ultrapure TLR4-specific LPS-EB) and this resulted in high levels of SEAP (**Figure 6A**). This activity could be reduced when cells were pretreated with a TLR4 antagonist (LPS-RS which binds to TLR4 but does not induce a downstream signal), or with TLR4 blocking antibodies (**Figure 6A**).

Using this system, cells were pretreated with antibodies and then treated with rAlt a 1. Directly supporting our data from experiments with TLR4-specific siRNAs and blocking antibodies in BEAS-2B cells, the HEK-hTLR4 cells but not corresponding HEK-null control cells were responsive to rAlt a 1 (**Figure 6B**). Furthermore, this response could be almost completely abolished by directly blocking the TLR4 receptor using both TLR4 blocking antibodies and the TLR4 antagonistic ligand, LPS-RS. Non-blocking control antibodies had no effect on rAlt a 1-induced SEAP. We also performed similar experiments in hTLR2 HEK-blue cells. Results of these experiments indicated that Alt a 1 induced SEAP activity was dependent upon TLR2 (**Figure 6C**).

The specific mechanism for how Alt a 1 triggers both TLR2 and TLR4 is unclear. One explanation could lie in the requirement of co-receptor molecules for the receptors, such as CD14 and MD2. Experiments focusing upon co-receptor molecules for both TLRs were explored in HEK-hTLR2 and HEK-hTLR4 cells. CD14 associates with both TLR2 and TLR4 upon signaling. Another receptor, MD2, is more specific to TLR4. Therefore, we tested to see if these adaptors/co-receptors may be important for signaling using CD14 and MD2 blocking antibodies first in hTLR4 HEK-blue cells.

When CD14 was blocked in hTLR4 HEK-blue cells, signaling appeared to be reduced only slightly and was not statistically significant (Figure S1 in Supplementary Material). This suggested that Alt a 1 may trigger immunity in a CD14-independent manner to a large degree through TLR4. Results of these experiments also suggested that MD2 may not be important for the ability of Alt a 1 to signal through TLR4.

By contrast, blocking CD14 in HEK-hTLR2-blue cells treated with Alt a 1 appeared to cause a small but significant reduction in SEAP (Figure S2 in Supplementary Material). This indicated CD14 may be required for optimal signaling by Alt a 1 *via* TLR2. Blocking MD2 had no effect on HEK-hTLR2-blue cells treated with Alt a 1 indicating unlike CD14, MD2 is most likely not involved in Alt a 1 induced signaling *via* TLR2.

Finally, we investigated the MyD88-dependent TLR5 receptor using a similar approach. To ensure that the conditions of our system were compatible with HEK-hTLR5 cells, we first used bacterial flagellin from *S. typhimurium* (FLA-ST), a canonical ligand for TLR5 as a positive control. As expected, FLA-ST induced robust TLR5-dependent SEAP activity. In contrast to HEK-hTLR2 and HEK-hTLR4, HEK-hTLR5 cells treated with Alt a 1 showed no response indicating that Alt a 1 does not trigger a TLR5–MyD88-dependent response (data not shown).

DISCUSSION

Alt a 1 is the most relevant allergen from the fungus *A. alternata*. Over 90% of patients sensitized to *Alternaria* typically have specific IgE to Alt a 1, indicating that it is a major allergen (29, 30). Sequence and structural studies have indicated that Alt a 1 is a species-specific allergen with no known cross reactivity with other allergens. Its sequence and β-barrel structure is unique among fungal allergens (16–20). Insights into its function have been hypothesized. Because Alt a 1 localizes to the cell wall of

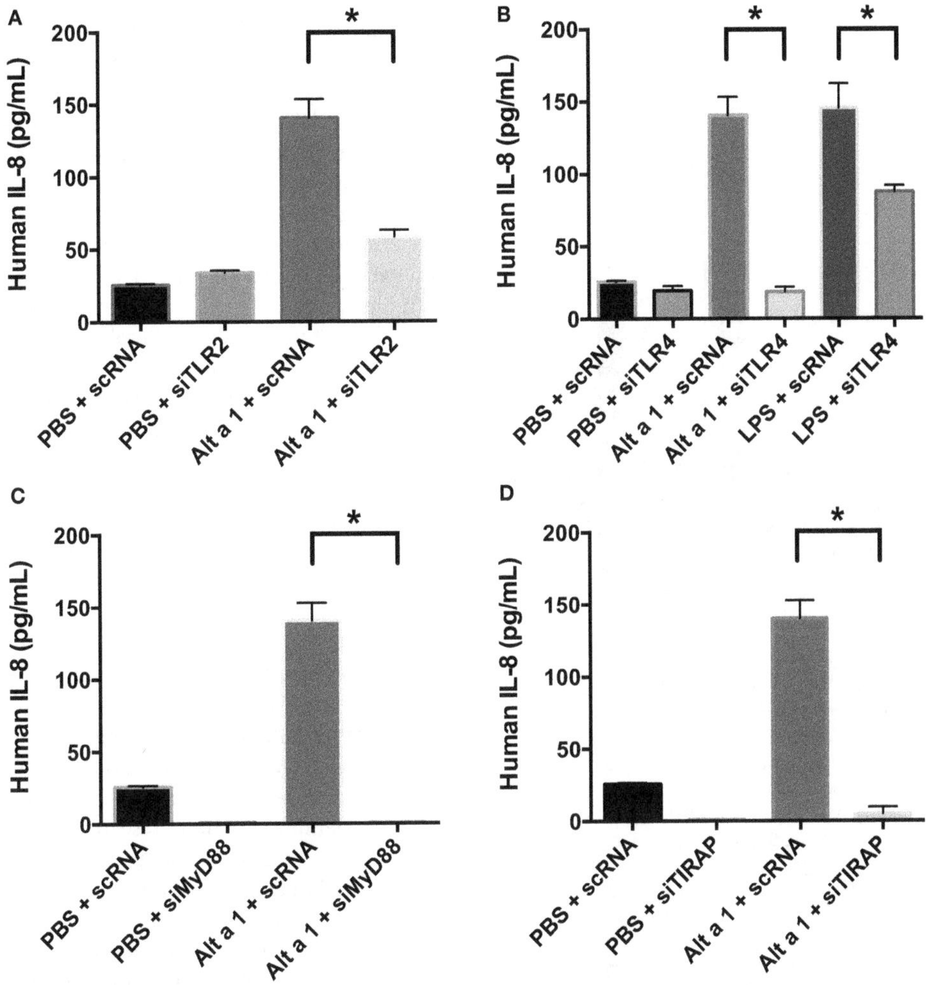

FIGURE 4 | Alt a 1 induces signaling in BEAS-2B cells *via* toll-like receptor (TLR)2, TLR4, MyD88, and TIRAP. 3.0×10^4 human BEAS-2B cells in DMEM + 10% FBS were cultured to 70% confluency in 24-well plates. The cells were transfected with 10 nM of either scrambled control or gene-specific siRNAs in serum-free Opti-MEM medium using Lipofectamine RNA iMAX Reagent according to the manufacturer's protocols. After 24 h, cells were treated with either 50 μg rAlt a 1 or an equivalent volume of PBS. Media was collected and assayed *via* BIOLEGEND IL-8 ELISAMAX. Data are represented as mean (SD). After testing for homogeneity of variances, Tukey's HSD was performed and adjusted (if applicable) ($^*p < 0.001$). **(A)** TLR2, **(B)** TLR4, **(C)** MyD88, and **(D)** TIRAP.

spores, it has been predicted to play a role in the stability of the spore (31). *Alternaria* spores isolated from schools, libraries, and offices have been shown to be capable of secreting detectable levels of Alt a 1 (32). On plants, this protein may play a role in the pathogenesis of *Alternaria* spp. (33). This protein has the potential to bind quercetin/flavonol like molecules of plant and fungal origin (34). Alt a 1 has been shown to be localized in the cytoplasm and cell wall of spores and secreted extremely rapidly in media of physiologically relevant pH especially slightly acidic conditions (34). This suggests that following spore inhalation, Alt a 1 may be secreted into the airways quite rapidly. Based on these recent secretion studies it is possible that all individuals are chronically exposed to Alt a 1 even in the absence of fungal colonization of the airways. Studies examining the importance of Alt a 1 beyond the scope of its capability of being used in diagnostic procedures have not been conducted (21).

In this study, we report for the first time that Alt a 1 induces innate immune responses in bronchial epithelial cells *in vitro*. A combination of cell lines and primary cells (BEAS-2B, NHBE, DHBE) with complementary experimental approaches were used to determine that at least some aspects of Alt a 1 signaling are dependent upon PRRs and adaptor molecules including TLR2, TLR4, MYD88, and TIRAP. Moreover, this is the first study to show that a single, highly purified molecule from *Alternaria* induces innate immune responses.

Previously, most immunological studies surrounding *Alternaria* have employed potent extracts consisting of a complex mixture of proteins and speculatively other molecules from *Alternaria* which could include mycotoxins, other secondary metabolites, and cell wall fragments such as chitin, mannans, and β-1,3-glucans. The complexity and inconsistency of extract composition has made it challenging to define specific components contributing to the

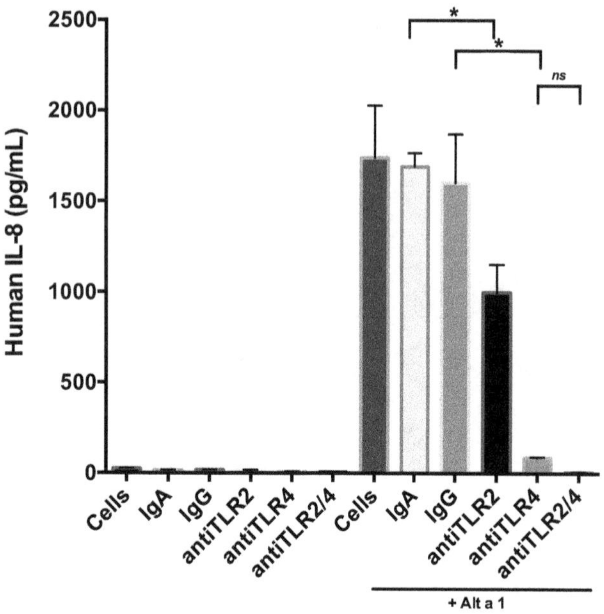

FIGURE 5 | Alt a 1 primarily induces innate immunity through toll-like receptor (TLR)4 in BEAS-2B cells. 2.5×10^5 BEAS-2B cells were grown in RPMI + FPS + 1% Pen Strep. Cells were washed 24 h before use. They were then starved for 6 h. The starve media was RPMI + 1% Pen Strep. Some cells were pretreated with 10 µg/mL anti-hTLR2-IgA, 10 µg/mL anti-hTLR4-IgG, 10 µg/mL human IgA2-control, or 10 µg/mL mouse-IgG1-control for 1 h, then given 50 µg rAlt a 1. Cells incubated for 24 h. Media was collected and assayed *via* BIOLEGEND IL-8 ELISAMAX. Data are represented as mean (SD). After testing for homogeneity of variances, Tukey's HSD was performed and adjusted (if applicable) ($^*p < 0.001$). The anti-hTLR2-IgA Alt a 1 treatment was compared to the Alt a 1-IgG treated control. The anti-hTLR4-IgG treatment was compared to the Alt a 1-IgG treated control. Alta1 + TLR2/4 treatment is significant when compared to the Alt a 1-IgG treated control or Alta1 + hTLR2 and is designated with an asterisk. However, Alta1 + hTLR2/4 is not significant when compared to Alta1 + TLR4.

proinflammatory nature of these products. It is widely accepted that different culture and extraction conditions can lead to the variability in airway cell response to extracts (22, 35). In addition, extracts can have widely different allergen content (36). Expression of fungal allergens can even vary by strain (37).

It has been reported in several studies that protease activities in *Alternaria* extracts, especially serine, aspartic, and cysteine protease activity, are potent inducers of cytokines *in vitro* and *in vivo* (38–40). Using inhibitors, it was preciously shown that serine proteases activity from *Alternaria* induced TSLP and IL-33, potentially playing an important role in the development of allergic inflammation, airway disease, and severe asthma exacerbations (38). Aspartic protease activity was shown to activate eosinophils leading to degranulation (39). Aspartic protease activity was shown to induce the release of several other cytokines, including IL-6 and IL-8 (40). Despite the evidence for the role of *Alternaria* proteases found in extracts to be potent inducers of cytokines, no single purified protease has been identified and correlated with these activities. It is important to note that Alt a 1 has not been reported to possess any protease activity. Alt a 1's enzymatic activity has been reported to be primarily esterase and phosphatase (14). While extracts have clearly defined a potential role that proteases play in the immune response of the airway to fungi, they have not allowed for the determination of the role that individual proteins of *Alternaria*, such as Alt a 1 may play in the context of allergic inflammation, sensitization, and development of more complex disorders such as asthma (41). It is interesting to speculate how Alt a 1 may contribute to the overall inflammatory response of *Alternaria* spores and hyphae in the context of other proinflammatory molecules found in *Alternaria* including proteases mentioned above, chitin, glucans, mannans, and other yet to be identified molecules. In this regard, we have created Alt a 1 knockout (KO) and overexpression mutants in *A. alternata* and have recently initiated *in vitro* and *in vivo* experiments comparing these mutants and wild-type (WT) spores for their ability to induce immune responses. Preliminary data from our lab indicate that mutant spores lacking Alt a 1 induce an overall lower innate immune response when compared to WT spores both *in vitro* (BEAS-2B cells) and in mouse *in vivo* models (Rumore et al., unpublished). Moreover, Alt a 1 overexpression mutants (secreting ~2.5 times as much Alt a 1 compared to WT) induce a dramatically higher innate immune response in these systems compared to Alt a 1 KO mutants or WT spores. Future experiments investigating the role of Alt a 1 in adaptive immunity *in vivo* are certainly warranted using these tools.

Although tremendous progress has been made over the past few decades regarding determining the mechanistic aspects of allergic inflammation, more research needs to be performed in innate immunity and its role in sensitization and exacerbation aspects of allergic diseases. Published studies have increasingly made it clear that TLRs are key players in innate immunity to a growing number of allergens. For example, the dust mite allergen, Der p 2, has been shown to mimic the activity of human and mouse MD2 in the presence of LPS to trigger a response through TLR4 (42) *in vitro* and *in vivo*. Der p 2 has been shown to induce TLR2–MYD88-dependent mediated innate immune signaling in nasal fibroblasts (43). In this study, we found the induction of several cytokines and chemokines by Alt a 1 in bronchial epithelial cells including GRO-a/b/g (CXCL1/2/3), IL-8, and MCP-1 (CCL2) and this was TLR2/4, MyD88, and TIRAP dependent. These cytokines and chemokines have been shown in many studies to play a role in monocyte, neutrophil, and fibroblast recruitment and angiogenesis in asthma and innate allergic inflammation (44–46). Studying if other cytokines and chemokines such as TSLP, IL-33, and IL-25 are induced by Alt a 1 and/or in different cell types may be the subject of future research. Our preliminary data strongly suggest that Alt a 1 is capable of inducing the release of IL-33 from NHBE cells and warrants further investigation in the future (data not shown).

More specifically, using gene knockdown approaches and complementary studies with blocking antibodies, we found that the ability of Alt a 1 to induce a potent cytokine response was dependent upon TLR2, TLR4, MyD88, and TIRAP. Treatment of engineered HEK-Blue Null, TLR2, TLR4, and TLR5 cells with Alt a 1 showed that TLR2 and TLR4-associated NF-κB signaling but not TLR5 is activated. Furthermore, incubation with TLR4 blocking antibodies and LPS-RS caused the abolishment of signaling

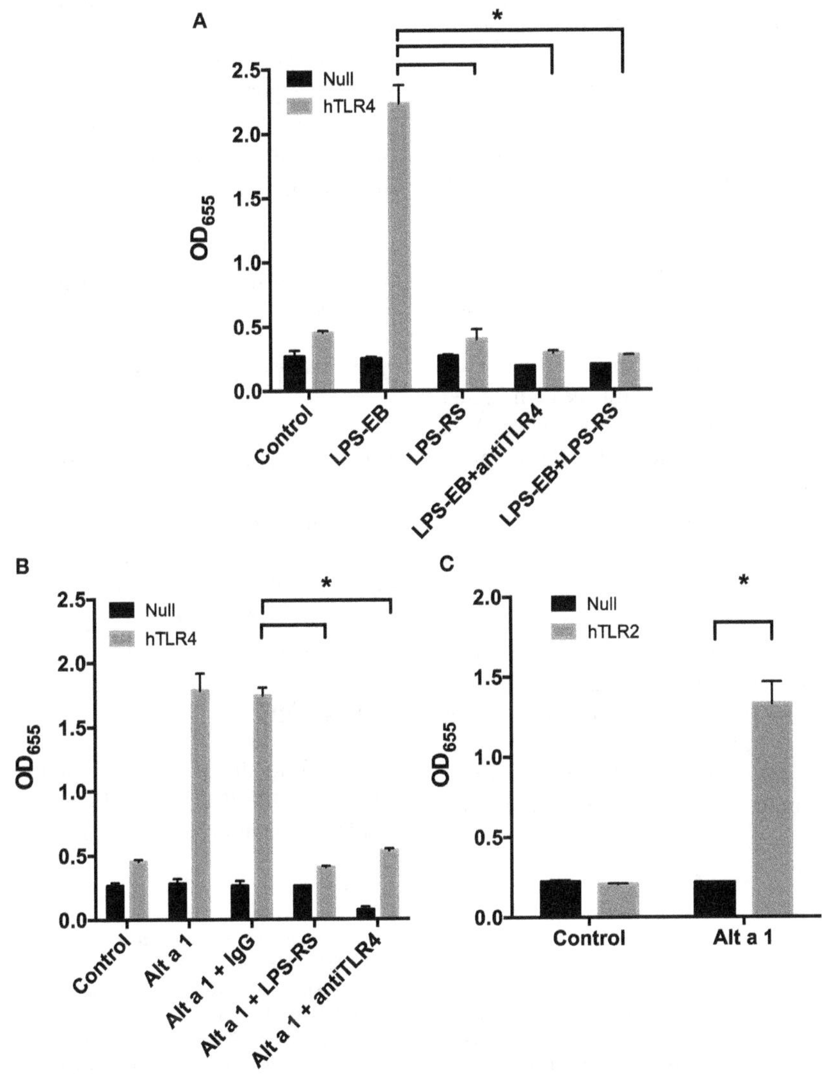

FIGURE 6 | Alt a 1 activates toll-like receptor (TLR)2/4-dependent NF-κB signaling in engineered human embryonic kidney (HEK) cells. 2.5 × 10^4 HEK-Blue hTLR4 **(A,B)**, HEK-Blue hTLR2 **(C)**, and HEK-Blue null cells **(A–C)** were plated in 96-well plates in 200 µL DMEM + 1% Pen/Strep/10% FBS. After 16 h at 37°C/5% CO_2, the media was removed from the cells. Cells were then starved for 2 h in DMEM + 1% Pen/Strep. **(A)** Cells were pretreated with 5 ng/mL ultrapure LPS-RS, 10 µg/mL anti-hTLR4-IgG, or 10 µg/mL mouse IgG 1 control for an hour. Then cells were treated with 5 ng/mL ultrapure LPS-EB. Cells incubated with treatments in the incubator for 24 h. Afterward 20 µL of the cell supernatant was added to 180 µL QUANTI-Blue reagent. After incubation for 3 h at 37°C, the plate was read at 655 nM room temperature. Data are represented as mean (SD). After testing for homogeneity of variances, Tukey's HSD was performed and adjusted (if applicable) (*$p < 0.001$). Comparisons shown are against LPS-EB (*$p < 0.001$). **(B)** Cells were pretreated with 5 ng/mL ultrapure LPS-RS, 10 µg/mL anti-hTLR4-IgG, or 10 µg/mL mouse IgG 1 control for an hour. Then cells were treated with 1 µg rAlt a 1. Cells incubated with treatments in the incubator for 24 h. Afterward, 20 µL of the cell supernatant was added to 180 µL QUANTI-Blue reagent. After incubation for 3 h at 37°C, the plate was read at 655 nM room temperature. Data are represented as mean (SD). After testing for homogeneity of variances, Tukey's HSD was performed and adjusted (if applicable) (*$p < 0.001$). Comparisons shown are against Alt a 1 + IgG (*$p < 0.001$). **(C)** Cells were treated with 1 µg rAlt a 1. Data are represented as mean (SD). After testing for homogeneity of variances, Tukey's HSD was performed and adjusted (if applicable) (*$p < 0.001$). Comparisons shown are against **(A)** LPS-EB, **(B)** Alt a 1 alone or Alt a 1 + IgG, and **(C)** Alt a 1 untreated null and hTLR2 cells and Alt a 1 treated null cells.

in both HEK-Blue TLR4 and human bronchial epithelial airway (BEAS-2B) cells. In contrast to studies with Der p 2, the MD2 mimic that presents LPS to TLR4, our studies suggest that Alt a 1 does not function as an MD2 mimic because it is structurally unrelated to MD2 or Der p 2. Furthermore, we had virtually undetectable amounts of LPS in our protein preparation. LPS was a requirement for Der p 2 signaling *via* TLR4 (42).

In addition to MD2 and CD14, another important protein in TLR4 signaling is lipopolysaccharide-binding protein (LBP). LBP is mainly found in the serum and has been found to facilitate TLR4 signaling by carrying LPS to the receptor. In a study by Kato et al. comparing gene expression profiles in the presence and absence of serum, it was found that induction of cytokines like IL-8 and members of the GRO family in PBMCs was not dependent upon

LBP being present, however, a subset of IFN-inducible genes was dependent upon LBP (47). The data from this study suggested that MyD88-dependent genes did not require LBP to be present but IRF-3 associated genes required LBP. In our experiments, we starved cells of serum prior to challenges with Alt a 1 and other ligands thus, most likely removing the vast majority of LBP present but still observed TLR4- and MyD88-dependent expression of cytokines like IL-8. If Alt a 1 functions as an LBP mimic, one would most likely not detect this in the context of our experimental design. As mentioned previously, we did not detect LPS in our protein preparations thus most likely ruling out the possibility that Alt a 1 could be an LPS carrier or binding protein mimicking MD2, CD14, or LBP. However, it is important to point out that even though our experiments using engineered HEK cells indicated that MD2 and CD14 are probably not major components of Alt a 1 induced signaling, overexpression of TLR2 and TLR4 receptors could mask the role of CD14 and MD2. Future experiments in BEAS-2B or other cell types are warranted to further elucidate the role of these adaptors in Alt a 1 induced immunity.

Another possibility to consider is contamination of our *Pichia*-produced protein preparations with ligands that may activate TLR2. However, there are no reports of *Pichia*-produced proteins harboring contaminants that activate TLR2. It has been shown that the allergen Der p 21 can induce IL-8 in BEAS-2B cells in a TLR2-dependent manner (48). However, rDer p 21 protein preparations used in this study were analyzed by MS and the authors did not report any contamination. The authors speculated that because Der p 21 is predicted to be a lipid binding protein it may carry an unknown ligand to TLR2. In the context of our study, it is possible that Alt a 1 directly binds to and activates TLR2 and TLR4 or liberates a ligand from the cell surface *via* its esterase and/or phosphatase enzymatic activity and will be the focus of future investigations.

Collectively, these findings provide new avenues for the study of allergic inflammation, the sensitization process, and the development of asthma and other allergic airway diseases especially to *Alternaria*.

AUTHOR CONTRIBUTIONS

TH and AR contributed equally to the manuscript (co-first authors), TH and AR designed and performed experiments, analyzed data, and contributed to writing of the paper, BH and XH designed and performed experiments and analyzed data, ML performed experiments and analyzed data, MC and SW created and provided experimental reagents critical for the study, LL and HK designed experiments and provided reagents, CL designed experiments, analyzed data, and contributed to writing of the paper.

FUNDING

Awards from the National Institute of Allergy and Infectious Diseases 5R01AI071106 to HK and CL, 5R21AI115986 to CL, and 1R21AI094071 to CL supported this research.

REFERENCES

1. Gergen PJ, Turkeltaub PC. The association of individual allergen reactivity with respiratory disease in a national sample: data from the second National Health and Nutrition Examination Survey, 1976-80 (NHANES II). *J Allergy Clin Immunol* (1992) 90:579–88. doi:10.1016/0091-6749(92)90130-T
2. Halonen M, Stern DA, Wright AL, Taussig LM, Martinez FD. *Alternaria* as a major allergen for asthma in children raised in a desert environment. *Am J Respir Crit Care Med* (1997) 155:1356–61. doi:10.1164/ajrccm.155.4.9105079
3. Salo PM, Arbes SJ Jr, Sever M, Jaramillo R, Cohn RD, London SJ, et al. Exposure to *Alternaria alternata* in US homes is associated with asthma symptoms. *J Allergy Clin Immunol* (2006) 118:892–8. doi:10.1016/j.jaci.2006.07.037
4. O'Hollaren MT, Yunginger JW, Offord KP, Somers MJ, O'Connell EJ, Ballard DJ, et al. Exposure to an aeroallergen as a possible precipitating factor in respiratory arrest in young patients with asthma. *N Engl J Med* (1991) 324:359–63. doi:10.1056/NEJM199102073240602
5. Andersson M, Downs S, Mitakakis T, Leuppi J, Marks G. Natural exposure to *Alternaria* spores induces allergic rhinitis symptoms in sensitized children. *Pediatr Allergy Immunol* (2003) 14:100–5. doi:10.1034/j.1399-3038.2003.00031.x
6. Peat JK, Tovey E, Mellis CM, Leeder SR, Woolcock AJ. Importance of house dust mite and *Alternaria* allergens in childhood asthma: an epidemiological study in two climatic regions of Australia. *Clin Exp Allergy* (1993) 23:812–20. doi:10.1111/j.1365-2222.1993.tb00258.x
7. Peat JK, Toelle BG, Gray EJ, Haby MM, Belousova E, Mellis CM, et al. Prevalence and severity of childhood asthma and allergic sensitisation in seven climatic regions of New South Wales. *Med J Aust* (1995) 163:22–6.
8. Hoffman DR. Mould allergens. In: Al-Doory Y, Domson JE, editors. *Mould Allergy*. Philadelphia: Lea and Febiger (1984). p. 104–16.
9. van Leeuwen WS. Bronchial asthma in relation to climate. *Proc R Soc Med* (1924) 17:19–26.
10. Sanchez H, Bush RK. A review of *Alternaria alternata* sensitivity. *Rev Iberoam Micol* (2001) 18:56–9.
11. Breitenbach M, Simon-Nobbe B. The allergens of *Cladosporium herbarum* and *Alternaria alternata*. *Chem Immunol* (2002) 81:48–72. doi:10.1159/000058862
12. Simon-Nobbe B, Probst G, Kajava AV, Oberkofler H, Susani M, Crameri R, et al. IgE-binding epitopes of enolases, a class of highly conserved fungal allergens. *J Allergy Clin Immunol* (2000) 106:887–95. doi:10.1067/mai.2000.110799
13. Weichel M, Schmid-Grendelmeier P, Flückiger S, Breitenbach M, Blaser K, Crameri R. Nuclear transport factor 2 represents a novel cross-reactive fungal allergen. *Allergy* (2003) 58:198–206. doi:10.1034/j.1398-9995.2003.23822.x
14. Barnes CS, Pacheco F, Landuyt J, Rosenthal D, Hu F, Portnoy J. Production of a recombinant protein from *Alternaria* containing the reported N-terminal of the Alt a1 allergen. *Adv Exp Med Biol* (1996) 409:197–203. doi:10.1007/978-1-4615-5855-2_26
15. Sáenz-de-Santamaría M, Guisantes JA, Martínez J. Enzymatic activities of *Alternaria alternata* allergenic extracts and its major allergen (Alt a 1). *Mycoses* (2006) 49:288–92. doi:10.1111/j.1439-0507.2006.01238.x
16. Twaroch TE, Curin M, Sterflinger K, Focke-Tejkl M, Swoboda I, Valenta R. Specific antibodies for the detection of *Alternaria* allergens and the identification of cross-reactive antigens in other fungi. *Int Arch Allergy Immunol* (2016) 170:269–78. doi:10.1159/000449415
17. Bowyer P, Fraczek M, Denning DW. Comparative genomics of fungal allergens and epitopes shows widespread distribution of closely related allergen and epitope orthologues. *BMC Genomics* (2006) 7:251. doi:10.1186/1471-2164-7-251
18. Crameri R. Structural aspects of fungal allergens. *Semin Immunopathol* (2014) 37:117–21. doi:10.1007/s00281-014-0458-0

19. Chruszcz M, Chapman MD, Osinski T, Solberg R, Demas M, Porebski PJ, et al. *Alternaria alternata* allergen Alt a 1: a unique β-barrel protein dimer found exclusively in fungi. *J Allergy Clin Immunol* (2012) 130:241–7.e9. doi:10.1016/j.jaci.2012.03.047
20. Wagner GE, Gutfreund S, Fauland K, Keller W, Valenta R, Zangger K. Backbone resonance assignment of Alt a 1, a unique β-barrel protein and the major allergen of *Alternaria alternata*. *Biomol NMR Assign* (2014) 8:229–31. doi:10.1007/s12104-013-9489-z
21. Asturias JA, Ibarrola I, Ferrer A, Andreu C, López-Pascual E, Quiralte J, et al. Diagnosis of *Alternaria alternata* sensitization with natural and recombinant Alt a 1 allergens. *J Allergy Clin Immunol* (2005) 115:1210–7. doi:10.1016/j.jaci.2005.02.012
22. Paris S, Fitting C, Ramirez E, Latgé JP, David B. Comparison of different extraction methods of *Alternaria* allergens. *J Allergy Clin Immunol* (1990) 85:941–8. doi:10.1016/0091-6749(90)90081-E
23. Aden E, Weber B, Bossert J, Teppke M, Frank E, Wahl R, et al. Standardization of *Alternaria alternata*: extraction and quantification of alt a 1 by using an mAb-based 2-site binding assay. *J Allergy Clin Immunol* (1999) 104:128–35. doi:10.1016/S0091-6749(99)70124-7
24. Implementing a Class of Permutation Tests. The coin Package | Hothorn. *J Stat Softw* (2017). Available from: https://www.jstatsoft.org/article/view/v028i08 (accessed January 8, 2017).
25. *An R Companion to Applied Regression* | SAGE Publications Inc (2017). Available from: https://us.sagepub.com/en-us/nam/an-r-companion-to-applied-regression/book233899 (accessed January 8, 2017).
26. Ritz C, Baty F, Streibig JC, Gerhard D. Dose-response analysis using R. *PLoS One* (2015) 10:e0146021. doi:10.1371/journal.pone.0146021
27. Hothorn T, Bretz F, Westfall P. Simultaneous inference in general parametric models. *Biom J* (2008) 50:346–63. doi:10.1002/bimj.200810425
28. Object-oriented computation of sandwich estimators. *J Stat Softw* (2017). Available from: https://www.jstatsoft.org/article/view/v016i09 (accessed January 8, 2017).
29. Yunginger JW, Jones RT, Nesheim ME, Geller M. Studies on *Alternaria* allergens. *J Allergy Clin Immunol* (1980) 66:138–47. doi:10.1016/0091-6749(80)90061-5
30. Kleine-Tebbe J, Worm M, Jeep S, Matthiesen F, Løwenstein H, Kunkel G. Predominance of the major allergen (Alt a I) in *Alternaria* sensitized patients. *Clin Exp Allergy* (1993) 23:211–8. doi:10.1111/j.1365-2222.1993.tb00884.x
31. Twaroch TE, et al. Predominant localization of the major *Alternaria* allergen Alt a 1 in the cell wall of airborne spores. *J Allergy Clin Immunol* (2012) 129:1148–9. doi:10.1016/j.jaci.2011.10.008
32. Skóra J, Otlewska A, Gutarowska B, Leszczyńska J, Majak I, Stępień Ł. Production of the allergenic protein Alt a 1 by *Alternaria* isolates from working environments. *Int J Environ Res Public Health* (2015) 12:2164–83. doi:10.3390/ijerph120202164
33. Cramer RA, Lawrence CB. Cloning of a gene encoding an Alt a 1 isoallergen differentially expressed by the necrotrophic fungus *Alternaria brassicicola* during *Arabidopsis* infection. *Appl Environ Microbiol* (2003) 69:2361–4. doi:10.1128/AEM.69.4.2361-2364.2003
34. Garrido-Arandia M, Silva-Navas J, Ramírez-Castillejo C, Cubells-Baeza N, Gómez-Casado C, Barber D, et al. Characterisation of a flavonoid ligand of the fungal protein Alt a 1. *Sci Rep* (2016) 6:33468. doi:10.1038/srep33468
35. Kim JH, Harvey LA, Evans AL, Byfield GE, Betancourt DA, Dean TR. Biological responses of Raw 264.7 macrophage exposed to two strains of *Stachybotrys chartarum* spores grown on four different wallboard types. *Inhal Toxicol* (2016) 28:303–12. doi:10.3109/08958378.2016.1170909
36. De Vouge MW, Thaker AJ, Zhang L, Muradia G, Rode H, Vijay HM. Molecular cloning of IgE-binding fragments of *Alternaria alternata* allergens. *Int Arch Allergy Immunol* (1998) 116:261–8. doi:10.1159/000023954
37. Martínez J, Gutiérrez A, Postigo I, Cardona G, Guisantes J. Variability of Alt a 1 expression by different strains of *Alternaria alternata*. *J Investig Allergol Clin Immunol* (2006) 16:279–82.
38. Snelgrove RJ, Gregory LG, Peiró T, Akthar S, Campbell GA, Walker SA, et al. *Alternaria*-derived serine protease activity drives IL-33–mediated asthma exacerbations. *J Allergy Clin Immunol* (2014) 134:583–92.e6. doi:10.1016/j.jaci.2014.02.002
39. Matsuwaki Y, Wada K, White TA, Benson LM, Charlesworth MC, Checkel JL, et al. Recognition of fungal protease activities induces cellular activation and eosinophil-derived neurotoxin release in human eosinophils. *J Immunol* (2009) 183:6708–16. doi:10.4049/jimmunol.0901220
40. Matsuwaki Y, Wada K, White T, Moriyama H, Kita H. *Alternaria* fungus induces the production of GM-CSF, interleukin-6 and interleukin-8 and calcium signaling in human airway epithelium through protease-activated receptor 2. *Int Arch Allergy Immunol* (2012) 158:19–29. doi:10.1159/000337756
41. Kustrzeba-Wójcicka I, Siwak E, Terlecki G, Wolańczyk-Mędrala A, Mędrala W. *Alternaria alternata* and its allergens: a comprehensive review. *Clin Rev Allergy Immunol* (2014) 47:354–65. doi:10.1007/s12016-014-8447-6
42. Trompette A, Divanovic S, Visintin A, Blanchard C, Hegde RS, Madan R, et al. Allergenicity resulting from functional mimicry of a toll-like receptor complex protein. *Nature* (2009) 457:585–8. doi:10.1038/nature07548
43. Chiou Y-L, Lin C-Y. Der p2 activates airway smooth muscle cells in a TLR2/MyD88-dependent manner to induce an inflammatory response. *J Cell Physiol* (2009) 220:311–8. doi:10.1002/jcp.21764
44. Keglowich L, Roth M, Philippova M, Resink T, Tjin G, Oliver B, et al. Bronchial smooth muscle cells of asthmatics promote angiogenesis through elevated secretion of CXC-chemokines (ENA-78, GRO-α, and IL-8). *PLoS One* (2013) 8:e81494. doi:10.1371/journal.pone.0081494
45. Singh SR, Sutcliffe A, Kaur D, Gupta S, Desai D, Saunders R, et al. CCL2 release by airway smooth muscle is increased in asthma and promotes fibrocyte migration. *Allergy* (2014) 69:1189–97. doi:10.1111/all.12444
46. Roy RM, Wüthrich M, Klein BS. Chitin elicits CCL2 from airway epithelial cells and induces CCR2-dependent innate allergic inflammation in the lung. *J Immunol* (2012) 189:2545–52. doi:10.4049/jimmunol.1200689
47. Kato A, Ogasawara T, Homma T, Saito H, Matsumoto K. Lipopolysaccharide-binding protein critically regulates lipopolysaccharide-induced IFN-beta signaling pathway in human monocytes. *J Immunol* (2004) 172(10):6185–94. doi:10.4049/jimmunol.172.10.6185
48. Pulsawat P, Theeraapisakkun M, Nony E, Le Mignon M, Jain K, Buaklin A, et al. Characterization of the house dust mite allergen Der p 21 produced in *Pichia pastoris*. *Protein Expr Purif* (2014) 101:8–13. doi:10.1016/j.pep.2014.05.001

11

Canonical Stimulation of the NLRP3 Inflammasome by Fungal Antigens Links Innate and Adaptive B-Lymphocyte Responses by Modulating IL-1β and IgM Production

Mohamed F. Ali, Harika Dasari, Virginia P. Van Keulen and Eva M. Carmona*

The Thoracic Diseases Research Unit and the Division of Pulmonary and Critical Care, Department of Medicine Mayo Clinic and Foundation, Rochester, MN, United States

***Correspondence:**
Eva M. Carmona
carmona.eva@mayo.edu

The NLRP3 inflammasome is activated in response to different bacterial, viral, and fungal pathogens and serves as modulator of different pattern recognition receptors signaling pathways. One of the main functions of NLRP3 is to participate in IL-1β maturation which is important in the host defense against *Pneumocystis* and other fungal infections. However, dysregulation of NLRP3 and IL-1β secretion are also implicated in the pathophysiology of many auto-inflammatory disorders. Often time's inflammatory flares are preceded by infectious illnesses questioning the role of infection in autoimmune exacerbations. However, we still do not fully understand the exact role that infection or even colonization plays as a trigger of inflammation. Herein, we investigated the role of NLRP3 in circulating B-lymphocytes following activation with two major microbial antigens (β-glucan and CpG). NLRP3 was determined essential in two independent B-lymphocytes processes: pro-inflammatory cytokine secretion and antibody regulation. Our results show that the β-glucan fungal cell wall carbohydrate stimulated B-lymphocytes to secrete IL-1β in a process partially mediated by Dectin-1 activation *via* SYK and the transcription factors NF-κB and AP-1. This IL-1β secretion was regulated by the NLRP3 inflammasome and was dependent on potassium efflux and Caspase-1. Interestingly, B-lymphocytes activated by unmethylated CpG motifs, found in bacterial and fungal DNA, failed to induce IL-1β. However, B-lymphocyte stimulation by CpG resulted in NLRP3 and Caspase-1 activation and the production and secretion of IgM antibodies. Furthermore, CpG-stimulated IgM secretion, unlike β-glucan-mediated IL-1β production, was mediated by the mammalian target of rapamycin (mTOR). Inhibition of NLRP3 and the mTOR pathway in CpG activated B-lymphocytes resulted in impaired IgM secretion suggesting their participation in antibody regulation. In conclusion, this study describes a differential response of NLRP3 to β-glucan and CpG antigens and identifies the NLRP3 inflammasome of human circulating B-lymphocytes as a modulator of the innate and adaptive immune systems.

Keywords: β-glucan, B-lymphocytes, inflammasome, fungi, CpG, NLRP3, IL-1β, IgM

INTRODUCTION

The host immune system greatly determines the severity of fungal diseases. In patients with an intact immune system, fungal infections are often clinically asymptomatic or manifest as a mild respiratory illness. In the immunocompromised host, however, fungal infections can disseminate and result in a life-threatening event with high morbidity and mortality. Fungal diseases are on the rise, likely as a result of increasing use of immunosuppressive agents to treat malignancies and autoimmune diseases. Better understanding of fungal immunity will help with the development of alternative antifungal therapeutic strategies that enhance specific aspects of host immunity.

B-lymphocytes, well-known players of the adaptive immune response, react to fungal pathogens by generating antibodies and by releasing inflammatory cytokines (1, 2). In the presence of T cells, B-lymphocyte responses are characterized by isotype class switch and generation of memory and long-lived plasma cells leading to the production of high affinity immunoglobulins (Igs) mostly of the IgG subtype. In the absence of T cells, B-lymphocytes still generate Igs but these are of low affinity and mostly IgM. T-cell independent activation of B-lymphocytes also results in the release of a variety of cytokines and chemokines which are mostly triggered by the activation of pattern recognition receptors (PRRs) such as toll-like receptors (TLRs) and C-lectin receptors (3). PRRs are expressed by most innate immune effector cells, including B-lymphocytes and play a critical role in the detection of pathogens by recognizing conserved pathogen-associated molecular patterns like β-glucan and CpG. β-glucans are highly immunogenic carbohydrates found in the cell wall of many fungi including *Aspergillus* spp., *Candida* spp., and *Pneumocystis* while CpG are highly immunoreactive unmethylated motifs found in bacterial and fungal DNA (4, 5). While each signal using specific PRRs, both have potent immunomodulatory properties and can activate B-lymphocytes directly without the participation of T cells. B-lymphocyte activation by β-glucan and CpG results in the secretion of a specific profile of pro-inflammatory cytokines and chemokines important for the orchestration and activation of monocytes, macrophages, and neutrophils and therefore essential for host defense against fungal and other infections (6–8).

The NLRP3 inflammasome is generally triggered by infection or tissue damage and participates in the processing of mature and bioactive IL-1β from its precursor and inactive form (pro-IL-1β) (9, 10). Since increased production of IL-1β is known to be important for the clearance of fungal infections and little is known about the contribution of B-lymphocytes to the innate immune fungal defense, we sought to investigate the role of NLRP3 activation in B-lymphocytes upon fungal β-glucan stimulation and compare it with B-lymphocyte responses to CpG.

The assembly of the inflammasome classically involves the recruitment of a Nod-like receptor (NLR), an adaptor protein (ASC) and a protease (pro-caspase-1). Depending on the stimuli, the activation of NLRP3 can follow a canonical pathway that involves caspase-1 activation or a non-canonical pathway that is independent of caspase-1. In the particular case of β-glucans, the data are contradictory and both pathways have been described (11–13). In B-lymphocytes, however, the participation of NLRP3 in cytokine regulation and other processes has not been well characterized.

Herein, we describe a dual function of the NLRP3 inflammasome in activated peripheral human B-lymphocytes as a modulator of IL-1β secretion as well as antibody production. While fungal β-glucans andCpG were both able to elicit activation of the NLRP3 inflammasome, the mechanisms of activation were divergent with β-glucan inducing IL-1β secretion and CpG an increase of IgM. Furthermore, CpG activation of NLRP3 was dependent on the activation of the mammalian target of rapamycin (mTOR) pathway while β-glucan activation was mTOR-independent.

MATERIALS AND METHODS

Reagents and Antibodies

Endotoxin-free buffers and reagents were scrupulously used in all experiments. Curdlan, Zymosan, and Laminarin were purchased from Sigma Chemical Co. (St. Louis, MO, USA). *Aspergillus fumigatus* β-glucan preparations were isolated as previously described (14). To ensure that all glucan preparations were free of endotoxin prior to use in culture, Curdlan, Zymosan, and *A. fumigatus* glucans were vigorously washed 10 times with distilled physiological saline, incubated rotating overnight with polymyxin B (Sigma, St. Louis, MO, USA) at 4°C, then vigorously washed again with distilled physiological saline. The final preparations were assayed for endotoxin with the limulus amebocyte lysate method using Pyrosate Rapid Endotoxin Detection Kit (Associates of Cape Cod, East Falmouth, MA, USA) and found to consistently contain less than 0.25 EU/ml. Glucans were pulse sonicated 10 times using a Branson digital sonifier (VWR Scientific, Radnor, PA, USA) at 35% amplitude immediately before addition to the cultures. The Erk 1/2 inhibitor (PD98059), SYK inhibitors (Piceatannol and R406), and NF-κB inhibitor (Bay11-7085) were all obtained from Calbiochem, Inc. (San Diego, CA, USA). AP-1 inhibitor (SR 11302) was from R&D Systems, Inc. (Minneapolis, MN, USA). Caspase inhibitors (Ac-YVAD-CMK and Ac-YVAD-CHO) were purchased from Cayman Chemical (Ann Arbor, MI, USA), VX-765 was from AdooQ Bioscience (Irvine, CA, USA), and Rapamycin was purchased from Selleck Chemicals (Houston, TX, USA). KCl and Adenosine 5′-triphosphate (ATP) were from Sigma and oxidized ATP (oxATP) and MCC950 were from EMD Millipore (Billerica, MA, USA). Phosphorothioate-protected CpG oligonucleotide (5′-TCGTCGTTTTGTCGTTTTGTCGTT-3′) ODN 2006 and *A. fumigatus* oligonucleotides; AF1 (5′-TCGTC GTTGTCGTCGTC-3′) and AF2 (5′-TCGTCGTTGTCGTC-3′) were commercially synthesized by Integrated DNA Technologies, Inc. For most of the experiments, we used CpG ODN 2006 (CpG) unless otherwise specified. Antibodies recognizing the inflammasome components caspase-1 and IL-1β were purchased from Santa Cruz Inc. (Dallas, TX, USA), while NLRP3, ASC, and the mTOR pathway antibodies; mTOR, phospho-mTOR, S6K, and phospho-S6K were from Cell Signaling Technology, Inc. (Danvers, MA, USA). The neutralizing antibody for Dectin-1 was purchased from AbD Serotec (Raleigh, NC, USA) and Isotype control antibody was from R&D Systems, Inc. (Minneapolis,

MN, USA). All other reagents were obtained from Sigma-Aldrich (St. Louis, MO, USA) unless specified otherwise.

Leukocyte Isolation and Culture

All methods were carried out in accordance with relevant guidelines and regulations. Human B-lymphocytes were isolated as previously described (7). Briefly, B-lymphocytes were isolated from acid citrate dextrose anticoagulated blood obtained from de-identified healthy volunteer platelet donors in accordance with the current regulations by the AABB and the US Food and Drug Administration (15) and by the Mayo Clinic Institutional Review Board (IRB). Ethics committee approval was not required according to the local and national and guidelines. Cells were isolated using RossetteSep B-cell enrichment cocktail according to the manufacturer's protocol (StemCell Technologies, Vancouver, BC, Canada). The enriched B-lymphocyte population was repeatedly observed to contain an average of 93.1% ± 2.3% B-lymphocytes. Sorting of human CD19+ B-lymphocytes into naïve (CD27−) and memory (CD27+) B-lymphocytes was performed using mouse anti-human CD27-APC-Vio770 and mouse anti-human CD19-PE antibodies from Miltenyi Biotec (San Diego, CA, USA), on a FACSAria II SORP flow cytometer running FACSDiva v 6.1.3 software.

RNA Isolation and Real-time qPCR Analysis

Total cellular RNA was isolated from B-lymphocytes using RNeasy Plus Universal Mini Kit (Qiagen) according to the manufacturer's instructions. For cDNA synthesis, total RNA concentrations and purity were determined using a Nanodrop ND-1000 spectrophotometer, and 1 μg RNA was used in a 20 μl reaction mixture using a Verso cDNA Synthesis Kit (Thermo Scientific). Quantitative real-time PCR was performed in 10 μl reaction in a 96-well plate using 2 μl of diluted cDNA with SYBR Premix Ex Taq (Clontech Laboratories, Inc.) on a ViiA7 Real-Time PCR Detection System (Life Technologies). The data were analyzed with ViiA7 software, version 1.2.4 (Life Technologies). Relative transcript expression of IL-1β was determined using the comparative Ct method, and was normalized to GAPDH transcripts of the same cDNA samples. The results were expressed as % of the target gene relative to that of GAPDH and plotted as the mean ± SEM. Experimental reproducibility was confirmed using three biological replicates from independent experiments which used B-lymphocytes from three different donors. The primers used for amplification were: IL-1β, 5′-ATGCACCTGTACGATCACTG-3′ and 5′-ACAAAGGACA TGGAGAACACC-3′; GAPDH, 5′-ACATCGCTCAGACACCA TG-3′ and 5′-TGTAGTTGAGGTCAATGAAGGG-3′.

Cytokines and IgM Detection

B-lymphocytes (4×10^5 cells/well in 96-well plates) were cultured with 1 μg/ml of CpG (ODN 2006), or with 1 μg/ml AF1, 1 μg/ml AF2, 200 μg/ml of Curdlan (Curd), 200 μg/ml Zymosan (Zym), 200 μg/ml or 200 μg/ml*A. fumigatus* β-glucan (AspG) in culture medium for 24 h for IL-1β and other cytokines and 5 days for IgM unless otherwise indicated. Cell supernatants were then analyzed for IL-1β, TNFα, IL-6, MMP7, and IgM production using human DuoSet ELISA kit for MMP-7 from R&D Systems, Inc. (Minneapolis, MN, USA), BD OptEIA human ELISA kit for IL-1β and Ready-Set-Go ELISA kit for TNFα, IL-6, and IgM from Thermo Fisher (Rochester, NY, USA). ELISAs were performed according to each manufacturer's instructions. Inhibitors [50 and 100 μM Caspase-1 inhibitors (VX-765 and YVAD.CMK), 50 mM KCl, 50 μM oxATP, 100 μM MCC950, 40 μM Piceatannol, 5 μM R406, 10 μM Bay11-7085, 10 μM SR11302 or 1 mg/ml Laminarin] and neutralizing antibodies (5 μg/ml anti-Dectin-1 IgG or mouse IgG) were incubated with B-lymphocytes for 1 h prior to addition of CpG or β-glucan preparations. Inhibitors were dissolved in dimethyl sulfoxide unless otherwise indicated. Solvents were added to all treatments to assure that solvents concentrations are the same in all treatment conditions.

Caspase-1 Activity Assay

Caspase-1 activity was determined by a Caspase-1 Fluorometric Assay (BioVision, Mountain View, CA, USA), according to the manufacturer's instruction. Briefly, 10^7 B-lymphocytes were stimulated with Curdlan and CpG in the presence of the caspase inhibitor YVAD-CMK, incubated at 37°C for 24 h and lysed with cell lysis buffer on ice for 10 min. Then, equal volumes of 2× reaction buffer and YVAD-AFC were added to the 200 μg of lysates in a 96-well plate and incubated for 2 h at 37°C. The samples were read on a Softmax microplate reader (Molecular Devices, Sunnyvale, CA, USA) with a 400 nm excitation filter and 505 nm emission filter. The caspase-1 activity is expressed relative to the unstimulated control.

Cellular Viability

Cell viability was assessed using the XTT Cell Proliferation Kit II (Roche Molecular Biochemicals, Indianapolis, IN, USA) according to the manufacturer's protocol. This assay measures the conversion of sodium-3′-[1-(phenylaminocarbonyl)-3, 4-tetrazolium]-bis(4-methoxy-6-nitro) benzenesulfonic acid hydrate (XTT) to a formazan dye through electron coupling in metabolically active mitochondria using the coupling reagent *N*-methyldibenzopyrazine methyl sulfate. Only metabolically active cells are capable of mediating this reaction, which is detected by absorbance of the dye at 450–500 nm. Briefly, 50 μl of the XTT labeling mixture was added to the 100 μl of growth medium containing B-lymphocytes and different concentrations of the inhibitors. The XTT labeling mixture was added in parallel samples 24 h after the addition of the various inhibitors. A set of blanks was also included that did not contain cells and was treated identically as the normal samples. In addition, a set of solvent controls was also included for each inhibitor. Absorbance was measured at 6 h after XTT addition. All treatments were performed in three replicates. Only inhibitor concentrations that elicited less than 20% net toxicity were used in these assays.

Preparation of Cell Lysates, Electrophoresis, and Immunoblotting

Total cellular proteins were obtained from B-lymphocytes following the described culture conditions. Briefly, the cells were washed with cold PBS twice and lysed in RIPA buffer (50 mM Tris–HCl pH 7.4, 15 mM NaCl, 0.25% deoxycholic acid, 1% NP-40) freshly supplemented with 1 mM phenylmethylsulfonyl fluoride, mammalian protease inhibitor mixture, 10 mM Na Fluoride, and 1 mM Na Orthovanadate. Cells were kept on ice for 15 min and then the lysates were centrifuged at 12,000 × *g* for 10 min at 4°C. The resultant soluble supernatant contained total cellular protein. Protein concentrations were determined with the Bio-Rad protein assay (Hercules, CA, USA) using BSA as the standard. Equal amounts of total cellular proteins were separated on SDS-10% polyacrylamide gels with Precision Plus Protein Dual Color Standards (Bio-Rad; Hercules, CA, USA) being used as the molecular weight standards. Proteins were transferred to Immobilon-P membranes (Millipore, Bedford, MA, USA). Membranes were then blocked at room temperature for 30 min with 1% BSA/TBST (TBS, pH 7.4, 1% BSA, 0.1% Tween 20) and incubated overnight at 4°C in a blocking solution containing primary antibodies at the appropriate dilutions. After washing with TBST, the membranes were incubated with horseradish peroxidase-conjugated secondary antibodies for 1 h. Immunoreactive bands were detected with SuperSignal West PicoChemiluminescent Substrate from Thermo Scientific (Rockford, IL, USA). Actin was used as loading control for the cell lysates and a non-specific protein for the cell supernatant.

Statistical Analyses

All data are presented as the mean ± SEM, from at least three independent experiments from different biological donors, unless otherwise specified. An experimental run included at least three different donors. The data were first analyzed using one-way ANOVA, the differences between the individual groups were compared using multiple comparisons post-test unless otherwise indicated. Statistical analysis was performed using GraphPad Prism Version 5 (GraphPad Software, La Jolla, CA, USA).

RESULTS

IL-1β Is Induced by Fungal β-Glucans in a T-Cell Independent Manner

B-lymphocytes respond to fungal β-glucans and bacterial DNA in a T-cell independent manner by releasing cytokines and chemokines important for the acute inflammatory response (8, 16). We have previously shown that β-glucan-stimulated peripheral human B-lymphocytes are a source of IL-8, IL-6, and TNFα (7). Additionally, supernatant from β-glucan-stimulated B-lymphocytes was able to significantly increase neutrophil chemotaxis suggesting the contribution of B-lymphocytes in the acute inflammatory process (7). To further understand the role of B-lymphocytes in fungal defense and since IL-1β has been shown to participate in fungal clearance and neutrophil recruitment (17, 18), freshly isolated peripheral B-lymphocytes from normal donors were stimulated with either β-glucan (Curdlan) or CpG (CpG ODN 2006) and assessed for IL-1β expression. RNA levels of IL-1β were significantly elevated in β-glucan-stimulated cells but not in those stimulated with CpG (**Figure 1A**). Protein levels of IL-1β were next confirmed in the cell supernatants by ELISA. As expected, β-glucan-stimulated cells secreted significant amounts of active IL-1β in a dose and time responsive manner (**Figures 1B,C**). The addition of β-glucan to CpG did not enhance IL-1β stimulation (**Figure 1D**). Furthermore, IL-1β secretion was not restricted to curdlan β-glucans as other β-glucan preparation such as zymosan and β-glucan from *Aspergillus* were also potent inducers of IL-1β (**Figure 1E**). Similarly, failure to induce IL-1β secretion was not restricted to CpG ODN 2006, since two different CpG motifs present in *A. fumigatus* DNA (AF1 and AF2) (4) also failed to stimulate IL-1β secretion (**Figure 1F**). The differential response of B-lymphocytes to β-glucan and CpG was intriguing, though similarly observed by our group in the setting of IL-8 and IgM (7). Our published studies demonstrated that β-glucan-induced IL-8 secretion had no effect on IgM while CpG stimulated IgM secretion did not participate in IL-8 secretion (7).

β-Glucan and CpG Induce Activation of the NLRP3 Inflammasome in Human Circulating B-Lymphocytes

The NLRP3 inflammasome is crucial for the processing of biologically inactive IL-1β (pro-IL-1β) into the mature and biologically active form (IL-1β). It was therefore important for us to determine its role in β-glucan-mediated IL-1β secretion. Protein expression of NLRP3, ASC, caspase-1, and pro-IL-1β as well as caspase-1 activity were therefore assessed and found to increase significantly upon β-glucan stimulation (**Figures 2A,C**). CpG stimulation did not induce pro-IL-1β, a required step needed for mature IL-1β production (**Figure 2B**). However, despite the lack of increase in pro-IL-1β, CpG also resulted in activation of the NLRP3 inflammasome (**Figures 2B,C**).

To further demonstrate that Caspase-1 and NLRP3 were indeed important in β-glucan-mediated IL-1β secretion and since primary human B-lymphocytes are not suitable for lentivirus infection or transfection with other forms of interfering RNA, IL-1β was measured in the cell supernatant of stimulated cells in the presence of different Caspase-1 and NLRP3 inhibitors. As shown in **Figures 2D–F**, the use of the caspase-1 inhibitors VX765 and YVAD-CMK, KCL, oxATP, and the specific NLRP3 inhibitor, MCC950 (19), resulted in significant decreases of IL-1β secretion, confirming the participation of the canonical NLRP3 inflammasome pathway in β-glucan-mediated IL-1β secretion. Absence of cell toxicity was confirmed for all the inhibitors as shown in Supplement S1 in Supplementary Material.

Since prior data suggested that in NLRP3 deficient mice IgM secretion and antibody production are impaired (8, 20–22), we hypothesized that NLRP3 may regulate IgM secretion. We and others have additionally shown that peripheral B-lymphocytes secrete IgM in response to CpG (ODN 2006) (7, 23) (Supplement S2 in Supplementary Material). To better understand the role of NLRP3 activation in CpG-stimulated B-lymphocytes we further investigated if IgM was also triggered in response to AF1 and AF2. As shown in **Figure 3A** IgM was similarly induced by all forms of CpG tested. Next, we evaluated IgM levels after CpG stimulation in the presence of different concentrations of MCC950. Interestingly, the levels of IgM decreased in the presence of MCC950 in a dose-dependent manner (**Figure 3B**; Supplement S3A

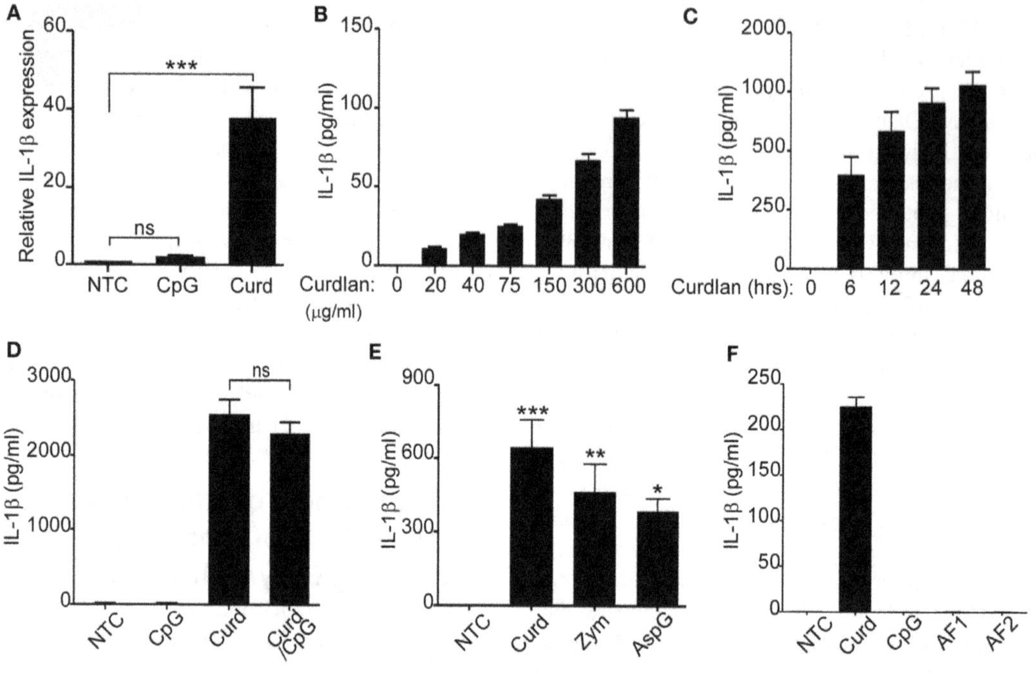

FIGURE 1 | Fungal β-glucans elicit IL-1β secretion in B-lymphocytes. Quantitative real-time PCR for IL-1β mRNA was determined in non-treated cells (NTC) or B-cells stimulated with CpG or Curdlan (Curd). Expression was normalized to GAPDH **(A)**. IL-1β levels were measured by ELISA in the cell supernatant of curdlan stimulated cells at different concentrations **(B)**, for different periods of time **(C)**, with CpG and Curdlan as indicated **(D)** with different β-glucan preparations: Curdlan, Zymosan (Zym), and *Aspergillus fumigatus* (AspG) **(E)** and with different CpG motifs from *A. fumigatus*: AF1 and AF2 **(F)**. Stimulation was done overnight unless otherwise indicated. 200 μg/ml β-glucan and 1 μg/ml CpG, AF1, and AF2 were used unless otherwise specified. Data are representative of at least three donors in each independent experiment ($n = 3$). $^{*}p < 0.05$, $^{**}p < 0.01$, $^{***}p < 0.0001$, ns, not significant ($p > 0.05$).

in Supplementary Material). To ensure that this effect was specific to inhibition of the NLRP3 inflammasome, IL-6, MMP-7, and TNFα were also assessed in the presence of MCC950. As shown in **Figure 3C,** none of the other cytokines and metalloproteases were affected by the presence of the inhibitor further supporting the specific role of the NLRP3 inflammasome in IgM secretion. Additionally, IgM release was also impaired in the presence of KCL, oxATP, and caspase inhibitors (**Figures 3D,E**; Supplement S3A in Supplementary Material), all well-known agents that affect the functioning of the NLRP3 inflammasome.

Dectin-1 and Syk-Participate in NLRP3 Activation by β-Glucans While CpG Signaling Activation of NLRP3 Regulates IgM *via* mTOR

Since the inflammasome was activated by both β-glucan and CpG and both are known to signal through very different PRRs, we next explored the specific signaling pathways that lead to IL-1β and IgM secretion upon β-glucan and CpG, respectively.

β-Glucans are known to signal predominantly through the C-lectin receptor Dectin-1 (6, 7, 24, 25) while CpG is the natural ligand for TLR9 (4, 26). Hence, we first explored the contribution of Dectin-1 in β-glucan-induced IL-1β signaling. B-lymphocytes were pre-incubated with either laminarin (a soluble β-glucan known to bind to Dectin-1 acting as a competitive inhibitor) or a specific Dectin-1 blocking antibody prior to β-glucan stimulation. IL-1β levels were significantly reduced in the presence of both, laminarin and the Dectin-1 antibody, confirming the role of Dectin-1 in β-glucan-mediated IL-1β secretion (**Figures 4A,B**). β-glucan-mediated IL-1β was also dependent on Syk and the transcription factors NF-κB and AP-1 (**Figures 4C,D**).

TLR9 is the main receptor for CpG motifs found in bacterial and fungal DNA (4, 26) and it is known that stimulation by CpG also involves mTOR (4, 6, 27–29). In contrast, β-glucan stimulation does not seem to require mTOR (6). Thus, to additionally understand the potential involvement of mTOR activation in IgM and IL-1β regulation, phosphorylation of mTOR and other mTOR-related proteins were assessed after cells were stimulated for different period of time with CpG or β-glucan. mTOR and other mTOR-related proteins (S6K, S6, and 4EBP1) tested were phosphorylated upon CpG but not after β-glucan stimulation with the exception of 4EBP1 which seemed to be phosphorylated by both (**Figure 5A**; Supplement S3B in Supplementary Material). β-glucan activation of 4EBP1 was inhibited in the presence of PD98059, a specific ERK1/2 inhibitor, and not by Rapamycin, a well-known mTOR inhibitor, suggesting that 4EBP1 activation, in β-glucan-stimulated cells, was mTOR-independent and required ERK1/2 (Supplement S4 in Supplementary Material), consistent with prior observations (30).

As our data suggested that NLRP3 regulates IgM *via* mTOR, we measured IgM levels after CpG-stimulation in the presence

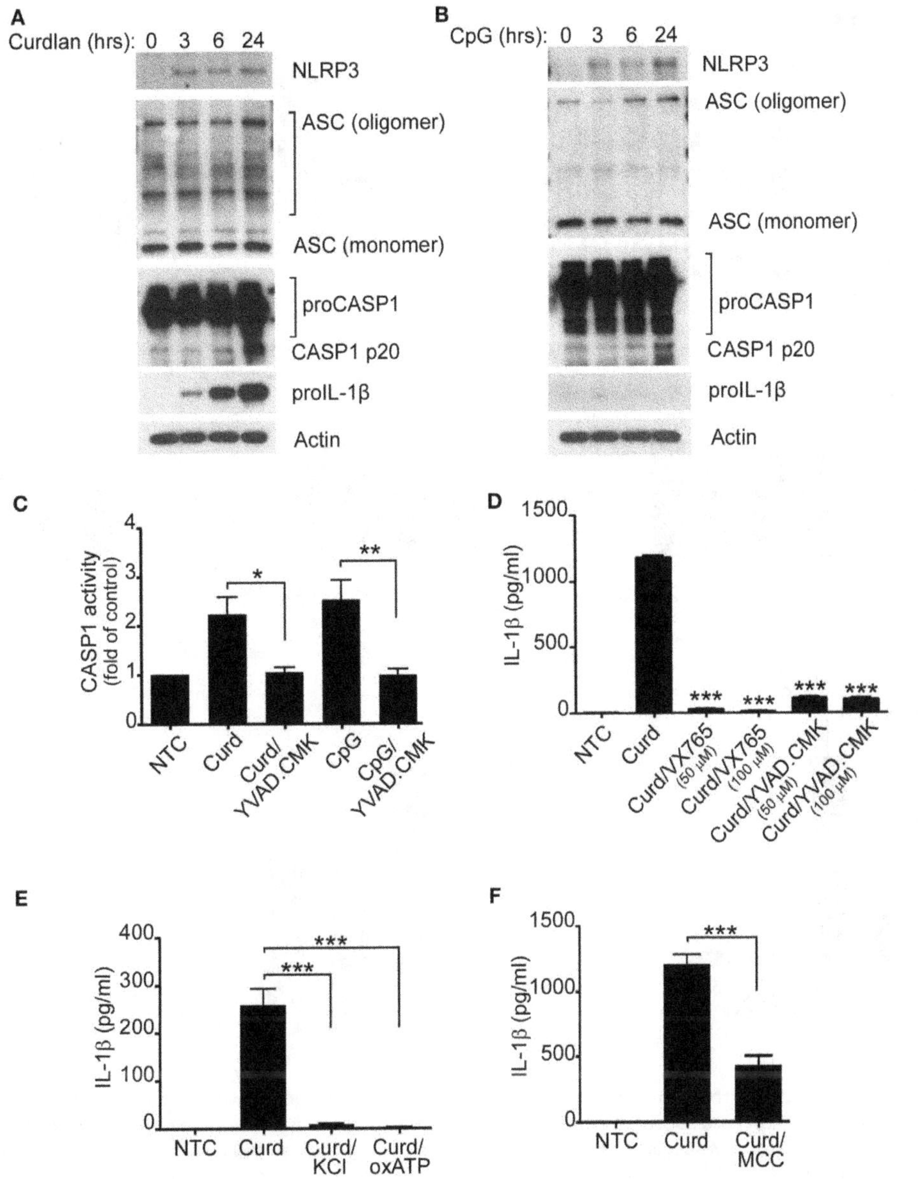

FIGURE 2 | IL-1β secretion requires the NLRP3 inflammasome. Immunoblot analysis of NLRP3, ASC, proCaspase-1, Caspase-1 p20, pro-IL-1β, and actin after curdlan **(A)** or CpG stimulation **(B)** for different periods of time, as indicated. **(C)** Capase1 activity was determined in unstimulated cells (NTC), after Curdlan (Curd) and CpG stimulation. In some cases, the stimulation was performed in the presence of the caspase inhibitor YVAD-CMK (50 μM) as indicated. IL-1β ELISA measured in the cell supernatant of NTC, after curdlan stimulation and after curdlan stimulation of cells pretreated with VX-765 and YVAD-CMK **(D)**, 50 mM KCL and 50 μM oxidized ATP (oxATP) **(E)** and 100 μM MCC950 **(F)** as indicated. 200 μg/ml curdlan and 1 μg/ml CpG were used for stimulation. Data are representative of at least three independent experiments. *$p < 0.05$, **$p < 0.01$, ***$p < 0.0001$.

and absence of Rapamycin. The use of Rapamycin resulted in significant reduction of IgM thus confirming the role of mTOR signaling in IgM regulation (**Figure 5B**; Supplement S3A in Supplementary Material). The levels of IgM in the presence of Rapamycin were comparably reduced to the levels of IgM after MCC950. In contrast, β-glucan stimulation of IL-1β, while reduced in the presence of MCC950, was not affected by the use of Rapamycin confirming that this is an mTOR-independent process (**Figure 5C**). Interestingly, Rapamycin inhibition of the NLRP3 inflammasome seemed to affect Caspase-1 activation as shown in **Figure 5D**. Similar observations were made for MCC950, consistent with prior published observations (31).

Memory B-Lymphocytes Are the Main Producers of IL-1β and IgM

Peripheral B-lymphocytes can be divided into naïve and memory cells. In order to further understand the subtype of B-lymphocytes responsible for the secretion of IL-1β and IgM,

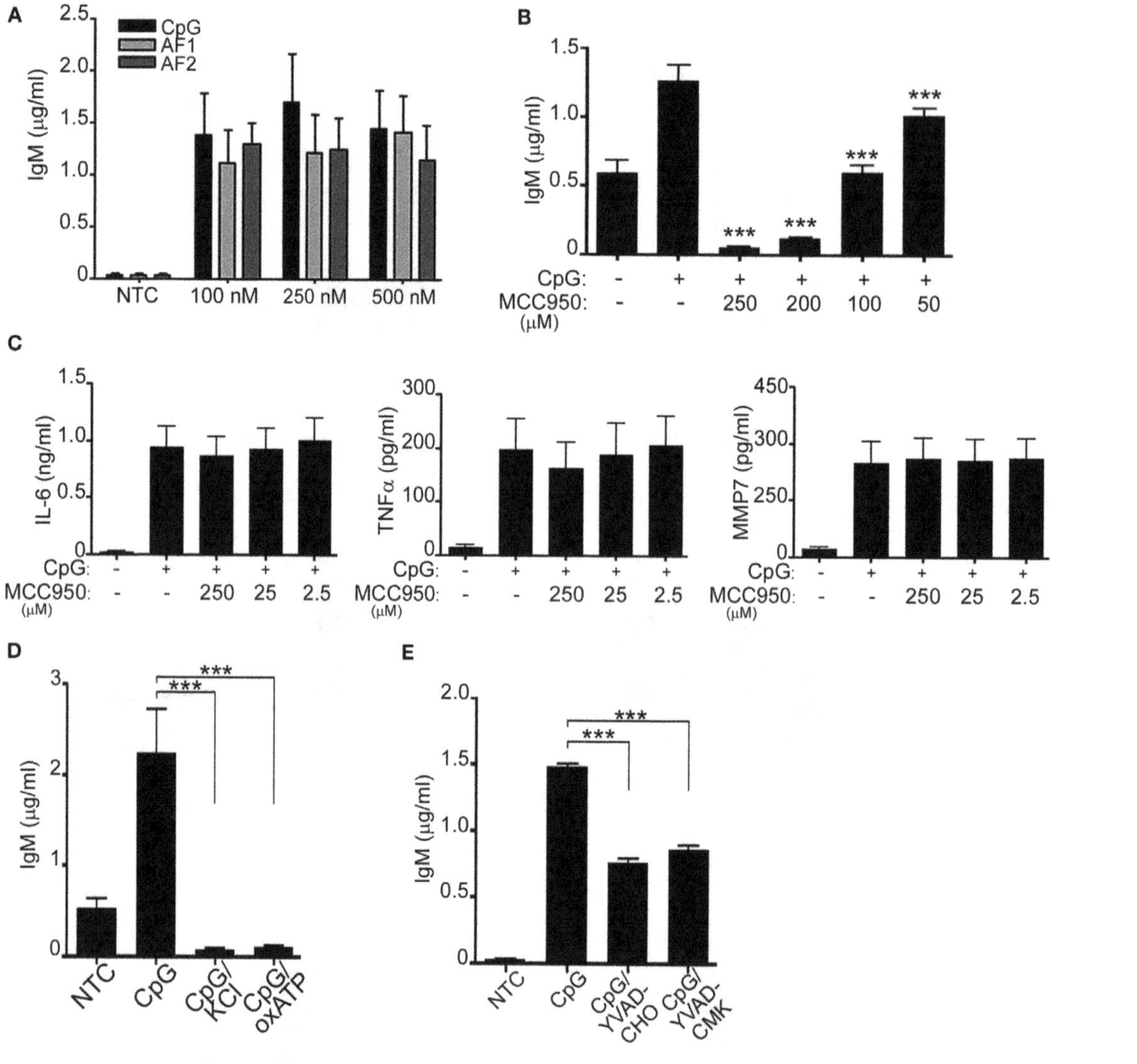

FIGURE 3 | CpG induces NLRP3-mediated antibody production. IgM **(A,B)**, IL-6, TNF-α, and MMP-7 **(C)** were measured by ELISA in the cell supernatant of unstimulated (NTC), CpG, AF1 and AF2 stimulated cells, and CpG stimulated cells in the presence of different concentrations of MCC950 as indicated. Cells were left untreated (NTC) or pre-incubated with 50 mM KCL, 50 µM oxidized ATP (oxATP) **(D)**, and the caspase-1 inhibitors, YVAD-CHO and YVAD-CMK, at a concentration of 50 µM each **(E)** prior to stimulation with CpG as indicated. 1 µg/ml CpG was used unless otherwise specified. Data are representative of at least three donors in each independent experiments ($n = 3$). $^{***}p < 0.0001$.

and since it is clearly established that naïve and memory cells produce different cytokine patterns upon stimulation (32, 33). We isolated B-lymphocytes by negative selection and then sorted them into $CD20^+CD27^-$ (naïve) and $CD20^+CD27^+$ (memory) cells. The two different subtypes of B-lymphocytes were independently stimulated with either β-glucan or CpG. IL-1β and IgM levels in the cell supernatant were then measured by ELISA. As **Figure 6A** shows, we observed that IL-1β was mostly secreted by memory cells whereas IgM production was greater from the sorted memory cells and significantly higher than naïve cells ($p < 0.001$), but was still seen at significant levels in the naïve cells upon CpG stimulation. Co-stimulation of the BCR receptor resulted in an increase in IgM secretion but it did not have a significant effect on IL-1β secretion (**Figure 6B**).

DISCUSSION

In this study, we demonstrate that in human peripheral B-lymphocytes the NLRP3 inflammasome is differentially activated by fungal β-glucan and CpG antigens. Activation of NLRP3 by fungal β-glucan resulted in the cleavage of pro-IL-1β into its active form. While this is a well-known function of the NLRP3 in other cell types such as macrophages and dendritic cells, its role in peripheral human B-lymphocytes was not yet clearly understood. Furthermore, herein we have shown that IL-1β secretion was mediated through the major β-glucan receptor Dectin-1 and required signaling through Syk, consistent with our prior observations of β-glucan signaling in B-lymphocytes and current knowledge in other immune cells (6, 7, 11, 34–36). IL-1β

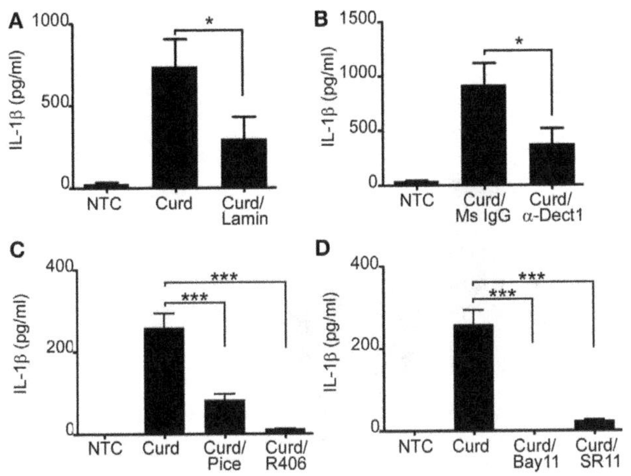

FIGURE 4 | Dectin-1 partially mediates IL-1β secretion and requires SYK and the transcriptions factors AP-1 and NF-κB. IL-1β ELISA measured in the cell supernatant of curdlan (Curd) stimulated cells in the presence or absence of 1 mg/ml Laminarin (Lamin) **(A)**, 5 μg/ml anti-dectin-1 antibody (α-Dect1) or 5 μg/ml isotype control (Ms IgG) **(B)**, 40 μM of the SYK inhibitor, piceatannol (pice) and 5 μM of the SYK inhibitor, R406 **(C)**, and 10 μM of the NF-κB inhibitor, Bay11, and 10 μM of the AP-1 inhibitor, SR11 **(D)**. Data are representative of at least three donors in each independent experiments ($n = 3$). *$p < 0.05$, ***$p < 0.0001$.

regulation was mediated by the transcription factors NF-κB and AP-1 known to be necessary for the transcription of pro-IL-1β (35, 37). Once pro-IL-1β is formed then subsequent activation of the NLRP3 inflammasome is necessary for the processing of the inactive pro-IL-1β into the active or mature form. Activation of the inflammasome *via* the canonical and non-canonical pathways has been described in other cell types (13, 35, 38). For instance, in dendritic cells, Dectin-1 participates not only in the activation of NF-κB and synthesis of pro-IL-1β by curdlan-activated dendritic cells but also in the production of mature IL-1β through a non-canonical inflammasome that recruits ASC and caspase-8 to the complex CARD-Malt-BCL10 (38). Caspase-8 has also been reported as an effector and regulator molecule of the canonical NLRP3 inflammasome that drives IL-1β production (13). Herein, we demonstrate that stimulation of B-lymphocytes with β-glucan and CpG resulted in the activation of the canonical NLRP3 pathway and involved both ASC and caspase-1 activation. Interestingly, while β-glucan-mediated IL-1β secretion via Dectin-1-Syk-NF-κB/AP-1 pathways and canonical NLRP3 activation, CpG stimulation of B-lymphocytes also resulted in the activation of the canonical NLRP3 inflammasome, but triggered the secretion of IgM and not IL-1β. The lack of IL-1β was likely due to the absence of pro-IL-1β which limited the production of the active form since no substrate was available.

Studies have shown that host immunity against disseminated *candida*, *aspergillosis*, and *pneumocystis* infection relies on IL-1β to clearly mount an adequate immune response, particularly in early stages of disease (17, 39–41). Impaired IL-1β secretion results in decreased recruitment of neutrophils, macrophages, and lymphocytes to the lungs, affecting the phagocytosis and killing of the fungi (17). IL-1β also acts by activating the release of other inflammatory cytokines, like IL-6 and TNFα as well as inducing Th17 polarization, all important mediators in antifungal defense (42). Furthermore, IL-1β is also involved in the pathogenesis of many inflammatory diseases such as familial mediterranean fever, familial cold-induced auto-inflammatory syndrome, steroid-resistant asthma, and rheumatoid arthritis (43–46). In most of these diseases, blocking IL-1β by monoclonal antibodies or blocking the NLRP3 inflammasome provide symptomatic relief and are currently the standard clinical treatment strategies. Understanding IL-1β regulation in B-lymphocytes offers a new way to potentially develop treatments that will continue to improve the clinical course of patients, not only during the acute infectious process, but potentially by ameliorating these chronic inflammatory conditions as well.

Over the last decade, microbiome studies have clearly demonstrated that the lower respiratory tract is colonized by many organisms and is not sterile as initially assumed. It is very likely that the lung microbiome, similar to the intestinal microbiome, plays an important role in maintaining the well-functioning defense mechanisms of the respiratory mucosa (47). It is also highly probable that bacterial and fungal antigens, through activation of PRRs, help to keep the immune system in a basal activation state that ultimately results in the well-being of the host. However, if this balance is disrupted, and the microbiota loses diversity, the more prevalent microbial antigens through the same PRR would have no regulatory negative feedback resulting in an exaggerated inflammatory response. In the clinical setting, single or paucity fungal colonization in the airway is not uncommon, particularly in immunosuppressed patients. While the clinical significance of this finding is unknown, in the majority of the cases it gets overlooked, as the thought is that it does not result in a clinically significant illness. While this may be true, our observations suggest that fungal antigens are potential triggers of IgM, IL-1β, and other inflammatory cytokines (IL-8, IL-6, and TNFα) that can potentially act as chronic stimuli for B-lymphocytes. Thus, it is important to recognize that fungal activated B-lymphocytes, while they can contribute to host protection against fungal diseases in the right clinical setting, they can also result in a source of chronic inflammation.

Contrary to what we observed in β-glucan-stimulated B-lymphocytes, our data also showed that CpG, while activating the NLRP3 inflammasome, did not result in IL-1β secretion, but upregulated IgM secretion *via* the mTOR signaling pathway (see proposed mechanism in **Figure 7**). The role of NLRP3 in antibody production has been suggested in animal models (8); however it has not been investigated in human B-lymphocytes. Herein, we showed that inhibition of NLRP3 decreased IgM production in a dose-dependent manner while not affecting the secretion of other cytokines such as TNF-α, IL-6, and MMP-7, suggesting that the production of IgM is seemingly controlled by the NLRP3 inflammasome.

The mTOR pathway is ubiquitously expressed in immune cells, including B-lymphocytes (48, 49). Upon activation it regulates important cell processes such as protein translation, cell growth and proliferation (50). mTOR functions as two signaling complexes, mTOR complex 1 (mTOR1) and mTOR complex 2 (mTOR2).

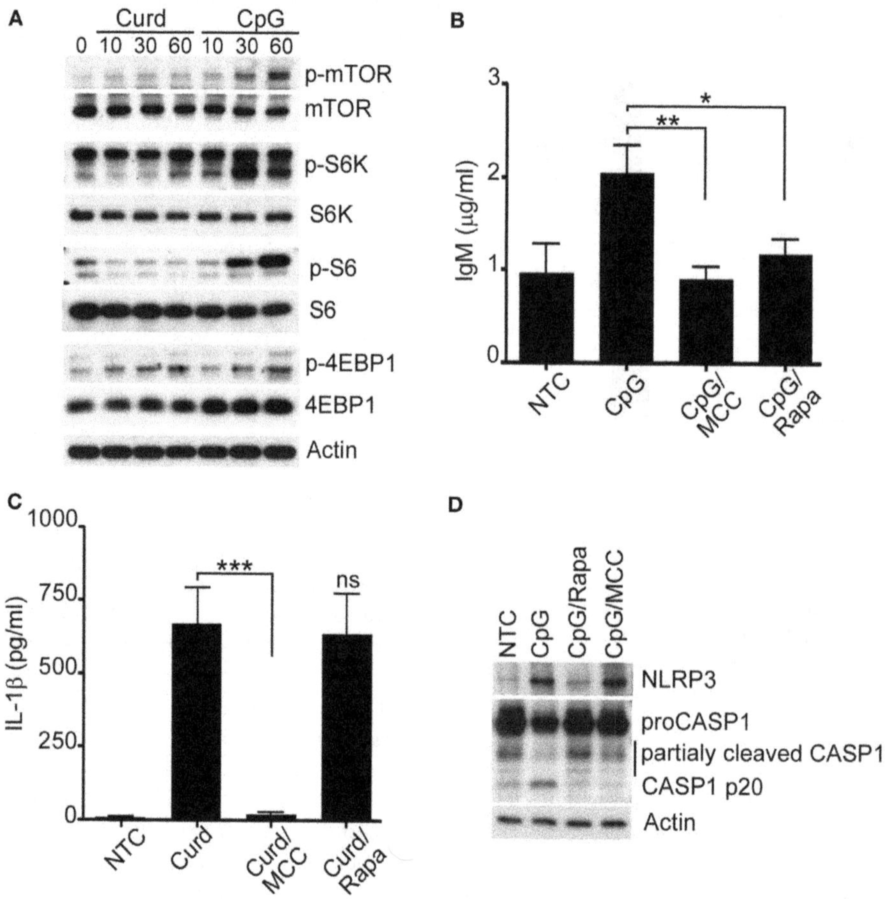

FIGURE 5 | Mammalian target of rapamycin (mTOR) regulates IgM production. **(A)** Immunoblot analysis of p-mTOR, p-S6K, p-S6, p-4EBP1 after curdlan (Curd) or CpG stimulation, for the indicated periods of time. Total mTOR, S6K, S6, 4EBP1 and actin were used as protein control. IgM **(B)** and IL-1β **(C)** ELISA were measured in the cell supernatant of unstimulated cells (NTC), CpG stimulated cells, and CpG stimulated cells in the presence of MCC950 (MCC) and Rapamycin (Rapa) for 24 h. **(D)** Immunoblot analysis of NLRP3, and Caspase-1 in NTC, after CpG stimulation in the presence and absence of MCC950 (MCC) and Rapamycin (Rapa). Actin was used as protein loading control. Cells were stimulated with 200 µg/ml curdlan and 1 µg/ml CpG and pre-incubated with 100 µM of MCC950 and 100 nM Rapamycin. Data are representative of at least three donors in each independent experiments ($n = 3$). $^{*}p < 0.05$, $^{**}p < 0.01$, $^{***}p < 0.0001$.

Activation of mTOR1 results in phosphorylation of p70-s6K (S6K), S6, and eukaryotic initiation factor 4E-binding protein (4E-BP1) which is important for the regulation of protein synthesis (50). Herein, we found phosphorylation of S6, S6K, and 4EBP-E after CpG stimulation. Furthermore, the use of Rapamycin, a well-described mTOR1 inhibitor, decreased IgM secretion. The use of Rapamycin also affected NLRP3 and caspase-1 activation, therefore impairing the function of NLRP3 inflammasome complex and suggesting that IgM regulation is not only mediated by NLRP3 but also by mTOR. Prior observations in macrophages also suggest that mTOR inhibition suppresses NLRP3 inflammasome activation in macrophages (31). In their study, mTOR regulated HK1-dependent glycolysis was critical for NLRP3 activation. While further investigations are needed in B-lymphocytes, studies to deeply understand the specific mechanism by which mTOR and NLRP3 are controlling antibody regulation in B-lymphocytes studies have shown that mTOR participates in the regulation of high affinity antibodies (51). Furthermore, in animal models, impaired mTOR signaling in follicular and marginal B-lymphocytes stimulated by LPS show a marked reduction of IgM and IgG (50, 52). That mTOR is important for germinal center formation is known (48) however, little is known about the unique function of mTOR in circulating human B-lymphocytes. Here, we have demonstrated the participation of mTOR in NLRP3 function and regulation of IgM. Interestingly, while β-glucans are able to trigger different cytokines and chemokines, they fail to induce IgM in human peripheral B-lymphocytes (7). These data differ from prior studies in murine models in which curdlan stimulation seemed to induce IgM secretion (8). While the differences seen between the two experimental models could be explained by the differences in the experimental methodology and the lack of β-glucan to induce proliferation in the human cells; herein, we have shown the inability of curdlan to trigger mTOR activation, a step found to be important for IgM secretion. Our observations are novel and raise awareness of the role of NLRP3 as regulator not only of IL-1β and IL-18 but also of IgM. Interestingly, despite NLRP3 activation, IL-18 was not induced by β-glucan or CpG in peripheral B-lymphocytes (7).

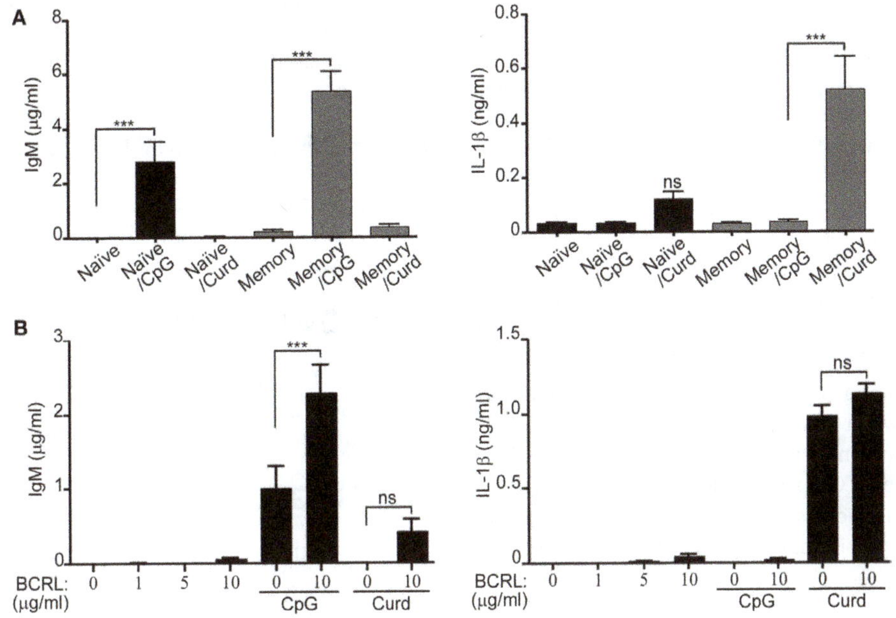

FIGURE 6 | Different levels of IL-1β and IgM secretion by stimulated naïve and memory B-lymphocytes. B-lymphocytes were isolated by negative selection, stained for 30 min with anti-CD20 and anti-CD27 antibodies, and sorted into ($CD20^{+}CD27^{+}$ and $CD20^{+}CD27^{-}$). Sorted cells were then plated at 2×10^{6}/ml and stimulated with CpG and curdlan (Curd) **(A)** or with B cell receptor ligand (BCRL) alone or in combination with CpG or curdlan **(B)** as indicated. IgM and IL-1β ELISA were measured in the cell supernatant 72 h later. 200 µg/ml curdlan and 1 µg/ml CpG were used unless otherwise specified. Data are representative of at least three donors in each independent experiment ($n = 2$) ***$p < 0.0001$, ns, not significant ($p > 0.05$).

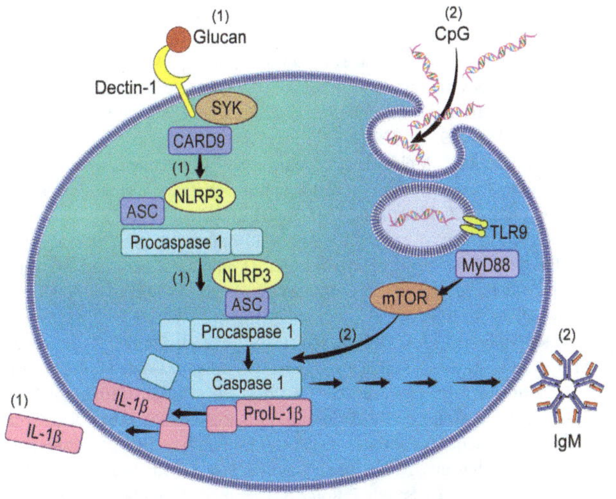

FIGURE 7 | Proposed mechanism of NLRP3 activation by β-glucan and CpG in circulating human B-lymphocytes. β-glucan and CpG activate NLRP3 in peripheral B-lymphocytes. While β-glucan activated B-lymphocytes secrete IL-1β *via* NLRP3 activation **(1)**, CpG does not induce IL-1β but IgM **(2)**. CpG-induced IgM *via* NLRP3 is mammalian target of rapamycin (mTOR)-dependent but not β-glucan-mediated IL-1β secretion.

Beyond their antibody-producing role, B-lymphocytes can affect the local immune environment through the release of cytokines and other proteins; however, how they modulate and contribute to the orchestration of the innate immune system is not clearly understood. Our group has recently shown that activated B-lymphocytes participate in the recruitment of neutrophils by releasing IL-8 and indirectly by contributing to the release of syndecan-4 *via* MMP-7 (6, 7). Syndecan proteins are expressed on the cell membrane and can be shed into the extracellular space by metalloproteases (53). Upon shedding they are free to bind to different cytokines participating in the regulation of cytokine influx and neutrophil recruitment (54–56). Herein, we further demonstrated that B-lymphocytes also contribute to the pool of IL-1β, a pro-inflammatory cytokine very important for antimicrobial host defense (42) and to the secretion of IgM antibodies. Naïve and memory B-lymphocytes play different roles in the regulation of the immune response by releasing different cytokine profiles (2). Here, we investigated the specific B-lymphocyte subtype responsible for IL-1β and IgM secretion and contrary to what we have observed with MMP-7, which was mostly released by naïve cells, memory cells were found to be the main source for both IL-1β and IgM (6). While the exact mechanisms by which different B-lymphocyte subtypes seem to preferentially secrete a specific cytokine milieu is not totally understood, these patterns are not fixed and can be influenced by the circumstances that surround their activation such as presence of T-lymphocytes and other inflammatory cells, by the integration of different signals from multiple receptors and by the proportion of the different B-lymphocytes compartments (2, 33, 57). These are important observations with therapeutic implications as B-lymphocyte reconstitution after Rituximab (B-lymphocyte depleted agent) treatment favors naïve B-lymphocytes (33). Increased numbers of naïve

B-lymphocytes, based on our observations, will result in a decrease of IL-1β and IgM levels potentially contributing to a less inflammatory milieu. How these changes may affect antimicrobial and anti-inflammatory host response need to be further investigated.

In summary, this study identified that the NLRP3 inflammasome is essential for two independent processes, pro-inflammatory cytokine secretion and antibody regulation. Whether NLRP3 activation resulted in cytokine or antibody regulation depended on the stimulating antigen with IL-1β secretion being triggered by fungal β-glucans and IgM by CpG. NLRP3 regulation was also differently regulated upon β-glucan or CpG antigens and was mTOR-independent when stimulated by β-glucans but mTOR-dependent upon CpG stimulation. The new role of the NLRP3 inflammasome and the mTOR pathway as regulators of IL-1β and IgM in activated B-lymphocytes studied here offers a potential new strategy to treat autoimmune disease in which IL-1β and pathogenic IgM antibodies may play a role, particularly if triggered by infectious agents. Further investigations are therefore needed to clarify the potential benefits of mTOR and NLRP3 inhibitors in these clinical settings.

AUTHOR CONTRIBUTIONS

Concept and design; data acquisition; and data interpretation/analysis: EC, MA, HD, and VV; manuscript drafting: EC, MA, and VV; manuscript review: all authors.

ACKNOWLEDGMENTS

We thank Dr. Peikert and Dr. Limper and all the members Dr. Limper's laboratory and the Mayo Clinic Thoracic Diseases Research Unit for their many helpful discussions.

FUNDING

Funded by NIH grants K08 (HL112849) to EC and funds from the Annenberg Foundation.

REFERENCES

1. Verma A, Wuthrich M, Deepe G, Klein B. Adaptive immunity to fungi. *Cold Spring Harb Perspect Med* (2014) 5:a019612. doi:10.1101/cshperspect.a019612
2. Lund FE. Cytokine-producing B lymphocytes-key regulators of immunity. *Curr Opin Immunol* (2008) 20:332–8. doi:10.1016/j.coi.2008.03.003
3. Mauri C, Bosma A. Immune regulatory function of B cells. *Annu Rev Immunol* (2012) 30:221–41. doi:10.1146/annurev-immunol-020711-074934
4. Ramirez-Ortiz ZG, Specht CA, Wang JP, Lee CK, Bartholomeu DC, Gazzinelli RT, et al. Toll-like receptor 9-dependent immune activation by unmethylated CpG motifs in *Aspergillus fumigatus* DNA. *Infect Immun* (2008) 76:2123–9. doi:10.1128/IAI.00047-08
5. Krieg AM. CpG motifs in bacterial DNA and their immune effects. *Annu Rev Immunol* (2002) 20:709–60. doi:10.1146/annurev.immunol.20.100301.064842
6. Ali MF, Dasari H, Van Keulen VP, Cornec D, Vasmatzis G, Peikert T, et al. Microbial antigens stimulate metalloprotease-7 secretion in human B-lymphocytes using mTOR-dependent and independent pathways. *Sci Rep* (2017) 7:3869. doi:10.1038/s41598-017-04199-2
7. Ali MF, Driscoll CB, Walters PR, Limper AH, Carmona EM. Beta-glucan-activated human B lymphocytes participate in innate immune responses by releasing proinflammatory cytokines and stimulating neutrophil chemotaxis. *J Immunol* (2015) 195:5318–26. doi:10.4049/jimmunol.1500559
8. Kumar H, Kumagai Y, Tsuchida T, Koenig PA, Satoh T, Guo Z, et al. Involvement of the NLRP3 inflammasome in innate and humoral adaptive immune responses to fungal beta-glucan. *J Immunol* (2009) 183:8061–7. doi:10.4049/jimmunol.0902477
9. Agostini L, Martinon F, Burns K, McDermott MF, Hawkins PN, Tschopp J. NALP3 forms an IL-1beta-processing inflammasome with increased activity in Muckle-Wells autoinflammatory disorder. *Immunity* (2004) 20:319–25. doi:10.1016/S1074-7613(04)00046-9
10. Franchi L, Eigenbrod T, Munoz-Planillo R, Nunez G. The inflammasome: a caspase-1-activation platform that regulates immune responses and disease pathogenesis. *Nat Immunol* (2009) 10:241–7. doi:10.1038/ni.1703
11. Gringhuis SI, den Dunnen J, Litjens M, van der Vlist M, Wevers B, Bruijns SC, et al. Dectin-1 directs T helper cell differentiation by controlling noncanonical NF-kappaB activation through Raf-1 and Syk. *Nat Immunol* (2009) 10:203–13. doi:10.1038/ni.1692
12. Gurung P, Kanneganti TD. Novel roles for caspase-8 in IL-1beta and inflammasome regulation. *Am J Pathol* (2015) 185:17–25. doi:10.1016/j.ajpath.2014.08.025
13. Antonopoulos C, Russo HM, El Sanadi C, Martin BN, Li X, Kaiser WJ, et al. Caspase-8 as an effector and regulator of NLRP3 inflammasome signaling. *J Biol Chem* (2015) 290:20167–84. doi:10.1074/jbc.M115.652321
14. Manners DJ, Masson AJ, Patterson JC. The heterogeneity of glucan preparations from the walls of various yeasts. *J Gen Microbiol* (1974) 80:411–7. doi:10.1099/00221287-80-2-411
15. Dietz AB, Bulur PA, Emery RL, Winters JL, Epps DE, Zubair AC, et al. A novel source of viable peripheral blood mononuclear cells from leukoreduction system chambers. *Transfusion* (2006) 46:2083–9. doi:10.1111/j.1537-2995.2006.01033.x
16. Klinman DM, Yi AK, Beaucage SL, Conover J, Krieg AM. CpG motifs present in bacteria DNA rapidly induce lymphocytes to secrete interleukin 6, interleukin 12, and interferon gamma. *Proc Natl Acad Sci U S A* (1996) 93:2879–83. doi:10.1073/pnas.93.7.2879
17. Chen W, Havell EA, Moldawer LL, McIntyre KW, Chizzonite RA, Harmsen AG. Interleukin 1: an important mediator of host resistance against *Pneumocystis carinii*. *J Exp Med* (1992) 176:713–8. doi:10.1084/jem.176.3.713
18. Vonk AG, Netea MG, van Krieken JH, Iwakura Y, van der Meer JW, Kullberg BJ. Endogenous interleukin (IL)-1 alpha and IL-1 beta are crucial for host defense against disseminated candidiasis. *J Infect Dis* (2006) 193: 1419–26. doi:10.1086/503363
19. Coll RC, Robertson AA, Chae JJ, Higgins SC, Munoz-Planillo R, Inserra MC, et al. A small-molecule inhibitor of the NLRP3 inflammasome for the treatment of inflammatory diseases. *Nat Med* (2015) 21:248–55. doi:10.1038/nm.3806
20. Eisenbarth SC, Colegio OR, O'Connor W, Sutterwala FS, Flavell RA. Crucial role for the Nalp3 inflammasome in the immunostimulatory properties of aluminium adjuvants. *Nature* (2008) 453:1122–6. doi:10.1038/nature06939
21. Kool M, Petrilli V, De Smedt T, Rolaz A, Hammad H, van Nimwegen M, et al. Cutting edge: alum adjuvant stimulates inflammatory dendritic cells through activation of the NALP3 inflammasome. *J Immunol* (2008) 181:3755–9. doi:10.4049/jimmunol.181.6.3755
22. Li H, Willingham SB, Ting JP, Re F. Cutting edge: inflammasome activation by alum and alum's adjuvant effect are mediated by NLRP3. *J Immunol* (2008) 181:17–21. doi:10.4049/jimmunol.181.1.17
23. Krieg AM, Yi AK, Matson S, Waldschmidt TJ, Bishop GA, Teasdale R, et al. Cpg motifs in bacterial-DNA trigger direct B-cell activation. *Nature* (1995) 374:546–9. doi:10.1038/374546a0
24. Brown GD, Taylor PR, Reid DM, Willment JA, Williams DL, Martinez-Pomares L, et al. Dectin-1 is a major beta-glucan receptor on macrophages. *J Exp Med* (2002) 196:407–12. doi:10.1084/jem.20020470

25. Carmona EM, Vassallo R, Vuk-Pavlovic Z, Standing JE, Kottom TJ, Limper AH. Pneumocystis cell wall beta-glucans induce dendritic cell costimulatory molecule expression and inflammatory activation through a Fas-Fas ligand mechanism. *J Immunol* (2006) 177:459–67. doi:10.4049/jimmunol.177.1.459
26. Hemmi H, Takeuchi O, Kawai T, Kaisho T, Sato S, Sanjo H, et al. A toll-like receptor recognizes bacterial DNA. *Nature* (2000) 408:740–5. doi:10.1038/35047123
27. Cao W, Manicassamy S, Tang H, Kasturi SP, Pirani A, Murthy N, et al. Toll-like receptor-mediated induction of type I interferon in plasmacytoid dendritic cells requires the rapamycin-sensitive PI(3)K-mTOR-p70S6K pathway. *Nat Immunol* (2008) 9:1157–64. doi:10.1038/ni.1645
28. Takeshita F, Leifer CA, Gursel I, Ishii KJ, Takeshita S, Gursel M, et al. Cutting edge: role of toll-like receptor 9 in CpG DNA-induced activation of human cells. *J Immunol* (2001) 167:3555–8. doi:10.4049/jimmunol.167.7.3555
29. Bauer S, Kirschning CJ, Hacker H, Redecke V, Hausmann S, Akira S, et al. Human TLR9 confers responsiveness to bacterial DNA via species-specific CpG motif recognition. *Proc Natl Acad Sci U S A* (2001) 98:9237–42. doi:10.1073/pnas.161293498
30. Kawabata K, Murakami A, Ohigashi H. Citrus auraptene targets translation of MMP-7 (matrilysin) via ERK1/2-dependent and mTOR-independent mechanism. *FEBS Lett* (2006) 580:5288–94. doi:10.1016/j.febslet.2006.08.072
31. Moon JS, Hisata S, Park MA, DeNicola GM, Ryter SW, Nakahira K, et al. mTORC1-induced HK1-dependent glycolysis regulates NLRP3 inflammasome activation. *Cell Rep* (2015) 12:102–15. doi:10.1016/j.celrep.2015.05.046
32. Perez-Andres M, Paiva B, Nieto WG, Caraux A, Schmitz A, Almeida J, et al. Human peripheral blood B-cell compartments: a crossroad in B-cell traffic. *Cytometry B Clin Cytom* (2010) 78(Suppl 1):S47–60. doi:10.1002/cyto.b.20547
33. Duddy M, Niino M, Adatia F, Hebert S, Freedman M, Atkins H, et al. Distinct effector cytokine profiles of memory and naive human B cell subsets and implication in multiple sclerosis. *J Immunol* (2007) 178:6092–9. doi:10.4049/jimmunol.178.10.6092
34. Kankkunen P, Teirila L, Rintahaka J, Alenius H, Wolff H, Matikainen S. (1,3)-beta-glucans activate both dectin-1 and NLRP3 inflammasome in human macrophages. *J Immunol* (2010) 184:6335–42. doi:10.4049/jimmunol.0903019
35. Gross O, Poeck H, Bscheider M, Dostert C, Hannesschlager N, Endres S, et al. Syk kinase signalling couples to the Nlrp3 inflammasome for anti-fungal host defence. *Nature* (2009) 459:433–6. doi:10.1038/nature07965
36. Carmona EM, Kottom TJ, Hebrink DM, Moua T, Singh RD, Pagano RE, et al. Glycosphingolipids mediate pneumocystis cell wall beta-glucan activation of the IL-23/IL-17 axis in human dendritic cells. *Am J Respir Cell Mol Biol* (2012) 47:50–9. doi:10.1165/rcmb.2011-0159OC
37. Roman J, Ritzenthaler JD, Fenton MJ, Roser S, Schuyler W. Transcriptional regulation of the human interleukin 1beta gene by fibronectin: role of protein kinase C and activator protein 1 (AP-1). *Cytokine* (2000) 12:1581–96. doi:10.1006/cyto.2000.0759
38. Gringhuis SI, Kaptein TM, Wevers BA, Theelen B, van der Vlist M, Boekhout T, et al. Dectin-1 is an extracellular pathogen sensor for the induction and processing of IL-1beta via a noncanonical caspase-8 inflammasome. *Nat Immunol* (2012) 13:246–54. doi:10.1038/ni.2222
39. Hise AG, Tomalka J, Ganesan S, Patel K, Hall BA, Brown GD, et al. An essential role for the NLRP3 inflammasome in host defense against the human fungal pathogen *Candida albicans*. *Cell Host Microbe* (2009) 5:487–97. doi:10.1016/j.chom.2009.05.002
40. Sainz J, Perez E, Gomez-Lopera S, Jurado M. IL1 gene cluster polymorphisms and its haplotypes may predict the risk to develop invasive pulmonary aspergillosis and modulate C-reactive protein level. *J Clin Immunol* (2008) 28:473–85. doi:10.1007/s10875-008-9197-0
41. Wojtowicz A, Gresnigt MS, Lecompte T, Bibert S, Manuel O, Joosten LA, et al. IL1B and DEFB1 polymorphisms increase susceptibility to invasive mold infection after solid-organ transplantation. *J Infect Dis* (2015) 211:1646–57. doi:10.1093/infdis/jiu636
42. Netea MG, Simon A, van de Veerdonk F, Kullberg BJ, Van der Meer JW, Joosten LA. IL-1beta processing in host defense: beyond the inflammasomes. *PLoS Pathog* (2010) 6:e1000661. doi:10.1371/journal.ppat.1000661
43. Chae JJ, Wood G, Masters SL, Richard K, Park G, Smith BJ, et al. The B30.2 domain of pyrin, the familial Mediterranean fever protein, interacts directly with caspase-1 to modulate IL-1beta production. *Proc Natl Acad Sci U S A* (2006) 103:9982–7. doi:10.1073/pnas.0602081103
44. Hoffman HM, Rosengren S, Boyle DL, Cho JY, Nayar J, Mueller JL, et al. Prevention of cold-associated acute inflammation in familial cold autoinflammatory syndrome by interleukin-1 receptor antagonist. *Lancet* (2004) 364:1779–85. doi:10.1016/S0140-6736(04)17401-1
45. Kim RY, Pinkerton JW, Essilfie AT, Robertson AAB, Baines KJ, Brown AC, et al. Role for NLRP3 inflammasome-mediated, IL-1beta-dependent responses in severe, steroid-resistant asthma. *Am J Respir Crit Care Med* (2017) 196:283–97. doi:10.1164/rccm.201609-1830OC
46. Brennan FM, McInnes IB. Evidence that cytokines play a role in rheumatoid arthritis. *J Clin Invest* (2008) 118:3537–45. doi:10.1172/JCI36389
47. Man WH, de Steenhuijsen Piters WA, Bogaert D. The microbiota of the respiratory tract: gatekeeper to respiratory health. *Nat Rev Microbiol* (2017) 15:259–70. doi:10.1038/nrmicro.2017.14
48. Limon JJ, Fruman DA. Akt and mTOR in B cell activation and differentiation. *Front Immunol* (2012) 3:228. doi:10.3389/fimmu.2012.00228
49. Donahue AC, Fruman DA. Distinct signaling mechanisms activate the target of rapamycin in response to different B-cell stimuli. *Eur J Immunol* (2007) 37:2923–36. doi:10.1002/eji.200737281
50. Powell JD, Pollizzi KN, Heikamp EB, Horton MR. Regulation of immune responses by mTOR. *Annu Rev Immunol* (2012) 30:39–68. doi:10.1146/annurev-immunol-020711-075024
51. Keating R, Hertz T, Wehenkel M, Harris TL, Edwards BA, McClaren JL, et al. The kinase mTOR modulates the antibody response to provide cross-protective immunity to lethal infection with influenza virus. *Nat Immunol* (2013) 14:1266–76. doi:10.1038/ni.2741
52. Benhamron S, Tirosh B. Direct activation of mTOR in B lymphocytes confers impairment in B-cell maturation and loss of marginal zone B cells. *Eur J Immunol* (2011) 41:2390–6. doi:10.1002/eji.201041336
53. Manon-Jensen T, Itoh Y, Couchman JR. Proteoglycans in health and disease: the multiple roles of syndecan shedding. *FEBS J* (2010) 277:3876–89. doi:10.1111/j.1742-4658.2010.07798.x
54. Endo K, Takino T, Miyamori H, Kinsen H, Yoshizaki T, Furukawa M, et al. Cleavage of syndecan-1 by membrane type matrix metalloproteinase-1 stimulates cell migration. *J Biol Chem* (2003) 278:40764–70. doi:10.1074/jbc.M306736200
55. Li Q, Park PW, Wilson CL, Parks WC. Matrilysin shedding of syndecan-1 regulates chemokine mobilization and transepithelial efflux of neutrophils in acute lung injury. *Cell* (2002) 111:635–46. doi:10.1016/S0092-8674(02)01079-6
56. Park PW, Foster TJ, Nishi E, Duncan SJ, Klagsbrun M, Chen Y. Activation of syndecan-1 ectodomain shedding by *Staphylococcus aureus* alpha-toxin and beta-toxin. *J Biol Chem* (2004) 279:251–8. doi:10.1074/jbc.M308537200
57. Gray D, Gray M, Barr T. Innate responses of B cells. *Eur J Immunol* (2007) 37:3304–10. doi:10.1002/eji.200737728

12

Exploitation of Scavenger Receptor, Macrophage Receptor with Collagenous Structure, by *Cryptococcus neoformans* Promotes Alternative Activation of Pulmonary Lymph Node CD11b^{+} Conventional Dendritic Cells and Non-Protective Th2 Bias

Jintao Xu[1,2†], Adam Flaczyk[2†], Lori M. Neal[1,2], Zhenzong Fa[2], Daphne Cheng[2], Mike Ivey[2], Bethany B. Moore[1,3], Jeffrey L. Curtis[1,2], John J. Osterholzer[1,2] and Michal A. Olszewski[1,2]*

[1] Division of Pulmonary and Critical Care Medicine, Department of Internal Medicine, University of Michigan Health System, Ann Arbor, MI, United States, [2] Department of Veterans Affairs Health System, VA Ann Arbor Healthcare System (VHA), Ann Arbor, MI, United States, [3] Department of Microbiology and Immunology, University of Michigan Medical School, Ann Arbor, MI, United States

***Correspondence:**
Michal A. Olszewski
olszewsm@umich.edu

[†]These authors have contributed equally to this work.

Macrophage receptor with collagenous structure (MARCO) contributes to fungal containment during the early/innate phase of cryptococcal infection; however, its role in adaptive antifungal immunity remains unknown. Using a murine model of cryptococcosis, we compared host adaptive immune responses in wild-type and MARCO$^{-/-}$ mice throughout an extended time course post-infection. Unlike in early infection, MARCO deficiency resulted in improved pulmonary fungal clearance and diminished cryptococcal dissemination during the efferent phase. Improved fungal control in the absence of MARCO expression was associated with enhanced hallmarks of protective Th1-immunity, including higher frequency of pulmonary TNF-α-producing T cells, increased cryptococcal-antigen-triggered IFN-γ and TNF-α production by splenocytes, and enhanced expression of M1 polarization genes by pulmonary macrophages. Concurrently, we found lower frequencies of IL-5- and IL-13-producing T cells in the lungs, impaired production of IL-4 and IL-10 by cryptococcal antigen-pulsed splenocytes, and diminished serum IgE, which were hallmarks of profoundly suppressed efferent Th2 responses in MARCO-deficient mice compared to WT mice. Mechanistically, we found that MARCO expression facilitated early accumulation and alternative activation of CD11b^{+} conventional DC (cDC) in the lung-associated lymph nodes (LALNs), which contributed to the progressive shift of the immune response from Th1 toward Th2 at the priming site (LALNs) and local infection site (lungs) during the efferent phase of cryptococcal infection. Taken together, our study shows that MARCO can be exploited by the fungal pathogen to promote accumulation and alternative activation of CD11b^{+} cDC in the LALN, which in turn alters Th1/Th2 balance to promote fungal persistence and dissemination.

Keywords: scavenger receptor macrophage receptor with collagenous structure, fungal persistence, Th2 response, CD11b^{+} conventional DC, *Cryptococcus neoformans*

INTRODUCTION

Cryptococcus neoformans is an environmental fungal pathogen that causes severe meningoencephalitis with mortality rates of up to 20–60%, despite the availability of antifungal drugs (1). Cryptococcal infections generally manifest in patients compromised due to HIV infection, cancer, or organ transplantation. However, up to 25% of cases reported in the United States and 60% of cases in China occur in patients without recognizable immune-deficiencies (2, 3). Furthermore, Cryptococci can persist within immune competent hosts for an extended period of time and can reactivate following immune-compromise (4). Increasing evidence suggests that both host immune dysfunction and immune modulation induced by *C. neoformans* contributes to fungal persistence (2, 5–8).

One major way through which *C. neoformans* promotes fungal persistence is by altering $CD4^+$ helper T (Th) cell polarization and subsequent macrophage activation status (9, 10). Virulence factors that contribute to the shift of host responses away from protective Th1 to non-protective Th2 bias correlate with invasive fungal disease severity [reviewed in Ref. (2, 11)]. The absence of protective Th1 cytokines (IFN-γ and TNF-α) and enhanced production of Th2 type cytokines (IL-4, IL-5, and IL-13) facilitate alternative activation of macrophages, which enable intracellular survival and growth of *C. neoformans* (12, 13). Th cell differentiation is orchestrated by antigen-presenting cells. During *C. neoformans* infection, pulmonary $CD11b^+$ conventional DC (cDC) are the primary cellular population responsible for non-protective Th2 cell polarization (14, 15). However, the factors that modulate the migration and activation of $CD11b^+$ cDC during fungal infection are not well understood. Although skewing of Th2 responses is one well-established effect of cryptococcal virulence factors (6–8, 12, 15), very few loopholes in the host immune system that can be exploited by *C. neoformans* to promote non-protective responses have been identified (15–17). Identification of host factors that contribute to non-protective responses and enable fungal persistence may reveal new targets for promoting effective T cell responses that are crucial for combat fungal infections.

Macrophage receptor with collagenous structure (MARCO) (human Gene ID: 8685) is a scavenger receptor that plays important roles in host defense against viral, bacterial, and parasitic infections (18). Our recent study showed that MARCO expression contributes to fungal containment during the innate phase of cryptococcal infection by enhancing production of pro-inflammatory cytokines and recruitment of mononuclear phagocytes to the infection sites (19). Besides its well-studied roles in antibacterial and antifungal innate immunity (20–24), the importance of MARCO in regulating adaptive immunity is being increasingly recognized. Notably, MARCO expression has been shown to regulate morphology, gene expression, and migration of dendritic cell (DC) upon stimulation; thus, MARCO may act as an important link for the initiation and polarization of adaptive responses (25–27). Recent studies support this paradigm and showed that MARCO is involved in the development of T cell-mediated immunity during tumor inflammation and allergic airway responses (28, 29). While the role of MARCO in modulation of adaptive immunity to fungi remains unclear, a previous study by our group demonstrated that another scavenger receptor, scavenger receptor-A (SR-A), can be exploited by *C. neoformans* to support Th2 immune polarization during infection (17). Thus, we hypothesized that MARCO also regulates T cell-mediated immunity during fungal infections, possibly through modulation of DC migration and/or activation.

In the current study, we focused on the roles of MARCO in the adaptive immune response during *C. neoformans* infection. Using a murine model of cryptococcosis, we found that MARCO expression shifts both local and systemic Th responses away from protective Th1 toward non-protective Th2 response with impaired classical activation of macrophages. Thus, MARCO expression contributes to fungal growth and dissemination during the efferent phase of cryptococcal infection. Mechanistically, we show that MARCO expression facilitates the accumulation and alternative activation of $CD11b^+$ cDC in the lung-associated lymph nodes (LALN) which promote the priming of a non-protective Th2 response in secondary lymphoid organs during *C. neoformans* infection.

MATERIALS AND METHODS

Mice

C57BL/6 mice (wild type) were obtained from Jackson Laboratories (Bar Harbor, ME, USA). MARCO-deficient ($MARCO^{-/-}$) mice, obtained initially from Dr. Lester Kobzik (21), were bred and housed under specific pathogen-free conditions in the Animal Care Facility at the VA Ann Arbor Healthcare System. Both male and female mice were between the ages of 6–12 week at the time of infection and were humanely euthanized by CO_2 inhalation at the time of data collection. All experiments were approved by the Institutional Animal Committee on Use and Care and the Veterans Administration Institutional Animal Care and Use Committee under protocol # 0512-025 and were carried out according to NIH guidelines and the Guide for the Care and Use of Laboratory Animals.

Cryptococcus neoformans

Cryptococcus neoformans strain 52D was recovered from 10% glycerol frozen stocks stored at −80°C and grown to stationary phase at 37°C using Sabouraud dextrose broth (1% Neopeptone, 2% dextrose; Difco, Detroit, MI, USA) on a shaker. The cultures were centrifuged and washed with non-pyrogenic saline (Travenol, Deerfield, IL, USA). Cells were counted *via* hemocytometer and diluted to 3.3×10^5 yeast/ml in sterile non-pyrogenic saline.

Intratracheal Inoculation of *C. neoformans*

Mice were anesthetized *via* intraperitoneal (i.p.) injection of ketamine (100 mg/kg body weight) plus xylazine (6.8 mg/kg) and were restrained on a foam plate. A small incision was made through the skin covering the trachea. The underlying salivary glands and muscles were separated. A 30-G needle was attached to a 1 ml tuberculin syringe with *C. neoformans* suspension (3.3×10^5 yeast/ml) and infection was performed by intratracheally injecting 30 μl (10^4 CFU) of inoculum into the lungs. After inoculation, the skin was closed with cyanoacrylate adhesive and the mice were monitored during recovery from the anesthesia.

Lung Leukocyte Isolation

The lungs from each mouse were excised, washed in RPMI 1640 and digested enzymatically as previously described (30). In brief, lungs were minced with scissors followed by Gentle MACS homogenization and incubated at 37°C for 35 min in 5 ml/mouse digestion buffer [RPMI 1640, 5% FBS, penicillin, and streptomycin (Invitrogen, Grand Island, NY, USA); 1 mg/ml collagenase A (Roche Diagnostics, Indianapolis, IN, USA); and 30 μg/ml DNase I]. The cell suspension and tissue fragments were further dispersed by Gentle MACS homogenization and were centrifuged. Erythrocytes in the cell pellets were lysed by addition of 3 ml NH_4Cl buffer (0.829% NH_4Cl, 0.1% $KHCO_3$, and 0.0372% Na_2EDTA, pH 7.4) for 3 min followed by a threefold excess of RPMI 1640. Cells were re-suspended and subjected to syringe dispersion and filtered through a sterile 100-μm nylon screen (Nitex, Kansas City, MO, USA). The filtrate was centrifuged for 30 min at 1,500 × *g* with no brake in the presence of 20% Percoll (Sigma) to separate leukocytes from cell debris and epithelial cells. Leukocyte pellets were re-suspended in complete RPMI 1640 media and enumerated on a hemocytometer after dilution in trypan blue (Sigma).

CFU Assay

For determination of fungal burden, small aliquots of digested lungs, spleens, and brains were collected. Series of 10-fold dilutions of the samples were plated on Sabouraud dextrose agar plates in duplicate 10-μl aliquots and incubated at room temperature. *C. neoformans* colonies were counted 2 days later and the number of CFU was calculated on a per-organ basis.

LALN Leukocyte Isolation

Individual LALN were excised and then dispersed using a 1-ml sterile syringe plunger and flushed through a 70-μm cell strainer (BD Falcon, Bedford, MA, USA) with complete media into a sterile tube. After being centrifuged at 2,500 rpm/min for 5 min, the supernatant was removed and the cell pellets were used for gene expression analysis by quantitative real-time RT-PCR (qRT-PCR) or flow cytometry.

Ag-Specific Cytokine Production by Splenocytes

Spleens were excised and dispersed using a 3-ml sterile syringe plunger and flushed through a 70-μm cell strainer (BD Falcon) with complete media. Isolated spleen cells were cultured in media with heat-killed *C. neoformans* in a ratio of 1:2 in 6-well plates with 2 ml complete RPMI 1640 medium at 37°C and 5% CO2 for 48 h. Supernatants were stored and analyzed for cytokine levels as described earlier. The Ag-specific cytokine production was quantified using a LEGENDplex cytometric bead array (CBA) kit (BioLegend, San Diego, CA, USA) following the manufacturer's specifications and read on an LSRII flow cytometer (Becton, Dickinson Immunocytometry Systems, Mountain View, CA, USA). Analysis was performed using BioLegend's LEGENDplex software.

Total Serum IgE

Serum was obtained from the blood samples collected by severing the vena cava of the mice before lung excision. Blood samples were then allowed to clot and were spun to separate serum. Serum samples were diluted 100-fold and assayed for total IgE levels using a mouse IgE sandwich ELISA kit (BioLegend, San Diego, CA, USA) following the manufacturer's specifications.

RT-qPCR

Total RNA from lung leukocytes was prepared using TRIzol reagent (Invitrogen), and first-strand cDNA was synthesized using Reverse Transcription Kit (Qiagen, Hilden, Germany) according to the manufacturer's instructions. Relative gene expression was quantified with SYBR green-based detection (Alkali Scientific) using a light cycler96 system (Roche) according to the manufacturer's protocols. Relative gene expression was normalized to 18S mRNA using the $2^{-\Delta Ct}$ method. Fold induction of gene expression was normalized to baseline expression in uninfected mice using the $2^{-\Delta\Delta Ct}$ method.

Abs and Flow Cytometric Analysis

Ab cell staining was performed as previously described (17). For extracellular staining, cells were washed in PBS then stained with Live Dead Fixable Aqua (Life Technologies) for 30 min. Cells were stained with extracellular antibodies (see below), washed, and fixed in 2% formaldehyde. For intracellular staining, the cells were stimulated with 50 ng/ml PMA and 1 μg/ml ionomycin (Millipore) for 6 h (lung and LALN leukocytes) or heat-killed *C. neoformans* for 24 h (spleen cells) prior to Ab staining. Brefeldin A and monensin (BioLegend) were added for the last 4 h. The cells were harvested, stained with extracellular, and subsequently intracellular antibodies (see below). Data were collected on a FACS LSR2 flow cytometer using FACSDiva software (Becton Dickinson Immunocytometry Systems, Mountain View, CA, USA) and analyzed using FlowJo software (Tree Star, San Carlos, CA, USA).

The following gating strategy was used to identify leukocyte subsets in the lungs. First, consecutive gates identified singlets, live cells and $CD45^+$ leukocytes. Next, a series of selective gates were used to identify neutrophils ($CD11b^+Ly6G^+$); eosinophils ($SSC^{high}CD11c^{low}/SiglecF^+$); Alveolar macrophages ($CD11c^{high}/SiglecF^+$); and $Ly6C^{high}$ monocytes ($CD11c^-/CD11b^+/Ly6C^{high}$). In cells expressing both CD11c and high levels of MHCII, autofluorescent (AF^+) exudate macrophages were distinguished from non-AF (AF^-) DCs. Thereafter, DC were further separated into moDC, $CD11b^+$ DC and $CD103^+$ DC as follows: moDC were gated as $CD11c^+MHCII^{high}CD64^+$ cells, then remaining $CD11c^+MHCII^{high}CD64^-$ cells were further divided into $CD11b^+$ DC and $CD103^+$ DC based on the expression of SIRPα and XCR1, respectively (31). A similar gating strategy was used for leukocytes in the LALN. To identify $CD4^+$ Th cells, singlet and live cells were first selected and the total numbers of $CD45^+$ leukocytes were identified. Next, the $CD3^+CD4^+$ cells were identified and the expression levels of specific cytokines (IFN-γ, TNF-α, IL-5, and IL-13) or transcriptional factors (Gata3) were evaluated. Total numbers of each cell population were calculated by multiplying the frequency of the population by the total number of leukocytes (the original hemocytometer count of total cells). Isotype control antibodies were used to set gates for positive events in all flow cytometric analyses.

Calculations and Statistics

All values are reported as mean ± SEM. Unpaired non-parametric test (Mann–Whitney) or two-way ANOVA with a Bonferroni *post hoc* test were used for comparisons of individual means. Statistical calculations were performed using GraphPad Prism version 6.00 (GraphPad Software, San Diego, CA, USA). Means with p values <0.05 were considered significantly different.

RESULTS

MARCO Expression Promotes Fungal Persistence and Systemic Dissemination during the Efferent Phase of *C. neoformans* Infection

Our previous study showed that MARCO contributes to fungal control during the early/afferent phase of *C. neoformans* infection (19). However, whether MARCO expression affects long-term adaptive immunity against *C. neoformans* is unclear. To explore the function of MARCO during the late/efferent phase of cryptococcal infection, we infected WT and MARCO$^{-/-}$ mice with *C. neoformans* strain 52D and analyzed the fungal burden at 35 days post infection (dpi). Whereas our prior results demonstrated that MARCO-deficient mice have increased fungal burden at the early stage of infection (19), we found that MARCO-deficient mice exhibit decreased pulmonary fungal burden at 35 dpi compared to WT mice (**Figure 1A**). Fungal burdens in spleen and brain were also lower in MARCO$^{-/-}$ mice compared to WT mice at 35 dpi (**Figure 1A**). We further evaluated the effects of MARCO on the kinetics of pulmonary fungal growth during the efferent phase of *C. neoformans* infection. While equivalent growth of yeast in the lungs was noted in WT and MARCO$^{-/-}$ mice at 21 dpi, MARCO deficiency resulted in lower fungal burden at 35 and 49 dpi (**Figure 1B**). Together, our results demonstrate that MARCO expression promotes pulmonary fungal persistence and systemic dissemination during the efferent phase of *C. neoformans* infection.

MARCO Expression Promotes Non-Protective Th2 Response in the Lungs during the Efferent Phase of *C. neoformans* Infection

T helper cell polarization in the lungs is strongly correlated with clearance and persistence during the efferent phase of *C. neoformans* infection (32). To determine how MARCO expression affects T cell-mediated responses in the lungs, we analyzed leukocyte populations in the infected lungs of WT and MARCO$^{-/-}$ mice using flow cytometry. The accumulation of total leukocytes and leukocyte subsets, including eosinophils, alveolar macrophages, and total DCs, in the infected lungs were similar between WT and MARCO$^{-/-}$ mice at 21, 35, and 49 dpi (Figure S1 in Supplementary Material).

We next examined the effect of MARCO on T cell polarization during *C. neoformans* infection. There was no difference in the accumulation of CD4$^+$ T cells in the lungs of *C. neoformans*-infected MARCO$^{-/-}$ and WT mice during the efferent phase of cryptococcal infection (**Figure 2A**). However, MARCO deficiency resulted in reduced *Il-5* and *Il-13* mRNA expression, but not *IFN-γ* and *TNF-α* mRNA expression, by total lung leukocytes isolated from infected mice at 35 dpi, suggesting an impaired Th2 response in MARCO-deficient mice (**Figure 2B**). Phenotypes of T helper cells were further analyzed by intracellular staining using

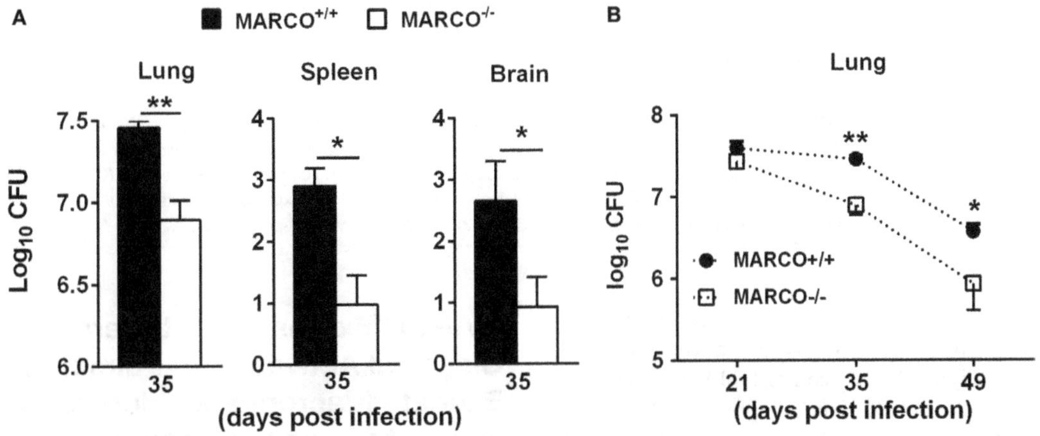

FIGURE 1 | Macrophage receptor with collagenous structure (MARCO) expression contributes to fungal growth and dissemination during the efferent phase of *Cryptococcus neoformans* infection. MARCO$^{+/+}$ and MARCO$^{-/-}$ mice were infected intratracheally with 10^4 *C. neoformans* 52D. **(A)** MARCO expression impaired fungal clearance in the lungs, spleens, and brains at 35 dpi during *C. neoformans* infection. **(B)** Kinetics of pulmonary fungal clearance in the MARCO$^{+/+}$ and MARCO$^{-/-}$ mice during efferent phase of *C. neoformans* infection. Results represent mean ± SEM from one of two separate matched experiments (n = 5 mice for each time point). $^*p < 0.05$, $^{**}p < 0.01$.

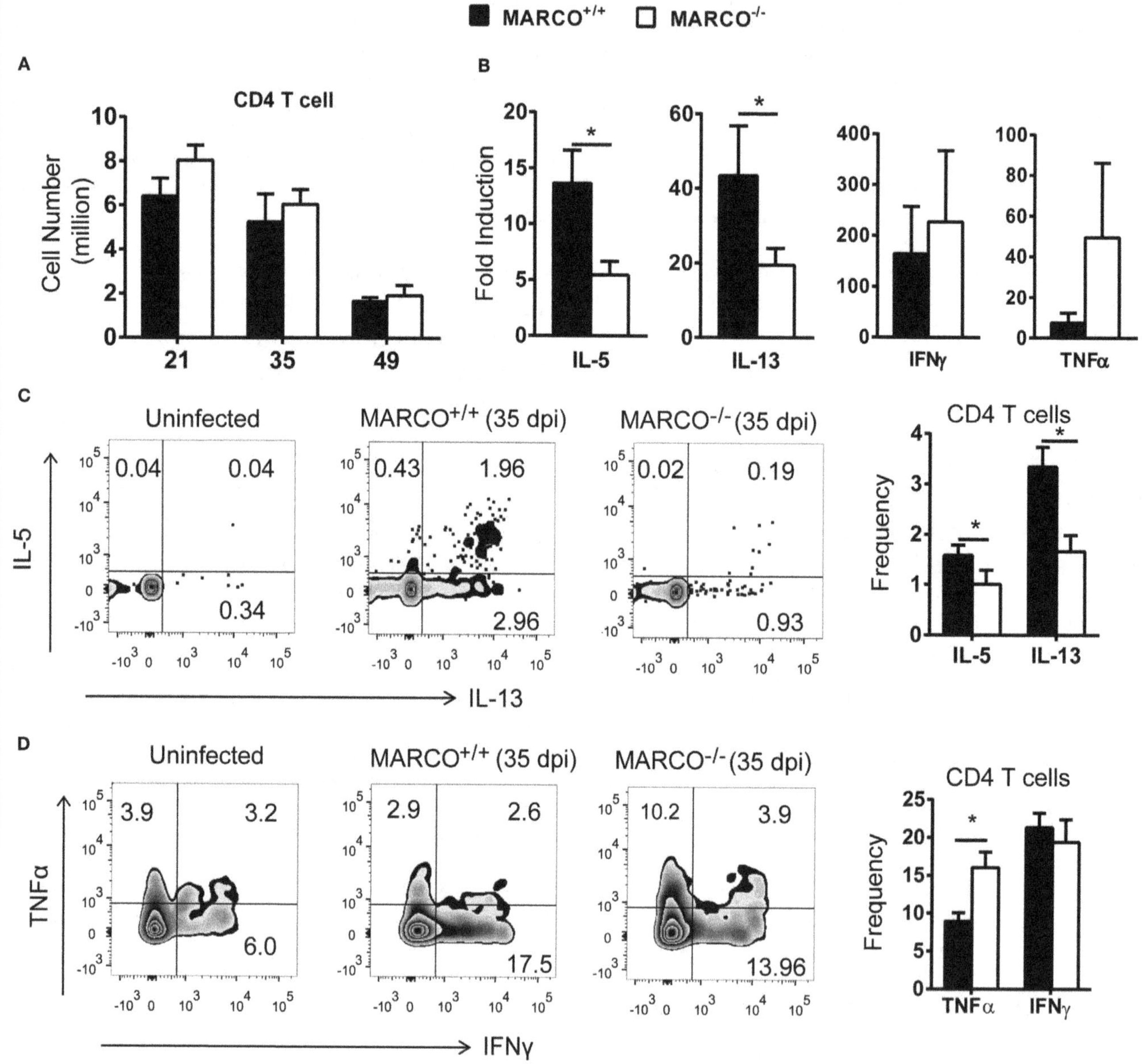

FIGURE 2 | Macrophage receptor with collagenous structure (MARCO) expression promotes Th2 response in the lungs during the efferent phase of *Cryptococcus neoformans* infection. **(A)** MARCO is dispensable for the accumulation of CD4+ T cells in the lungs of *C. neoformans*-infected mice. **(B)** MARCO expression facilitates *IL-5* and *IL-13* but not *IFN-γ* and *TNF-α* mRNA expression by total lung leukocytes at 35 dpi during *C. neoformans* infection. **(C)** MARCO expression promotes IL-5 and IL-13 production by CD4+ T cells in the lungs of *C. neoformans*-infected mice. **(D)** MARCO expression inhibits TNF-α production by CD4+ T cells in the lungs of *C. neoformans*-infected mice. Results represent mean ± SEM ($n = 5$) from one of at least two independent experiments. *$p < 0.05$.

flow cytometry. Frequencies of CD4 T cells expressing IL-5 and IL-13 were significantly lower in MARCO$^{-/-}$ mice compared to WT mice at 35 dpi (**Figure 2C**). By contrast, MARCO deficiency led to higher frequencies of CD4+ T cells expressing TNF-α albeit without affecting those expressing INF-γ at 35 dpi (**Figure 2D**). Collectively, our data demonstrated that MARCO expression did not affect accumulation of lung myeloid or lymphoid cells but altered the balance of T cell polarization away from protective Th1 responses toward non-protective Th2 responses in the lungs during the efferent phase of *C. neoformans* infection.

MARCO Expression Interferes with Classical Activation of Pulmonary Exudate Macrophages during the Efferent Phase of *C. neoformans* Infection

The balance of Th1/Th2 cytokines influences macrophage activation status and their subsequent fungicidal activities (33, 34). Exudate macrophages derived from recruited monocytes during infection have been shown to be the most efficient effector cells in killing *C. neoformans* (35). We next sought to determine whether

MARCO expression affects the activation status of pulmonary macrophages during the efferent phase of *C. neoformans* infection. Equivalent recruitment of exudate macrophages was noted between infected MARCO$^{-/-}$ and WT mice during the efferent phase of *C. neoformans* infection (**Figure 3A**). However, MARCO deficiency resulted in augmented mRNA expression of *iNOS* but not *Arg1* by lung macrophages at 35 dpi (**Figure 3B**). Moreover, we found that MARCO deficiency resulted in significantly increased expression of CD80 and CD86 by exudate macrophages at 35 dpi (**Figures 3C,D**), consistent with improved pulmonary fungal clearance in these mice. Interestingly, expression of CD80, CD86, iNOS, and Arg1 by alveolar macrophages was similar between infected MARCO$^{-/-}$ and WT mice (not shown). Thus, consistent with the diminished efferent Th1 responses, MARCO expression is associated with impaired classical activation of exudate macrophages in the lungs during the efferent phase of *C. neoformans* infection.

MARCO Expression Enhances Non-Protective and Opposes Protective Systemic Responses during the Efferent Phase of *C. neoformans* Infection

Since MARCO affected extra-pulmonary *C. neoformans* dissemination, we next studied its effects on systemic immune responses during the efferent phase of cryptococcal infection. To accomplish this, we evaluated the cytokine production by splenocytes of infected MARCO$^{-/-}$ and WT mice in response to cryptococcal antigen. Consistent with results from the lungs, production of non-protective cytokines, including IL-4 and IL-10, was lower by splenocytes from MARCO$^{-/-}$ compared to WT mice at 21 dpi (**Figure 4A**). The concentration of serum IgE, a hallmark of systemic Th2 response, was also significantly lower in MARCO$^{-/-}$ mice compared to WT mice at 21 and 35 dpi (**Figure 4B**). Furthermore, MARCO deficiency led to elevated production of beneficial Th1 cytokines such as IFN-γ (21 and 35 dpi) and TNF-α (35 dpi) by splenocytes in response to cryptococcal antigen stimulation (**Figure 4C**). We next investigated whether T cells were the major source of antigen-triggered IFN-γ production in splenocyte cultures using intracellular flow cytometric analysis. We identified increased frequencies of IFN-γ-producing CD8$^+$ T cells in MARCO$^{-/-}$ mice compared to WT mice (**Figure 4D**). We also observed a similar, strong trend in increased frequencies of IFN-γ-producing CD4$^+$ T cells in MARCO$^{-/-}$ mice compared to WT mice ($p = 0.1$) (**Figure 4D**), which became significant when splenocyte culture were stimulated with PMA and ionomycin (data not shown). Interestingly, we also found a higher frequency of non-T cell populations (CD4$^-$CD8$^-$) producing IFN-γ in antigen stimulated splenocyte cultures from MARCO$^{-/-}$ mice compared to those from WT mice (**Figure 4D**). These results indicate that MARCO expression also broadly affects IFN-γ production by cells outside the T cell compartment. Collectively, we found that MARCO expression promotes a systemic shift away from protective responses toward non-protective responses during the efferent phase of *C. neoformans* infection.

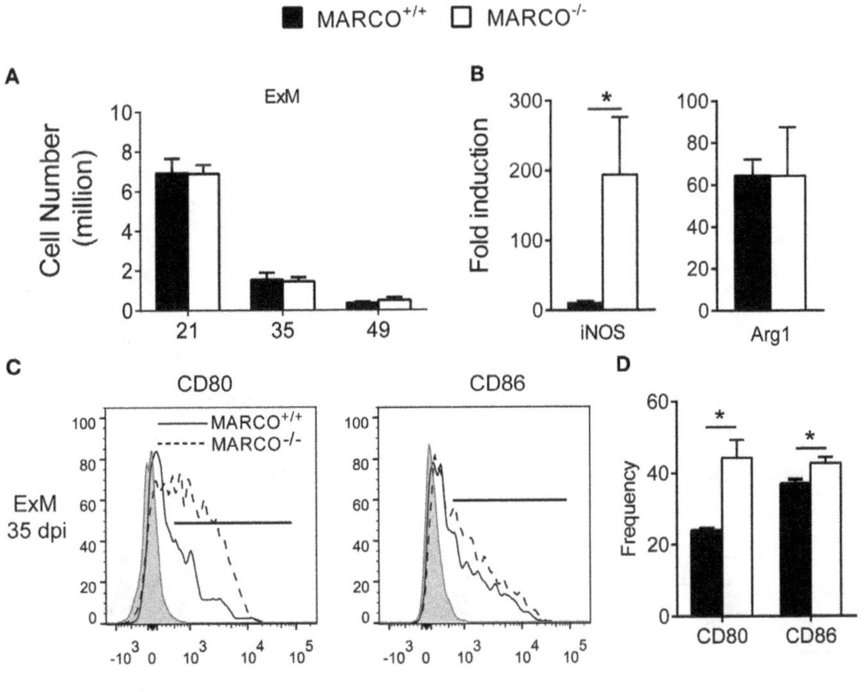

FIGURE 3 | Macrophage receptor with collagenous structure (MARCO) expression impairs classical activation of macrophages in the lungs during the efferent phase of *Cryptococcus neoformans* infection. **(A)** Accumulation of exudate macrophages was not affected by MARCO deletion during *C. neoformans* infection. **(B)** MARCO impairs iNOS expression by adherent macrophages from lungs of infected mice at 35 dpi. **(C,D)** MARCO impairs expression of CD80 and CD86 by lung exudate macrophages at 35 dpi. Results represent mean ± SEM ($n = 5$) from one of two independent experiments. *$p < 0.05$. ExM, exudate macrophages.

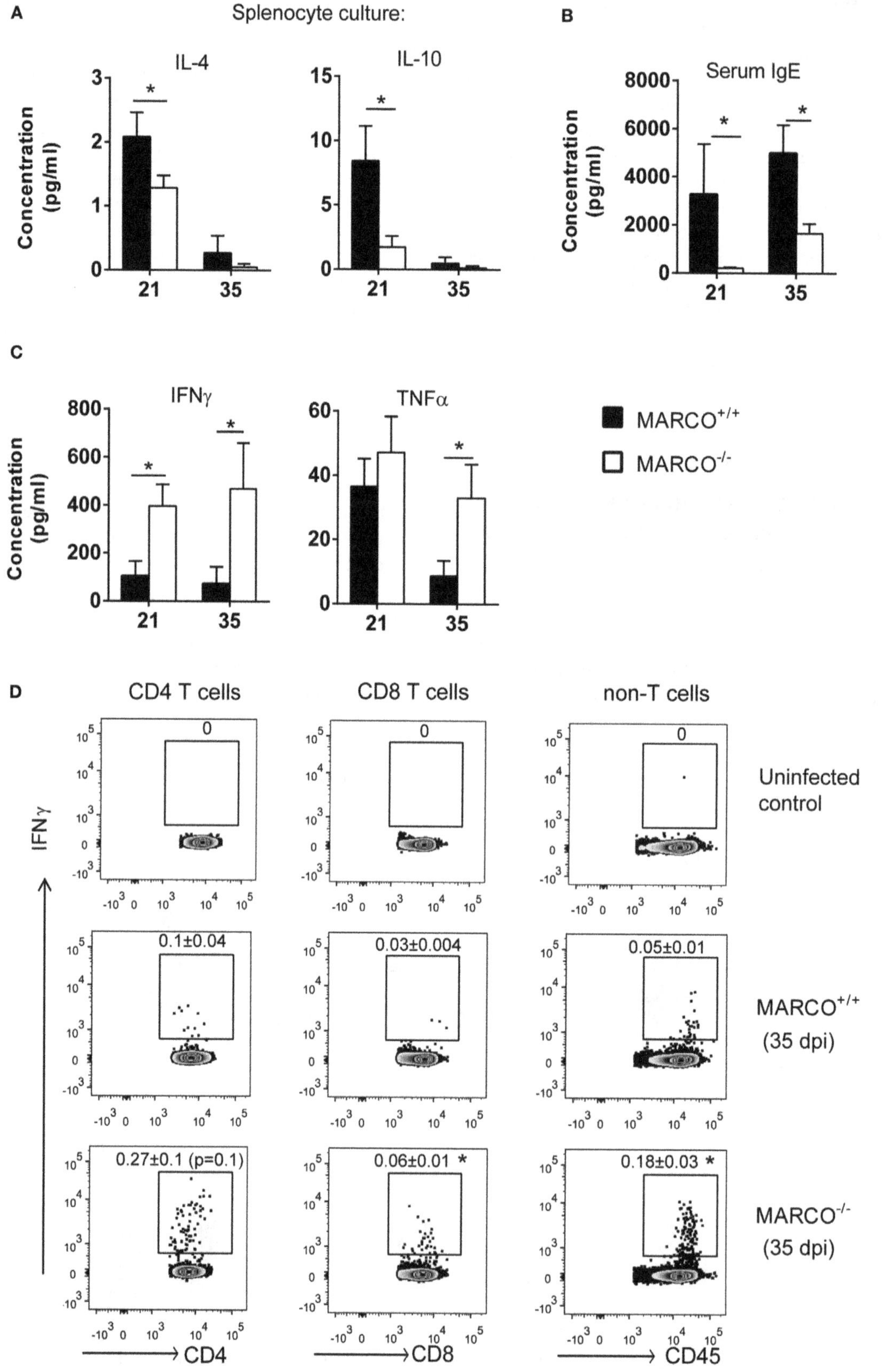

FIGURE 4 | Continued

FIGURE 4 | Continued
Macrophage receptor with collagenous structure (MARCO) expression promotes systemic Th2 response and inhibits Th1 response during the efferent phase of *Cryptococcus neoformans* infection. Spleen leukocytes were isolated from infected MARCO$^{-/-}$ and MARCO$^{+/+}$ mice at 21 and 35 dpi. After stimulated with heat-killed *C. neoformans* for 48 h, cytokine production in the supernatant of cell cultures was analyzed by cytometric bead assay. **(A)** MARCO expression increases IL-4 and IL-10 production by spleen leukocytes at 21 dpi. **(B)** MARCO expression significantly increases serum IgE level in mice infected with *C. neoformans*. **(C)** MARCO expression inhibits production of IFN-γ and TNF-α by spleen leukocytes at 21 or 35 dpi. **(D)** MARCO expression inhibits production of IFN-γ by CD4^{+} T cells, CD8^{+} T cells and non-T cells (CD4^{-}CD8^{-}) at 35 dpi. Splenocytes were stimulated with heat-killed *C. neoformans* and analyzed by intracellular flow cytometry. Results represent mean ± SEM ($n > 4$). $^{*}p < 0.05$.

MARCO Expression Contributes to Th2 Priming in the LALNs during *C. neoformans* Infection

We next dissected the mechanisms by which MARCO modulates Th polarization. T cells are primed in the draining lymph nodes and their polarization is orchestrated by distinct DC subsets during *C. neoformans* infection (36). We, thus, looked at the priming of T cells in the LALN at 10 dpi, an early time point at the onset of T cell polarization. Though MARCO deficiency had no effect on the T cell expansion in LALNs at 10 dpi (**Figure 5A**), we found reduced expression of *IL-13* by the LALN leukocytes of infected MARCO$^{-/-}$ mice compared to WT mice (**Figure 5B**). Furthermore, expression of *IFN-γ* and the transcription factors *T-bet* and *Eomesodermin* by LALN leukocytes were similar between MARCO$^{-/-}$ and WT mice (**Figure 5B** and data not shown). To further assess whether MARCO promotes Th2 priming in the LALN during *C. neoformans* infection, we performed intracellular staining for cytokines and transcription factors in LALN leukocytes. Consistent with our gene expression analysis, we found that MARCO deficiency resulted in reduced frequencies of LALN CD4^{+} T cells expressing Th2-associated cytokine IL-13 and transcriptional factor Gata3 at 10 dpi (**Figure 5C**). By contrast, MARCO deficiency had no effect on IFN-γ expression by CD4^{+} T cells in the LALN at 10 dpi. Thus, MARCO expression enhances early Th2 priming but appears to have little or no effect on early Th1 priming in the LALN during *C. neoformans* infection.

MARCO Expression Promotes Accumulation of CD11b^{+} cDC in the LALN during *C. neoformans* Infection

Pulmonary CD11b^{+} cDC have been shown to orchestrate the development of non-protective Th2 responses during cryptococcal infection (15). To test whether MARCO expression affects the accumulation of DC in the LALN, we analyzed leukocyte populations in the LALN of infected MARCO$^{-/-}$ and WT mice at 10 dpi. While total leukocyte accumulation in the LALN was not altered in MARCO-deficient mice, MARCO expression significantly promoted the accumulation of migratory DC (CD11c^{+}MHCII^{high}) in the LALN of infected mice (**Figures 6A,B**). We further explored whether MARCO affected the accumulation of specific DC subsets in the LALN during *C. neoformans* infection. Notably, MARCO deficiency selectively impaired accumulation of CD11b^{+} cDC, but had no effect on the accumulation of CD103^{+} cDC and moDC subsets in the LALN of *C. neoformans*-infected mice (**Figure 6C**). Thus, MARCO expression is critical for the accumulation of CD11b^{+} cDC in the LALN during *C. neoformans* infection.

MARCO Expression Promotes Alternative Activation and Inhibits Classical Activation of CD11b^{+} cDC in LALNs during *C. neoformans* Infection

The activation status of DC in the LALN can be influenced by fungal virulence factors and plays a vital role in the control of T cell polarization (16, 37). We further assessed the effect of MARCO on the activation status of CD11b^{+} cDC in the LALN during *C. neoformans* infection by analyzing the expression of classical activation markers (CD80 and CD86) as well as alternative activation marker (CD206) on CD11b^{+} cDC. We found that MARCO deficiency led to increased expression of CD80 and CD86 and decreased expression of CD206 by CD11b^{+} cDC in the LALN at 10 dpi (**Figures 7A,B**). Interestingly, MARCO deficiency had no effect on the activation status of CD103^{+} cDC and moDC in LALN of infected mice (not shown). These data show that MARCO expression specifically promotes alternative activation and inhibits classical activation of CD11b^{+} cDC in the LALN. Collectively, this MARCO-dependent accumulation and alternative activation of CD11b^{+} cDC in the LALN may represent a critical mechanism through which MARCO promotes the development of a stronger Th2 response and downregulates the Th1 response, leading to fungal persistence during the efferent phase of *C. neoformans* infection (**Figure 8**).

DISCUSSION

Although our previous study demonstrated that scavenger receptor MARCO is involved in the phagocytosis of *C. neoformans* by lung leukocytes and early recruitment of myeloid cells, the function of MARCO in the later stages of adaptive antifungal immunity remains unknown. Here, we demonstrated that MARCO expression ultimately promotes fungal persistence and dissemination by directly or indirectly contributing to the development of non-protective responses during cryptococcal infection. Our immunological analysis mechanistically linked these effects during the adaptive phase with increased pulmonary and systemic Th2 responses and impaired classical activation of macrophages in the lungs. We further show that the upstream accumulation and alternative activation of CD11b^{+} cDC in LALN of *C. neoformans*-infected mice provides a likely mechanism through which *C. neoformans* exploits MARCO to trigger a shift to Th2 responses. Collectively, our study uncovers novel

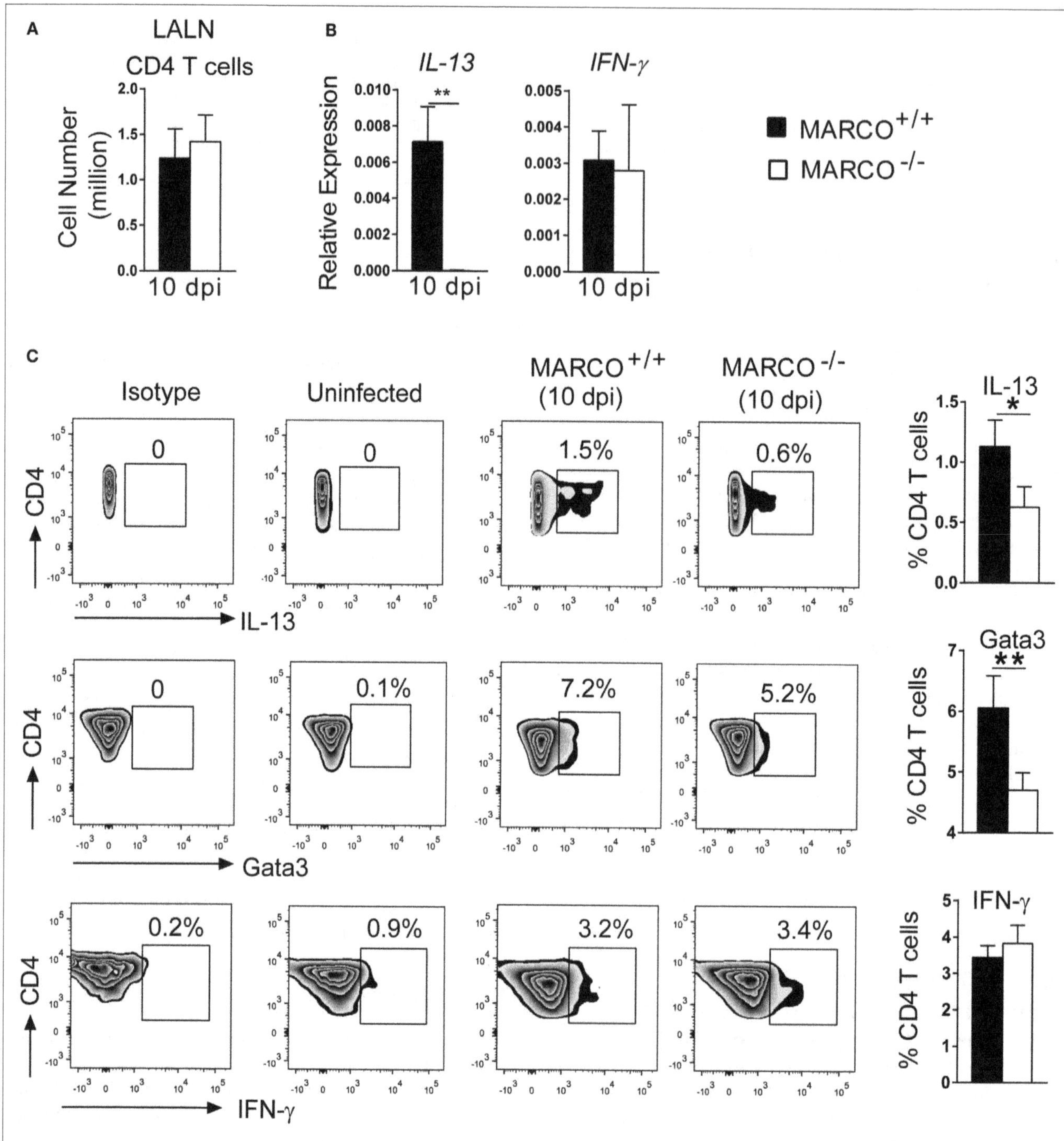

FIGURE 5 | Macrophage receptor with collagenous structure (MARCO) promotes Th2 response in the LALN of *Cryptococcus neoformans*-infected mice. **(A)** MARCO is dispensable for accumulation of $CD4^+$ T cells in the LALN of *C. neoformans*-infected mice at 10 dpi. **(B)** Expression of IL-13 and IFN-γ by total LALN leukocytes from infected $MARCO^{-/-}$ and $MARCO^{+/+}$ mice at 10 dpi were analyzed by RT-qPCR. Note that MARCO enhanced mRNA expression of IL-13 but not IFN-γ by total LALN leukocytes. Expression of each target gene was normalized to the 18S housekeeping gene. **(C)** MARCO expression promotes IL-13 and Gata3 but not IFN-γ protein production by $CD4^+$ T cells in the LALN of *C. neoformans*-infected mice. Results represent mean ± SEM ($n = 5$) with similar results from two independent experiments. $^*p < 0.05$.

cellular and molecular pathway through which *C. neoformans* evades host defenses and induces non-protective antifungal immunomodulation.

Our current study revealed the novel observation that MARCO expression significantly promotes fungal persistence and extra-pulmonary dissemination during the efferent phase of

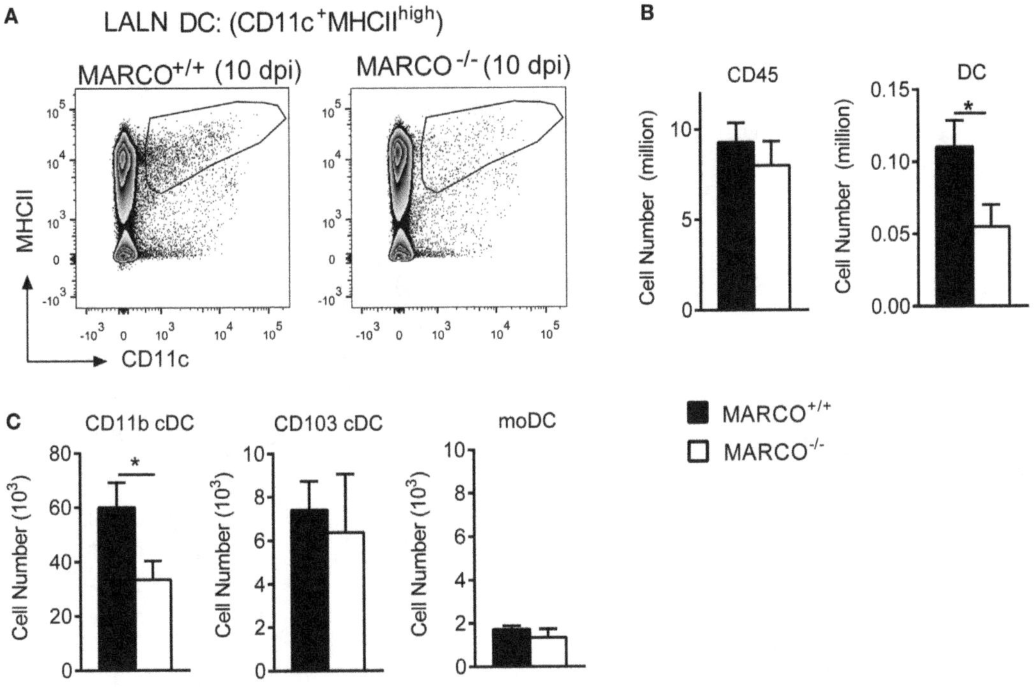

FIGURE 6 | Macrophage receptor with collagenous structure (MARCO) expression promotes the accumulation of CD11b+ cDC in the lung-associated lymph node (LALN) of *Cryptococcus neoformans*-infected mice. **(A,B)** MARCO expression promotes the accumulation of dendritic cell (DC) but not total leukocytes in LALN of *C. neoformans*-infected mice at 10 dpi. **(C)** MARCO expression promotes the accumulation of CD11b+ cDC but not CD103+ cDC and moDC. Results represent mean ± SEM ($n = 5$), with similar results from two independent experiments. $^*p < 0.05$. cDC, conventional dendritic cells; moDC, monocytes-derived dendritic cells.

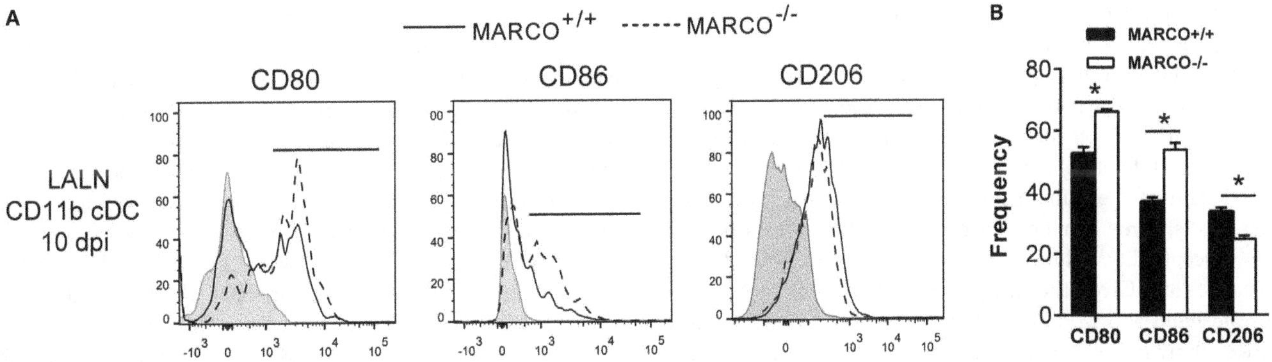

FIGURE 7 | Macrophage receptor with collagenous structure (MARCO) expression promotes alternative activation and inhibits classical activation of CD11b+ conventional DC (cDC) in the lung-associated lymph node (LALN) of *Cryptococcus neoformans*-infected mice. **(A)** Surface expression of CD80, CD86, and CD206 by CD11b+ cDC was analyzed by flow cytometry. **(B)** Bar graphs represent percentage of CD11b+ cDC expressing CD80, CD86, and CD206. Note that CD11b+ cDC from infected MARCO+/+ mice exhibited higher expression of CD80 and CD86 but lower levels of CD206 compared to CD11b+ cDC from infected MARCO-/- mice. Results represent mean ± SEM ($n = 5$), with similar results from two independent experiments. $^*p < 0.05$.

C. neoformans infection. Interestingly, our previous study demonstrated that MARCO orchestrates innate defenses and contributes to fungal containment during initial response to cryptococcal infection by promoting early inflammatory cytokine production in the lungs and phagocytosis by myeloid cells (19). These results show that, in the grand scheme, the initial benefits of MARCO expression during the innate phase were gradually replaced by the non-protective effects induced by MARCO during the efferent phase of *C. neoformans* infection. Collectively, we found that MARCO can play distinct functions in host defenses to pathogens, protective during the relatively short innate phase and then non-protective during subsequent efferent phase.

Distinct roles of specific factors in innate versus adaptive responses, while rare, are not unique to MARCO and can be found in other immune receptors, such as T-cell immunoglobulin domain and mucin domain 3 (TIM3), which was shown to

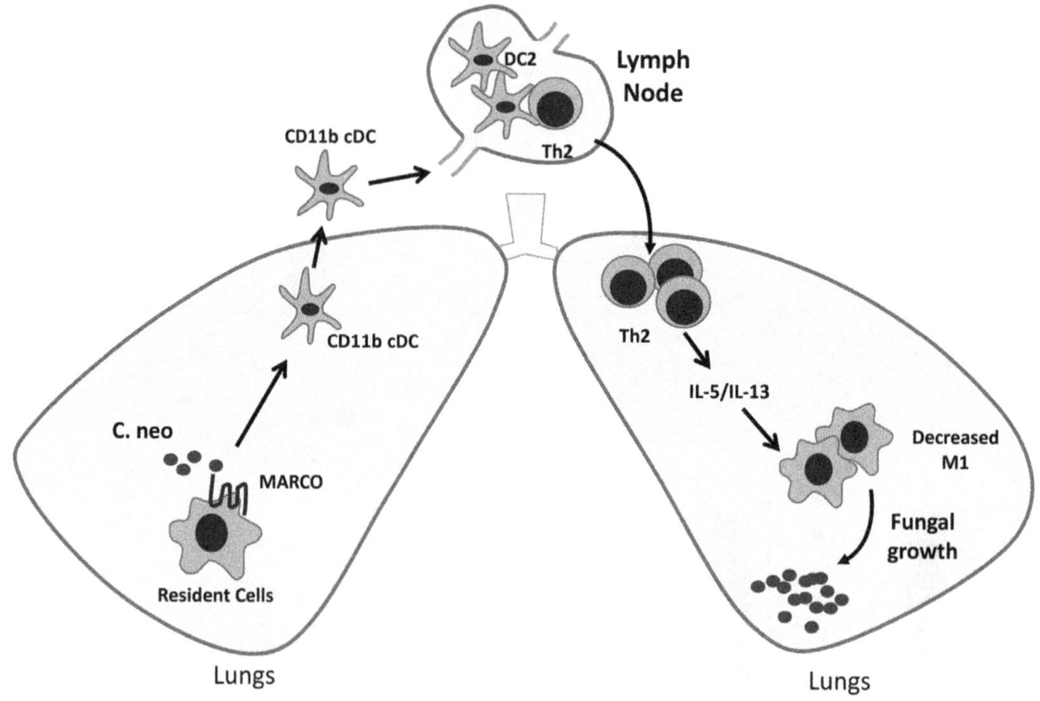

FIGURE 8 | Roles of macrophage receptor with collagenous structure (MARCO) in orchestrating adaptive immunity during fungal infection. MARCO expression contributes to accumulation of CD11b+ conventional DC (cDC) and their alternative activation in the lung-associated lymph node (LALN), which promotes the development of Th2 responses in the LALN and lungs during *Cryptococcus neoformans* infection. Thus, efferent control of fungal growth was impaired along with increased production of type 2 cytokines IL-5 and IL-13, and alternative activation of effector cells in the lungs of MARCO$^{+/+}$ mice.

promote pro-inflammatory innate responses while restraining Th1 responses (38). While it is not uncommon for pathogens to exploit loopholes in the signaling cascades of the immune system and hijack protective pathways, our results showing dual roles of MARCO during cryptococcal infection may provide insights that explain why different genetic variants of MARCO differentially affect health of the human population. In human pulmonary tuberculosis, some genetic variants of MARCO are associated with susceptibility, while other variants are associated with resistance (39). Given the similarities of pathogenicity between *C. neoformans* and *M. tuberculosis* (both can survive and grow intracellularly in the alveolar macrophages and require Th1-cell help for their eradication), it is possible that these distinct variants may affect the magnitude of protective versus non-protective effects of MARCO. Another element of pathogenesis shared by *C. neoformans* and *M. tuberculosis* is their ability to induce latent infections (40, 41). Since, non-protective elements of the immune response contribute to cryptococcal persistence (42, 43), MARCO and other factors exploited by *C. neoformans* may in fact contribute to the development of cryptococcal latency. Thus, possible contribution of MARCO expression to long-term latency of *C. neoformans* infection and whether genetic variants of MARCO are associated with susceptibility to cryptococcosis in humans warrants further study.

The effects of MARCO in the development of adaptive immunity were less well explored compared to its well-studied innate functions in control of infections such as *Mycobacterium tuberculosis, Streptococcus pneumonia, and Leishmania major* (21–23). In this study, we showed that MARCO expression can be later exploited by *C. neoformans* to modulate T cell polarization during the efferent phase of infection. Consistent with the higher fungal burden in WT mice, MARCO expression led to enhancement of non-protective Th2 responses, diminished protective Th1 responses, and impaired classical activation of macrophages in the lungs during the efferent phase of *C. neoformans* infection (**Figure 8**). Interestingly, while the effects of MARCO on induction of systemic and pulmonary Th2 bias were similar (Th2 cytokine production in lungs and spleen and corresponding changes in serum IgE level), divergent functions of MARCO were found when it comes to IFN-γ production. MARCO expression was associated with diminished expression of IFN-γ by both T cells and non-T cells in the spleens, while we did not observe any effects of MARCO on IFN-γ production by the lung and LALN cells. Thus, while our current study substantially advances our understanding of the role of MARCO as an important modulator of host adaptive immunity during fungal infections, future studies are needed to fully characterize the mechanisms by which MARCO plays divergent roles in different organs of the infected host.

Molecular and cellular mechanisms of non-protective Th2 response development during *C. neoformans* infection are incompletely understood. Pathogen virulence factors, such as capsule, chitin, urease, and other lipid mediators, promote Th2 responses during *C. neoformans* infection (8, 44, 45), however, host signaling pathways exploited by fungal pathogens that contribute to Th2 development are less studied. Though critical roles of pulmonary CD11b$^+$ cDC in Th2 response development during *C. neoformans* infection was demonstrated (15), the underlying mechanisms are not fully elucidated. In our study, we demonstrated that the upstream Th2 priming in the draining lymph nodes was enhanced by MARCO expression. More importantly, our results showed that the accumulation and alternative activation of CD11b$^+$ cDC also depended on MARCO expression. Thus, the increased accumulation and alternative activation of CD11b$^+$ cDC is likely a crucial mechanism by which *C. neoformans* exploits MARCO to promote the Th2 response and downregulate Th1 response during infection. However, at this time, we cannot rule out that other possible cell subsets affected by *C. neoformans* in a MARCO-dependent fashion might also enhance non-protective Th2 responses.

The current study demonstrates that MARCO exhibits some interesting similarities and differences during fungal infections when compared with our previous study on the role of another scavenger receptor, SR-A (17). While our studies demonstrated that *C. neoformans* can exploit multiple scavenger receptors to facilitate its survival in the host by triggering the same type of immunomodulation, there are significant differences between the effects of SR-A and MARCO on DC activation. SR-A promotes the early production of type 2 cytokines in both the lungs and LALN during the afferent phase of *C. neoformans* infection and globally contributed to the alternative activation of DC at both sites (17). By contrast, MARCO contributes to increased early IFN-γ production and classical activation of moDC in the lungs (19), at the same time selectively enhances the accumulation and alternative activation of CD11b$^+$cDC in the LALN of *C. neoformans*-infected mice. These seemingly discrepant effects within mucosal sites and regional lymph nodes demonstrate that MARCO signaling is likely contextual, depending on DC subsets and/or effects of local micro-environments. While future studies are needed to clarify this, our studies indicate that both MARCO and SR-A can promote Th2 polarization during cryptococcal infection possibly *via* different mechanisms.

In summary, our novel findings show that MARCO facilitates cryptococcal persistence in the host through promoting non-protective Th2 responses during the efferent phase of *C. neoformans* infection. We identify MARCO-dependent accumulation and alternative activation of CD11b$^+$ cDC as one mechanism explaining these effects. Thus, this study substantially advances our understanding about the roles of MARCO in the adaptive phase of antifungal immunity.

AUTHOR CONTRIBUTIONS

JX and AF contributed to experimental design, experimental work, data analysis, and manuscript writing. LN, ZF, DC, and MI contributed to experimental work and manuscript editing. BBM, JC, and JO contributed to write and edit manuscript. MO contributed to secure funding, oversee the project, design framework, and experimental work.

ACKNOWLEDGMENTS

MO, JO, and JC were supported by VA Merit grants (I01BX000656, BX002120-01 and I01CX000911, respectively). In addition, MO was supported by VA RCS award (IK6BX003615). BM was supported by NIH grant AI117229, HL127805, and HL119682. LN was supported by T-32 research training grant T32HL07749. The authors wish to thank Enze Xing, Guolei Zhao, Xueli Gao, and Jessica Kolbe for technical assistance and the UROP program at the University of Michigan for their support of undergraduate research.

REFERENCES

1. Brown GD, Denning DW, Gow NA, Levitz SM, Netea MG, White TC. Hidden killers: human fungal infections. *Sci Transl Med* (2012) 4:165rv113. doi:10.1126/scitranslmed.3004404
2. Olszewski MA, Zhang Y, Huffnagle GB. Mechanisms of cryptococcal virulence and persistence. *Future Microbiol* (2010) 5:1269–88. doi:10.2217/fmb.10.93
3. Fang W, Fa Z, Liao W. Epidemiology of *Cryptococcus* and cryptococcosis in China. *Fungal Genet Biol* (2015) 78:7–15. doi:10.1016/j.fgb.2014.10.017
4. Spitzer ED, Spitzer SG, Freundlich LF, Casadevall A. Persistence of initial infection in recurrent *Cryptococcus neoformans* meningitis. *Lancet* (1993) 341:595–6. doi:10.1016/0140-6736(93)90354-J
5. Wager CML, Wormley FL Jr. Is development of a vaccine against *Cryptococcus neoformans* feasible? *PLoS Pathog* (2015) 11:e1004843. doi:10.1371/journal.ppat.1004843
6. He X, Lyons DM, Toffaletti DL, Wang F, Qiu Y, Davis MJ, et al. Virulence factors identified by *Cryptococcus neoformans* mutant screen differentially modulate lung immune responses and brain dissemination. *Am J Pathol* (2012) 181:1356–66. doi:10.1016/j.ajpath.2012.06.012
7. Qiu Y, Davis MJ, Dayrit JK, Hadd Z, Meister DL, Osterholzer JJ, et al. Immune modulation mediated by cryptococcal laccase promotes pulmonary growth and brain dissemination of virulent *Cryptococcus neoformans* in mice. *PLoS One* (2012) 7:e47853. doi:10.1371/journal.pone.0047853
8. Osterholzer JJ, Surana R, Milam JE, Montano GT, Chen G-H, Sonstein J, et al. Cryptococcal urease promotes the accumulation of immature dendritic cells and a non-protective T2 immune response within the lung. *Am J Pathol* (2009) 174:932–43. doi:10.2353/ajpath.2009.080673
9. Rohatgi S, Pirofski LA. Host immunity to *Cryptococcus neoformans*. *Future Microbiol* (2015) 10:565–81. doi:10.2217/fmb.14.132
10. Voelz K, May RC. Cryptococcal interactions with the host immune system. *Eukaryot Cell* (2010) 9:835–46. doi:10.1128/EC.00039-10
11. Gibson JF, Johnston SA. Immunity to *Cryptococcus neoformans* and *C. gattii* during cryptococcosis. *Fungal Genet Biol* (2015) 78:76–86. doi:10.1016/j.fgb.2014.11.006
12. Müller U, Stenzel W, Köhler G, Werner C, Polte T, Hansen G, et al. IL-13 induces disease-promoting type 2 cytokines, alternatively activated macrophages and allergic inflammation during pulmonary infection of mice with *Cryptococcus neoformans*. *J Immunol* (2007) 179:5367–77. doi:10.4049/jimmunol.179.8.5367
13. Zhang Y, Wang F, Tompkins KC, McNamara A, Jain AV, Moore BB, et al. Robust Th1 and Th17 immunity supports pulmonary clearance but cannot prevent systemic dissemination of highly virulent *Cryptococcus neoformans* H99. *Am J Pathol* (2009) 175:2489–500. doi:10.2353/ajpath.2009.090530
14. Iwasaki A, Medzhitov R. Control of adaptive immunity by the innate immune system. *Nat Immunol* (2015) 16:343–53. doi:10.1038/ni.3123
15. Wiesner DL, Specht CA, Lee CK, Smith KD, Mukaremera L, Lee ST, et al. Chitin recognition via chitotriosidase promotes pathologic type-2 helper T cell responses to cryptococcal infection. *PLoS Pathog* (2015) 11:e1004701. doi:10.1371/journal.ppat.1004701

16. Valdez PA, Vithayathil PJ, Janelsins BM, Shaffer AL, Williamson PR, Datta SK. Prostaglandin E2 suppresses antifungal immunity by inhibiting interferon regulatory factor 4 function and interleukin-17 expression in T cells. *Immunity* (2012) 36:668–79. doi:10.1016/j.immuni.2012.02.013
17. Qiu Y, Dayrit JK, Davis MJ, Carolan JF, Osterholzer JJ, Curtis JL, et al. Scavenger receptor A modulates the immune response to pulmonary *Cryptococcus neoformans* infection. *J Immunol* (2013) 191:238–48. doi:10.4049/jimmunol.1203435
18. Canton J, Neculai D, Grinstein S. Scavenger receptors in homeostasis and immunity. *Nat Rev Immunol* (2013) 13:621–34. doi:10.1038/nri3515
19. Xu J, Flaczyk A, Neal LM, Fa Z, Eastman AJ, Malachowski AN, et al. Scavenger receptor MARCO orchestrates early defenses and contributes to fungal containment during cryptococcal infection. *J Immunol* (2017) 198:3548–57. doi:10.4049/jimmunol.1700057
20. Areschoug T, Gordon S. Scavenger receptors: role in innate immunity and microbial pathogenesis. *Cell Microbiol* (2009) 11:1160–9. doi:10.1111/j.1462-5822.2009.01326.x
21. Arredouani M, Yang Z, Ning Y, Qin G, Soininen R, Tryggvason K, et al. The scavenger receptor MARCO is required for lung defense against pneumococcal pneumonia and inhaled particles. *J Exp Med* (2004) 200:267–72. doi:10.1084/jem.20040731
22. Gomes IN, Palma LC, Campos GO, Lima JGB, De Almeida TF, De Menezes JP, et al. The scavenger receptor MARCO is involved in *Leishmania major* infection by CBA/J macrophages. *Parasite Immunol* (2009) 31:188–98. doi:10.1111/j.1365-3024.2009.01093.x
23. Bowdish DM, Sakamoto K, Kim M-J, Kroos M, Mukhopadhyay S, Leifer CA, et al. MARCO, TLR2, and CD14 are required for macrophage cytokine responses to mycobacterial trehalose dimycolate and *Mycobacterium tuberculosis*. *PLoS Pathog* (2009) 5:e1000474. doi:10.1371/journal.ppat.1000474
24. Dorrington MG, Roche AM, Chauvin SE, Tu Z, Mossman KL, Weiser JN, et al. MARCO is required for TLR2-and Nod2-mediated responses to *Streptococcus pneumoniae* and clearance of pneumococcal colonization in the murine nasopharynx. *J Immunol* (2013) 190:250–8. doi:10.4049/jimmunol.1202113
25. Kissick HT, Dunn LK, Ghosh S, Nechama M, Kobzik L, Arredouani MS. The scavenger receptor MARCO modulates TLR-induced responses in dendritic cells. *PLoS One* (2014) 9:e104148. doi:10.1371/journal.pone.0104148
26. Grolleau A, Misek DE, Kuick R, Hanash S, Mulé JJ. Inducible expression of macrophage receptor MARCO by dendritic cells following phagocytic uptake of dead cells uncovered by oligonucleotide arrays. *J Immunol* (2003) 171:2879–88. doi:10.4049/jimmunol.171.6.2879
27. Granucci F, Petralia F, Urbano M, Citterio S, Di Tota F, Santambrogio L, et al. The scavenger receptor MARCO mediates cytoskeleton rearrangements in dendritic cells and microglia. *Blood* (2003) 102:2940–7. doi:10.1182/blood-2002-12-3651
28. Komine H, Kuhn L, Matsushita N, Mulé JJ, Pilon-Thomas S. Examination of MARCO activity on dendritic cell phenotype and function using a gene knockout mouse. *PLoS One* (2013) 8:e67795. doi:10.1371/journal.pone.0067795
29. Arredouani MS, Franco F, Imrich A, Fedulov A, Lu X, Perkins D, et al. Scavenger receptors SR-AI/II and MARCO limit pulmonary dendritic cell migration and allergic airway inflammation. *J Immunol* (2007) 178:5912–20. doi:10.4049/jimmunol.178.9.5912
30. Olszewski MA, Huffnagle GB, McDonald RA, Lindell DM, Moore BB, Cook DN, et al. The role of macrophage inflammatory protein-1 alpha/CCL3 in regulation of T cell-mediated immunity to *Cryptococcus neoformans* infection. *J Immunol* (2000) 165:6429–36. doi:10.4049/jimmunol.165.11.6429
31. Guilliams M, Lambrecht B, Hammad H. Division of labor between lung dendritic cells and macrophages in the defense against pulmonary infections. *Mucosal Immunol* (2013) 6:464–73. doi:10.1038/mi.2013.14
32. Wozniak KL, Hardison S, Olszewski M, Wormley FL Jr. Induction of protective immunity against cryptococcosis. *Mycopathologia* (2012) 173:387–94. doi:10.1007/s11046-011-9505-8
33. Hardison SE, Herrera G, Young ML, Hole CR, Wozniak KL, Wormley FL Jr. Protective immunity against pulmonary cryptococcosis is associated with STAT1-mediated classical macrophage activation. *J Immunol* (2012) 189:4060–8. doi:10.4049/jimmunol.1103455
34. Flaczyk A, Duerr CU, Shourian M, Lafferty EI, Fritz JH, Qureshi ST. IL-33 signaling regulates innate and adaptive immunity to *Cryptococcus neoformans*. *J Immunol* (2013) 191:2503–13. doi:10.4049/jimmunol.1300426
35. Osterholzer JJ, Chen G-H, Olszewski MA, Zhang Y-M, Curtis JL, Huffnagle GB, et al. Chemokine receptor 2-mediated accumulation of fungicidal exudate macrophages in mice that clear cryptococcal lung infection. *Am J Pathol* (2011) 178:198–211. doi:10.1016/j.ajpath.2010.11.006
36. Eastman AJ, Osterholzer JJ, Olszewski MA. Role of dendritic cell-pathogen interactions in the immune response to pulmonary cryptococcal infection. *Future Microbiol* (2015) 10:1837–57. doi:10.2217/fmb.15.92
37. Xu J, Eastman AJ, Flaczyk A, Neal LM, Zhao G, Carolan J, et al. Disruption of early tumor necrosis factor alpha signaling prevents classical activation of dendritic cells in lung-associated lymph nodes and development of protective immunity against cryptococcal infection. *MBio* (2016) 7:e00510–16. doi:10.1128/mBio.00510-16
38. Anderson AC, Anderson DE, Bregoli L, Hastings WD, Kassam N, Lei C, et al. Promotion of tissue inflammation by the immune receptor Tim-3 expressed on innate immune cells. *Science* (2007) 318:1141–3. doi:10.1126/science.1148536
39. Bowdish DM, Sakamoto K, Lack NA, Hill PC, Sirugo G, Newport MJ, et al. Genetic variants of MARCO are associated with susceptibility to pulmonary tuberculosis in a Gambian population. *BMC Med Genet* (2013) 14:47. doi:10.1186/1471-2350-14-47
40. Alanio A, Vernel-Pauillac F, Sturny-Leclère A, Dromer F. *Cryptococcus neoformans* host adaptation: toward biological evidence of dormancy. *MBio* (2015) 6:e02580–14. doi:10.1128/mBio.02580-14
41. Getahun H, Matteelli A, Chaisson RE, Raviglione M. Latent *Mycobacterium tuberculosis* infection. *N Engl J Med* (2015) 372:2127–35. doi:10.1056/NEJMra1405427
42. Arora S, Olszewski MA, Tsang TM, McDonald RA, Toews GB, Huffnagle GB. Effect of cytokine interplay on macrophage polarization during chronic pulmonary infection with *Cryptococcus neoformans*. *Infect Immun* (2011) 79:1915–26. doi:10.1128/IAI.01270-10
43. Hernandez Y, Arora S, Erb-Downward JR, McDonald RA, Toews GB, Huffnagle GB. Distinct roles for IL-4 and IL-10 in regulating T2 immunity during allergic bronchopulmonary mycosis. *J Immunol* (2005) 174:1027–36. doi:10.4049/jimmunol.174.2.1027
44. Almeida GM, Andrade RM, Bento CA. The capsular polysaccharides of *Cryptococcus neoformans* activate normal CD4+ T cells in a dominant Th2 pattern. *J Immunol* (2001) 167:5845–51. doi:10.4049/jimmunol.167.10.5845
45. Vecchiarelli A, Pietrella D, Lupo P, Bistoni F, McFadden DC, Casadevall A. The polysaccharide capsule of *Cryptococcus neoformans* interferes with human dendritic cell maturation and activation. *J Leukoc Biol* (2003) 74:370–8. doi:10.1189/jlb.1002476

13

Tissue-Resident Macrophages in Fungal Infections

Shengjie Xu[1] *and Mari L. Shinohara*[1,2]*

[1] *Department of Immunology, Duke University School of Medicine, Durham, NC, United States,* [2] *Department of Molecular Genetics and Microbiology, Duke University School of Medicine, Durham, NC, United States*

Correspondence:
Mari L. Shinohara
mari.shinohara@duke.edu

Invasive fungal infections result in high morbidity and mortality. Host organs targeted by fungal pathogens vary depending on the route of infection and fungal species encountered. *Cryptococcus neoformans* infects the respiratory tract and disseminates throughout the central nervous system. *Candida albicans* infects mucosal tissues and the skin, and systemic *Candida* infection in rodents has a tropism to the kidney. *Aspergillus fumigatus* reaches distal areas of the lung once inhaled by the host. Across different tissues in naïve hosts, tissue-resident macrophages (TRMs) are one of the most populous cells of the innate immune system. Although they function to maintain homeostasis in a tissue-specific manner during steady state, TRMs may function as the first line of defense against invading pathogens and may regulate host immune responses. Thus, in any organs, TRMs are uniquely positioned and specifically programmed to function. This article reviews the current understanding of the roles of TRMs during major fungal infections.

Keywords: tissue-resident macrophages, fungal infections, microglia, alveolar macrophages, *Candida*, *Cryptococcus*, *Aspergillus*

INTRODUCTION

Macrophages were initially discovered in the late nineteenth century by Metchnikoff and named for its phagocytic activity as "devouring cells" in Greek (1, 2). They are capable of engulfing and digesting cellular debris, foreign substances, and microorganisms, which are critical for tissue remodeling and immune defense against pathogens. Based on the morphology, function, origin, and kinetics of these phagocytes, macrophages were categorized into the "mononuclear phagocytes system (MPS)" (3). Even after a century since the discovery of macrophages, research efforts have continuously focused on the origins and functions of macrophages for their significant impact on tissue homeostasis and disease pathogenesis.

Tissue-resident macrophages (TRMs) consist of heterogeneous subsets of macrophages distributed in tissues across the body and contribute to tissue homeostasis and immunosurveillance (4, 5). Depending on which organs they reside, some TRMs have specific names, such as alveolar macrophages (AMs) (lung), microglia (brain), Kupffer cells (liver), renal macrophages (kidney), and osteoclasts (skeletal system). As such specific names indicate, TRMs are considered to have specific functions due to various tissue microenvironments (6, 7). This mini-review provides an outline of several major TRMs in fungal infections, mainly focusing on murine studies, by which a majority of mechanistic insights about TRMs have been obtained.

ORIGINS OF TRMs

Developmental Origins of TRMs

Tissue-resident macrophages used to be considered as cells derived from circulating monocytes during the early establishment of the MPS (3). However, a series of recent studies drastically changed this notion, particularly through the technical advancement of *in vivo* cellular lineage-tracing by employing the "fate-mapping" technique using the mouse Cre-lox genetic system. Such *in vivo* lineage-tracing approaches have shown, for example, that microglia arise early in mouse development and are derived from primitive macrophages in the yolk sac (YS) (8). These studies suggested that microglia are ontogenically distinct from monocyte-derived macrophages (MDMs), which are of the hematopoietic origin. In addition to microglia, F4/80^{hi} Kupffer cells and epidermal Langerhans cells were demonstrated to be YS-derived and do not require Myb, a transcription factor required for the development of hematopoietic stem cells (HSCs) (9). By employing the conditional CX_3CR1 fate-mapping system, another study showed that origins of Kupffer cells, AMs, splenic, and peritoneal macrophages, are also embryonic, at least in part (10). Introduction of fate-mapping markers other than CX_3CR1 further clarified that TRMs in many tissues consist of mixed populations of the embryonic (YS and/or fetal liver) and the BM hematopoietic origins, except for microglia that are exclusively of the YS-origin (11–13).

A majority of TRMs are self-maintained throughout adult life with minimal contribution from circulating monocytes (14). However, populations of TRMs can also be replaced. For example, intestinal macrophages in mouse neonates are derived from YS and fetal liver, but do not persist into adulthood and are replaced by MDMs around the time of weaning (15). Cardiac macrophages are established from YS and fetal monocyte progenitors, but disruption of homeostasis replaces the population with MDMs (11). These murine studies strongly suggested that TRMs, in general, are derived from diverse precursors including YS macrophages, fetal liver monocytes, and even circulating HSC-derived monocytes; and ontogenic origins of TRMs greatly vary depending on tissues.

TRMs Reflecting Organ-Specific Microenvironments

Tissue-resident macrophages develop locally and adapt to tissue microenvironments during embryogenesis and beyond. Distinct gene expression patterns were identified among local TRMs from various tissues (6, 7, 16, 17), and are often reflected at the epigenetic level, particularly indicated by differential histone marks on the enhancer landscape (6, 7). Multiple pieces of evidence have suggested that such tissue-specific patterns of gene expression in TRMs are influenced by tissue-specific environmental factors, including heme (18), retinoic acid (6, 17), and TGF-β (6, 19). Interestingly, macrophage "precursors" derived from YS, fetal liver, and adult monocytes appear to have the plasticity to become certain TRMs, based on tissue-specific gene expression profiles. For example, macrophages precursors from various origins develop into functional and self-maintaining AMs, when transplanted to an empty alveolar niche (20). However, once differentiated into organ-specific macrophages, TRMs, except for Kupffer cells, cannot efficiently colonize the empty AM niche (20), suggesting that the plasticity would be lost after the precursor stage. Thus, functions of TRMs are actively shaped by their local tissue microenvironment.

TRMs IN ANTIFUNGAL RESPONSES

Critical steps to protect hosts from infections include; early recognition of the fungi, activation of host immunity, and killing of the spores and vegetative fungal cells to contain fungal dissemination (21–24). During early stages of fungal infections, infected hosts rely on tissue-resident "cells," not necessarily TRMs alone, to function as the first line of defense. Here, despite the tissue-specific functions of TRMs from various organs, a general expectation for TRMs is to function as immune sentinels to detect infections at the front line. In fact, TRMs express a wide array of cell surface receptors that sense intruding microbes and produce chemokines and cytokines to recruit and activate other cell subsets for further help (25, 26). However, do TRMs always work to protect hosts? We will visit this topic in the following subsections. As some backgrounds for this section, we would like to mention that TRMs are not considered to play a role in T cell priming with microbe-derived antigens in draining lymph nodes because they are not migratory cells (27). It is also of note that CCR2$^+$ inflammatory MDMs play critical role in fungal clearance (28–32). Here, CCR2$^+$ MDMs are recruited from circulation by chemoattractants secreted by sentinel cells. In the following subsections and **Table 1**, we focus on the early interaction of TRMs with fungi.

Lung—AMs

Because lungs are exposed to the outer environment, they constantly inhale microbes, which enter the distal airway to bronchioles and alveoli. AMs are lung-resident macrophages considered to be largely derived from fetal liver monocytes (10, 13, 51) and represent more than 90% of leukocytes in a bronchoalveolar lavage in healthy animals (52). Since fungal infections through the pulmonary route have been intensively studied, AMs may be the best-documented TRMs in fungal infections. Here, we discuss AMs and two major pulmonary fungal pathogens, *Cryptococcus neoformans* and *Aspergillus fumigatus*, which can cause serious invasive cryptococcosis and aspergillosis, respectively (21, 53–55).

C. neoformans spores and *A. fumigatus* conidia enter into the lungs by inhalation and encounter lung-resident cells first, including AMs. Although AMs are not effective in antigen presentation to T cells due to their low level of costimulatory molecules (56), AMs are considered to be at the first line of immune defense against pulmonary pathogens (57). AMs express complement receptor 3 (CR3) and Fcγ receptors (FcγR) to opsonize and phagocytose *C. neoformans* spores (33, 34, 58, 59). Phagocytosis of *C. neoformans* spores is enhanced by extracellular sphingosine-1-phosphate, which upregulates FcγR expression on AMs (35). In *A. fumigatus* infection, AMs can trap dormant *A. fumigatus* conidia with pseudopods and endocytose

TABLE 1 | Tissue-resident macrophage antifungal response.

Cell type	Fungal pathogen	Macrophage responses	Experimental approaches
Alveolar macrophages	*C. neoformans*	Take up spores which are opsonized by complement and antibodies through CR3 and Fcγ receptors (33, 34) mediated by S1PR2 (35)	Stimulating adherent murine bronchoalveolar lavage (BAL) cells in tissue culture (35)
		Produce TNFα, CXCL1, CXCL2, CCL2, and IL-1β (36)	Stimulating adherent murine BAL cells in tissue culture (36)
	A. fumigatus	Trap *A. fumigatus* conidia by pseudopods and take up conidia in actin-dependent manner (37)	Stimulating MH-S murine AM cell line in tissue culture (38)
		Kill *A. fumigatus* conidia through phagolysosome acidification (37) and production of reactive oxidant species (39)	Stimulating adherent murine BAL cells in tissue culture (39)
		Bind and uptake *A. fumigatus* conidia through SP-A and SP-D (40)	Stimulating BAL cells from aspergillosis patients in tissue culture (40)
		Detect cell wall β-1,3-glucans through Dectin-1 (41) and NOD2 receptors (42)	Murine *A. fumigatus* pulmonary infection model: AMs identified as $CD45^+Ly6G^-$ $CD11c^+$ cells (41)
		Induce proinflammatory cytokines and chemokines (38)	Stimulating MH-S cell line and adherent murine BAL cells in tissue culture (38)
Microglia	*C. albicans*	Detect cell wall β-glucan through Dectin-1 and activate Syk, Vav1, and PI3K (43) required for phagocytosis (44), and superoxide production (45)	Stimulating murine microglia primary cell culture and BV-2 microglial cell line (43)
		Increase CD11b expression and change morphology (46)	Invasive murine candidiasis model: evaluating $MHC\text{-}II^+Iba1^+$ microglia *in situ* or $CD45^+CD11b^+MHC\text{-}II^+$ microglia by flow cytometry (46)
	C. neoformans	Produce chemokines, MCP-1, MIP-1α, and MIP-1β through FcR-mediated activation by antibody-bound *C. neoformans* (47)	Stimulating human fetal microglia cells with *C. neoformans* and antifungal antibodies in tissue culture (47)
		Require IFNγ or LPS priming to eliminate *C. neoformans* through nitric oxide production (48)	Stimulating BV-2 microglial cell line (48)
	A. fumigatus	Require complement system for phagocytosis of *A. fumigatus* conidia (49, 50)	Stimulating human primary microglia in tissue culture (50)
Kidney macrophages	*C. albicans*	Internalize conidia and pseudohyphae (29)	Invasive murine candidiasis model: evaluating $CX3CR1^+$ renal macrophages *in situ* (29)
		Produce chemokines, CXCL1, and CXCL2 (25)	Invasive murine candidiasis model: evaluating $SSC^{lo}CD45^+Ly6G^-CD11b^+F4/80^{hi}$ renal macrophages by flow cytometry (25)

conidia in an actin-dependent manner (37, 60). Although neutrophils are the main population involved in complement-dependent opsonization, phagocytosis, and killing of the fungi (61, 62), AMs can also kill internalized *A. fumigatus* conidia by detection of conidia swelling and the endosome–phagosome fusion, resulting in acidification of the organelles (37). Activation of NADPH oxidase in AMs was also reported (39), suggesting AMs to gain an "M1" phenotype. Alternatively, another study showed that *A. fumigatus* infection promotes AMs to gain an alternative activated macrophage phenotype, or also known as the M2 phenotype, based on upregulation of M2 macrophage markers, such as gene transcripts encoding arginase-1 (Arg1), Ym1, and CD206 (63). Interestingly, the study did not observe the induction of *Nos2*, a major M1 macrophage marker (63). It was suggested that Arg1-expressing AMs potentially deprive L-arginine, a substrate of arginase. Since L-arginine is an essential nutrient source of fungi, the expression of Arg1 may result in inhibiting fungal growth through arginine deprivation (63). These studies suggested the presence of multiple mechanisms by which AMs protects hosts from fungal infections.

Failure in the initial clearance of invaded fungi allows them to take advantage of the humid and nutrient-rich milieu in the lung to disseminate. As the next layer to contain fungal dissemination, inflammatory neutrophils and monocytes need to be recruited in the lung. Here, it is possible that AMs play a sentinel role to recruit such inflammatory cells by secreting cytokines and chemokines to fight against fungi. For example, dectin-1 on AMs detects β-glucans on the fungal cell surface (41, 64) and stimulates the production of proinflammatory cytokines TNFα, IL-6, and IL-18 (65). Intracellular receptor NOD2 in AMs can also induce the synthesis of cytokines, such as IL-12, IFN-γ, GM-CSF, CCL2/MCP-1, CXCL2/MIP-2, and CXCL1/KC (38, 42). It is of note that the majority of these studies on cytokine and chemokine expression were performed with isolated AMs or cell lines in tissue culture. Thus, *in vivo* protein expression patterns of AMs to *A. fumigatus* and *C. neoformans* infections need to be studied.

Neutrophil chemoattractants, such as CXCL1 and CXCL2, have a great impact on the host protection from *A. fumigatus* infection (66, 67), and the main source of the chemoattractants in *A. fumigatus* infection was reported to be epithelial cells, rather than AMs (68). Indeed, AM depletion by clodronate does not alter neutrophil recruitment and host mortality in pulmonary *A. fumigatus* infection (69). Thus, a role of AMs in

A. fumigatus may be minor. In contrast in *C. neoformans* infection, AMs highly express CXCL1 and CXCL2, as well as TNFα (36), but *C. neoformans* can survive in AMs and contribute to latent infection (70). However, it is puzzling that depletion of AMs and DCs "together," by using CD11c-DTR mice (AMs and DCs are CD11c positive), resulted in more neutrophil infiltration in the lung 4 days after *C. neoformans* infection and enhanced mortality with severe lung inflammation (71). Although it is not clear which cell type, DCs, or AMs, is dominant in inhibiting neutrophil recruitment in the lung, questions that can be brought up are how DCs and/or AMs inhibit neutrophil recruitment and whether the inhibition occurs only under some conditions. Since it is technically difficult to deplete AMs alone, we still need to wait to understand if and how AMs are detrimental or protective in fungal infections.

Central Nervous System (CNS)—Microglia

Fungal infections in the CNS are usually secondary to infections in peripheral tissues. Yet, once fungal pathogens reach to the CNS, it can be fatal to hosts. Some species of *Candida*, *Cryptococcus*, and *Aspergillus* can cause life-threatening CNS infections in immunocompromised patients (72–74). Microglia reside in the CNS parenchyma and are poised to provide the first line of defense against invading pathogens. Through the expression of various pattern-recognition receptors, microglia can recognize a wide range of pathogens that colonize the CNS (75, 76). In this section, we discuss responses of microglia during CNS infection by these fungi.

Candida albicans commonly colonizes the mucocutaneous locations in the host, and can also invade the bloodstream to cause systemic candidiasis. Innate immunity is the dominant protective mechanism against disseminated candidiasis. Microglia detect β-glucans through dectin-1, resulting in phosphorylation of Syk (43), and activation of Vav1 and PI3K, which are required for phagocytosis and superoxide production (45). However, dectin-1 stimulation alone is not sufficient for microglia to induce cytokines or chemokine production (43). This suggests a unique mechanism of dectin-1 signaling in microglia distinct from other types of TRMs and MDMs, in which dectin-1 signaling is sufficient for production of cytokines and chemokines. Microglia are also found in the retina and activated by invasive candidiasis, resulting in enhanced expression of cell surface CD11b, and morphological change (46), as well as phagocytosis of *C. albicans* conidia through dectin-1 activation (44).

In contrast to *Candida*, *C. neoformans* spores are not effectively cleared by microglia. Thus, microglia require other immune cells and mechanisms to effectively combat *C. neoformans* infection in the CNS (77, 78). Opsonization of *C. neoformans* spores by antibodies plays a critical role in the induction of cytokine and chemokine expression in microglia (48). For example, opsonizing antibodies induce microglial expression of chemokines, such as CCL2/MCP-1, CCL3/MIP-1α, and CCL4/MIP-1β, but the response is also known to be inhibited by cryptococcal capsular polysaccharides (47). In addition to antibodies, LPS and IFNγ promote the killing of opsonized and unopsonized *C. neoformans* by augmenting nitric oxide production without inducing phagocytosis in a microglial cell line (48). Another study showed that IFNγ is required for enhanced anticryptococcal responses when microglia are activated by intracranial injection of IL-2 and a CD40 agonistic antibody (79). Taken together, IFNγ appears to be critical for microglia to respond to *C. neoformans*.

Aspergillus fumigatus also causes meningitis, but little is known about responses of microglia to *A. fumigatus*. One study showed that CR3 expression of microglia is reduced by an *A. fumigatus*-derived protease, resulting in a significant decrease in phagocytosis by primary human microglia (49). The high frequency of host mortality by cerebral aspergillosis suggests that antifungal responses of microglia are not efficient, although it might be possible that IFNγ also enhances the response against *Aspergillus* by microglia.

Taken together, these studies suggest that microglia are not efficient in fungal clearance. Although it is not clear why microglia are not effective cells among the MPS, the specific microenvironment of the CNS, which is known as an immune-privileged site, may be involved in shaping the character of microglia. The CNS is isolated from other peripheral organs because it is separated from blood circulation by the blood–brain barrier. The physical separation of the CNS from the immune system in the rest of organs, at least in part, may contribute to the specific development and functions of microglia, distinct from the rest of TRMs.

Kidney—Renal Macrophages

In healthy kidneys, immune cells are rarely found except for resident DCs and macrophages (80). Renal macrophages are found in the tubulointerstitium (81), a compartment of the kidney bounded by the vasculature and nephrons, and comprising about 80% of kidney volume (80). Renal macrophages in adult mice are largely derived from fetal liver monocytes (11, 82) and have been extensively studied due to their involvement in immune homeostasis (83–85) and host defense against infections (29, 86).

The kidney is a main target organ in murine systemic candidiasis (87, 88), but not necessarily a primary target in human systemic candidiasis (89). Nevertheless, host resistance heavily depends on the immune system in the kidney. For example, renal macrophages, as well as possibly splenic and liver macrophage, are considered to be protective in host defense against *Candida* (29, 87, 90). CX_3CR1-deficient mice are susceptible to *Candida* infection, possibly due to reduced numbers of kidney-resident and -infiltrated macrophages (91). As early as 2 h after *Candida* infection, renal macrophages elicit their protective responses by internalizing conidia and encasing pseudohyphal elements (91). In addition to their phagocytic ability, renal macrophages isolated from naïve mice are shown to kill *Candida* conidia in tissue culture (91). Besides their endogenous fungal-killing ability, kidney $F4/80^{hi}$ macrophages also recruit neutrophils by secreting high levels of chemokine CXCL2 in the first 24 h of systemic *Candida* infection in an autophagy-dependent manner (25), indeed playing a role as immune sentinels. In summary, kidney macrophages are important players in fungal clearance in murine candidiasis model.

CLOSING REMARKS

Our knowledge on TRMs identities and functions has been greatly expanded in the last decade. Depending on the physical locations and fungal pathogens, TRMs respond in different ways. Tissue-specific factors may also have impacts on the antifungal outcome of TRMs. However, there are still many unanswered questions and technical hurdles to further advance the field. Here, we close our discussion with six questions.

(A) *Do the functions of TRMs from various organs share something in common?* Because TRMs are shaped by tissue-specific environments to acquire unique intracellular gene expression profile and assisted by tissue factors to enhance their antifungal response, previous studies have focused on the dissimilarity among TRMs from various organs. Yet, all TRMs are expected to play a similar role in maintaining immune surveillance and behaving as sentinels when infections occur. Thus, despite their organ-specific environments, TRMs could potentially share some functions, particularly as sentinels during infections. (B) *To which extent can result from tissue culture experiments be applied to TRMs' functions in vivo?* Majority of functional studies on TRMs have been performed in tissue culture or even with cell lines. It is not clear if *ex vivo* behaviors of TRMs reflect those *in vivo*. (C) *Do human TRMs behave similarly to murine TRMs?* Due to the technical limits to isolate TRMs from humans, a majority of TRM studies have been carried out by using animals. Therefore, it is again not clear if and to what extent TRMs from human and murine share similar responses. (D) *Are TRMs involved in allowing fungi to switch from commensal/non-pathogenic to pathogenic?* TRMs' involvement in the switching might be possible because of the localization of TRMs in tissues where commensal fungi are homed. (E) *Are TRMs heterogeneous if they are within a single organ?* For example, the presence of microglia subsets has been identified (92, 93). It is intriguing to explore possible cellular subsets within TRMs in a single tissue and their possibly distinct functions. To answer the question, new technologies, such as single-cell sequencing or CyTOF would be very powerful tools to answer the question. (F) *How can we "specifically" deplete a certain TRM population?* One of the most significant technical challenges in studying TRMs may be depleting a certain population of TRMs. Clodronate-liposome is used to deplete TRMs, but it is not specific depletion. There are genetically modified mice and antagonists of certain receptors used to particularly deplete microglia. However, what is the best method to deplete AMs or Kupffer cells, for example? These are at least several questions and challenges to overcome to better understand TRMs in fungal infections and even other pathogenic conditions.

AUTHOR CONTRIBUTIONS

All authors listed have made a substantial, direct, and intellectual contribution to the work and approved it for publication.

ACKNOWLEDGMENTS

We thank M. Elizabeth Deerhake and William E. Barclay for critical reading and editing of the manuscript. This study was supported by an NIH grant to M.L.S. (R01-AI088100).

REFERENCES

1. Cavaillon JM. The historical milestones in the understanding of leukocyte biology initiated by Elie Metchnikoff. *J Leukoc Biol* (2011) 90:413–24. doi:10.1189/jlb.0211094
2. Kaufmann SH. Immunology's foundation: the 100-year anniversary of the Nobel Prize to Paul Ehrlich and Elie Metchnikoff. *Nat Immunol* (2008) 9:705–12. doi:10.1038/ni0708-705
3. van Furth R, Cohn ZA, Hirsch JG, Humphrey JH, Spector WG, Langevoort HL. The mononuclear phagocyte system: a new classification of macrophages, monocytes, and their precursor cells. *Bull World Health Organ* (1972) 46:845–52.
4. Taylor PR, Martinez-Pomares L, Stacey M, Lin HH, Brown GD, Gordon S. Macrophage receptors and immune recognition. *Annu Rev Immunol* (2005) 23:901–44. doi:10.1146/annurev.immunol.23.021704.115816
5. Varol C, Mildner A, Jung S. Macrophages: development and tissue specialization. *Annu Rev Immunol* (2015) 33:643–75. doi:10.1146/annurev-immunol-032414-112220
6. Gosselin D, Link VM, Romanoski CE, Fonseca GJ, Eichenfield DZ, Spann NJ, et al. Environment drives selection and function of enhancers controlling tissue-specific macrophage identities. *Cell* (2014) 159:1327–40. doi:10.1016/j.cell.2014.11.023
7. Lavin Y, Winter D, Blecher-Gonen R, David E, Keren-Shaul H, Merad M, et al. Tissue-resident macrophage enhancer landscapes are shaped by the local microenvironment. *Cell* (2014) 159:1312–26. doi:10.1016/j.cell.2014.11.018
8. Ginhoux F, Greter M, Leboeuf M, Nandi S, See P, Gokhan S, et al. Fate mapping analysis reveals that adult microglia derive from primitive macrophages. *Science* (2010) 330:841–5. doi:10.1126/science.1194637
9. Schulz C, Gomez Perdiguero E, Chorro L, Szabo-Rogers H, Cagnard N, Kierdorf K, et al. A lineage of myeloid cells independent of Myb and hematopoietic stem cells. *Science* (2012) 336:86–90. doi:10.1126/science.1219179
10. Yona S, Kim KW, Wolf Y, Mildner A, Varol D, Breker M, et al. Fate mapping reveals origins and dynamics of monocytes and tissue macrophages under homeostasis. *Immunity* (2013) 38:79–91. doi:10.1016/j.immuni.2012.12.001
11. Epelman S, Lavine KJ, Beaudin AE, Sojka DK, Carrero JA, Calderon B, et al. Embryonic and adult-derived resident cardiac macrophages are maintained through distinct mechanisms at steady state and during inflammation. *Immunity* (2014) 40:91–104. doi:10.1016/j.immuni.2013.11.019
12. Guilliams M, De Kleer I, Henri S, Post S, Vanhoutte L, De Prijck S, et al. Alveolar macrophages develop from fetal monocytes that differentiate into long-lived cells in the first week of life via GM-CSF. *J Exp Med* (2013) 210:1977–92. doi:10.1084/jem.20131199
13. Hoeffel G, Chen J, Lavin Y, Low D, Almeida FF, See P, et al. C-Myb(+) erythro-myeloid progenitor-derived fetal monocytes give rise to adult tissue-resident macrophages. *Immunity* (2015) 42:665–78. doi:10.1016/j.immuni.2015.03.011
14. Hashimoto D, Chow A, Noizat C, Teo P, Beasley MB, Leboeuf M, et al. Tissue-resident macrophages self-maintain locally throughout adult life with minimal contribution from circulating monocytes. *Immunity* (2013) 38:792–804. doi:10.1016/j.immuni.2013.04.004
15. Bain CC, Bravo-Blas A, Scott CL, Gomez Perdiguero E, Geissmann F, Henri S, et al. Constant replenishment from circulating monocytes maintains the macrophage pool in the intestine of adult mice. *Nat Immunol* (2014) 15:929–37. doi:10.1038/ni.2967
16. Gautier EL, Shay T, Miller J, Greter M, Jakubzick C, Ivanov S, et al. Gene-expression profiles and transcriptional regulatory pathways that underlie the identity and diversity of mouse tissue macrophages. *Nat Immunol* (2012) 13:1118–28. doi:10.1038/ni.2419
17. Okabe Y, Medzhitov R. Tissue-specific signals control reversible program of localization and functional polarization of macrophages. *Cell* (2014) 157:832–44. doi:10.1016/j.cell.2014.04.016
18. Haldar M, Kohyama M, So Alex Y-L, Kc W, Wu X, Briseño Carlos G, et al. Heme-mediated SPI-C induction promotes monocyte differentiation into iron-recycling macrophages. *Cell* (2014) 156:1223–34. doi:10.1016/j.cell.2014.01.069
19. Butovsky O, Jedrychowski MP, Moore CS, Cialic R, Lanser AJ, Gabriely G, et al. Identification of a unique TGF-beta-dependent molecular and functional signature in microglia. *Nat Neurosci* (2014) 17:131–43. doi:10.1038/nn.3599

20. van de Laar L, Saelens W, De Prijck S, Martens L, Scott CL, Van Isterdael G, et al. Yolk sac macrophages, fetal liver, and adult monocytes can colonize an empty niche and develop into functional tissue-resident macrophages. *Immunity* (2016) 44:755–68. doi:10.1016/j.immuni.2016.02.017
21. Buchanan KL, Murphy JW. What makes *Cryptococcus neoformans* a pathogen? *Emerg Infect Dis* (1998) 4:71–83. doi:10.3201/eid0401.980109
22. Hasenberg M, Behnsen J, Krappmann S, Brakhage A, Gunzer M. Phagocyte responses towards *Aspergillus fumigatus*. *Int J Med Microbiol* (2011) 301: 436–44. doi:10.1016/j.ijmm.2011.04.012
23. Schaffner A, Douglas H, Braude A. Selective protection against conidia by mononuclear and against mycelia by polymorphonuclear phagocytes in resistance to *Aspergillus*. Observations on these two lines of defense in vivo and in vitro with human and mouse phagocytes. *J Clin Invest* (1982) 69:617–31. doi:10.1172/JCI110489
24. Shoham S, Levitz SM. The immune response to fungal infections. *Br J Haematol* (2005) 129:569–82. doi:10.1111/j.1365-2141.2005.05397.x
25. Kanayama M, Inoue M, Danzaki K, Hammer G, He YW, Shinohara ML. Autophagy enhances NFkappaB activity in specific tissue macrophages by sequestering A20 to boost antifungal immunity. *Nat Commun* (2015) 6:5779. doi:10.1038/ncomms6779
26. Zhang L, Wang CC. Inflammatory response of macrophages in infection. *Hepatobiliary Pancreat Dis Int* (2014) 13:138–52. doi:10.1016/S1499-3872(14)60024-2
27. Mildner A, Jung S. Development and function of dendritic cell subsets. *Immunity* (2014) 40:642–56. doi:10.1016/j.immuni.2014.04.016
28. Hohl TM, Rivera A, Lipuma L, Gallegos A, Shi C, Mack M, et al. Inflammatory monocytes facilitate adaptive CD4 T cell responses during respiratory fungal infection. *Cell Host Microbe* (2009) 6:470–81. doi:10.1016/j.chom.2009.10.007
29. Lionakis MS, Swamydas M, Fischer BG, Plantinga TS, Johnson MD, Jaeger M, et al. CX3CR1-dependent renal macrophage survival promotes *Candida* control and host survival. *J Clin Invest* (2013) 123:5035–51. doi:10.1172/JCI71307
30. Ngo LY, Kasahara S, Kumasaka DK, Knoblaugh SE, Jhingran A, Hohl TM. Inflammatory monocytes mediate early and organ-specific innate defense during systemic candidiasis. *J Infect Dis* (2014) 209:109–19. doi:10.1093/infdis/jit413
31. Serbina NV, Jia T, Hohl TM, Pamer EG. Monocyte-mediated defense against microbial pathogens. *Annu Rev Immunol* (2008) 26:421–52. doi:10.1146/annurev.immunol.26.021607.090326
32. Shi C, Pamer EG. Monocyte recruitment during infection and inflammation. *Nat Rev Immunol* (2011) 11:762–74. doi:10.1038/nri3070
33. Griffin FM Jr. Roles of macrophage Fc and C3b receptors in phagocytosis of immunologically coated *Cryptococcus neoformans*. *Proc Natl Acad Sci U S A* (1981) 78:3853–7. doi:10.1073/pnas.78.6.3853
34. Zaragoza O, Taborda CP, Casadevall A. The efficacy of complement-mediated phagocytosis of *Cryptococcus neoformans* is dependent on the location of C3 in the polysaccharide capsule and involves both direct and indirect C3-mediated interactions. *Eur J Immunol* (2003) 33:1957–67. doi:10.1002/eji.200323848
35. McQuiston T, Luberto C, Del Poeta M. Role of sphingosine-1-phosphate (S1P) and S1P receptor 2 in the phagocytosis of *Cryptococcus neoformans* by alveolar macrophages. *Microbiology* (2011) 157:1416–27. doi:10.1099/mic.0.045989-0
36. Guillot L, Carroll SF, Homer R, Qureshi ST. Enhanced innate immune responsiveness to pulmonary *Cryptococcus neoformans* infection is associated with resistance to progressive infection. *Infect Immun* (2008) 76:4745–56. doi:10.1128/IAI.00341-08
37. Ibrahim-Granet O, Philippe B, Boleti H, Boisvieux-Ulrich E, Grenet D, Stern M, et al. Phagocytosis and intracellular fate of *Aspergillus fumigatus* conidia in alveolar macrophages. *Infect Immun* (2003) 71:891–903. doi:10.1128/IAI.71.2.891-903.2003
38. Dubourdeau M, Athman R, Balloy V, Huerre M, Chignard M, Philpott DJ, et al. *Aspergillus fumigatus* induces innate immune responses in alveolar macrophages through the MAPK pathway independently of TLR2 and TLR4. *J Immunol* (2006) 177:3994–4001. doi:10.4049/jimmunol.177.6.3994
39. Philippe B, Ibrahim-Granet O, Prevost MC, Gougerot-Pocidalo MA, Sanchez Perez M, Van der Meeren A, et al. Killing of *Aspergillus fumigatus* by alveolar macrophages is mediated by reactive oxidant intermediates. *Infect Immun* (2003) 71:3034–42. doi:10.1128/IAI.71.6.3034-3042.2003
40. Madan T, Eggleton P, Kishore U, Strong P, Aggrawal SS, Sarma PU, et al. Binding of pulmonary surfactant proteins A and D to *Aspergillus fumigatus* conidia enhances phagocytosis and killing by human neutrophils and alveolar macrophages. *Infect Immun* (1997) 65:3171–9.
41. Hohl TM, Van Epps HL, Rivera A, Morgan LA, Chen PL, Feldmesser M, et al. *Aspergillus fumigatus* triggers inflammatory responses by stage-specific beta-glucan display. *PLoS Pathog* (2005) 1:e30. doi:10.1371/journal.ppat.0010030
42. Zhang HJ, Qu JM, Shao CZ, Zhang J, He LX, Yuan ZH. *Aspergillus fumigatus* conidia upregulates NOD2 protein expression both in vitro and in vivo. *Acta Pharmacol Sin* (2008) 29:1202–8. doi:10.1111/j.1745-7254.2008.00860.x
43. Shah VB, Huang Y, Keshwara R, Ozment-Skelton T, Williams DL, Keshvara L. Beta-glucan activates microglia without inducing cytokine production in dectin-1-dependent manner. *J Immunol* (2008) 180:2777–85. doi:10.4049/jimmunol.180.5.2777
44. Maneu V, Yanez A, Murciano C, Molina A, Gil ML, Gozalbo D. Dectin-1 mediates in vitro phagocytosis of *Candida albicans* yeast cells by retinal microglia. *FEMS Immunol Med Microbiol* (2011) 63:148–50. doi:10.1111/j.1574-695X.2011.00829.x
45. Shah VB, Ozment-Skelton TR, Williams DL, Keshvara L. Vav1 and PI3K are required for phagocytosis of beta-glucan and subsequent superoxide generation by microglia. *Mol Immunol* (2009) 46:1845–53. doi:10.1016/j.molimm.2009.01.014
46. Maneu V, Noailles A, Megias J, Gomez-Vicente V, Carpena N, Gil ML, et al. Retinal microglia are activated by systemic fungal infection. *Invest Ophthalmol Vis Sci* (2014) 55:3578–85. doi:10.1167/iovs.14-14051
47. Goldman D, Song X, Kitai R, Casadevall A, Zhao ML, Lee SC. *Cryptococcus neoformans* induces macrophage inflammatory protein 1alpha (MIP-1alpha) and MIP-1beta in human microglia: role of specific antibody and soluble capsular polysaccharide. *Infect Immun* (2001) 69:1808–15. doi:10.1128/IAI.69.3.1808-1815.2001
48. Blasi E, Barluzzi R, Mazzolla R, Tancini B, Saleppico S, Puliti M, et al. Role of nitric oxide and melanogenesis in the accomplishment of anticryptococcal activity by the BV-2 microglial cell line. *J Neuroimmunol* (1995) 58:111–6. doi:10.1016/0165-5728(95)00016-U
49. Rambach G, Hagleitner M, Mohsenipour I, Lass-Florl C, Maier H, Wurzner R, et al. Antifungal activity of the local complement system in cerebral aspergillosis. *Microbes Infect* (2005) 7:1285–95. doi:10.1016/j.micinf.2005.04.014
50. Rambach G, Dum D, Mohsenipour I, Hagleitner M, Wurzner R, Lass-Florl C, et al. Secretion of a fungal protease represents a complement evasion mechanism in cerebral aspergillosis. *Mol Immunol* (2010) 47:1438–49. doi:10.1016/j.molimm.2010.02.010
51. Kopf M, Schneider C, Nobs SP. The development and function of lung-resident macrophages and dendritic cells. *Nat Immunol* (2015) 16:36–44. doi:10.1038/ni.3052
52. Lohmann-Matthes ML, Steinmuller C, Franke-Ullmann G. Pulmonary macrophages. *Eur Respir J* (1994) 7:1678–89.
53. Denning DW. Invasive aspergillosis. *Clin Infect Dis* (1998) 26:781–803; quiz 804–5. doi:10.1086/513943
54. Hohl TM, Feldmesser M. *Aspergillus fumigatus*: principles of pathogenesis and host defense. *Eukaryot Cell* (2007) 6:1953–63. doi:10.1128/EC.00274-07
55. Latge JP. *Aspergillus fumigatus* and aspergillosis. *Clin Microbiol Rev* (1999) 12:310–50.
56. Chelen CJ, Fang Y, Freeman GJ, Secrist H, Marshall JD, Hwang PT, et al. Human alveolar macrophages present antigen ineffectively due to defective expression of B7 costimulatory cell surface molecules. *J Clin Invest* (1995) 95:1415–21. doi:10.1172/JCI117796
57. Fels AO, Cohn ZA. The alveolar macrophage. *J Appl Physiol (1985)* (1986) 60:353–69.
58. Luo Y, Cook E, Fries BC, Casadevall A. Phagocytic efficacy of macrophage-like cells as a function of cell cycle and Fcgamma receptors (FcgammaR) and complement receptor (CR)3 expression. *Clin Exp Immunol* (2006) 145:380–7. doi:10.1111/j.1365-2249.2006.03132.x
59. Luo Y, Tucker SC, Casadevall A. Fc- and complement-receptor activation stimulates cell cycle progression of macrophage cells from G1 to S. *J Immunol* (2005) 174:7226–33. doi:10.4049/jimmunol.174.11.7226

60. Marr KA, Koudadoust M, Black M, Balajee SA. Early events in macrophage killing of *Aspergillus fumigatus* conidia: new flow cytometric viability assay. *Clin Diagn Lab Immunol* (2001) 8:1240–7. doi:10.1128/CDLI.8.6.1240-1247.2001
61. Braem SG, Rooijakkers SH, van Kessel KP, de Cock H, Wosten HA, van Strijp JA, et al. Effective neutrophil phagocytosis of *Aspergillus fumigatus* is mediated by classical pathway complement activation. *J Innate Immun* (2015) 7:364–74. doi:10.1159/000369493
62. Jaillon S, Peri G, Delneste Y, Fremaux I, Doni A, Moalli F, et al. The humoral pattern recognition receptor PTX3 is stored in neutrophil granules and localizes in extracellular traps. *J Exp Med* (2007) 204:793–804. doi:10.1084/jem.20061301
63. Bhatia S, Fei M, Yarlagadda M, Qi Z, Akira S, Saijo S, et al. Rapid host defense against *Aspergillus fumigatus* involves alveolar macrophages with a predominance of alternatively activated phenotype. *PLoS One* (2011) 6:e15943. doi:10.1371/journal.pone.0015943
64. Dague E, Alsteens D, Latge JP, Dufrene YF. High-resolution cell surface dynamics of germinating *Aspergillus fumigatus* conidia. *Biophys J* (2008) 94:656–60. doi:10.1529/biophysj.107.116491
65. Gersuk GM, Underhill DM, Zhu L, Marr KA. Dectin-1 and TLRs permit macrophages to distinguish between different *Aspergillus fumigatus* cellular states. *J Immunol* (2006) 176:3717–24. doi:10.4049/jimmunol.176.6.3717
66. Braedel S, Radsak M, Einsele H, Latge JP, Michan A, Loeffler J, et al. *Aspergillus fumigatus* antigens activate innate immune cells via toll-like receptors 2 and 4. *Br J Haematol* (2004) 125:392–9. doi:10.1111/j.1365-2141.2004.04922.x
67. Mehrad B, Wiekowski M, Morrison BE, Chen SC, Coronel EC, Manfra DJ, et al. Transient lung-specific expression of the chemokine KC improves outcome in invasive aspergillosis. *Am J Respir Crit Care Med* (2002) 166:1263–8. doi:10.1164/rccm.200204-367OC
68. Jhingran A, Kasahara S, Shepardson KM, Junecko BA, Heung LJ, Kumasaka DK, et al. Compartment-specific and sequential role of MyD88 and CARD9 in chemokine induction and innate defense during respiratory fungal infection. *PLoS Pathog* (2015) 11:e1004589. doi:10.1371/journal.ppat.1004589
69. Mircescu MM, Lipuma L, van Rooijen N, Pamer EG, Hohl TM. Essential role for neutrophils but not alveolar macrophages at early time points following *Aspergillus fumigatus* infection. *J Infect Dis* (2009) 200:647–56. doi:10.1086/600380
70. McQuiston TJ, Williamson PR. Paradoxical roles of alveolar macrophages in the host response to *Cryptococcus neoformans*. *J Infect Chemother* (2012) 18:1–9. doi:10.1007/s10156-011-0306-2
71. Osterholzer JJ, Milam JE, Chen GH, Toews GB, Huffnagle GB, Olszewski MA. Role of dendritic cells and alveolar macrophages in regulating early host defense against pulmonary infection with *Cryptococcus neoformans*. *Infect Immun* (2009) 77:3749–58. doi:10.1128/IAI.00454-09
72. Goodman JS, Kaufman L, Koenig MG. Diagnosis of cryptococcal meningitis. Value of immunologic detection of cryptococcal antigen. *N Engl J Med* (1971) 285:434–6. doi:10.1056/NEJM197108192850804
73. Gottfredsson M, Perfect JR. Fungal meningitis. *Semin Neurol* (2000) 20:307–22. doi:10.1055/s-2000-9394
74. Kleinschmidt-DeMasters BK. Central nervous system aspergillosis: a 20-year retrospective series. *Hum Pathol* (2002) 33:116–24. doi:10.1053/hupa.2002.30186
75. Kielian T. Toll-like receptors in central nervous system glial inflammation and homeostasis. *J Neurosci Res* (2006) 83:711–30. doi:10.1002/jnr.20767
76. Larsen PH, Holm TH, Owens T. Toll-like receptors in brain development and homeostasis. *Sci STKE* (2007) 2007:e47. doi:10.1126/stke.4022007pe47
77. Aguirre K, Miller S. MHC class II-positive perivascular microglial cells mediate resistance to *Cryptococcus neoformans* brain infection. *Glia* (2002) 39:184–8. doi:10.1002/glia.10093
78. Hill JO, Aguirre KM. CD4+ T cell-dependent acquired state of immunity that protects the brain against *Cryptococcus neoformans*. *J Immunol* (1994) 152:2344–50.
79. Zhou Q, Gault RA, Kozel TR, Murphy WJ. Protection from direct cerebral *Cryptococcus* infection by interferon-gamma-dependent activation of microglial cells. *J Immunol* (2007) 178:5753–61. doi:10.4049/jimmunol.178.9.5753
80. Kaissling B, Hegyi I, Loffing J, Le Hir M. Morphology of interstitial cells in the healthy kidney. *Anat Embryol (Berl)* (1996) 193:303–18. doi:10.1007/BF00186688
81. Hume DA, Gordon S. Mononuclear phagocyte system of the mouse defined by immunohistochemical localization of antigen F4/80. Identification of resident macrophages in renal medullary and cortical interstitium and the juxtaglomerular complex. *J Exp Med* (1983) 157:1704–9. doi:10.1084/jem.157.5.1704
82. Hoeffel G, Chen J, Lavin Y, Low D, Almeida Francisca F, See P, et al. C-Myb+ erythro-myeloid progenitor-derived fetal monocytes give rise to adult tissue-resident macrophages. *Immunity* (2015) 42:665–78. doi:10.1016/j.immuni.2015.03.011
83. Cao Q, Wang Y, Wang XM, Lu J, Lee VW, Ye Q, et al. Renal F4/80+ CD11c+ mononuclear phagocytes display phenotypic and functional characteristics of macrophages in health and in adriamycin nephropathy. *J Am Soc Nephrol* (2015) 26:349–63. doi:10.1681/ASN.2013121336
84. Ginhoux F, Jung S. Monocytes and macrophages: developmental pathways and tissue homeostasis. *Nat Rev Immunol* (2014) 14:392–404. doi:10.1038/nri3671
85. Kim MG, Boo CS, Ko YS, Lee HY, Cho WY, Kim HK, et al. Depletion of kidney CD11c+ F4/80+ cells impairs the recovery process in ischaemia/reperfusion-induced acute kidney injury. *Nephrol Dial Transplant* (2010) 25:2908–21. doi:10.1093/ndt/gfq183
86. Hochheiser K, Heuser C, Krause TA, Teteris S, Ilias A, Weisheit C, et al. Exclusive CX3CR1 dependence of kidney DCs impacts glomerulonephritis progression. *J Clin Invest* (2013) 123:4242–54. doi:10.1172/JCI70143
87. Lionakis MS, Lim JK, Lee CC, Murphy PM. Organ-specific innate immune responses in a mouse model of invasive candidiasis. *J Innate Immun* (2011) 3:180–99. doi:10.1159/000321157
88. Spellberg B, Ibrahim AS, Edwards JE Jr, Filler SG. Mice with disseminated candidiasis die of progressive sepsis. *J Infect Dis* (2005) 192:336–43. doi:10.1086/430952
89. Lionakis MS. New insights into innate immune control of systemic candidiasis. *Med Mycol* (2014) 52:555–64. doi:10.1093/mmy/myu029
90. Hebecker B, Vlaic S, Conrad T, Bauer M, Brunke S, Kapitan M, et al. Dual-species transcriptional profiling during systemic candidiasis reveals organ-specific host-pathogen interactions. *Sci Rep* (2016) 6:36055. doi:10.1038/srep36055
91. Lionakis MS, Netea MG. *Candida* and host determinants of susceptibility to invasive candidiasis. *PLoS Pathog* (2013) 9:e1003079. doi:10.1371/journal.ppat.1003079
92. Hickey WF, Kimura H. Perivascular microglial cells of the CNS are bone marrow-derived and present antigen in vivo. *Science* (1988) 239:290–2. doi:10.1126/science.3276004
93. Keren-Shaul H, Spinrad A, Weiner A, Matcovitch-Natan O, Dvir-Szternfeld R, Ulland TK, et al. A unique microglia type associated with restricting development of Alzheimer's disease. *Cell* (2017) 169:1276–90.e17. doi:10.1016/j.cell.2017.05.018

14

Regulation of C-Type Lectin Receptor-Mediated Antifungal Immunity

Juan Tang[1†], Guoxin Lin[2,3†], Wallace Y. Langdon[4], Lijian Tao[1] and Jian Zhang[2]*

[1] Department of Nephrology, Xiangya Hospital, Central South University, Changsha, Hunan, China, [2] Department of Pathology, The University of Iowa, Iowa City, IA, United States, [3] Department of Anesthesiology, The Third Xiangya Hospital, Central South University, Changsha, Hunan, China, [4] School of Biological Sciences, University of Western Australia, Perth, WA, Australia

***Correspondence:**
Jian Zhang
jian-zhang@uiowa.edu

[†] These authors have contributed equally to this work.

Of all the pathogen recognition receptor families, C-type lectin receptor (CLR)-induced intracellular signal cascades are indispensable for the initiation and regulation of antifungal immunity. Ongoing experiments over the last decade have elicited diverse CLR functions and novel regulatory mechanisms of CLR-mediated-signaling pathways. In this review, we highlight novel insights in antifungal innate and adaptive-protective immunity mediated by CLRs and discuss the potential therapeutic strategies against fungal infection based on targeting the mediators in the host immune system.

Keywords: C-type lectin receptor, fungal infection, signaling pathways, posttranslational modifications, immunity

INTRODUCTION

Fungi are ubiquitously present in the mucosal and epidermal surfaces in healthy individuals and often cause infections in immune-compromised patients. These include HIV-positive patients, recipients of organ transplants, and cancer patients treated with chemotherapy. In healthy individuals, fungal infections can also develop including vulvovaginal candidiasis, tinea pedis, fungal keratitis, and chromoblastomycosis (1–6). Invasive fungal infections, particularly with *Candida albicans* (*C. albicans*), demonstrate high mortality rates and kill more than 1.5 million people worldwide annually (7). Moreover, other identified pathogenic fungi such as *Aspergillus fumigatus* (*A. fumigatus*), *C. auris*, and *Cryptococcus gattii* (*C. gattii*) also pose a great threat to public health (1, 8, 9). Toxicity and resistance to the limited number of antifungal agents that are currently available contributes to high morbidity and mortality associated with fungal sepsis. Therefore, there is an urgent need to better understand the immune response during fungal infection and develop new immuno-therapeutic approaches.

C-type lectin receptors (CLRs), including transmembrane and soluble forms, are characterized by containing at least one C-type lectin-like domain (CTLD). They have been shown to recognize both endogenous and exogenous ligands (10). As the most important pattern recognition receptor (PRR) family for the detection of fungi, CLRs are recognized to play a critical role in tailoring immune responses against fungal exposure (11–14). In this review, we will focus on the roles and mechanisms of membrane-bound CLR-mediated-signaling pathways in host defense against fungal infections, with an emphasis on *C. albicans*. *C. albicans* is the most common fungal species isolated from biofilms, formed either on implanted devices or on human tissues, which become pathogenic in immune-compromised patients. We will also discuss the role of posttranslational modifications (PTMs) of CLR-signaling pathway components in anti-fungal immunity. In addition, we will also summarize the recent progress on the potential host-derived immune therapies for disseminated candidiasis.

FUNGAL RECOGNITION

The pathogen-associated molecular patterns (PAMPs) on the fungal cell wall are crucial for the initiation of innate immune responses against fungal pathogens. The fungal cell wall is predominantly composed of carbohydrate polymers interspersed with glycoproteins (15–17). The three major components, found in almost all fungi, are β-glucans, which are anchored in the inner core of the cell wall, chitin, which is a robust β-1,4-linked homopolymer of N-acetylglucosamine (GlcNac) located in the inner cell wall, and mannans, which are localized in the outer layer of the fungal yeast cell wall. The central core of the cell wall is branched β-1,3/1,6-glucans that are linked to chitin *via* β-1,4 linkages (15, 18). Mannans are chains of up to several hundred mannoses that are added to fungal proteins *via* N- or O-linkages. Mannoproteins can covalently attach to glucans or chitin *via* either their sugar residues or glycosylphosphatidylinositol (17). In addition, O-linked glycoproteins containing mannobiose-rich structures from *Malassezia* function as distinct ligands to induce immune responses (19). Another crucial component on the fungal cell wall is melanin, which is involved in fungal virulence, resistance to antifungal drugs, and protection against insults from the environment (20, 21).

The recognition of PAMPs expressed in pathogens involves four families of PRRs, including Toll-like receptors (TLRs), NOD-like receptors (NLRs), retinoic acid-inducible gene I (RIG-I)-like receptors (RLRs), and CLRs, each of which shows notable differences regarding pathogen recognitions, signal transduction, and intracellular downstream pathways (14, 22). Among these PRRs, CLRs have been shown to be essential for fungal recognition, either alone or in conjunction with TLRs (23–25). The family of CLRs comprises a subset of CTLD-containing proteins, including some Ca^{2+}-dependent and Ca^{2+}-independent carbohydrate-binding membrane-bound receptors. They are preferentially expressed by myeloid cells (26, 27). Ca^{2+}-dependent carbohydrate binding is the most common CTLD function in vertebrates. Under these circumstances, the CTLD is therefore named as a carbohydrate recognition domain (CRD) (27). CLRs can recognize an array of molecules such as carbohydrates, proteins, and lipids.

Several PRRs have been reported to recognize β-glucans, including Dectin-1, complement receptor 3 (CR3), and three members of the scavenger receptor family, CD5, CD36, and SCARF1 (28–33). Recent studies have revealed that Dectin-2, Dectin-3, macrophage mannose receptor (MR), macrophage-inducible C-type lectin (Mincle), and dendritic cell (DC)-specific ICAM3-grabbing non-integrin (DC-SIGN) can recognize mannans and mannoproteins (12, 13, 34–37). It has been shown that Dectin-1 specifically recognizes β-1, 3-glucans (11, 38), whereas Dectin-2 and Dectin-3 specifically recognize α-mannans (12, 13). The receptor(s) that recognizes chitin is still unknown, although NOD2, MR, and TLR9 were proposed to recognize chitin (39).

CLRs IN ANTIFUNGAL IMMUNE RESPONSE

The major CLRs that are recognized to be involved in antifungal immune responses are Dectin-1, Dectin-2, Dectin-3, MR, Mincle, and DC-SIGN. Dectin-1, Dectin-2, Dectin-3, Mincle, and DC-SIGN share a similar molecular structure consisting of a CRD, a stalk region, a transmembrane domain, and a cytoplasmic domain (40–42). By contrast, MR is composed of an amino terminal cysteine-rich domain, a single fibronectin type II domain, eight CRDs, a transmembrane domain, and a cytoplasmic tail (43, 44) (**Figure 1**). These CLRs can be divided into two main groups based on their intracellular-signaling motifs: CLRs with immunoreceptor tyrosine-based activation motifs (ITAMs) or ITAM-like (also named hem-ITAM) domains and CLRs containing non-immunoreceptor tyrosine-based motifs such as MR and DC-SIGN (27, 45). The activation of these receptors can transduce intracellular-signaling pathways directly through integral ITAM-like motif(s) within the cytoplasmic tails (such as Dectin-1), or indirectly through association with ITAM-containing FcR-γ chains, including Dectin-2, Dectin-3, and Mincle (25, 27, 46). Upon ligand binding, the activation of receptors induces the tyrosine phosphorylation of ITAM-like/ITAM motif(s) by Src family kinases, leading to the recruitment and activation of Syk kinase. This subsequently initiates downstream-signaling pathways. The activation of Syk signaling requires its interaction with two phosphorylated tyrosines within ITAM-like/ITAM motifs. However, unlike canonical ITAM motifs within FcR-γ adaptors which contain a repeat of YxxI/L, the ITAM-like motif located in the cytoplasmic tail of Dectin-1 has only a single YxxI/L; thus, the signaling from Syk may involve the receptor dimerization of Dectin-1 containing a single phosphotyrosine (25, 47) (**Figure 1**). Signals from the CLRs initiate and modulate not only innate immune responses but also the development of adaptive immunity, especially T_H1 and T_H17 responses, which are crucial for the control of fungal infections. The role of Dectin-1, Dectin-2, and Dectin-3 in antifungal immunity is of considerable interest and has been extensively studied during the last decade.

Signaling Pathways Mediated by Dectin-1

Dectin-1 (encoded by *Clec7a*), which is mostly expressed by myeloid phagocytes (macrophages, DCs, and neutrophils), recognizes β-1,3-glucans in a calcium-independent manner (40). The engagement of Dectin-1 by β-1,3-glucans induces the activation of Src protein tyrosine kinase (PTK). Src phosphorylates the single cytoplasmic ITAM-like domain of Dectin-1, which subsequently results in the recruitment and activation of Syk (25, 48, 49). The activated Syk then phosphorylates protein kinase C δ (PKC-δ), which phosphorylates caspase activation and recruitment domain-containing protein 9 (CARD9) (50, 51). This facilitates complex formation with Bcl-10 and MALT1 (51, 52), thus eliciting NF-κB activation (24, 51) (**Figure 1**). In addition, Dectin-1-induced activation of extracellular signal-regulated protein kinase (ERK) is also mediated through CARD9, which links Ras-GRF1 to H-Ras (53). In addition to the Syk-dependent pathways, signaling from Dectin-1 also involves Syk-independent pathways mediated by Raf-1, resulting in noncanonical NF-κB activation by collaboration with the Syk-dependent NF-κB-inducing kinase (NIK) pathway (24). The activation of NF-κB and ERK mediates the inflammatory responses against fungal infections and directs T_H1/T_H17 differentiation for antifungal immunity (24, 54–56).

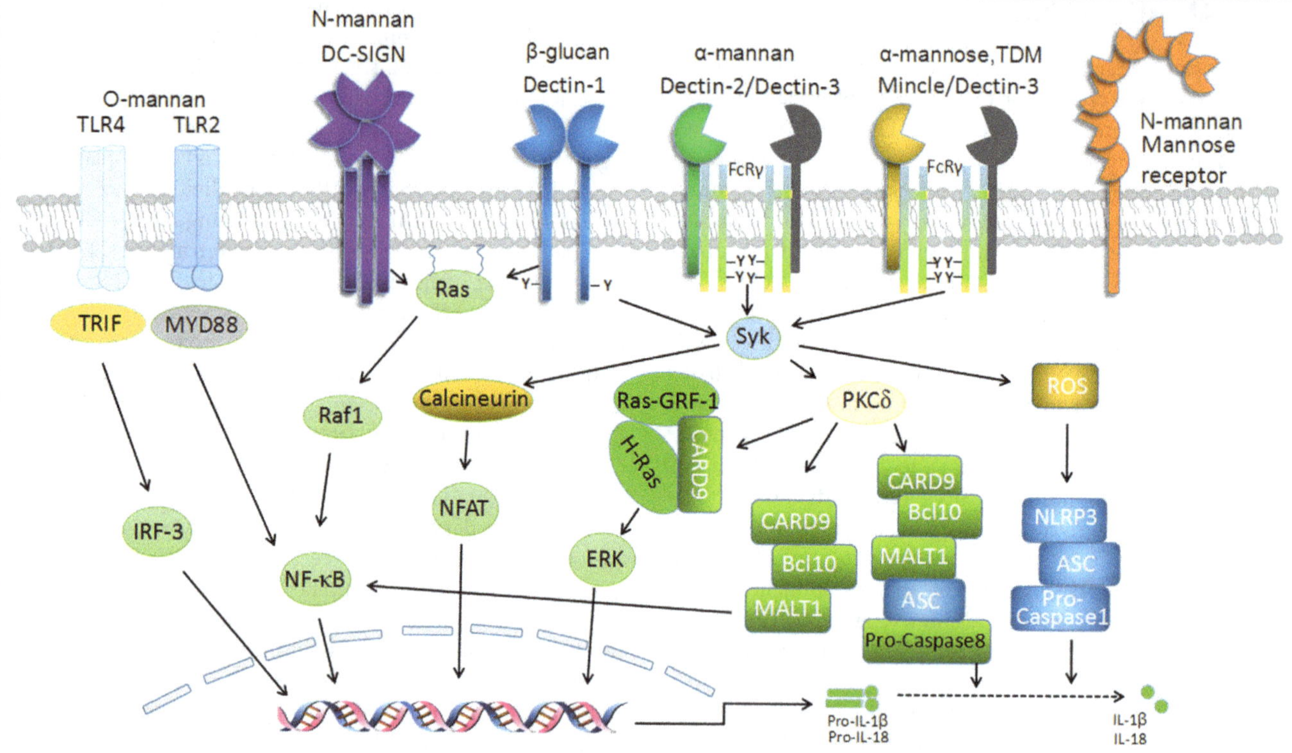

FIGURE 1 | C-type lectin receptor (CLR) signaling in fungal recognition. Schematic representation of the transmembrane CLRs associated with antifungal immunity and their intracellular-signaling networks. The recognition of fungal components by several CLRs, including Dectin-1, Dectin-2, Dectin-3, macrophage-inducible C-type lectin (Mincle), and dendritic cell-specific ICAM3-grabbing non-integrin (DC-SIGN), induces downstream signaling *via* Syk-dependent and Raf-1-dependent pathways to mediate antifungal immunity. Dectin-1 homodimers, Dectin-2-Dectin-3 heterodimers, and Mincle-Dectin-3 heterodimers couple with immunoreceptor tyrosine-based activation motif (ITAM)-like and FcR-γ-associated ITAM motifs, respectively, to recruit Syk to initiate downstream signaling, which leads to reactive oxygen species (ROS) production and caspase activation and recruitment domain-containing protein 9 (CARD9)/Bcl-10/MALT1 complex-mediated activation of NF-κB pathway. ROS triggers NLRP3 inflammasome assembly and activation, which cleave pro-IL-1β and pro-IL-18 into mature forms to elicit protective roles in anti-fungi immunity. Dectin-1-signaling pathway also induces Syk-dependent activation of Ras-GRF1, which recruits H-Ras *via* the CARD9 adaptor and ultimately leads to extracellular signal-regulated protein kinase (ERK) activation. Furthermore, signaling by Syk results in nuclear factor of activated T cells (NF-AT) activation in a calcineurin-dependent fashion, which integrates with NF-κB signaling to regulate gene transcription. Moreover, Dectin-1-signaling activation seems to be essential for the formation of noncanonical caspase-8 inflammasome, which is responsible for active IL-1β production.

Dectin-1 signaling induces numerous signaling events characterized by phagocytosis, respiratory burst, and the production of various inflammatory mediators, including cytokines, chemokines, and inflammatory lipids (40, 47, 57, 58). It is well established that the production of IL-1β, together with IL-6 and IL-23, is essential for antifungal immune responses partly through priming adaptive immunity to differentiate CD4⁺ T cells to T_H1/T_H17 cells (24, 56, 59). Moreover, the production of type I interferons (IFNs) can be induced after fungal recognition and require Dectin-1/Syk signaling and transcription factor IRF5 involvement (49). In mouse models, enhanced IFN-β secretion is critical for protection from fungal challenge (49, 60). Importantly, consistent with animal studies, type I IFNs exert a protective role against *C. albicans* infection in humans (61). Dectin-1 signaling also triggers the activation of nuclear factor of activated T cells (NF-AT) through the Syk/calcineurin pathway, leading to the production of inflammatory cytokines, such as IL-2, IL-10, and IL-12 p70, and the regulation of T cell development and differentiation (62–64) (**Figure 1**).

CARD9 is considered to be essential for tailoring immune responses to fungal pathogens (51). The survival of *Card9*$^{-/-}$ mice is greatly impaired following systemic *C. albicans* infection (51, 53). In addition, NF-κB-mediated cytokine production is severely defective in the absence of CARD9 (51, 53). Notably, human CARD9 deficiency, which is referred to as an autosomal-recessive disorder, is associated with a spectrum of fungal diseases caused by various fungal pathogens (65). Currently, 16 human CARD9 mutations, including nonsense and missense mutations, have been reported in patients worldwide (66). CARD9 mutations result in the impairment of mucosal fungal defense, partly by inhibiting T_H17-induced immune responses, which are responsible for the susceptibility to chronic mucocutaneous candidiasis (67). However, the underlying mechanism regarding how human CARD9 mutations affect T_H17 immunity deserves further investigation.

Strikingly, CARD9 serves as the only currently known human gene in regulating the dissemination of *C. albicans* to the central nervous system (CNS). CARD9 deficiency in both mice and humans results in vulnerability to fungal infection in the CNS, owing to impaired neutrophil accumulation in the fungal-infected CNS, which correlates with the lack of CXC-chemokine induction (68). Consistent with these findings, decreased neutrophil recruitment to the lungs was reported in *Card9*$^{-/-}$ mice infected with *A. fumigatus* (69). CARD9 deficiency may also predispose to extrapulmonary *A. fumigatus* infection in humans as a result of impaired neutrophil recruitment (70). Nevertheless, the CARD9-dependent-protective role seems less necessary for pulmonary mold infections. Thus, future studies are required to decipher the role of CARD9 in other immune cells to explain its "organ-specific" and "species-specific" function in antifungal immunity. Moreover, the effects of genetic mutations in CARD9-coupled receptors (Dectin-1, Dectin-2, and Dectin-3) and CARD9-binding partners (MALT1 and Bcl-10) in human antifungal host defense require more in-depth studies.

Vav proteins, the key upstream regulators of CARD9, are critical in CLR/CARD9-induced-inflammatory responses similar to CARD9 (71). Indeed, humans with polymorphisms in *DECTIN-1 and VAV3* show increased susceptibility to invasive *C. albicans* infection (71, 72). Interestingly, one recent study illustrated that neutrophilic myeloid-derived suppressor cells (MDSCs) are induced *in vitro* upon infection with various *Candida* species, which functionally inhibit T cell responses *via* Dectin-1/CARD9 signaling and subsequently suppress ROS generation, indicating that CARD9 seems to function as a negative modulator in fungal immune response (73). It is unknown whether this is true *in vivo*. The contribution of MDSCs to fungal infections requires further investigation.

Signaling Pathways Mediated by Dectin-2, Dectin-3, and Mincle

Dectin-2 (encoded by *Clec4n*), Dectin-3 (MCL, encoded by *Clec4d*), and Mincle (encoded by *Clec4e*) belong to the Dectin-2 family of CLRs, whose encoding genes are grouped closely at the telomeric end of the NK-gene cluster. They all have a single extracellular CTLD, short cytoplasmic tails, and trigger intracellular signaling indirectly through association with the ITAM-containing FcR-γ chain (55, 74–76). Signaling from Dectin-2, Dectin-3, and Mincle is mediated *via* the Syk/PKCδ-dependent CARD9/Bcl-10/MALT1 pathway, resulting in the activation of the transcription factor NF-κB and the subsequent production of inflammatory cytokines and chemokines (13, 75, 77). Dectin-2 recognizes high-mannose structures and binds *Candida* α-mannans in a calcium-dependent manner (12, 78). It can also recognize O-linked mannobiose-rich glycoprotein from *Malassezia*, glycans containing mannose from house dust mite extracts (19, 79). Dectin-2 has been implicated in the defense against numerous pathogens, including *C. albicans, C. neoformans, A. fumigatus, Saccharomyces cerevisiae, Paracoccidioides brasiliensis, Histoplasma capsulatum, Microsporum audouinii, Trichophyton rubrum, Mycobacterium tuberculosis,* and *Schistosoma mansoni* (75, 78, 80). Dectin-2 and Dectin-3 can form heterodimers to recognize the hyphal forms of *C. albicans* to induce pro-inflammatory production (13), although the involvement of Dectin-3 in *C. neoformans* infection is still controversial (81).

Mice deficient for Dectin-2 are highly susceptible to systemic candidiasis (12). Further study indicates that Dectin-2 and Dectin-3, two similar CLRs, form a constitutive heterodimeric PRR for sensing α-mannans on the surface of *C. albicans* and induce Syk-mediated activation of NF-κB to combat fungal invasion (13). Blocking either Dectin-2 or Dectin-3 with antibodies dramatically eliminates NF-κB-mediated-inflammatory responses upon *C. albicans* stimulation. The genetic deletion of Dectin-3, or mice receiving Dectin-3-blocking antibodies, showed high susceptibility to systemic candidiasis (13). Therefore, Dectin-2 coupled with Dectin-3 displays protective antifungal immunity in animal models. Recently, two studies also showed that Dectin-3 is constitutively expressed in myeloid cells and functions as an FcR-γ-coupled receptor for sensing trehalose-6,6'-dimycolate (TDM), a potent mycobacterial adjuvant (76, 82). In addition, Dectin-3 is also essential for inducing Mincle expression upon TDM stimulation (82). Dectin-3 has been shown to interact with Mincle *via* the stalk region of Dectin-3, thus enhancing the protein expression of Mincle (83).

Emerging evidence showed that the engagement of the T_H17/IL-17 pathway plays a critical role in host defense against mucosal fungal infection (84). Both Dectin-2 and Dectin-3 are of great importance for T_H17 cell differentiation in host defense against *C. albicans* or *Blastomyces dermatitidis* (12, 85). Furthermore, PI3K-δ, a proximal Syk-dependent-signaling intermediate downstream of Dectin-2, plays an important role in the generation of T_H2 and T_H17 immunities against infection with *Dermatophagoides farina* (*D. farina*) (86). In addition, a recent study showed that NF-κB subunit c-Rel-dependent cytokine induction relies on the Dectin-2/MALT1-signaling cascade to trigger T_H17-polarizing cytokines IL-1β and IL-23 secretion, thus possessing T_H17-protective immunity against pathogenic fungal invasion (52). The expression of IL-17RC on humans and murine neutrophils has been identified in a Dectin-2-dependent pathway (87). Dectin-2-induced autocrine IL-17 secretion has also been implicated with ROS generation and fungal killing (87).

Mincle has been shown to recognize *mycobacteria, C. albicans, Malasezzia,* and *Fonsecaea species* (36, 88–90). It is the sensor for α-mannose, glycolipid trehalose-6, 6′-dimycolate (TDM), and the self-ribonucleoprotein SAP-130 (74, 88, 91). Mincle is expressed constitutively at low levels in myeloid cells, and its expression is dependent on Dectin-3 (76, 83, 92). The expression pattern of Mincle suggests that it may not be the major fungal recognition receptor. In support of this notion, although mice lacking Mincle display increased fungal burden in the kidneys, the survival rate of *Mincle*$^{-/-}$ mice is similar to wild-type mice upon systemic *C. albicans* infection (89). It has been shown that Mincle is not a phagocytic receptor but modestly potentiates pro-inflammatory cytokine production (89). Mincle has been shown to inhibit Dectin-1-induced T_H1 responses to *F. monophora* infection by inducing IRF1 degradation through the E3 ubiquitin ligase Mdm2, which impairs the polarization of T_H1 cells. Defective T_H1 responses contribute to the chronic infection of *F. monophora* which causes chromoblastomycosis, a chronic fungal skin infection (93). In addition, Mincle has been demonstrated to specifically recognize *Malassezia* species and play a crucial role in host defense against this fungus (36).

Other Fungal Recognition Receptors

MR (CD206, encoded by *Mrc1*): MR recognizes N-linked mannan of infectious *Candida* and mediates endocytosis and phagocytosis (94). Recent studies indicate that MR might promote the secretion of pro-inflammatory cytokines through the activating intracellular signal cascades. Although non-ITAM motifs are identified within the MR, a recent study reports that human MR becomes tyrosine phosphorylated upon *M. tuberculosis* (*M. tb*) infection, and this phosphorylation mediates a sequential association of Grb-2 and SHP-1 (95), suggesting that human MR itself can transduce downstream signaling. However, no known signaling motifs in murine MR have been identified, and no signaling has been induced directly from murine MR in response to fungal infections. Using human peripheral blood mononuclear cells, MR was found to be the main receptor pathway for the induction of T_H17 cells by *C. albicans in vitro* (34). However, the importance of MR in fungal recognition is challenged by the fact that normal host defense is not altered during systemic candidiasis or *Pneumocystis carinii* infection in *Mr*$^{-/-}$ mice (96). In support of this, MR is also not required for resistance to *Coccidioides immitis* infection (97). Therefore, MR may not be the major fungal recognition receptor in mice. It is possible that the human and murine MRs may behave differently. This notion is supported by a recent report that human but not mouse MR signaling induced by *M. tb* regulates macrophage recognition and vesicle trafficking (95).

DC-SIGN (encoded by *Cd209a*): DC-SIGN is a transmembrane receptor for pathogen binding and uptake, which is mainly expressed in a subset of macrophages and DCs (98, 99). It has been demonstrated that DC-SIGN can bind and internalize soluble ligands effectively, which facilitates antigen processing and presentation to T cells (100). DC-SIGN has a high affinity to detect varied carbohydrate-based ligands, including mannose structures and fucose-bearing glycans, to recognize diverse organisms including HIV-1, *M. tb*, *Helicobacter pylori*, or fungi such as *C. albicans*, *A. fumigatus*, and *C. tropicum* (35, 37, 101–103). The polymorphisms of both Dectin-1 and DC-SIGN were reported to associate with invasive pulmonary Aspergillosis infection (104). It has been demonstrated that DC-SIGN can recognize *Candida* mannan and that *N*-linked mannosyl residues are essential for this interaction (37). In particular, the *N*-mannosylation is required for the binding, phagocytosis, and immune sensing of *C. albicans* by human DCs (37). Upon high-mannose recognition, the signalosome leads to Raf-1 activation and subsequent p65 acetylation, which facilitates gene-transcriptional expression, especially amplifying TLR-induced cytokine production such as IL-10, IL-6, and IL-12 (23). However, DC-SIGN in collaboration with MR seems to suppress Dectin-1-mediated T_H17 responses, but potentiate T_H1 responses in β-glucan- or *M. tb*-treated DCs (105). Moreover, DC-SIGN, which contains abundant galactomannan, is also found to play an important role in the recognition and binding of *A. fumigatus* conidia in human DCs (103). The ligation of DC-SIGN by the glycoprotein fimbriae of *Porphyromonas gingivalis* promotes the evasion of antibacterial autophagy and lysosome fusion, resulting in intracellular persistence in myeloid DCs, whereas TLR2 activation can overcome autophagy evasion and pathogen persistence in DCs (106). However, the importance of DC-SIGN in antifungal immunity has not been verified by a gene-targeting approach.

CD23 (encoded by *Fcer2a*): CD23 is the low-affinity receptor for IgE and is also a novel CLR which binds to α-mannans and β-glucans (107). A recent study illustrated that c-Jun N-terminal kinase 1 (JNK1) deficiency exerts a protective effect in systemic candidiasis. The expression of CD23 is negatively regulated through a Dectin-1-induced NF-AT pathway (107). Antifungal effector NOS2 is dramatically augmented through the recognition of α-mannans and β-glucans with CD23 in mice lacking JNK1. Likewise, the genetic deletion of CD23 abrogates the protection of *Jnk1*$^{-/-}$ mice from disseminated candidiasis. JNK inhibitors boost antifungal innate immunity *in vivo* and *in vitro* (107). Taken together, JNK inhibition may also be a novel therapeutic strategy to combat disseminated candidiasis (**Figure 2**).

CR3 (Mac-1, $\alpha_{M\beta2}$, or CD11b/CD18): CR3 is mainly expressed in leukocytes. CR3 consists of an I domain and a specific lectin domain, which bind to protein ligands such as iC3b, fibronectin and ICAM-1, and complement deposited on β-1,6-glucans (108). CR3 has been shown to cooperate with Dectin-1 for the detection of β-glucans and the regulation of innate immune responses during fungal pathogen exposure (109). Recent studies identified that CR3 and Dectin-1 collaboratively induce cytokine responses in macrophages in an Syk/JNK/AP-1 manner upon disseminated *H. capsulatum* infection (110), which further facilitates fungal-adaptive immune responses. Still, the underlying molecular mechanisms of crosstalk among other fungal PRRs will be of great interest for future investigations.

Collaboration between CLRs and TLRs

There is emerging evidence that signaling from CLRs in collaboration with other PRRs, especially TLRs, is indispensable for optimal antifungal immunity. It has been reported that the cooperative interaction between Dectin-1 and TLR2 or TLR4 synergistically facilitates the production of TNF, IL-23, and IL-10, but reduces IL-12 (59, 111). Dectin-1/TLR2 can amplify MR-mediated Th17 responses and IL-17 production upon *C. albicans* infection (34). In addition, DC-SIGN modulates the signaling from multiple TLRs on human DCs through activating Raf-1-dependent acetylation of NF-κB, which can promote the transcription of IL-10 and enhance antifungal-inflammatory response (23).

Recent studies have shown the importance of costimulation of Mincle and TLRs in protective antifungal response to *F. pedrosoi*, the most common fungus associated with chromoblastomycosis. Normally, *F. pedrosoi* is recognized by CLRs, but not TLRs, leading to the defective production of costimulatory cytokines and impaired fungal clearance. Intriguingly, the exogenous application of TLR7 ligand, imiquimod, restores the induction of inflammatory responses mediated *via* both Syk/CARD9- and MyD88-dependent-signaling pathways, as well as facilitates *F. pedrosoi* clearance in mice (90). In support of this finding, the topical administration of imiquimod to several patients with chromoblastomycosis also results in rapid infection resolution and greatly improved the lesions (112).

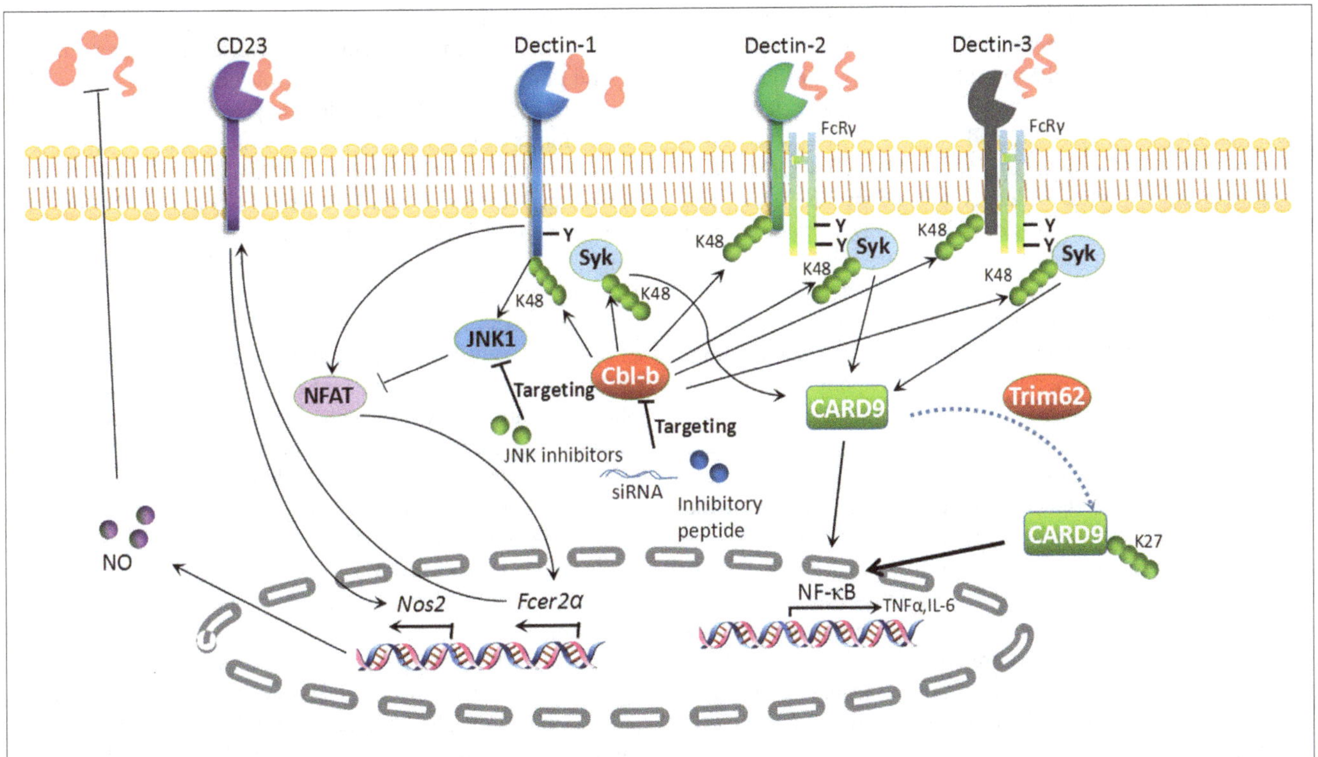

FIGURE 2 | Potential targets in antifungal immunity. K48-linked polyubiquitination of Dectin-1, Dectin-2, Dectin-3, and Syk is mediated by the E3 ubiquitin ligase Cbl-b, which results in the degradation of these molecules. Subsequently, the pro-inflammatory cytokines are impaired in the presence of Cbl-b. The inhibition of Cbl-b with an inhibitory peptide or *Cbl-b* siRNA can boost antifungal immunity, which provides a potential treatment strategy for fungal invasion. CD23 is a novel C-type lectin receptor for fungal recognition, which is elevated in parallel with NO production in *Jnk1*$^{-/-}$ mice. The inhibition of c-Jun N-terminal kinase 1 (JNK1) has revealed its potential as a therapeutic target for enhancing antifungal immunity. TRIM62, another E3 ubiquitin ligase, is responsible for K27-linked polyubiquitination of caspase activation and recruitment domain-containing protein 9 (CARD9) to elicit its antifungal immunity. TRIM62 or CARD9 variants appear to be potential therapeutic targets for fungal infections.

INFLAMMASOMES IN ANTIFUNGAL IMMUNITY

Emerging evidence shows that the engagement of inflammasomes plays a critical role in host defense against fungal infection, which can lead to the processing and activation of IL-1β and IL-18 (113). Both cytokines are implicated in mediating antifungal cellular responses, especially the promotion of adaptive T_H1/T_H17 responses.

NLRP3 has been proposed to be the main inflammasome involved in protective fungal immunity (114). Several CLRs and TLRs can induce the priming of inflammasomes and the activation of NF-κB *via* the recognition of fungal PAMPs, resulting in the expression of pro-IL-1β and pro-IL-18 (115–117). Both Dectin-1/Syk- and TLR2/MYD88-signaling pathways have been shown to induce NLRP3 priming in murine macrophages infected with *C. albicans* (114). In addition, the production of pro-IL-1β in response to *A. fumigatus, M. canis, Malassezia* spp., *P. brasiliensis*, and *C. neoformans* requires Dectin-1/Syk-dependent signaling (118–122). A more recent study indicates that Dectin-2 is the primary receptor for NLRP3 inflammasome activation in DCs in response to *H. capsulatum* (117). It is unknown whether Dectin-2 and other CLRs such as Dectin-3, Mincle, and MR are also involved in the activation of inflammasomes.

The canonical NLRP3 inflammasome can be triggered by ROS, K^+ efflux, and lysosomal cathepsins release induced by various fungal species. Upon infection with *C. albicans* and *A. fumigatus*, it has been shown that the activation of the NLRP3 inflammasome requires transition from the yeast to the filamentous phase (123), which may be attributed to the differential exposure of β-glucans on the fungal surface and thus the differential recognition by Dectin-1 (124). Upon phagocytosis by host macrophages, *C. albicans* filaments trigger lysosomal rupture, which is required for the particulate activation of the NLRP3 inflammasome (124, 125). In addition, *C. albicans*-secreted aspartic proteases Sap2 and Sap6 are thought to activate the caspase-1-dependent NLRP3 inflammasome by inducing ROS production and K^+ efflux (126). Recent evidence has shown that NLRP3 coupling with AIM2 receptors is required to activate caspase-1- and caspase-8-dependent inflammasomes and induce protective antifungal responses in DCs challenged with *A. fumigatus* (127). Mice deficient in both NLRP3 and AIM2 are more susceptible to invasive Aspergillosis than mice lacking a single inflammasome receptor, suggesting the importance of cooperative activation and dual cytoplasmic surveillance of these two inflammasomes against *A. fumigatus* infection (127). Interestingly, mucosal *Candida* infection induces the activation of an NLRC4-dependent inflammasome, which can utilize caspase-1 to process IL-1β and IL-18 (128). The NLRC4 inflammasome protects against mucosal fungal overgrowth and facilitates inflammatory cytokine secretion and neutrophil influx in a murine model of oropharyngeal candidiasis (128).

Recently, an NLR-independent and caspase-8-dependent inflammasome have been identified (115). It seems that Dectin-1 signaling induces the formation of a CARD9/Bcl-10/MALT1/caspase-8/ASC complex which is dependent on Syk (115). Interestingly, caspase-8 in this complex is only partially cleaved to generate a p43 intermediate, which averts the triggering of caspase-3 and apoptosis (115). Dectin-1-mediated activation of caspase-8 appears to be involved in the cleavage of pro-IL-1β and the production of its bioactive form to defend against fungi (115). A subsequent study reported that this noncanonical caspase-8 inflammasome can be activated and modulated by Tec, an intracellular non-receptor PTK, which acts as a novel signaling mediator between Dectin-1/Syk and PLC-γ2 in macrophages upon infection with *Candida* (116). The genetic ablation or the chemical inhibition of Tec results in a dramatic reduction of inflammatory responses and protects from fatal fungal sepsis (116). Interestingly, it has been shown that caspase-8, coordinating with caspase-1, plays a crucial role in promoting NLRP3 inflammasome-dependent maturation of IL-1β mediated by Dectin-1 and CR3 in DCs during β-glucan sensing and *C. albicans* infection (109). In addition, the same group also showed that there is crosstalk between CR3 and Dectin-1 during *H. capsulatum* yeast infection in macrophage TNF and IL-6 responses in an Syk/JNK/AP-1-dependent manner (110). However, it was reported that *H. capsulatum* α-(1,3)-glucan blocks innate immune recognition by Dectin-1 (129). The importance of Dectin-1 in *H. capsulatum* infection, in particular *in vivo*, remains to be determined. Furthermore, the role of caspase-8 in controlling antifungal immunity has not been confirmed by a gene-targeting approach.

CLR-MEDIATED PTMS IN ANTIFUNGAL IMMUNITY

Recent literature has shed additional light on novel molecules engaged in antifungal immunity and PTMs in CLR-signaling cascades, thus opening new avenues for innovative therapeutic approaches (107, 130–133). It has been increasingly recognized that PTMs serve as modulators to tailor fungal evasion by targeting innate sensors, adaptors, signaling components, and transcription factors. Subsequently, PTMs regulate the activation, survival, and stability of potent proteins by linking covalent bonds to functional groups (134). To date, several PTMs including phosphorylation and ubiquitination have been characterized in the regulation of immune responses against fungi.

Protein Kinases and Phosphatases in Antifungal Innate Immunity

Two major cytoplasmic kinase families in innate cells, including the Src family kinases and the Syk, are involved in intracellular-signaling cascades upon fungal pathogen exposure. Signaling involving the phosphorylation of tyrosine residues within the ITAM(s) by Src family kinases leads to the recruitment and activation of Syk, which then phosphorylates phospholipase Cγ2 (PLC-γ2). Activated PLC-γ2 initiates the hydrolysis of membrane-bound phosphatidylinositol-3,4,5-triphosphate (PIP_3) to soluble inositol triphosphate (IP_3) and diacylglycerol, both of which result in the influx of calcium and the activation of PKC-δ, the latter mediating the phosphorylation of CARD9 and the subsequent activation of the CARD9/Bcl-10/MALT1 complex. Downstream signaling through the Syk/PLCγ2 pathway from Dectin-1 and Dectin-2 involves the activation of NF-κB, ERK, and NF-AT (24, 53, 135, 136).

Numerous studies have shown that the balance between phosphorylation and dephosphorylation is of great importance in orchestrating fungal immune responses. In addition to Src kinases phosphorylating ITAM(s) within Dectin-1 and FcR-γ, recent literature has shown that two members of Src family kinases, Fyn and Lyn, facilitate the *cryptococcal*-killing capacity in NK cells by mediating PI3K/ERK1/2-signaling activity, which further directs the traffic of perforin-containing granules to synapses for pathogen clearance (137). Whether other Src family kinases are involved in the regulation of fungal invasion remains to be determined.

The CARD9/Bcl-10/MALT1 complex in Dectin-1 signaling upon *Candida* infection has been known to activate the IKK complex, leading to the phosphorylation of IκB and the activation of all canonical NF-κB subunits including p50, p65, and c-Rel (24, 51, 138). Importantly, Syk activation in response to Dectin-1 stimulation is also able to activate noncanonical subunits of NF-κB (p52 and RelB) through NIK and IKKα, leading to the nuclear translocation of p52–RelB dimers (24). In addition, Dectin-1 signaling can induce Syk-independent phosphorylation and activation of Raf-1 *via* Ras. Activated Ras leads to the activation of Raf-1, which then phosphorylates NF-κB p65, and facilitates p65–RelB dimer formation that sequesters active RelB and potentiates T_H1 responses by inducing IL-12p40 and IL-1β (24). Interestingly, another group recently found that Dectin-1 stimulated with *C. albicans* triggers Syk-dependent phosphorylation of Ras-GRF1, which mediates the recruitment and activation of H-Ras through CARD9 alone, but not the CARD9/Bcl-10/MALT1 complex, leading to the phosphorylation and activation of ERK, but not NF-κB and subsequent pro-inflammatory responses (53). This suggests that upon Dectin-1 signaling, CARD9 is required for ERK activation but is dispensable for NF-κB activation.

CLR (Dectin-1, Dectin-2/3, or Mincle) signaling has been reported to phosphorylate and activate SHP-2, which is able to recruit Syk to Dectin-1 or to the adaptor FcR-γ, thus resulting in the activation of Syk and downstream signaling and mediate antifungal innate immune responses and T_H17 responses (139). In addition, the phosphatase SHIP-1 has been recently identified to co-localize with Dectin-1-phosphorylated hem-ITAM and to negatively modulate ROS production in a Dectin/Syk/PI3K/PDK1/NADPH oxidase-dependent manner in response to *C. albicans* infection (140). Thus, a novel role of SHIP-1 in selectively controlling the balance of effectors in the Syk/PI3K pathway has been identified. Phosphatase and tensin homolog deleted on chromosome 10 also serves as a negative modulator to regulate the PGE2/cAMP/PKA-signaling cascade *via* blocking F-actin-mediated cytoskeletal remodeling and dephosphorylating cofilin-1 during immune defense against pathogenic *C. albicans* (141). Therefore, phosphorylation- and dephosphorylation-mediated protein kinases and phosphatases are crucial for controlling antifungal immunity.

Ubiquitin Ligases and Deubiquitinating Enzymes in Antifungal Innate Immunity

PTM of target proteins by polyubiquitination has been intensively studied in numerous biological systems (142–146). Seven lysine residues in ubiquitin determine the specific type of polyubiquitination. Lysine 48 (K48)-linked polyubiquitination is involved in proteasome-mediated protein degradation, whereas lysine 63-linked polyubiquitination is usually engaged in signal pathway transmission (145). In addition to K48- and K63-linked polyubiquitination, K6-, K11-, K27-, K29-, and K33-linked polyubiquitination are being exploited to address their roles in immune responses and inflammatory diseases (145). Recently, a number of studies have highlighted an important role for ubiquitination of the CLR-signaling pathway in fungal immunity (130–133).

TRIM62

TRIM62, also named DEAR1, is a member of the TRIM/RBCC family, which includes proteins with conserved RING finger, B-box, and coiled-coil domains (147). It has been well established that CARD9 positively modulates host immune responses following fungal infection. TRIM62 has been shown to function as a CARD9-binding component and to mediate K27-linked polyubiquitination of CARD9 at K125 to facilitate its protective role in anti-fungi immune responses (130). Similar to *Card9*$^{-/-}$ mice, *Trim62*$^{-/-}$ mice also show increased susceptibility, as well as impaired cytokine responses, in a *C. albicans* infection model (130). Therefore, TRIM62 acts as a positive regulator essential for CARD9-mediated antifungal immunity. TRIM62 or CARD9 variants are therefore potential therapeutic targets for fungal infections (**Figure 2**).

Cbl-b

Cbl-b is a member of Cbl family RING finger E3 ubiquitin ligases (142, 148). Several other groups including ours identified RING finger-type E3 ubiquitin ligase Cbl-b as a key E3 ubiquitin ligase mediating host antifungal innate immunity (131–133). The genetic deletion of Cbl-b renders mice less susceptible to systemic *C. albicans* infection, which is in line with the hyperproduction of pro-inflammatory cytokines TNF-α and IL-6, the robust release of reactive oxygen species (ROS), and improved fungal killing. At the molecular level, Cbl-b targets Dectin-1, Dectin-2, Dectin-3, and SYK for K48-linked polyubiquitination and proteasome-mediated degradation, which further facilitates its anti-inflammatory response (131–133). Interestingly, Cbl-b small-inhibitory peptides and *Cbl-b*-specific siRNA provide protective efficacy against disseminated candidiasis (131, 132). Therefore, targeting Cbl-b may be a potential therapeutic strategy for disseminated candidiasis (**Figure 2**).

A20

A20 is a deubiquitination enzyme which is pivotal for tailoring innate immune responses by inhibiting the NF-κB-signaling cascade (149). IKKγ and TRAF6 activities are dampened in a non-catalytic manner by A20 (149, 150). A recent study showed that A20 is removed by autophagy, which further boosts NF-κB capacity in F4/80^{hi} tissue-resident macrophages to facilitate the pathogen clearance during disseminated *Candida* infection (151).

CONCLUSION

Much progress has been made to unveil the underlying mechanisms of fungal immunity. CLRs are considered to be pivotal in orchestrating innate and adaptive immunity against fungal pathogens based on animal and some human genetic studies. The discovery of novel molecules such as Cbl-b and JNK in anti-fungi immune responses has laid the foundation for potential treatment strategies. Yet, the exact crosstalk between innate and adaptive antifungal immunities, and the yet-to-be-defined PTMs, needs to be resolved in future studies. Moreover, translational studies of newly identified molecular targets are essential for future clinical application. Thus, the studies described in this review provide direction for the rational design of therapeutic strategies in disseminated candidiasis; however, further translational studies with animal models remain to be performed before moving forward into clinical application.

AUTHOR CONTRIBUTIONS

JT, GL, and JZ conceptualized the scope of the review; JT, GL, and JZ wrote the review; and LT and WYL edited the review.

FUNDING

This work is supported by the US National Institutes of Health (grants R01 AI090901, AI121196, and 123253; all to Jian Zhang) and the American Heart Association (AHA Great Rivers Associate Grant-in-Aid grant 16GRT2699004 to Jian Zhang).

REFERENCES

1. Brown GD, Denning DW, Levitz SM. Tackling human fungal infections. *Science* (2012) 336(6082):647. doi:10.1126/science.1222236
2. Gudlaugsson O, Gillespie S, Lee K, Vande Berg J, Hu J, Messer S, et al. Attributable mortality of nosocomial candidemia, revisited. *Clin Infect Dis* (2003) 37(9):1172–7. doi:10.1086/378745
3. Alter SJ, McDonald MB, Schloemer J, Simon R, Trevino J. Common child and adolescent cutaneous infestations and fungal infections. *Curr Probl Pediatr Adolesc Health Care* (2018) 48(1):3–25. doi:10.1016/j.cppeds.2017.11.001
4. Falagas ME, Betsi GI, Athanasiou S. Probiotics for prevention of recurrent vulvovaginal candidiasis: a review. *J Antimicrob Chemother* (2006) 58(2):266–72. doi:10.1093/jac/dkl246
5. Ansari Z, Miller D, Galor A. Current thoughts in fungal keratitis: diagnosis and treatment. *Curr Fungal Infect Rep* (2013) 7(3):209–18. doi:10.1007/s12281-013-0150-110.1007/s12281-013-0150-1
6. Seyedmousavi S, Netea MG, Mouton JW, Melchers WJ, Verweij PE, de Hoog GS. Black yeasts and their filamentous relatives: principles of pathogenesis and host defense. *Clin Microbiol Rev* (2014) 27(3):527–42. doi:10.1128/CMR.00093-13

7. Brown GD, Denning DW, Gow NA, Levitz SM, Netea MG, White TC. Hidden killers: human fungal infections. *Sci Transl Med* (2012) 4(165):165rv13. doi:10.1126/scitranslmed.3004404
8. Byrnes EJ III, Li W, Lewit Y, Ma H, Voelz K, Ren P, et al. Emergence and pathogenicity of highly virulent *Cryptococcus gattii* genotypes in the northwest United States. *PLoS Pathog* (2010) 6(4):e1000850. doi:10.1371/journal.ppat.1000850
9. Sears D, Schwartz BS. *Candida auris*: an emerging multidrug-resistant pathogen. *Int J Infect Dis* (2017) 63:95–8. doi:10.1016/j.ijid.2017.08.017
10. Geijtenbeek TB, Gringhuis SI. Signalling through C-type lectin receptors: shaping immune responses. *Nat Rev Immunol* (2009) 9(7):465–79. doi:10.1038/nri2569
11. Taylor PR, Tsoni SV, Willment JA, Dennehy KM, Rosas M, Findon H, et al. Dectin-1 is required for beta-glucan recognition and control of fungal infection. *Nat Immunol* (2007) 8(1):31–8. doi:10.1038/Ni1408
12. Saijo S, Ikeda S, Yamabe K, Kakuta S, Ishigame H, Akitsu A, et al. Dectin-2 recognition of alpha-mannans and induction of Th17 cell differentiation is essential for host defense against *Candida albicans*. *Immunity* (2010) 32(5):681–91. doi:10.1016/j.immuni.2010.05.001
13. Zhu LL, Zhao XQ, Jiang C, You Y, Chen XP, Jiang YY, et al. C-type lectin receptors dectin-3 and dectin-2 form a heterodimeric pattern-recognition receptor for host defense against fungal infection. *Immunity* (2013) 39(2):324–34. doi:10.1016/j.immuni.2013.05.017
14. Dambuza IM, Brown GD. C-type lectins in immunity: recent developments. *Curr Opin Immunol* (2015) 32:21–7. doi:10.1016/j.coi.2014.12.002
15. Gow NAR, Latge J-P, Munro CA. The fungal cell wall: structure, biosynthesis, and function. *Microbiol Spectr* (2017) 5(3). doi:10.1128/microbiolspec.FUNK-0035-2016
16. Latge JP. The cell wall: a carbohydrate armour for the fungal cell. *Mol Microbiol* (2007) 66(2):279–90. doi:10.1111/j.1365-2958.2007.05872.x
17. Levitz SM. Innate recognition of fungal cell walls. *PLoS Pathog* (2010) 6(4):e1000758. doi:10.1371/journal.ppat.1000758
18. Bowman SM, Free SJ. The structure and synthesis of the fungal cell wall. *Bioessays* (2006) 28(8):799–808. doi:10.1002/bies.20441
19. Ishikawa T, Itoh F, Yoshida S, Saijo S, Matsuzawa T, Gonoi T, et al. Identification of distinct ligands for the C-type lectin receptors Mincle and dectin-2 in the pathogenic fungus *Malassezia*. *Cell Host Microbe* (2013) 13(4):477–88. doi:10.1016/j.chom.2013.03.008
20. Gomez BL, Nosanchuk JD. Melanin and fungi. *Curr Opin Infect Dis* (2003) 16(2):91–6. doi:10.1097/01.aco.0000065076.06965.04
21. Nosanchuk JD, Stark RE, Casadevall A. Fungal melanin: what do we know about structure? *Front Microbiol* (2015) 6:1463. doi:10.3389/fmicb.2015.01463
22. Kawai T, Akira S. The roles of TLRs, RLRs and NLRs in pathogen recognition. *Int Immunol* (2009) 21(4):317–37. doi:10.1093/intimm/dxp017
23. Gringhuis SI, den Dunnen J, Litjens M, van Het Hof B, van Kooyk Y, Geijtenbeek TB. C-type lectin DC-SIGN modulates toll-like receptor signaling *via* Raf-1 kinase-dependent acetylation of transcription factor NF-kappaB. *Immunity* (2007) 26(5):605–16. doi:10.1016/j.immuni.2007.03.012
24. Gringhuis SI, den Dunnen J, Litjens M, van der Vlist M, Wevers B, Bruijns SC, et al. Dectin-1 directs T helper cell differentiation by controlling noncanonical NF-kappaB activation through Raf-1 and Syk. *Nat Immunol* (2009) 10(2):203–13. doi:10.1038/ni.1692
25. Rogers NC, Slack EC, Edwards AD, Nolte MA, Schulz O, Schweighoffer E, et al. e Sousa: Syk-dependent cytokine induction by dectin-1 reveals a novel pattern recognition pathway for C type lectins. *Immunity* (2005) 22(4):507–17. doi:10.1016/j.immuni.2005.03.004
26. Zelensky AN, Gready JE. The C-type lectin-like domain superfamily. *FEBS J* (2005) 272(24):6179–217. doi:10.1111/j.1742-4658.2005.05031.x
27. Sancho D, Reis C. e Sousa: signaling by myeloid C-type lectin receptors in immunity and homeostasis. *Annu Rev Immunol* (2012) 30:491–529. doi:10.1146/annurev-immunol-031210-101352
28. Brown GD, Gordon S. Immune recognition. A new receptor for beta-glucans. *Nature* (2001) 413(6851):36–7. doi:10.1038/35092620
29. Ross GD, Cain JA, Myones BL, Newman SL, Lachmann PJ. Specificity of membrane complement receptor type three (CR3) for beta-glucans. *Complement* (1987) 4(2):61–74. doi:10.1159/000463010
30. Xia Y, Vetvicka V, Yan J, Hanikyrova M, Mayadas T, Ross GD. The beta-glucan-binding lectin site of mouse CR3 (CD11b/CD18) and its function in generating a primed state of the receptor that mediates cytotoxic activation in response to iC3b-opsonized target cells. *J Immunol* (1999) 162(4): 2281–90.
31. Vera J, Fenutria R, Canadas O, Figueras M, Mota R, Sarrias MR, et al. The CD5 ectodomain interacts with conserved fungal cell wall components and protects from zymosan-induced septic shock-like syndrome. *Proc Natl Acad Sci U S A* (2009) 106(5):1506–11. doi:10.1073/pnas.0805846106
32. Brown GD, Taylor PR, Reid DM, Willment JA, Williams DL, Martinez-Pomares L, et al. Dectin-1 is a major beta-glucan receptor on macrophages. *J Exp Med* (2002) 196(3):407–12. doi:10.1084/Jem.20020470
33. Means TK, Mylonakis E, Tampakakis E, Colvin RA, Seung E, Puckett L, et al. Evolutionarily conserved recognition and innate immunity to fungal pathogens by the scavenger receptors SCARF1 and CD36. *J Exp Med* (2009) 206(3):637–53. doi:10.1084/jem.20082109
34. van de Veerdonk FL, Marijnissen RJ, Kullberg BJ, Koenen HJ, Cheng SC, Joosten I, et al. The macrophage mannose receptor induces IL-17 in response to *Candida albicans*. *Cell Host Microbe* (2009) 5(4):329–40. doi:10.1016/j.chom.2009.02.006
35. Cambi A, Gijzen K, de Vries J, Torensma R, Joosten B, Adema GJ, et al. The C-type lectin DC-SIGN (CD209) is an antigen-uptake receptor for *Candida albicans* on dendritic cells. *Eur J Immunol* (2003) 33(2):532–8. doi:10.1002/immu.200310029
36. Yamasaki S, Matsumoto M, Takeuchi O, Matsuzawa T, Ishikawa E, Sakuma M, et al. C-type lectin Mincle is an activating receptor for pathogenic fungus, *Malassezia*. *Proc Natl Acad Sci U S A* (2009) 106(6):1897–902. doi:10.1073/pnas.0805177106
37. Cambi A, Netea MG, Mora-Montes HM, Gow NA, Hato SV, Lowman DW, et al. Dendritic cell interaction with *Candida albicans* critically depends on N-linked mannan. *J Biol Chem* (2008) 283(29):20590–9. doi:10.1074/jbc.M709334200
38. Saijo S, Fujikado N, Furuta T, Chung SH, Kotaki H, Seki K, et al. Dectin-1 is required for host defense against *Pneumocystis carinii* but not against *Candida albicans*. *Nat Immunol* (2007) 8(1):39–46. doi:10.1038/ni1425
39. Wagener J, Malireddi RK, Lenardon MD, Koberle M, Vautier S, MacCallum DM, et al. Fungal chitin dampens inflammation through IL-10 induction mediated by NOD2 and TLR9 activation. *PLoS Pathog* (2014) 10(4):e1004050. doi:10.1371/journal.ppat.1004050
40. Brown GD. Dectin-1: a signalling non-TLR pattern-recognition receptor. *Nat Rev Immunol* (2006) 6(1):33–43. doi:10.1038/Nri1745
41. Graham LM, Brown GD. The dectin-2 family of C-type lectins in immunity and homeostasis. *Cytokine* (2009) 48(1–2):148–55. doi:10.1016/j.cyto.2009.07.010
42. Guo Y, Feinberg H, Conroy E, Mitchell DA, Alvarez R, Blixt O, et al. Structural basis for distinct ligand-binding and targeting properties of the receptors DC-SIGN and DC-SIGNR. *Nat Struct Mol Biol* (2004) 11(7):591–8. doi:10.1038/nsmb784
43. Kruskal BA, Sastry K, Warner AB, Mathieu CE, Ezekowitz RA. Phagocytic chimeric receptors require both transmembrane and cytoplasmic domains from the mannose receptor. *J Exp Med* (1992) 176(6):1673–80. doi:10.1084/jem.176.6.1673
44. Boskovic J, Arnold JN, Stilion R, Gordon S, Sim RB, Rivera-Calzada A, et al. Structural model for the mannose receptor family uncovered by electron microscopy of Endo180 and the mannose receptor. *J Biol Chem* (2006) 281(13):8780–7. doi:10.1074/jbc.M513277200
45. Svajger U, Anderluh M, Jeras M, Obermajer N. C-type lectin DC-SIGN: an adhesion, signalling and antigen-uptake molecule that guides dendritic cells in immunity. *Cell Signal* (2010) 22(10):1397–405. doi:10.1016/j.cellsig.2010.03.018
46. Kerrigan AM, Brown GD. Syk-coupled C-type lectins in immunity. *Trends Immunol* (2011) 32(4):151–6. doi:10.1016/j.it.2011.01.002
47. Goodridge HS, Reyes CN, Becker CA, Katsumoto TR, Ma J, Wolf AJ, et al. Activation of the innate immune receptor dectin-1 upon formation of a 'phagocytic synapse'. *Nature* (2011) 472(7344):471–5. doi:10.1038/nature10071
48. Leibundgut-Landmann S, Osorio F, Brown GD, Reis C. e Sousa: stimulation of dendritic cells *via* the dectin-1/Syk pathway allows priming of cytotoxic T-cell responses. *Blood* (2008) 112(13):4971–80. doi:10.1182/blood-2008-05-158469

49. del Fresno C, Soulat D, Roth S, Blazek K, Udalova I, Sancho D, et al. Interferon-beta production *via* dectin-1-Syk-IRF5 signaling in dendritic cells is crucial for immunity to *C. albicans*. *Immunity* (2013) 38(6):1176–86. doi:10.1016/j.immuni.2013.05.010
50. Strasser D, Neumann K, Bergmann H, Marakalala MJ, Guler R, Rojowska A, et al. Syk kinase-coupled C-type lectin receptors engage protein kinase C-sigma to elicit Card9 adaptor-mediated innate immunity. *Immunity* (2012) 36(1):32–42. doi:10.1016/j.immuni.2011.11.015
51. Gross O, Gewies A, Finger K, Schafer M, Sparwasser T, Peschel C, et al. Card9 controls a non-TLR signalling pathway for innate anti-fungal immunity. *Nature* (2006) 442(7103):651–6. doi:10.1038/nature04926
52. Gringhuis SI, Wevers BA, Kaptein TM, van Capel TM, Theelen B, Boekhout T, et al. Selective C-Rel activation *via* Malt1 controls anti-fungal T(H)-17 immunity by dectin-1 and dectin-2. *PLoS Pathog* (2011) 7(1):e1001259. doi:10.1371/journal.ppat.1001259
53. Jia XM, Tang B, Zhu LL, Liu YH, Zhao XQ, Gorjestani S, et al. CARD9 mediates dectin-1-induced ERK activation by linking Ras-GRF1 to H-Ras for antifungal immunity. *J Exp Med* (2014) 211(11):2307–21. doi:10.1084/jem.20132349
54. LeibundGut-Landmann S, Gross O, Robinson MJ, Osorio F, Slack EC, Tsoni SV, et al. e Sousa: Syk- and CARD9-dependent coupling of innate immunity to the induction of T helper cells that produce interleukin 17. *Nat Immunol* (2007) 8(6):630–8. doi:10.1038/ni1460
55. Robinson MJ, Osorio F, Rosas M, Freitas RP, Schweighoffer E, Gross O, et al. e Sousa: dectin-2 is a Syk-coupled pattern recognition receptor crucial for Th17 responses to fungal infection. *J Exp Med* (2009) 206(9):2037–51. doi:10.1084/jem.20082818
56. Zielinski CE, Mele F, Aschenbrenner D, Jarrossay D, Ronchi F, Gattorno M, et al. Pathogen-induced human TH17 cells produce IFN-gamma or IL-10 and are regulated by IL-1beta. *Nature* (2012) 484(7395):514–8. doi:10.1038/nature10957
57. Goodridge HS, Underhill DM, Touret N. Mechanisms of Fc receptor and dectin-1 activation for phagocytosis. *Traffic* (2012) 13(8):1062–71. doi:10.1111/j.1600-0854.2012.01382.x
58. Underhill DM, Rossnagle E, Lowell CA, Simmons RM. Dectin-1 activates Syk tyrosine kinase in a dynamic subset of macrophages for reactive oxygen production. *Blood* (2005) 106(7):2543–50. doi:10.1182/blood-2005-03-1239
59. Dennehy KM, Willment JA, Williams DL, Brown GD. Reciprocal regulation of IL-23 and IL-12 following co-activation of dectin-1 and TLR signaling pathways. *Eur J Immunol* (2009) 39(5):1379–86. doi:10.1002/Eji.200838543
60. Bourgeois C, Majer O, Frohner IE, Lesiak-Markowicz I, Hildering KS, Glaser W, et al. Conventional dendritic cells mount a type I IFN response against *Candida* spp. requiring novel phagosomal TLR7-mediated IFN-beta signaling. *J Immunol* (2011) 186(5):3104–12. doi:10.4049/jimmunol.1002599
61. Smeekens SP, Ng A, Kumar V, Johnson MD, Plantinga TS, van Diemen C, et al. Functional genomics identifies type I interferon pathway as central for host defense against *Candida albicans*. *Nat Commun* (2013) 4:1342. doi:10.1038/ncomms2343
62. Goodridge HS, Simmons RM, Underhill DM. Dectin-1 stimulation by *Candida albicans* yeast or zymosan triggers NFAT activation in macrophages and dendritic cells. *J Immunol* (2007) 178(5):3107–15. doi:10.4049/jimmunol.178.5.3107
63. Fric J, Zelante T, Wong AY, Mertes A, Yu HB, Ricciardi-Castagnoli P. NFAT control of innate immunity. *Blood* (2012) 120(7):1380–9. doi:10.1182/blood-2012-02-404475
64. Macian F. NFAT proteins: key regulators of T-cell development and function. *Nat Rev Immunol* (2005) 5(6):472–84. doi:10.1038/nri1632
65. Lanternier F, Pathan S, Vincent QB, Liu L, Cypowyj S, Prando C, et al. Deep dermatophytosis and inherited CARD9 deficiency. *N Engl J Med* (2013) 369(18):1704–14. doi:10.1056/NEJMoa1208487
66. Drummond RA, Lionakis MS. Mechanistic insights into the role of C-type lectin receptor/CARD9 signaling in human antifungal immunity. *Front Cell Infect Microbiol* (2016) 6:39. doi:10.3389/fcimb.2016.00039
67. Glocker EO, Hennigs A, Nabavi M, Schaffer AA, Woellner C, Salzer U, et al. A homozygous CARD9 mutation in a family with susceptibility to fungal infections. *N Engl J Med* (2009) 361(18):1727–35. doi:10.1056/NEJMoa0810719
68. Drummond RA, Collar AL, Swamydas M, Rodriguez CA, Lim JK, Mendez LM, et al. CARD9-dependent neutrophil recruitment protects against fungal invasion of the central nervous system. *PLoS Pathog* (2015) 11(12):e1005293. doi:10.1371/journal.ppat.1005293
69. Jhingran A, Kasahara S, Shepardson KM, Junecko BA, Heung LJ, Kumasaka DK, et al. Compartment-specific and sequential role of MyD88 and CARD9 in chemokine induction and innate defense during respiratory fungal infection. *PLoS Pathog* (2015) 11(1):e1004589. doi:10.1371/journal.ppat.1004589
70. Rieber N, Gazendam RP, Freeman AF, Hsu AP, Collar AL, Sugui JA, et al. Extrapulmonary *Aspergillus* infection in patients with CARD9 deficiency. *JCI Insight* (2016) 1(17):e89890. doi:10.1172/jci.insight.89890
71. Roth S, Bergmann H, Jaeger M, Yeroslaviz A, Neumann K, Koenig PA, et al. Vav proteins are key regulators of Card9 signaling for innate antifungal immunity. *Cell Rep* (2016) 17(10):2572–83. doi:10.1016/j.celrep.2016.11.018
72. Fischer M, Spies-Weisshart B, Schrenk K, Gruhn B, Wittig S, Glaser A, et al. Polymorphisms of dectin-1 and TLR2 predispose to invasive fungal disease in patients with acute myeloid leukemia. *PLoS One* (2016) 11(3):e0150632. doi:10.1371/journal.pone.0150632
73. Rieber N, Singh A, Oz H, Carevic M, Bouzani M, Amich J, et al. Pathogenic fungi regulate immunity by inducing neutrophilic myeloid-derived suppressor cells. *Cell Host Microbe* (2015) 17(4):507–14. doi:10.1016/j.chom.2015.02.007
74. Yamasaki S, Ishikawa E, Sakuma M, Hara H, Ogata K, Saito T. Mincle is an ITAM-coupled activating receptor that senses damaged cells. *Nat Immunol* (2008) 9(10):1179–88. doi:10.1038/ni.1651
75. Sato K, Yang XL, Yudate T, Chung JS, Wu J, Luby-Phelps K, et al. Dectin-2 is a pattern recognition receptor for fungi that couples with the Fc receptor gamma chain to induce innate immune responses. *J Biol Chem* (2006) 281(50):38854–66. doi:10.1074/jbc.M606542200
76. Miyake Y, Toyonaga K, Mori D, Kakuta S, Hoshino Y, Oyamada A, et al. C-type lectin MCL is an FcRgamma-coupled receptor that mediates the adjuvanticity of mycobacterial cord factor. *Immunity* (2013) 38(5):1050–62. doi:10.1016/j.immuni.2013.03.010
77. Kerscher B, Willment JA, Brown GD. The dectin-2 family of C-type lectin-like receptors: an update. *Int Immunol* (2013) 25(5):271–7. doi:10.1093/intimm/dxt006
78. McGreal EP, Rosas M, Brown GD, Zamze S, Wong SY, Gordon S, et al. The carbohydrate-recognition domain of dectin-2 is a C-type lectin with specificity for high mannose. *Glycobiology* (2006) 16(5):422–30. doi:10.1093/glycob/cwj077
79. Barrett NA, Maekawa A, Rahman OM, Austen KF, Kanaoka Y. Dectin-2 recognition of house dust mite triggers cysteinyl leukotriene generation by dendritic cells. *J Immunol* (2009) 182(2):1119–28. doi:10.4049/jimmunol.182.2.1119
80. Ritter M, Gross O, Kays S, Ruland J, Nimmerjahn F, Saijo S, et al. da Costa: schistosoma mansoni triggers dectin-2, which activates the Nlrp3 inflammasome and alters adaptive immune responses. *Proc Natl Acad Sci U S A* (2010) 107(47):20459–64. doi:10.1073/pnas.1010337107
81. Campuzano A, Castro-Lopez N, Wozniak KL, Leopold Wager CM, Wormley FL Jr. Dectin-3 is not required for protection against *Cryptococcus neoformans* infection. *PLoS One* (2017) 12(1):e0169347. doi:10.1371/journal.pone.0169347
82. Zhao XQ, Zhu LL, Chang Q, Jiang C, You Y, Luo T, et al. C-type Lectin receptor dectin-3 mediates trehalose 6,6'-dimycolate (TDM)-induced Mincle expression through CARD9/Bcl10/MALT1-dependent nuclear factor (NF)-kappaB activation. *J Biol Chem* (2014) 289(43):30052–62. doi:10.1074/jbc.M114.588574
83. Miyake Y, Masatsugu OH, Yamasaki S. C-type lectin receptor MCL facilitates Mincle expression and signaling through complex formation. *J Immunol* (2015) 194(11):5366–74. doi:10.4049/jimmunol.1402429
84. Hernandez-Santos N, Gaffen SL. Th17 cells in immunity to *Candida albicans*. *Cell Host Microbe* (2012) 11(5):425–35. doi:10.1016/j.chom.2012.04.008
85. Wang H, Li M, Lerksuthirat T, Klein B, Wuthrich M. The C-type lectin receptor MCL mediates vaccine-induced immunity against infection with *Blastomyces dermatitidis*. *Infect Immun* (2015) 84(3):635–42. doi:10.1128/IAI.01263-15
86. Lee MJ, Yoshimoto E, Saijo S, Iwakura Y, Lin X, Katz HR, et al. Phosphoinositide 3-kinase delta regulates dectin-2 signaling and the generation of Th2 and Th17 immunity. *J Immunol* (2016) 197(1):278–87. doi:10.4049/jimmunol.1502485

87. Taylor PR, Roy S, Leal SM Jr, Sun Y, Howell SJ, Cobb BA, et al. Activation of neutrophils by autocrine IL-17A-IL-17RC interactions during fungal infection is regulated by IL-6, IL-23, RORgammat and dectin-2. *Nat Immunol* (2014) 15(2):143–51. doi:10.1038/ni.2797
88. Ishikawa E, Ishikawa T, Morita YS, Toyonaga K, Yamada H, Takeuchi O, et al. Direct recognition of the mycobacterial glycolipid, trehalose dimycolate, by C-type lectin Mincle. *J Exp Med* (2009) 206(13):2879–88. doi:10.1084/jem.20091750
89. Wells CA, Salvage-Jones JA, Li X, Hitchens K, Butcher S, Murray RZ, et al. The macrophage-inducible C-type lectin, Mincle, is an essential component of the innate immune response to *Candida albicans*. *J Immunol* (2008) 180(11):7404–13. doi:10.4049/jimmunol.180.11.7404
90. Sousa Mda G, Reid DM, Schweighoffer E, Tybulewicz V, Ruland J, Langhorne J, et al. Restoration of pattern recognition receptor costimulation to treat chromoblastomycosis, a chronic fungal infection of the skin. *Cell Host Microbe* (2011) 9(5):436–43. doi:10.1016/j.chom.2011.04.005
91. Bugarcic A, Hitchens K, Beckhouse AG, Wells CA, Ashman RB, Blanchard H. Human and mouse macrophage-inducible C-type lectin (Mincle) bind *Candida albicans*. *Glycobiology* (2008) 18(9):679–85. doi:10.1093/glycob/cwn046
92. Kerscher B, Wilson GJ, Reid DM, Mori D, Taylor JA, Besra GS, et al. Mycobacterial receptor, Clec4d (CLECSF8, MCL), is coregulated with Mincle and upregulated on mouse myeloid cells following microbial challenge. *Eur J Immunol* (2016) 46(2):381–9. doi:10.1002/eji.201545858
93. Wevers BA, Kaptein TM, Zijlstra-Willems EM, Theelen B, Boekhout T, Geijtenbeek TB, et al. Fungal engagement of the C-type lectin Mincle suppresses dectin-1-induced antifungal immunity. *Cell Host Microbe* (2014) 15(4):494–505. doi:10.1016/j.chom.2014.03.008
94. Porcaro I, Vidal M, Jouvert S, Stahl PD, Giaimis J. Mannose receptor contribution to *Candida albicans* phagocytosis by murine E-clone J774 macrophages. *J Leukoc Biol* (2003) 74(2):206–15. doi:10.1189/jlb.1202608
95. Rajaram MVS, Arnett E, Azad AK, Guirado E, Ni B, Gerberick AD, et al. *M. tuberculosis*-initiated human mannose receptor signaling regulates macrophage recognition and vesicle trafficking by FcRgamma-chain, Grb2, and SHP-1. *Cell Rep* (2017) 21(1):126–40. doi:10.1016/j.celrep.2017.09.034
96. Lee SJ, Zheng NY, Clavijo M, Nussenzweig MC. Normal host defense during systemic candidiasis in mannose receptor-deficient mice. *Infect Immun* (2003) 71(1):437–45. doi:10.1128/IAI.71.1.437-445.2003
97. Viriyakosol S, Jimenez Mdel P, Saijo S, Fierer J. Neither dectin-2 nor the mannose receptor is required for resistance to *Coccidioides immitis* in mice. *Infect Immun* (2014) 82(3):1147–56. doi:10.1128/IAI.01355-13
98. van Kooyk Y, Geijtenbeek TB. DC-SIGN: escape mechanism for pathogens. *Nat Rev Immunol* (2003) 3(9):697–709. doi:10.1038/nri1182
99. Tassaneetrithep B, Burgess TH, Granelli-Piperno A, Trumpfheller C, Finke J, Sun W, et al. DC-SIGN (CD209) mediates dengue virus infection of human dendritic cells. *J Exp Med* (2003) 197(7):823–9. doi:10.1084/jem.20021840
100. Engering A, Geijtenbeek TB, van Vliet SJ, Wijers M, van Liempt E, Demaurex N, et al. The dendritic cell-specific adhesion receptor DC-SIGN internalizes antigen for presentation to T cells. *J Immunol* (2002) 168(5):2118–26. doi:10.4049/jimmunol.168.5.2118
101. Hodges A, Sharrocks K, Edelmann M, Baban D, Moris A, Schwartz O, et al. Activation of the lectin DC-SIGN induces an immature dendritic cell phenotype triggering Rho-GTPase activity required for HIV-1 replication. *Nat Immunol* (2007) 8(6):569–77. doi:10.1038/ni1470
102. Gringhuis SI, den Dunnen J, Litjens M, van der Vlist M, Geijtenbeek TB. Carbohydrate-specific signaling through the DC-SIGN signalosome tailors immunity to *Mycobacterium tuberculosis*, HIV-1 and *Helicobacter pylori*. *Nat Immunol* (2009) 10(10):1081–8. doi:10.1038/ni.1778
103. Serrano-Gomez D, Leal JA, Corbi AL. DC-SIGN mediates the binding of *Aspergillus fumigatus* and keratinophylic fungi by human dendritic cells. *Immunobiology* (2005) 210(2–4):175–83. doi:10.1016/j.imbio.2005.05.011
104. Sainz J, Lupianez CB, Segura-Catena J, Vazquez L, Rios R, Oyonarte S, et al. Dectin-1 and DC-SIGN polymorphisms associated with invasive pulmonary Aspergillosis infection. *PLoS One* (2012) 7(2):e32273. doi:10.1371/journal.pone.0032273
105. Zenaro E, Donini M, Dusi S. Induction of Th1/Th17 immune response by *Mycobacterium tuberculosis*: role of dectin-1, Mannose receptor, and DC-SIGN. *J Leukoc Biol* (2009) 86(6):1393–401. doi:10.1189/jlb.0409242
106. El-Awady AR, Miles B, Scisci E, Kurago ZB, Palani CD, Arce RM, et al. Porphyromonas gingivalis evasion of autophagy and intracellular killing by human myeloid dendritic cells involves DC-SIGN-TLR2 crosstalk. *PLoS Pathog* (2015) 10(2):e1004647. doi:10.1371/journal.ppat.1004647
107. Zhao X, Guo Y, Jiang C, Chang Q, Zhang S, Luo T, et al. JNK1 negatively controls antifungal innate immunity by suppressing CD23 expression. *Nat Med* (2017) 23(3):337–46. doi:10.1038/nm.4260
108. Brown GD. Innate antifungal immunity: the key role of phagocytes. *Annu Rev Immunol* (2011) 29:1–21. doi:10.1146/annurev-immunol-030409-101229
109. Ganesan S, Rathinam VAK, Bossaller L, Army K, Kaiser WJ, Mocarski ES, et al. Caspase-8 modulates dectin-1 and complement receptor 3-driven IL-1beta production in response to beta-glucans and the fungal pathogen, *Candida albicans*. *J Immunol* (2014) 193(5):2519–30. doi:10.4049/jimmunol.1400276
110. Huang JH, Lin CY, Wu SY, Chen WY, Chu CL, Brown GD, et al. CR3 and dectin-1 collaborate in macrophage cytokine response through association on lipid rafts and activation of Syk-JNK-AP-1 pathway. *PLoS Pathog* (2015) 11(7):e1004985. doi:10.1371/journal.ppat.1004985
111. Brown GD, Herre J, Williams DL, Willment JA, Marshall ASJ, Gordon S. Dectin-1 mediates the biological effects of beta-glucans. *J Exp Med* (2003) 197(9):1119–24. doi:10.1084/Jem.20021890
112. de Sousa Mda G, Belda W Jr, Spina R, Lota PR, Valente NS, Brown GD, et al. Topical application of imiquimod as a treatment for chromoblastomycosis. *Clin Infect Dis* (2014) 58(12):1734–7. doi:10.1093/cid/ciu168
113. Tavares AH, Burgel PH, Bocca AL. Turning up the heat: inflammasome activation by fungal pathogens. *PLoS Pathog* (2015) 11(7):e1004948. doi:10.1371/journal.ppat.1004948
114. Hise AG, Tomalka J, Ganesan S, Patel K, Hall BA, Brown GD, et al. An essential role for the NLRP3 inflammasome in host defense against the human fungal pathogen *Candida albicans*. *Cell Host Microbe* (2009) 5(5):487–97. doi:10.1016/j.chom.2009.05.002
115. Gringhuis SI, Kaptein TM, Wevers BA, Theelen B, van der Vlist M, Boekhout T, et al. Dectin-1 is an extracellular pathogen sensor for the induction and processing of IL-1beta *via* a noncanonical caspase-8 inflammasome. *Nat Immunol* (2012) 13(3):246–54. doi:10.1038/ni.2222
116. Zwolanek F, Riedelberger M, Stolz V, Jenull S, Istel F, Koprulu AD, et al. The non-receptor tyrosine kinase Tec controls assembly and activity of the non-canonical caspase-8 inflammasome. *PLoS Pathog* (2014) 10(12):e1004525. doi:10.1371/journal.ppat.1004525
117. Chang TH, Huang JH, Lin HC, Chen WY, Lee YH, Hsu LC, et al. Dectin-2 is a primary receptor for NLRP3 inflammasome activation in dendritic cell response to *Histoplasma capsulatum*. *PLoS Pathog* (2017) 13(7):e1006485. doi:10.1371/journal.ppat.1006485
118. Tavares AH, Magalhaes KG, Almeida RD, Correa R, Burgel PH, Bocca AL. NLRP3 inflammasome activation by *Paracoccidioides brasiliensis*. *PLoS Negl Trop Dis* (2013) 7(12):e2595. doi:10.1371/journal.pntd.0002595
119. Guo C, Chen M, Fa Z, Lu A, Fang W, Sun B, et al. Acapsular *Cryptococcus neoformans* activates the NLRP3 inflammasome. *Microbes Infect* (2014) 16(10):845–54. doi:10.1016/j.micinf.2014.08.013
120. Said-Sadier N, Padilla E, Langsley G, Ojcius DM. *Aspergillus fumigatus* stimulates the NLRP3 inflammasome through a pathway requiring ROS production and the Syk tyrosine kinase. *PLoS One* (2010) 5(4):e10008. doi:10.1371/journal.pone.0010008
121. Mao L, Zhang L, Li H, Chen W, Wang H, Wu S, et al. Pathogenic fungus *Microsporum canis* activates the NLRP3 inflammasome. *Infect Immun* (2014) 82(2):882–92. doi:10.1128/IAI.01097-13
122. Kistowska M, Fenini G, Jankovic D, Feldmeyer L, Kerl K, Bosshard P, et al. *Malassezia* yeasts activate the NLRP3 inflammasome in antigen-presenting cells *via* Syk-kinase signalling. *Exp Dermatol* (2014) 23(12):884–9. doi:10.1111/exd.12552
123. Joly S, Ma N, Sadler JJ, Soll DR, Cassel SL, Sutterwala FS. Cutting edge: *Candida albicans* hyphae formation triggers activation of the Nlrp3 inflammasome. *J Immunol* (2009) 183(6):3578–81. doi:10.4049/jimmunol.0901323
124. Gow NA, van de Veerdonk FL, Brown AJ, Netea MG. *Candida albicans* morphogenesis and host defence: discriminating invasion from colonization. *Nat Rev Microbiol* (2011) 10(2):112–22. doi:10.1038/nrmicro2711
125. Krysan DJ, Sutterwala FS, Wellington M. Catching fire: *Candida albicans*, macrophages, and pyroptosis. *PLoS Pathog* (2014) 10(6):e1004139. doi:10.1371/journal.ppat.1004139

126. Pietrella D, Pandey N, Gabrielli E, Pericolini E, Perito S, Kasper L, et al. Secreted aspartic proteases of *Candida albicans* activate the NLRP3 inflammasome. *Eur J Immunol* (2013) 43(3):679–92. doi:10.1002/eji.201242691
127. Karki R, Man SM, Malireddi RK, Gurung P, Vogel P, Lamkanfi M, et al. Concerted activation of the AIM2 and NLRP3 inflammasomes orchestrates host protection against *Aspergillus* infection. *Cell Host Microbe* (2015) 17(3):357–68. doi:10.1016/j.chom.2015.01.006
128. Tomalka J, Ganesan S, Azodi E, Patel K, Majmudar P, Hall BA, et al. A novel role for the NLRC4 inflammasome in mucosal defenses against the fungal pathogen *Candida albicans*. *PLoS Pathog* (2011) 7(12):e1002379. doi:10.1371/journal.ppat.1002379
129. Rappleye CA, Eissenberg LG, Goldman WE. *Histoplasma capsulatum* alpha-(1,3)-glucan blocks innate immune recognition by the beta-glucan receptor. *Proc Natl Acad Sci U S A* (2007) 104(4):1366–70. doi:10.1073/pnas.0609848104
130. Cao Z, Conway KL, Heath RJ, Rush JS, Leshchiner ES, Ramirez-Ortiz ZG, et al. Ubiquitin ligase TRIM62 regulates CARD9-mediated anti-fungal immunity and intestinal inflammation. *Immunity* (2015) 43(4):715–26. doi:10.1016/j.immuni.2015.10.005
131. Xiao Y, Tang J, Guo H, Zhao Y, Tang R, Ouyang S, et al. Targeting CBLB as a potential therapeutic approach for disseminated candidiasis. *Nat Med* (2016) 22(8):906–14. doi:10.1038/nm.4141
132. Wirnsberger G, Zwolanek F, Asaoka T, Kozieradzki I, Tortola L, Wimmer RA, et al. Inhibition of CBLB protects from lethal *Candida albicans* sepsis. *Nat Med* (2016) 22(8):915–23. doi:10.1038/nm.4134
133. Zhu LL, Luo TM, Xu X, Guo YH, Zhao XQ, Wang TT, et al. E3 ubiquitin ligase Cbl-b negatively regulates C-type lectin receptor-mediated antifungal innate immunity. *J Exp Med* (2016) 213(8):1555–70. doi:10.1084/jem.20151932
134. Leach MD, Brown AJ. Posttranslational modifications of proteins in the pathobiology of medically relevant fungi. *Eukaryot Cell* (2012) 11(2):98–108. doi:10.1128/EC.05238-11
135. Kingeter LM, Lin X. C-type lectin receptor-induced NF-kappaB activation in innate immune and inflammatory responses. *Cell Mol Immunol* (2012) 9(2):105–12. doi:10.1038/cmi.2011.58
136. Gorjestani S, Yu M, Tang B, Zhang D, Wang D, Lin X. Phospholipase Cgamma2 (PLCgamma2) is key component in dectin-2 signaling pathway, mediating anti-fungal innate immune responses. *J Biol Chem* (2011) 286(51):43651–9. doi:10.1074/jbc.M111.307389
137. Oykhman P, Timm-McCann M, Xiang RF, Islam A, Li SS, Stack D, et al. Requirement and redundancy of the Src family kinases Fyn and Lyn in perforin-dependent killing of *Cryptococcus neoformans* by NK cells. *Infect Immun* (2013) 81(10):3912–22. doi:10.1128/IAI.00533-13
138. Dennehy KM, Ferwerda G, Faro-Trindade I, Pyz E, Willment JA, Taylor PR, et al. Syk kinase is required for collaborative cytokine production induced through dectin-1 and toll-like receptors. *Eur J Immunol* (2008) 38(2):500–6. doi:10.1002/Eji.200737741
139. Deng Z, Ma S, Zhou H, Zang A, Fang Y, Li T, et al. Tyrosine phosphatase SHP-2 mediates C-type lectin receptor-induced activation of the kinase Syk and anti-fungal TH17 responses. *Nat Immunol* (2015) 16(6):642–52. doi:10.1038/ni.3155
140. Blanco-Menendez N, Del Fresno C, Fernandes S, Calvo E, Conde-Garrosa R, Kerr WG, et al. SHIP-1 couples to the dectin-1 hemITAM and selectively modulates reactive oxygen species production in dendritic cells in response to *Candida albicans*. *J Immunol* (2015) 195(9):4466–78. doi:10.4049/jimmunol.1402874
141. Serezani CH, Kane S, Medeiros AI, Cornett AM, Kim SH, Marques MM, et al. PTEN directly activates the actin depolymerization factor cofilin-1 during PGE2-mediated inhibition of phagocytosis of fungi. *Sci Signal* (2012) 5(210):ra12. doi:10.1126/scisignal.2002448
142. Liu Q, Zhou H, Langdon WY, Zhang J. E3 ubiquitin ligase Cbl-b in innate and adaptive immunity. *Cell Cycle* (2014) 13(12):1875–84. doi:10.4161/cc.29213
143. Liu YC. Ubiquitin ligases and the immune response. *Annu Rev Immunol* (2004) 22:81–127. doi:10.1146/annurev.immunol.22.012703.104813
144. Reyes-Turcu FE, Ventii KH, Wilkinson KD. Regulation and cellular roles of ubiquitin-specific deubiquitinating enzymes. *Annu Rev Biochem* (2009) 78:363–97. doi:10.1146/annurev.biochem.78.082307.091526
145. Zinngrebe J, Montinaro A, Peltzer N, Walczak H. Ubiquitin in the immune system. *EMBO Rep* (2014) 15(1):28–45. doi:10.1002/embr.201338025
146. Bhoj VG, Chen ZJ. Ubiquitylation in innate and adaptive immunity. *Nature* (2009) 458(7237):430–7. doi:10.1038/nature07959
147. Huang F, Xiao H, Sun BL, Yang RG. Characterization of TRIM62 as a RING finger E3 ubiquitin ligase and its subcellular localization. *Biochem Biophys Res Commun* (2013) 432(2):208–13. doi:10.1016/j.bbrc.2013.02.012
148. Zhang J. Ubiquitin ligases in T cell activation and autoimmunity. *Clin Immunol* (2004) 111(3):234–40. doi:10.1016/j.clim.2004.02.003
149. Shembade N, Ma A, Harhaj EW. Inhibition of NF-kappaB signaling by A20 through disruption of ubiquitin enzyme complexes. *Science* (2010) 327(5969):1135–9. doi:10.1126/science.1182364
150. Skaug B, Chen J, Du F, He J, Ma A, Chen ZJ. Direct, noncatalytic mechanism of IKK inhibition by A20. *Mol Cell* (2011) 44(4):559–71. doi:10.1016/j.molcel.2011.09.015
151. Kanayama M, Inoue M, Danzaki K, Hammer G, He YW, Shinohara ML. Autophagy enhances NFkappaB activity in specific tissue macrophages by sequestering A20 to boost antifungal immunity. *Nat Commun* (2015) 6:5779. doi:10.1038/ncomms6779

15

NOD-Like Receptor P3 Inflammasome Controls Protective Th1/Th17 Immunity against Pulmonary Paracoccidioidomycosis

*Claudia Feriotti[1], Eliseu Frank de Araújo[1], Flavio Vieira Loures[1], Tania Alves da Costa[1], Nayane Alves de Lima Galdino[1], Dario Simões Zamboni[2] and Vera Lucia Garcia Calich[1]**

[1]Department of Immunology, University of São Paulo, São Paulo, Brazil, [2]Department of Cell Biology, School of Medicine of Ribeirão Preto, University of São Paulo, São Paulo, Brazil

***Correspondence:**
Vera Lucia Garcia Calich
vlcalich@icb.usp.br

The NOD-like receptor P3 (NLRP3) inflammasome is an intracellular multimeric complex that triggers the activation of inflammatory caspases and the maturation of IL-1β and IL-18, important cytokines for the innate immune response against pathogens. The functional NLRP3 inflammasome complex consists of NLRP3, the adaptor protein apoptosis-associated speck-like protein, and caspase-1. Various molecular mechanisms were associated with NLRP3 activation including the presence of extracellular ATP, recognized by the cell surface P2X7 receptor (P2X7R). Several pattern recognition receptors on innate immune cells recognize *Paracoccidioides brasiliensis* components resulting in diverse responses that influence adaptive immunity and disease outcome. However, the role of NLRP3 inflammasome was scantily investigated in pulmonary paracoccidioidomycosis (PCM), leading us to use an intratracheal (i.t.) model of infection to study the influence of this receptor in anti-fungal immunity and severity of infection. For *in vivo* studies, *C57BL/6* mice deficient for several NLRP3 inflammasome components (*Nlrp3*$^{-/-}$, *Casp1/11*$^{-/-}$, *Asc*$^{-/-}$) as well as deficient for ATP receptor (*P2x7r*$^{-/-}$) were infected *via* i.t. with *P. brasiliensis* and several parameters of immunity and disease severity analyzed at the acute and chronic periods of infection. Pulmonary PCM was more severe in *Nlrp3*$^{-/-}$, *Casp1/11*$^{-/-}$, *Asc*$^{-/-}$, and *P2x7r*$^{-/-}$ mice as demonstrated by the increased fungal burdens, mortality rates and tissue pathology developed. The more severe disease developed by NLRP3, ASC, and Caspase-1/11 deficient mice was associated with decreased production of IL-1β and IL-18 and reduced inflammatory reactions mediated by PMN leukocytes and activated $CD4^+$ and $CD8^+$ T cells. The decreased T cell immunity was concomitant with increased expansion of $CD4^+CD25^+$Foxp3 regulatory T (Treg) cells. Characterization of intracellular cytokines showed a persistent reduction of $CD4^+$ and $CD8^+$ T cells expressing IFN-γ and IL-17 whereas those producing IL-4 and TGF-β appeared in increased frequencies. Histopathological studies showed that all deficient mouse strains developed more severe lesions containing elevated numbers of budding yeast cells resulting in increased mortality rates. Altogether, these findings led us to conclude that the activation of the NLRP3 inflammasome has a crucial role in the immunoprotection against pulmonary PCM by promoting the expansion of Th1/Th17 immunity and reducing the suppressive control mediated by Treg cells.

Keywords: pulmonary paracoccidioidomycosis, NOD-like receptor P3 inflammasome, Th1/Th17 immunity, regulatory T cells, immunoregulation

INTRODUCTION

Paracoccidioides brasiliensis is the etiological agent of paracoccidioidomycosis (PCM), the most prevalent systemic mycosis in Latin America (1). The pattern recognition receptors (PRRs) expressed on phagocytic cells recognize pathogen-associated molecular patterns (PAMPs) on *P. brasiliensis* surface and regulate the innate and adaptive phases of immunity. The different signaling pathways used by these PRRs to activate immune cells result in different patterns of cell activation, production of diverse pools of cytokines and chemokines triggering diverse immune mechanisms. In human PCM and experimental models, the prevalent expansion of Th1/Th17 cells with reduced expansion of Treg cells characterize the benign disease, whereas elevated proliferation of Th2/Th9 and Treg cells is associated with severe PCM (2–11).

The toll-like receptors (TLRs) play a crucial role in the recognition of fungal pathogens such as *P. brasiliensis*, *Candida albicans*, *Aspergillus fumigatus*, *Cryptococcus neoformans*, and others (8, 12–16). TLR2 and TLR4 sense *P. brasiliensis* mediated by MyD88-dependent signaling that leads to cytokines production by alveolar and peritoneal macrophages (6, 7, 17, 18). These components were also seen to control the adaptive immunity and severity of disease developed by *P. brasiliensis* infected mice (6, 7, 18). In addition, C-type lectin receptors (CLRs) like mannose receptor (MR) and dectin-1 as well as the complement receptors 3 play an important role in *P. brasiliensis* recognition and activation of immune cells (8, 19–22). Altogether, these studies have demonstrated that in pulmonary PCM, as in other infectious pathologies, PRRs are key elements that govern protective immunity, which must be tightly controlled by anti-inflammatory mechanisms as those mediated by Treg cells and their products (5–7).

The NOD-like receptor P3 (NLRP3) belongs to the NOD family of cytosolic PRRs that detect intracellular PAMPs well as danger signals, named danger associated molecular patterns (DAMPs). Under cell activation, components of NLR family can aggregate into large cytoplasmic complexes called inflammasomes (23). The members of this family have a LRR (leucine-rich repeat) domain in the C-terminal structure, a nucleotide-binding and oligomerization domain containing a neuronal apoptosis inhibitory protein, and a N-terminal caspase recruitment domain (CARD) or pyrin (PYD) domain. In the canonical pathway of NLRP3 inflammasome activation, NLRP3 oligomerization is initiated through the apoptosis-associated speck-like protein (ASC) containing C-terminal CARD that is recruited to the complex *via* NLRP3-PYD-ASC-PYD interaction. ASC associates with procaspase-1 *via* CARD interaction, leading to caspase-1 activation that promotes the processing of pro-IL-1β and pro-IL-18 into their mature forms (24–26). The NLRP3 inflammasome is activated by a large repertoire of PAMPs and DAMPs, including ATP, uric acid crystals, silica, aluminum hydroxide, asbestos, reactive oxygen species (ROS), and bacterial or viral RNA (27, 28). Besides the canonical pathway, a non-canonical pathway that utilizes caspase-11 has been shown to activate NLRP3 inflammasome (29, 30). The non-canonical NLRP3 inflammasome can be directly activated by LPS derived from Gram-negative bacteria and by some fungi, which are delivered into the cytosol and activate caspase-11. This, in turn, triggers the opening of the pannexin-1 channel that induces the K + efflux required for NLRP3 inflammasome activation and release of mature IL-1β (30, 31). The first signal for pro-IL-1β processing is through pro-IL-1β and NLRP3 expression mediated by NF-kB transcription that is potentially activated by TLRs and CLRs, and the second signal is the proteolytic processing of pro-caspase-1 by activated NLRP3 (25). NLRP3 is the NLR mostly involved in the immunity against fungal infections (32–34). In *C. albicans* infection, the canonical and non-canonical pathways of NLRP3 inflammasome activation were shown to be essential for mediating IL-1β secretion (29, 35). *In vivo* studies of disseminated *C. albicans* infection showed that NLRP3, Syk, ASC, and caspase-1 are fundamental to control disease severity and regulate the adaptive antifungal immune response through the induction of Th1 and Th17 development (36, 37). In an invasive pulmonary model of aspergillosis, NLRP3 and AIM2 were required to engage the inflammasome to trigger innate immune responses against *A. fumigatus*; mice lacking both AIM2 and NLRP3, but not mice lacking a single inflammasome receptor, were hyper susceptible to invasive aspergillosis (38). The pioneer study of Tavares et al. demonstrated that following *P. brasiliensis* infection, the production of mature IL-1β by bone marrow-derived dendritic cells depends on NLRP3 and caspase-1 activation (39), although the fungal molecules associated with this process are still unknown. However, K + efflux, ROS generation, lysosomal acidification, and cathepsin B release to the cytosol were seen to be required to the NLRP3 inflammasome activation by *P. brasiliensis* (39). Furthermore, a recent work of our lab showed that a dectin-1-Syk mediated mechanism controls NLRP3 inflammasome activation by *P. brasiliensis* infected macrophages of resistant A/J mice (21). In another study using a murine model of systemic PCM induced by intravenous infection, the susceptibility of NLRP3 and caspase-1 knockout mice to *P. brasiliensis* infection was evaluated and their increased susceptibility was associated with reduced IL-18 production and Th1 immunity (40).

Because the human disease is thought to be acquired by the pulmonary route, and diverse routes of infection induce different patterns of immunity and disease severity (41), in the present study, we sought to investigate the role of NLRP3 inflammasome in the pulmonary infection caused by *P. brasiliensis*. Therefore, several C57BL/6 mouse strains deficient for NLRP3 inflammasome components (*Nlrp3*$^{-/-}$, *Casp1/11*$^{-/-}$, *Asc*$^{-/-}$ mice) as well as deficient for the ATP receptor (*P2x7r*$^{-/-}$ mice) were intratracheally infected with 1×10^6 *P. brasiliensis* yeasts and compared with their wild type (WT) controls. Several parameters of pulmonary infection and immune response were evaluated at the acute and chronic phases of the disease. Our results indicated that NLRP3 inflammasome plays a crucial role in the control of the innate and adaptive immunity against *P. brasiliensis* infection. This control was associated with IL-1β and IL-18 secretion induced by caspase-1 activity starting at an early phase of infection. The activation of NLRP3 inflammasome was seen to be essential to control fungal growth and activate protective T cell immunity. This protective inflammatory response was composed of increased numbers of PMN leukocytes and activated $CD4^+$ and $CD8^+$ T lymphocytes that migrate to the site of infection. Furthermore, NLRP3 inhibited the expansion and migration of regulatory T (Treg) cells resulting in a well-balanced and protective Th1/Th17 immunity.

MATERIALS AND METHODS

Mice

Wild type (*WT*), *Nlrp3*$^{-/-}$, *Casp1/11*$^{-/-}$, *P2x7r*$^{-/-}$, and *Asc*$^{-/-}$ *C57BL/6* mouse strains were obtained from our Isogenic Unit (Immunology Department of Institute of Biomedical Sciences of University of São Paulo, Brazil). *Casp1/11*$^{-/-}$ mice (42) were provided by Dr. Flavell, R. (Howard Hughes Medical Institute, Yale University School of Medicine), *Asc*$^{-/-}$ mice (43) were provided by Dr. Zamboni, D. S. (University of São Paulo, Ribeirão Preto, São Paulo, Brazil), *Nlrp3*$^{-/-}$ mice (44) and *P2x7r*$^{-/-}$ (45) mice were obtained from Jackson Laboratories and used at 8–11 weeks of age. Specific pathogen free mice were fed with sterilized laboratory chow and water *ad libitum*. Animal experiments were performed in strict accordance with the Brazilian Federal Law 11,794 establishing procedures for the scientific use of animals, and the State Law establishing the Animal Protection Code of the State of São Paulo. All efforts were made to minimize suffering, and all animal procedures were approved by the Ethics Committee on Animal Experiments of the Institute of Biomedical Sciences of University of São Paulo (Proc.76/04/CEUA).

Fungus

Paracoccidioides brasiliensis (Pb 18 strain), isolated from a young patient in 1929, was maintained by weekly subcultivation in semisolid Fava Netto's medium at 35°C (46). Yeast cells were collected, washed, and adjusted to 20×10^6 cells/mL. Viability was determined with Janus Green B vital dye (Merck Frankfurter Straße, Darmstadt, GER) and was always higher than 85%. The presence of LPS in all used solutions was determined by the Limulus amebocyte lysate chromogenic assay (Sigma-Aldrich, St. Louis, MO, USA) and always showed LPS levels <0.015 EU/mL.

Intratracheal Fungal Infection

Mice were anesthetized and submitted to intratracheal (i.t.) *P. brasiliensis* infection as previously described (47). Briefly, after intraperitoneal injection of ketamine (90 mg/kg) and xylazine (10 mg/kg), animals were infected with 1×10^6 Pb18 yeast cells, contained in 50 μL of PBS, by surgical i.t. inoculation, which allowed dispensing of the fungal cells directly into the lungs. The skin was then sutured, and mice were placed under a heat lamp until they recovered from anesthesia.

Colony Forming Units (CFUs) Assays

To assess the viable number of CFU in target organs, lungs, and livers from *C57BL/6*, *Nlrp3*$^{-/-}$, *Casp1/11*$^{-/-}$, *P2x7*r$^{-/-}$ and *Asc*$^{-/-}$ mice were aseptically removed, weighted, and homogenized in 5 ml PBS using tissue grinders as previously described (48). In brief, 100 μL aliquots of 50- and 100-fold dilutions from organ homogenates were plated onto petri dishes containing brain heart infusion agar (Difco) supplemented with 5% *P. brasiliensis* 192 culture filtrate and 4% (v/v) horse serum (Instituto Butantan, São Paulo, Brazil) and incubated at 36°C. The fungal counting started at day 5 after plating, which is the period when the fungus starts to grow. Thereafter, the counting was performed daily and number of CFUs per gram of tissue determined.

Mortality Rates

Mortality studies were done with groups of 8 *C57BL/6*, *Nlrp3*$^{-/-}$, *Casp1/11*$^{-/-}$, *P2xR7*$^{-/-}$, and *Asc*$^{-/-}$ mice inoculated i.t. with 1×10^6 yeast cells. Deaths were registered daily and experiments were repeated twice.

Histopathological Analysis

Histopathological analysis of lungs and livers was performed as previously described (49). Briefly, lungs and livers from *C57BL/6*, *Nlrp3*$^{-/-}$, *Casp1/11*$^{-/-}$, *P2x7r*$^{-/-}$, and *Asc*$^{-/-}$ mice were fixed in formalin (10%) and embedded in paraffin. Tissues sections were stained with hematoxylin–eosin (H&E) for analysis of the lesions and Grocott for fungal evaluation. Morphometrical analysis was performed using Nikon DXM 1200c digital camera and Nikon NIS Elements AR 2.30 software. Results were expressed as the mean ± SD for the total area of lesions.

Cytokines Detection

The levels of IL-1β, IL-18, TNF-α, and IL-6 were measured in lung homogenates by ELISA with antibodies pairs purchased from eBioscience according to the manufacturer's protocol. The absorbance values were determined using a spectrophotometric plate reader (VersaMax, Molecular Devices).

Flow Cytometry Analysis

Cells obtained from lung homogenates at 48 h, 2, 4, and 10 weeks after i.t. infection were isolated as previously described (50). In brief, the lungs were excised, minced, and digested with collagenase (1 mg/ml, Sigma) and DNase (30 μg/mL, Sigma) in RPMI buffer (5% fetal calf serum, Sigma). Leukocytes were isolated with Percoll (20%, Sigma). The numbers of leukocytes were adjusted to 1×10^6 cells/mL and suspended in staining buffer (PBS, 2% fetal calf serum and 0.1% NaN3). Fc receptors were blocked using unlabeled anti-CD16/32 antibodies (1 μg/ml; BD Biosciences), and cells were stained for 20 min at 4°C with the monoclonal antibodies diluted at optimal concentration: pacific blue (PB)-labeled anti-CD45, anti-CD25, anti-IL-1β, anti-F4/80 (5 μg/ml); phycoerythrin (PE)-labeled anti-CD4, anti-Ly6G, anti-Syk kinase (2 μg/ml); PECy7-labeled anti-CD8, anti-CD4, anti-IL-4 (2 μg/ml); allophycocyanin (APC)-labeled anti-CD44, anti-FoxP3, anti-CD8, anti-CD86, anti-IFN-γ (5 μg/ml); APC-Cy7-labeled, anti-CD45 (2 μg/ml); Brilliant Violet 510 (BV)-labeled anti-IL-17 (2 μg/ml); peridinin chlorophyll protein (PerCP)-labeled anti-TGF-β, anti-CD62L, anti-MHCII (2 μg/ml); fluorescein isothiocyanate-labeled anti-CD11b, anti-CD3 (5 μg/ml); (from BD Biosciences or BioLegend). Cells were washed twice with staining buffer, fixed with 1% paraformaldehyde (Sigma), and acquired using a FACSCanto II equipment and software FlowJo (Tree-Star).

Intracellular Cytokines Measurement

The intracellular detection of cytokines was performed as previously described (49). Briefly, cells were labeled for surface molecules with monoclonal antibodies: anti-CD45, anti-CD8 (PB), anti-CD4 (PE), and anti-CD25 (PB) (BD Biosciences). For intracellular staining, cells were treated with Cytofix/Cytoperm kit (BD Biosciences), according to manufacturer's protocol and labeled with anti-IL-1β (PECY7), anti-IFN-γ (APC), anti-IL-17 (BV), anti-IL-4 (PECy7), anti-TGF-β (PerCP) monoclonal antibodies. For Treg characterization, plots were gated on $CD4^+CD25^+$ cells. Cells were fixed with 1% paraformaldehyde (Sigma) and acquired at 50,000 events using a FACSCanto II equipment and FACSDiva software (BD Biosciences) using software FlowJo (Tree-Star).

RNA Isolation and cDNA Synthesis

Lungs were homogenized in TRIzol reagent using tissue grinders. RNA isolation and purification was performed as described (49) using Ultraclean Tissue & Cells RNA Isolation Kit (MO BIO Laboratories) according to the manufacturer's protocol. RNA concentration was assessed on a NanoDrop ND-1000 spectrophotometer. c-DNA synthesis was performed using the High Capacity RNA-to-cDNA kit (Applied Biosystems) following the manufacturer's instructions.

Real-time Quantitative Polymerase Chain Reaction

The cDNA was amplified using TaqMan Universal PCR Master Mix (Applied Biosystems) according to manufacturer's protocol. The primers used were: IL-1β Mm01336189_m1; IL-18 Mm00434225_m1; ASC (Pycard) Mm00445747_ g1; Syk (Sykb) Mm01333032_m1; Casp-1 Mm00438023_m1; Nlrp3 Mm00840904_m1 (Applied Biosystems). Data were normalized to GAPDH gene expression. TaqMan PCR assays were performed on a MxP3000P QPCR System, and data were developed using the MxPro QPCR software (Stratagene). The average threshold cycle (CT) values of samples were normalized to CT value of GAPDH gene. The relative expression was determined by the $2^{-\Delta\Delta}$CT method.

Statistics

Values represent means ± SD. Comparison among multiple groups was done with ANOVA non-pared test, and multiple comparisons according Bonferroni Differences between survivals were compared by log-rank test. All statistical analyses were performed using the software GraphPad Prism (GraphPad Software, Inc.).

RESULTS

NLRP3 Inflammasome Controls the Pulmonary and Hepatic Fungal Loads of Mice i.t. Infected with *P. brasiliensis* Yeasts

To evaluate the function of NLRP3 inflammasome in pulmonary PCM, we first investigated the control of fungal burdens by WT and NLRP3 inflammasome deficient (*Nlrp3*$^{-/-}$, *Casp1/11*$^{-/-}$, and *Asc*$^{-/-}$) mice i.t. infected with (1×10^6) yeasts cells. Mice deficient for the ATP receptor (*P2x7r*$^{-/-}$) were also studied. Lung and liver of mice were excised, macerated, and the homogenates were diluted at 1:100 and plated in Petri dishes. The fungal counting started at day 5 after plating, which is the period when the fungus starts to grow. Thereafter, the counting was performed daily. The degree of infection was analyzed from the acute to the late phases (48 h, 2, 4, and 10 weeks) of infection. In the acute phase (48 h p.i.), no differences in the pulmonary and hepatic fungal loads between WT and NLRP3 deficient mice were seen. In contrast, increased fungal recovery at weeks 2, 4, and 10 of infection were observed in the lungs of *Nlrp3*$^{-/-}$, *Casp1/11*$^{-/-}$, *P2x7r*$^{-/-}$, and *Asc*$^{-/-}$ mice, that was more prominent at 10 weeks of infection (**Figure 1A**). At weeks 4 and 10 after infection increased, fungal burdens were seen in the liver of all deficient mice (**Figure 1B**). These data demonstrate that NLRP3 played an important role in the control of pulmonary fungal load and its dissemination to the liver.

P. brasiliensis Infection Induces the Expression of mRNA from NLRP3-Inflammasome Related Components That Is Abolished in *Nlrp3*$^{-/-}$, *Casp1/11*$^{-/-}$, and *Asc*$^{-/-}$ Mice

The activation of NLRP3 inflammasome requires two steps, the first mediated by PRRs and NFkB activation. Pathogen components, which are TLRs agonists as well as inflammatory cytokines such as TNF-α and IL-1β can trigger NFκB activation through diverse signaling pathways (51, 52). Therefore, caspase-1 can trigger NFkB activity *via* activity of pro-inflammatory cytokines produced by ASC-dependent inflammasome activation. Additionally, recent studies have shown that caspase-1 and ASC can direct NFkB activation, and this process is independent on the enzymatic activity of caspase-1 (52, 53). Indeed, caspase-1 can trigger TLR2- and TLR4-mediated NFκB activation *via* MyD88 adaptor like (MAL) for signal transduction (54). This led us to hypothesize that the absence of NLRP3 components might reduce the mRNA expression of cytokines and other NLRP3-related components. Therefore, the expression of IL-1β, IL-18, NLRP3, Caspase-1, ASC, and Syk mRNA was characterized in lung macerates of *WT*, *Nlrp3*$^{-/-}$, *Casp1/11*$^{-/-}$, and *Asc*$^{-/-}$ mice at week 4 after infection. Increased expression of IL-1β, IL-18, NLRP3, Caspase-1, ASC, and Syk mRNA was detected in the lungs of WT mice compared to knockouts mice and uninfected mice as a control (**Figures 2A,B**) demonstrating that *P. brasiliensis* infection induces an increased synthesis of components associated with NLRP3 inflammasome. In addition, the increased expression of Syk mRNA suggests the contribution of this enzyme in the activation process of NLRP3 as shown in our previous study (21).

Secretion of IL-1β and IL-18 but Not TNF-α and IL-6 Depends on NLRP3 Activation

The cytokines levels in lung homogenates of *WT*, *Nlrp3*$^{-/-}$, *Casp1/11*$^{-/-}$, *P2x7r*$^{-/-}$, and *Asc*$^{-/-}$ mice were analyzed at 48 h, 2, 4, and 10 weeks of *P. brasiliensis* infection. High levels of IL-1β

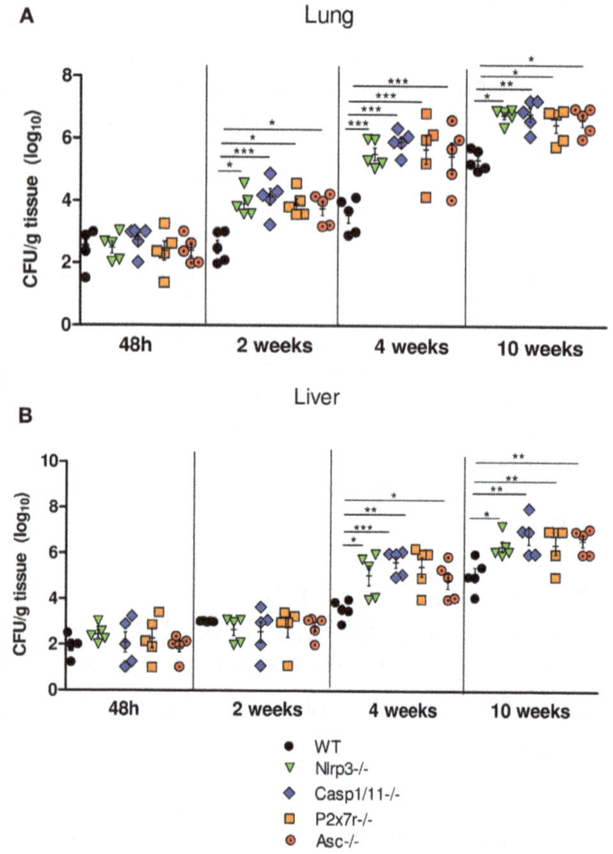

FIGURE 1 | NOD-like receptor P3 (NLRP3) inflammasome controls the pulmonary and hepatic fungal loads of mice i.t. infected with *P. brasiliensis* yeasts. Disease severity was assessed by a CFU assay using macerated lungs **(A)** and livers **(B)** of *WT* mice, *Nlrp3*$^{-/-}$, *Casp1/11*$^{-/-}$, *P2x7r*, and *Asc*$^{-/-}$ mice infected with 1 × 10^6 yeasts cells *via* i.t. at 48 h, 2, 4, and 10 weeks of infection. Data are expressed as the number of CFU/g tissue of an experiment using five mice. Equivalent results were obtained in a second experiment using the same number of infected animals (*$P < 0.05$, **$P < 0.01$, and ***$P < 0.001$).

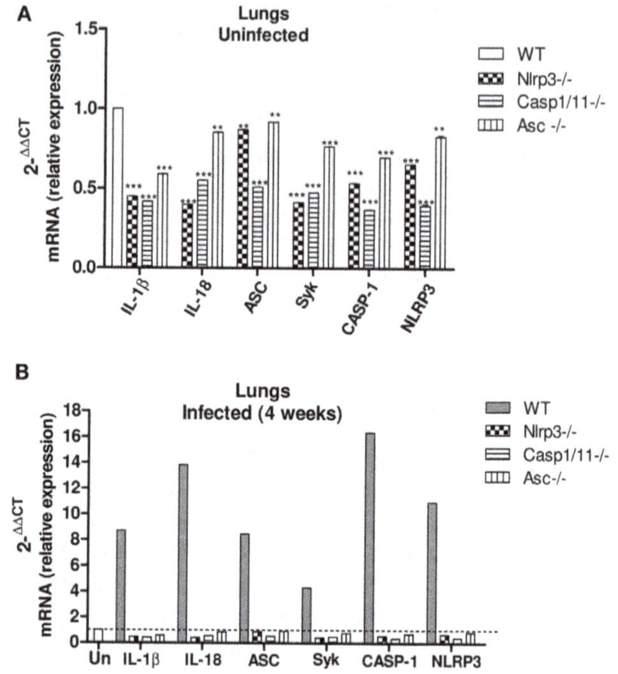

FIGURE 2 | *Paracoccidioides brasiliensis* infection induces an increased expression of mRNA from NLRP3 inflammasome-related components, which is abolished in *Nlrp3*$^{-/-}$, *Casp1/11*$^{-/-}$, and *Asc*$^{-/-}$ mice. Real-time quantitative polymerase chain reaction analysis of the IL-1β, IL-18, Asc, Casp-1, Nlrp3, and Syk genes expression in the lung macerates of *Nlrp3*$^{-/-}$, *Casp1/11*$^{-/-}$, *Asc*$^{-/-}$, and WT uninfected mice **(A)** and at week 4 of infection **(B)**.

and IL-18 secretion were observed in the lungs of *WT* mice at all postinfection periods studied, but a more robust production was observed at weeks 4 and 10 postinfection. Equivalent reduced levels of these cytokines were detected in the lung supernatants of *Nlrp3*$^{-/-}$, *Casp1/11*$^{-/-}$, *P2x7r*$^{-/-}$, and *Asc*$^{-/-}$ mice (**Figures 3A,B**). From 48 h up to 10 weeks of infection a modest increase of TNF-α and IL-6 secretion was observed in the lungs of all mouse strains studied, but no significant differences were observed at any period of infection (**Figures 3C,D**). These findings showed that in pulmonary PCM, TNF-α, and IL-6 production is independent on NLRP3 activation.

NLRP3 Induces Increased Influx of PMN Leukocytes, into the Lungs of *P. brasiliensis* Infected Mice

The pulmonary cellular infiltrates in *WT*, *Nlrp3*$^{-/-}$, *Casp1/11*$^{-/-}$, and *Asc*$^{-/-}$ mice were analyzed by flow cytometry at several periods of *P. brasiliensis* infection (**Figure 4A**). An increased influx of total leukocytes characterized as CD45$^+$ cells was detected in the lungs of *WT* mice compared with *Nlrp3*$^{-/-}$, *Casp1/11*$^{-/-}$, and *Asc*$^{-/-}$ mice, which was more expressive in the acute phase (48 h) of infection (**Figure 4B**). After 48 h and 2 weeks of infection, a high number of CD11b$^+$F4/80$^+$ macrophages were seen in the lungs of infected mice, that decreases at later periods, but no significant differences between *WT* and deficient mice were detected (**Figure 4C**). Interestingly, an increased influx of GR1$^+$Ly6G$^+$ PMN cells was seen in the lungs of *WT* mice in comparison with *Nlrp3*$^{-/-}$, *Casp1/11*$^{-/-}$, and *Asc*$^{-/-}$ mice at 48 h, 2 and 4 weeks of infection (**Figure 4D**). These data showed that NLRP3 actively regulates the cell infiltration that occurs in the lungs of *P. brasiliensis* infected mice.

NLRP3 Induces Increased Influx of Activated CD4$^+$ and CD8$^+$ T Cells into the Lungs of Infected Mice

The profile of CD4$^+$ cell activation was characterized by flow cytometry (**Figure 5A**). From week 2 onward, CD4$^+$ T lymphocytes appeared in increased numbers in the lungs of WT when compared with *Nlrp3*$^{-/-}$, *Casp1/11*$^{-/-}$, and *Asc*$^{-/-}$ mice (**Figure 5B**). The subpopulations of naïve (CD4$^+$CD44^{low}CD62L^{high}) and effector/memory (CD4$^+$CD44^{high}CD62L^{low}) T cells were also determined. Our data showed increased numbers of naïve CD4$^+$ T cells in the lungs of *Nlrp3*$^{-/-}$, *Casp1/11*$^{-/-}$, and *Asc*$^{-/-}$ compared with WT mice at weeks 2, 4, and 10 of infection (**Figure 5C**). In

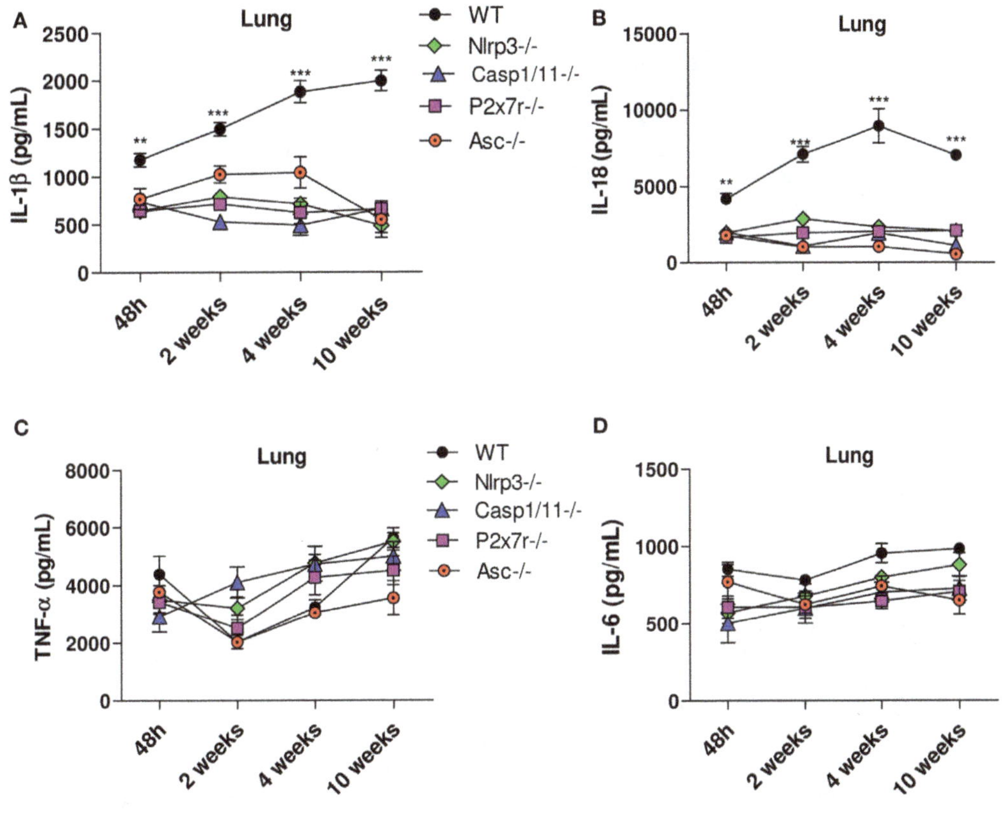

FIGURE 3 | Secretion of IL-1β and IL-18 but not TNF-α and IL-6 is controlled by NLRP3 inflammasome activation. The supernatants of macerated lungs from *WT*, *Nlrp3*$^{-/-}$, *Casp1*$^{-/-}$ *P2x7r*$^{-/-}$, and *Asc*$^{-/-}$ mice infected *via* i.t. with 1 × 10^6 *Paracoccidioides brasiliensis* yeasts were used to assess IL-1β, IL-18, TNF-α and IL-6 production by ELISA. Levels of IL-1β and IL-18 **(A,B)** and TNF-α and IL-6 **(C,D)** in the lungs of mice 48 h, 2, 4, and 10 weeks after infection with *P. brasiliensis* yeasts. Data represents one of two independent experiments using five mice per group (n = 5). Experiment was performed in triplicates represented as Mean ± SEM (**P < 0.01 and ***P < 0.001 compared with deficient mice).

contrast, WT mice presented increased numbers of pulmonary effector/memory CD4$^+$ T cells at the same postinfection periods (**Figure 5D**). When the presence of activated CD8$^+$ T cells was evaluated, an increased number of activated CD8$^+$CD69$^+$ T cells were detected in the lungs of WT mice at weeks 2, 4, and 10 of infection. In contrast, *Nlrp3*$^{-/-}$, *Casp1/11*$^{-/-}$, and *Asc*$^{-/-}$ mice had diminished numbers of activated CD8+ CD9+ T cells at 2 and 4 weeks that were totally abolished at 10 weeks of infection (**Figures 5E,F**).

NLRP3 Inhibits the Presence of Treg Cells into the Lungs of Infected Mice

Regulatory T cells were characterized by the CD4$^+$CD25$^+$FOXP3$^+$ phenotype as shown in the **Figure 6A**. An increased number of Treg cells was observed in the lungs of *Nlrp3*$^{-/-}$, *Casp1/11*$^{-/-}$, and *Asc*$^{-/-}$ at 4 and 10 weeks of infection, compared with WT mice, which also showed increased number of these cells, although lower than NLRP3 components deficient mice (**Figure 6B**). These data showed that NLRP3 played a role in the control of adaptive immunity to *P. brasiliensis* infection by increasing the number of activated T cells in WT mice, as shown in **Figure 5D**, and reducing the presence of Treg cells that migrate to the lung of WT mice.

NLRP3 Signaling Induces a Prevalent Expansion CD4$^+$ and CD8$^+$ T Cells Expressing IFN-γ and IL-17 with Concomitant Reduction of IL-4$^+$ and TGF-β T Cells

We have further studied the expression of intracellular pro-IL-1β, IFN-γ, IL-4, IL-17, and TGF-β cytokines by CD4$^+$ and CD8$^+$ T cells in the lungs of infected *WT*, *Nlrp3*$^{-/-}$, *Casp1/11*$^{-/-}$, and *ASC*$^{-/-}$ mice at 48 h, 2, 4, and 10 weeks of infection. Our data showed that in the acute phase of infection (48 h) there was an elevated frequency of CD4$^+$ and CD8$^+$ T cells expressing intracellular pro-IL-1β, IFN-γ, and IL-4 in the lungs of WT and deficient (*Nlrp3*$^{-/-}$, *Casp1/11*$^{-/-}$, and *ASC*$^{-/-}$) mice, but no significant differences were observed between the mouse strains. At this period, no significant expression of IL-17 and TGF-β was detected in CD4$^+$ and CD8$^+$ T cells (**Figures 7A,E**). From 2 to 10 weeks of infection, increased frequencies of IFN-γ$^+$ and IL-17$^+$ CD4$^+$ T cells were seen in the lungs of *WT* mice when compared with *Nlrp3*$^{-/-}$, *Casp1/11*$^{-/-}$, and *Asc*$^{-/-}$ mice. In contrast, there was an increased percentage of IL-4$^+$ and TGF-β$^+$ CD4$^+$ T cells in the lungs of *Nlrp3*$^{-/-}$, *Casp1/11*$^{-/-}$, and *Asc*$^{-/-}$ compared with WT mice (**Figures 7B–D**). Generally,

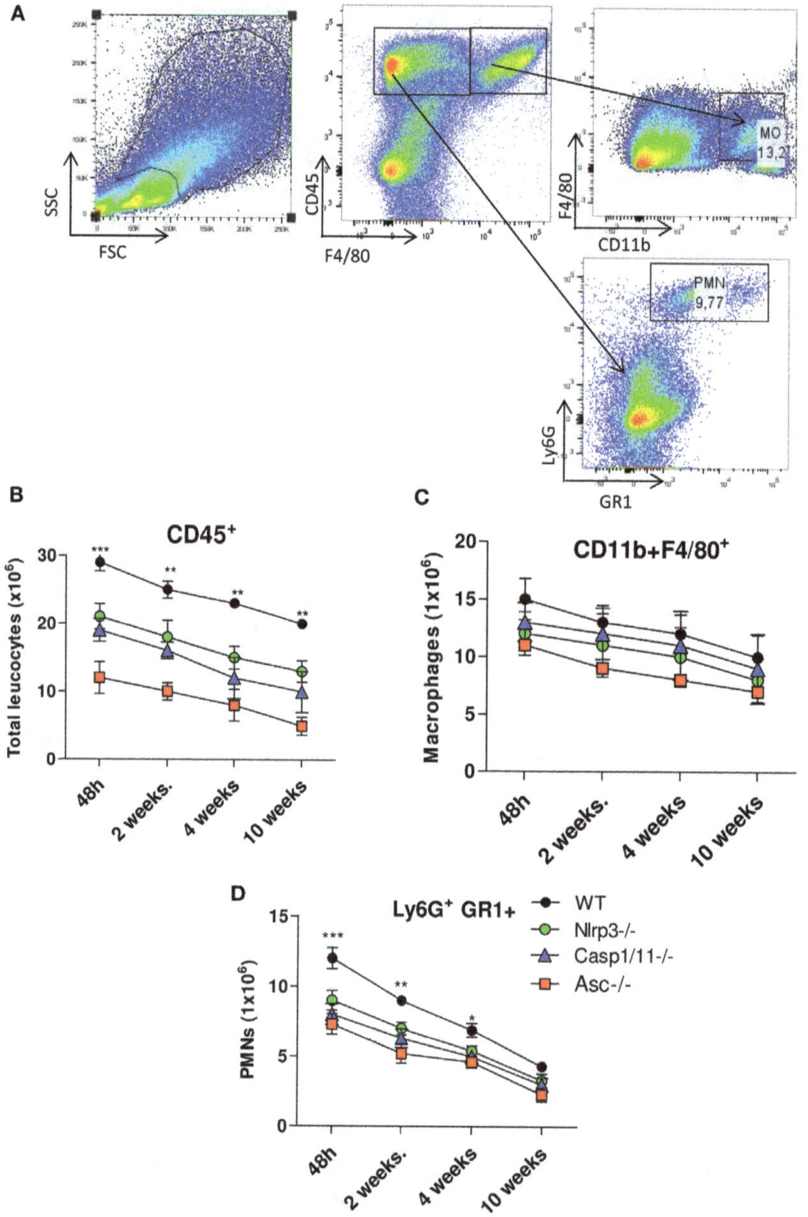

FIGURE 4 | Activation of NLRP3 inflammasome induces increased influx of PMN leukocytes into the lungs of *Paracoccidioides brasiliensis* infected mice. Inflammatory cell infiltrates in the lungs of *WT*, *Nlrp3*$^{-/-}$, *Casp1*$^{-/-}$, and *Asc*$^{-/-}$ mice infected with 1 × 10^6 *P. brasiliensis* yeasts were analyzed at different postinfection periods (48 h, 2, 4, and 10 weeks) by flow cytometry. **(A)** Gates strategy using WT cells, **(B)** total leukocytes, **(C)** macrophages, and **(D)** PMN leukocytes were phenotyped by anti-CD45, F4/80, CD11b, GR1, and anti-Ly6G fluorochromes-labeled antibodies. Data represents one of two independent experiments using five mice per group ($n = 5$). Experiment was performed in triplicates represented as Mean ± SEM ($^*P < 0.05$, $^{**}P < 0.01$, and $^{***}P < 0.001$, compared with deficient mice).

CD8$^+$ T cells appeared in decreased frequencies when compared with CD4$^+$ T cells, but a similar profile of cytokines expression was observed in both T cell subpopulations (**Figures 7E–H**). Interestingly, differences in IL-17 synthesis by CD8 T cell were only seen at week 10 postinfection. These data showed that NLRP3 played an important role in the polarization of type-1 and type-17 T cell responses in WT mice resulting in a better control of *P. brasiliensis* infection. In contrast, *Nlrp3*$^{-/-}$, *Casp1/11*$^{-/-}$, and *Asc*$^{-/-}$ mice showed a prevalent Th2/Th3/Treg profile of response that was unable to control the fungal infection.

P. brasiliensis Infected *Nlrp3*$^{-/-}$, *Casp1/11*$^{-/-}$, *P2x7r*$^{-/-}$, and *Asc*$^{-/-}$ Mice Show Increased Tissue Pathology and Decreased Survival Rates

To better clarify the importance of NLRP3 in the severity of *P. brasiliensis* infection, the histopathological analysis of the

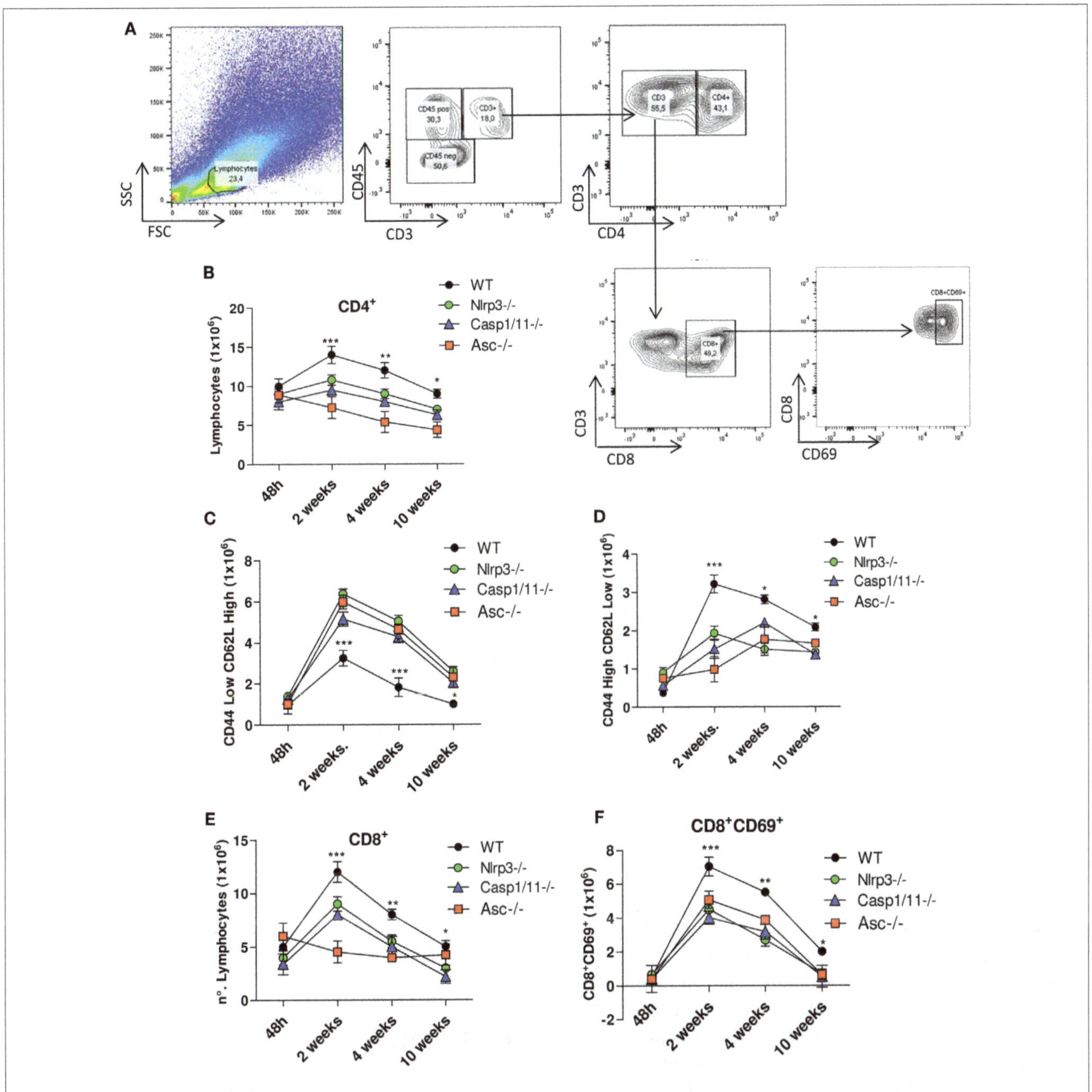

FIGURE 5 | NOD-like receptor P3 (NLRP3) inflammasome induces the migration of activated CD4+ and CD8+ T cells into the lungs of *Paracoccidioides brasiliensis* infected mice. Inflammatory cell infiltrates in the lungs of *WT*, *Nlrp3*$^{-/-}$, *Casp1*$^{-/-}$, and *Asc*$^{-/-}$ mice infected with 1 × 10^6 *P. brasiliensis* yeasts were analyzed at different postinfection periods (48 h, 2, 4, and 10 weeks) by flow cytometry. **(A)** Gates strategy using lung leukocytes from WT mice. **(B)** CD4$^+$ T cells were characterized using anti-CD4 labeled antibodies. **(C)** Naïve (CD44^{low}CD62L^{high}) and **(D)** memory/effector (CD44^{high}CD62L^{low}) CD4$^+$ T lymphocytes were characterized using adequate gates and fluorochromes-labeled anti-CD4, CD44, and CD62L antibodies. **(E)** CD8$^+$ and **(F)** CD8$^+$CD69$^+$-activated T cells were characterized using anti-CD8 and CD69 fluorochromes-labeled antibodies. Data represents one of two independent experiments using five mice per group (n = 5). Experiment was performed in triplicates represented as Mean ± SEM (*P < 0.05, **P < 0.01, and ***P < 0.001, compared with deficient mice).

lung tissues of *WT* and *Nlrp3*$^{-/-}$, *Casp1/11*$^{-/-}$, *P2x7*$^{-/-}$, and *Asc*$^{-/-}$ mice was performed at weeks 4 and 10 of i.t. infection. The histological sections were stained with hematoxylin-eosin (H&E) for cellular identification and with Groccot stain for fungal identification and localization in the tissue (**Figure 8**). The degree of infection was evaluated based in the size and morphology of lung lesions as well as fungal presence and intensity of inflammatory infiltrates. At 4 weeks of infection, less extensive and severe pulmonary lesions were observed in the lungs of *WT* in comparison with *Nlrp3*$^{-/-}$, *Casp1/11*$^{-/-}$, *P2x7r*$^{-/-}$, and *Asc*$^{-/-}$ mice. The lungs of WT mice showed an inflammatory process that spread over the entire area of the

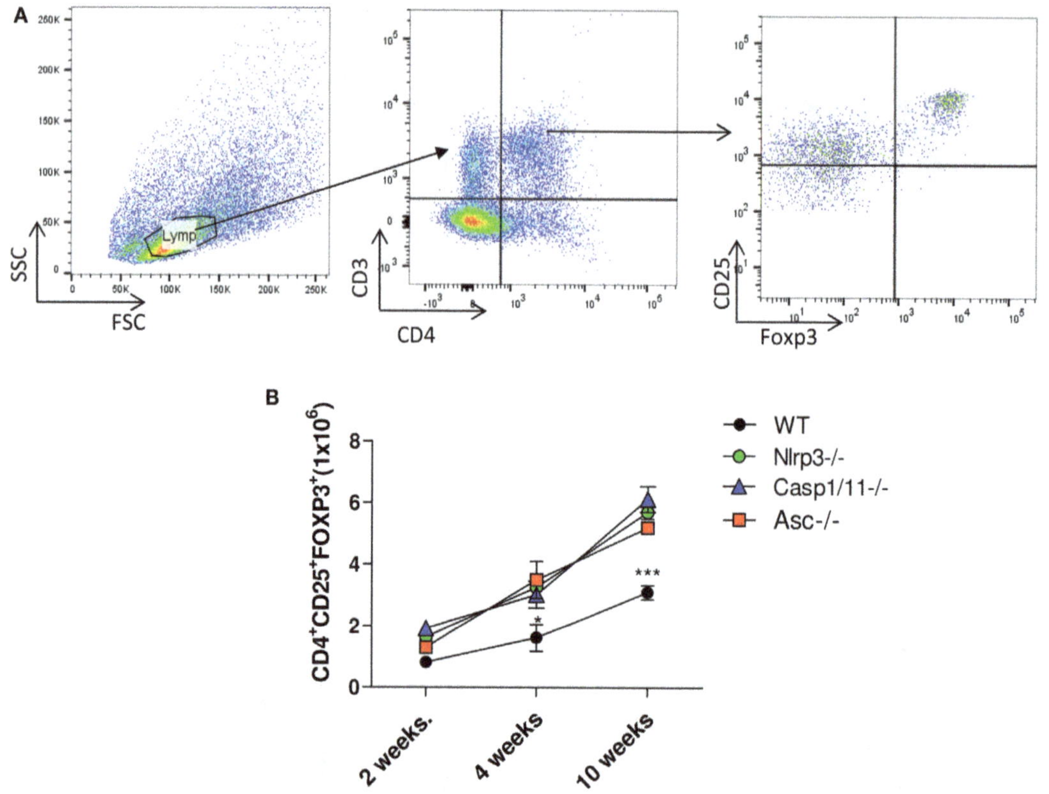

FIGURE 6 | NOD-like receptor P3 (NLRP3) inflammasome inhibits the presence of regulatory T (Treg) cells in the lungs of infected mice. The number of Treg cells ($CD4^+CD25^+FOXP3^+$) was determined in the lungs of *WT*, *Nlrp3*$^{-/-}$, *Casp1/11*$^{-/-}$, and *Asc*$^{-/-}$ mice infected with 1×10^6 *Paracoccidioides brasiliensis* yeasts at different postinfection periods (48 h, 2, 4, and 10 weeks) by flow cytometry. **(A)** Gates strategy using lung leukocytes from WT mice. **(B)** Treg cells ($CD4^+CD25^+FOXP3^+$) were characterized using adequate gates and fluorochromes-labeled anti CD4, CD25, and FOXP3 antibodies. Data represents one of two independent experiments using five mice per group ($n = 5$). Experiment was performed in triplicates represented as Mean ± SEM ($^*P < 0.05$, $^{**}P < 0.01$, and $^{***}P < 0.001$, compared with deficient mice).

organ. Large fungal loads were restricted to the center of lesions. The granulomas were large and coalescent, but there were some preserved organ areas. In *Nlrp3*$^{-/-}$, *Casp1/11*$^{-/-}$, *P2x7r*$^{-/-}$, and *Asc*$^{-/-}$ mice the extension and cellularity of the lesions as well as the presence of fungi were larger than in *WT* mice (**Figure 8A**). By 10 weeks of infection (**Figure 8B**), a similar pattern of lesions was detected, but at higher intensity. In comparison with week 4, a higher content of fungi within the granulomas and increased necrotic areas were seen at this postinfection period. In summary, the pathology developed by *Nlrp3*$^{-/-}$, *Casp1/11*$^{-/-}$, *P2x7r*$^{-/-}$, and *Asc*$^{-/-}$ mice was much more severe than that presented by *WT* mice corroborating the data of the increased fungal burden and impaired T cell immunity demonstrated by these mouse strains.

The extent of lesions areas in the lungs (**Figures 9A,B**) reveals that mice deficient for NLRP3, Caspase-1/11, P2X7R, and ASC showed significantly larger lesions occupying higher tissue area than those present in WT animals. Mortality studies were done with groups of eight mice i.t. infected with one million *P. brasiliensis* yeasts. Infected mice were monitored daily for a period of 250 days to determine the survival time. As can be seen, *Nlrp3*$^{-/-}$, *Casp1/11*$^{-/-}$, *P2x7r*$^{-/-}$, and *Asc*$^{-/-}$ mice had a significantly shorter survival time than WT mice (**Figure 9C**), further confirming the crucial importance of NLRP3 in the immunoprotection of pulmonary PCM.

DISCUSSION

The role of NLRP3 inflammasome and the cooperation of TLRs and CLRs in the modulation of immune response against *P. brasiliensis* infection in macrophages and dendritic cells have been studied in our lab (8, 15, 18, 22). Using our murine model of resistance and susceptibility to PCM, it was verified that the activation of NLRP3 inflammasome by *P. brasiliensis* infection of macrophages from resistant A/J mice is dependent on dectin-1-Syk signaling (21). Other studies showed the role of TLR2, TLR4, dectin-1, and MyD88 signaling in the secretion of pro-inflammatory cytokines (IL-1β, TNF-α, and IL-6) and control of protective Th1/Th17 immune responses (5, 18, 20). Mice and patients infected with *P. brasiliensis* secrete IL-1β and IL-18, suggesting that NLRP3 is an important player in the recognition of this fungal pathogen (55, 56). The role of NLRP3 using *in vivo* models of PCM were less explored; however, a recent study using

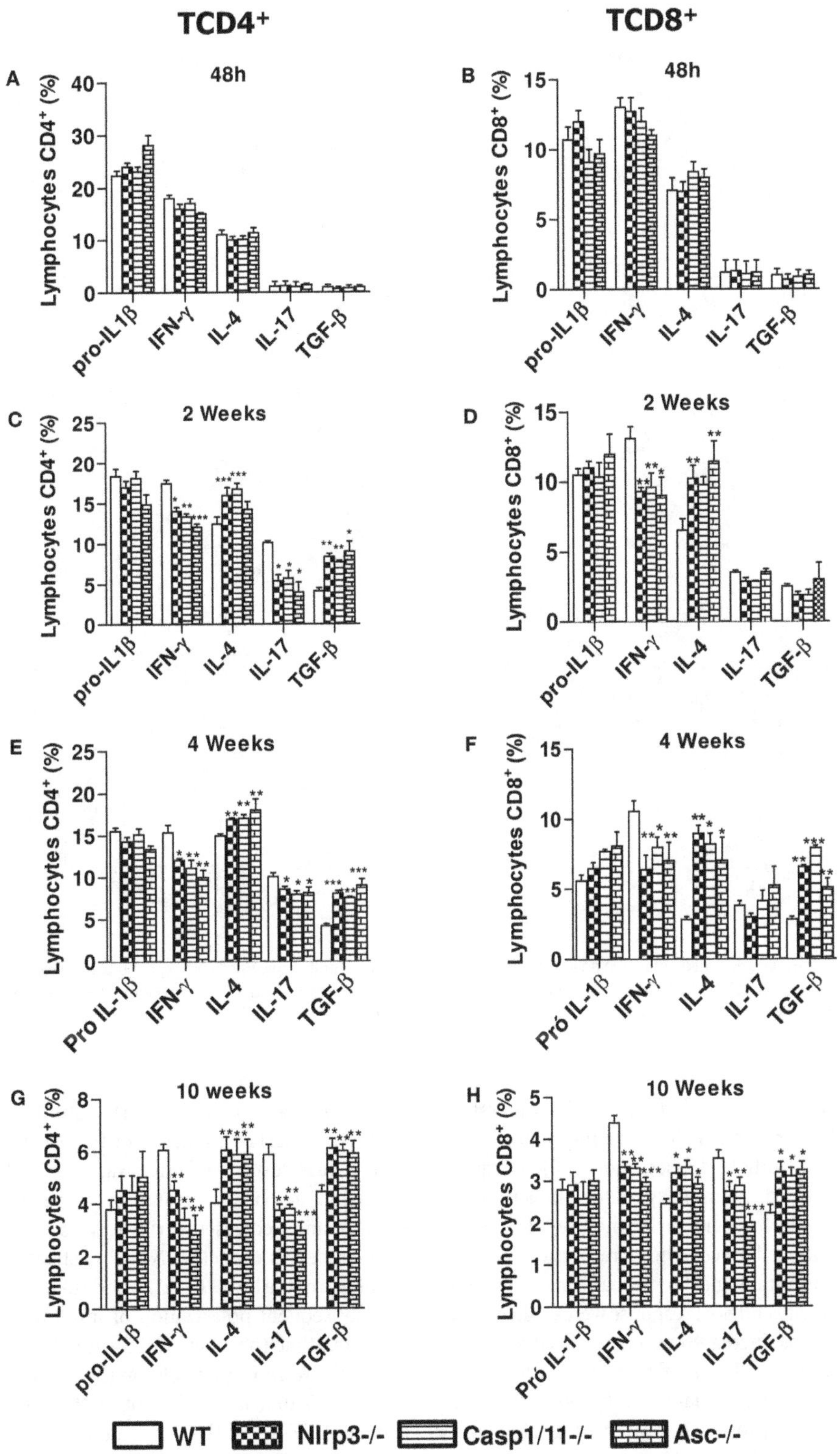

FIGURE 7 | NOD-like receptor P3 (NLRP3) inflammasome induces a Th1/Th17 profile of immune response. Intracellular cytokine analysis from inflammatory infiltrates of lungs of *WT*, *Nlrp3*$^{-/-}$, *Casp1/11*$^{-/-}$, and *Asc*$^{-/-}$ mice infected with 1 × 10^6 *Paracoccidioides brasiliensis* yeasts was performed at 48 h **(A,E)**, 2 weeks **(B,F)**, 4 weeks **(C,G)**, and 10 weeks **(D,H)** by flow cytometry. CD4+ and CD8+ T cells were labeled with anti-CD4 and anti-CD8 antibodies, permeabilized and intracellular cytokines determined using fluorochromes-labeled anti- IL-1β, IFN-γ, IL-4, IL-17, and TGF-β antibodies. Data represents one of two independent experiments using five mice per group (n = 5). Experiment was performed in triplicates represented as Mean ± SEM (*P < 0.05, **P < 0.01, and ***P < 0.001, compared with WT mice).

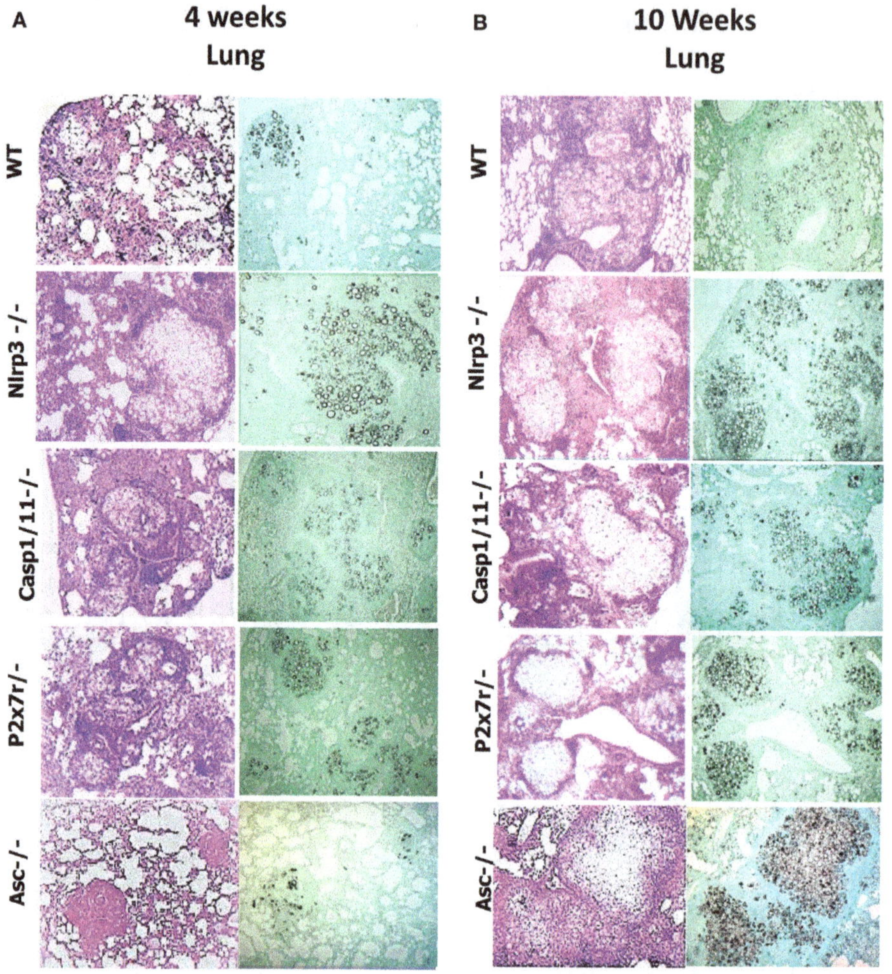

FIGURE 8 | NOD-like receptor P3 (NLRP3) inflammasome activation leads to less severe lung pathology. Photomicrographs of lungs of *WT*, *Nlrp3*$^{-/-}$, *Casp1/11*$^{-/-}$, *P2x7r*$^{-/-}$, and *Asc*$^{-/-}$ mice infected i.t. with 1 × 10^6 *Paracoccidioides brasiliensis* yeasts after 4 and 10 weeks of infection. **(A,B)** Histological lung sections were stained with hematoxylin–eosin [H&E, left panels of **(A,B)**] or Groccot [right panels of **(A,B)**].

mice systemically infected with *P. brasiliensis* demonstrated that NLRP3 controls host resistance by inducing a prevalent Th1 immunity associated with IL-18 secretion (40). Because human PCM is acquired by the pulmonary route of infection, in the present study, we sought to characterize the role of NLRP3 inflammasome in i.t. infected mice whose response involves pulmonary-mediated immunological mechanisms. Several parameters of disease severity and host response were evaluated at several postinfection periods. Increased numbers of viable yeasts were recovered from lungs and livers of *Nlrp3*$^{-/-}$, *Casp1/11*$^{-/-}$, *P2x7r*$^{-/-}$, and *Asc*$^{-/-}$ mice. Our CFU data corroborate with those of Ketelut-Carneiro et al. that found increased fungal loads in the lungs and livers of *Asc*$^{-/-}$ and *Casp1/11*$^{-/-}$ mice infected by the i.v. route (40). Our study has also revealed for the first time the importance of the purinergic P2X7 receptor (P2X7R) in NLRP3 activation by *P. brasiliensis* infection, in agreement with recent studies that demonstrated the participation of this receptor in the activation of the NLRP3 inflammasome and immunity against intracellular infections caused by *Mycobacterium*, *Chlamydia*, *Leishmania*, and *Toxoplasma* (57–60). In our pulmonary model of PCM, a marked influence of P2X7R in the immune response and disease severity of mice was clearly shown by the deficient fungicidal activity, decreased cytokines production, high tissue damage and decreased survival rates developed by P2X7R deficient mice. As expected, NLRP3 activation exerted a profound influence in the levels of IL-1β and IL-18 present in the lung tissue and subsequent polarization of immune response. This finding indicates that the new equilibrium in the pool of pulmonary cytokines were responsible by the diverse immunity developed by NLRP3 deficient mice, once the levels of other cytokines such as TNF-α and IL-6 remained in the control levels. It is well known that IL-1β and IL-18 contribute to the induction of the adaptive immune response by stimulation of T cell proliferation, differentiation of Th1/Th17 immunity and increased activity of NKT cytotoxic cells (61). NLRP3 and pro-IL-1β mRNAs are highly expressed in the first signal of NLRP3 activation, as a result of the engagement of PRRs and PAMPs on phagocytes (25, 62). Our findings demonstrated that the genetic deficiency

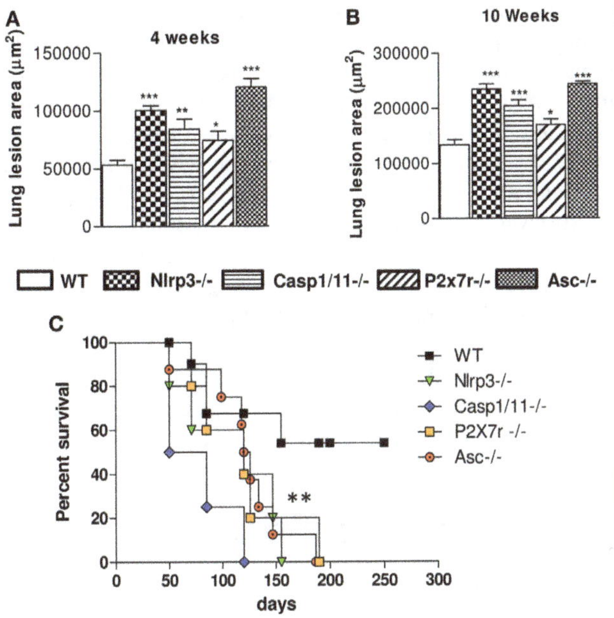

FIGURE 9 | NOD-like receptor P3 (NLRP3) inflammasome activation determines decreased pulmonary pathology and increased survival rates of *Paracoccidioides brasiliensis* infected mice. The total areas of lung lesions were calculated in the periods of 4 **(A)** and 10 weeks **(B)** after infection. Data are expressed as the mean ± SEM of triplicates from two independent experiments. **(C)** The mortality studies were conducted with groups of 8 *WT*, *Nlrp3*$^{-/-}$, *Casp1/11* $^{-/-}$, *Asc*$^{-/-}$, and *P2x7r*$^{-/-}$ mice i.t. infected with 1 × 10^6 *P. brasiliensis.* Mice were monitored daily for a period of 250 days to determine the survival time (*$P < 0.05$, **$P < 0.01$, and ***$P < 0.001$, compared with WT mice).

of NLRP3, Casp1/11, and Asc totally impaired the expression of IL-1β, IL-18, NLRP3, Casp1, and ASC mRNA in the lungs of infected mice at week 4 of infection. Besides the control of NLRP3 inflammasome components, *P. brasiliensis* infection induced an increased expression of Syk, confirming our previous studies demonstrating the crucial role of dectin-1-Syk signaling in the activation of this receptor (21). It is well known that the definition of the inflammatory infiltrates that accompanies an infectious process helps to define the type and intensity of the established immune response. Here, the expression of NLRP3 inflammasome-associated components was concomitant with increased infiltration of PMNs but not macrophages into the lungs of mice, indicating the selective influence of NLRP3 activation on this important effector cell in fungal infections. PMN-rich inflammatory reactions characterize the function of Th17 cells that, besides the typical production of IL-17 and IL-22, are committed with the secretion of chemokines involved in the migration and activation of PMN leukocytes (8, 63–66). In agreement, an enhanced differentiation of Th17 and Tc17 cells were seen during the infection of NLRP3 sufficient mice. The NLRP3 inflammasome activation has also induced an increased influx and activation of CD4$^+$ and CD8$^+$ T cells to the lungs of mice that were probably involved in the control of fungal loads, and subsequent control of lung pathology. Indeed, decreased numbers of CD4$^+$- and CD8$^+$-activated T cells were consistently seen in the lungs of *Nlrp3*$^{-/-}$, *Casp1/11*$^{-/-}$, and *Asc*$^{-/-}$ mice that developed increased fungal burdens associated with increased lung pathology and mortality rates. In pulmonary PCM, both T cell subsets participate in the protective mechanisms, with an intense and prominent contribution of CD8$^+$ T cells (67, 68). Although in less number, CD8$^+$ T cells were here shown to participate in the immunity associated with NLRP3 activation, a relevant observation added to the role of this receptor in the host defense mechanisms against *P. brasiliensis* infection.

The caspase-1-dependent cytokines exert important effects in the initiation of the adaptive Th1 and Th17 cellular responses to fungal infections (37). IL-1β has been suggested to promote inflammatory diseases by inducing the expansion of differentiated T cells (69) and has been implicated, alone or in combination with IL-6 and TGF-β, in driving murine and human Th17 priming and phenotype stabilization (66, 69). IL-18 was initially discovered as an IFN-γ-inducing factor, which together with IL-12 promotes the development of Th1 cells (70). Here, we assessed the intracellular cytokines production to define the effect of NLRP3 activation in the Th1, Th2, and Th17 defense mechanisms of *P. brasileinsis* infected mice. A new balance of Th cells subsets was seen in the absence of NLRP3 inflammasome components: an increased expression of IL-4 and TGF-β that accompanied a reduced number of IFN-γ$^+$ and IL-17$^+$ CD4$^+$ and CD8$^+$ T cells. In murine PCM, we previously demonstrated that IL-4 can exert protective or deleterious roles, depending on the mouse strain studied (71). It can dampen excessive inflammatory reactions of B10.A mice but suppresses the protective Th1 immunity of *C57BL/6* mice. A recent report showed that IL-4 suppresses NLRP3-dependent caspase-1activation and subsequent IL-1β secretion (72). These data show a mutual control between NLRP3 inflammasome and IL-4, as here observed. Our study also showed a clear association between NLRP3 activation and decreased synthesis of TGF-β and Treg cells development suggesting that the predominant pro-inflammatory milieu produced by this receptor significantly reduced the regulatory anti-inflammatory mechanisms. Interestingly, in a model of chronic kidney disease, the expression of NLRP3 was linked to the control of TGF-β-dependent signaling (73) although in our model enhanced TGF-β expressing cells were allied with absence of NLRP3 activation.

The analysis of intracellular cytokines revealed that NLRP3 played an important role in the induction of Th1 and Th17 responses with concomitant reduction of Th2/Treg expansion, a process of immune regulation associated with regressive disease in both humans and experimental models of PCM (2, 3, 5–8, 10). In addition, an important contribution of CD8$^+$ T cells to IL-17 and IFN-γ production was also seen. Although no studies have directly addressed the role of IL-17 in PCM, several indirect findings clearly demonstrated that a well-balanced production of pro- and anti-inflammatory cytokines is crucial to determine a protective immunity. The evaluation of cytokines production by patients with polar forms of PCM has shown that the prevalent synthesis of Th1/Th17 cytokines characterized the mild forms of chronic PCM, whereas an elevated production of IL-4 and IL-9, associated with high numbers of Treg cells, were linked with the severe forms of the disease (10). Our previous studies have also demonstrated that a balanced differentiation of Th1/Th17/Treg cells is fundamental to achieve immunoprotection in pulmonary PCM. Indeed, the absence of TLR2 signaling induces excessive pathology associated with increased Th17 differentiation an impaired Treg development (6). In contrast, in TLR4 deficiency the excessive proliferation of Treg cells and reduced Th17 differentiation led to more severe disease (7). Importantly, the absence of dectin-1 signaling induced a critical reduction in all IL-17 secreting cells, particularly IL-17^{+}CD8^{+} T cells and a severe PCM (20). These findings, and those here reported clearly indicate that the equilibrium in the expansion of T cell subpopulations is fundamental to immunoprotection against PCM.

The findings here reported are in contrast with those of Ketelut-Carneiro et al. showing that an enhanced Th1 immunity controlled by increase production of IL-18 was responsible by the protective role of NLRP3 inflammasome in a murine model of PCM (40). These discrepancies, however, could be attributed to the route of infection used. Indeed, the study of Ketelut-Carneiro et al. used i.v. infected mice (40), whereas our studies were done with i.t. infected animals. In this aspect, our previous studies have clearly shown the influence of the route of infection in the severity of the disease and immune response of *P. brasiliensis* infected mice (41). We verified that the s.c. route induces a self-healing infection in several mouse strains allied with elevated delayed hypersensitivity reactions. Interestingly, the previous s.c. infection of B10.A mice led to immunoprotection or disease exacerbation depending on the route of fungal challenge. Immunoprotection was achieved after intraperitoneal challenge and was associated with persistent cell-mediated immunity and a mixed type-1/type-2 immunity. Exacerbated disease was found after intravenous challenge and was linked with anergy of cellular immunity and prevalent type-2 immune response (41). In contrast to the prevalent Th1/Th17 immunity induced by NLRP3 inflammasome activation in *WT* mice, *Nlrp3*$^{-/-}$, *Casp1/11*$^{-/-}$, and *Asc*$^{-/-}$ mice showed increase expansion and migration of Treg cells to the site of infection that possibly have contributed to the deficient control of fungal loads and non-protective inflammatory reactions. In agreement, the survival studies showed increased mortality rates among *Nlrp3*$^{-/-}$, *Casp1/11*$^{-/-}$, *Asc*$^{-/-}$, and *P2x7r*$^{-/-}$ mice accompanying increased fungal burdens and areas of lung lesions. In conclusion, the more efficient immunity mediated by Th1 and Th17 cells associated with NLRP3 inflammasome activation is highly protective to pulmonary PCM and this intracellular receptor appears to be significantly involved in the control of signaling pathways that led to the integration of innate and adaptive host immune responses to *P. brasiliensis* infection.

AUTHOR CONTRIBUTIONS

Conceived and designed experiments: VC and CF. Contributed with reagent: DZ. Performed the experiments: CF, TC, EA, FL, and NG. Analyzed the data: CF, VC, FL, EA, and DZ. Wrote the paper: CF and VC.

ACKNOWLEDGMENTS

We thank Paulo Albe for processing the histological samples. This work was supported by Fundação de Amparo à Pesquisa do Estado de São Paulo (FAPESP, grants 2013/23536-3 and 2013/02396-9) and Conselho Nacional de Pesquisas (CNPq, grants 471317/2012-8 and 306812/2014-2).

REFERENCES

1. Brummer E, Castaneda E, Restrepo A. Paracoccidioidomycosis: an update. *Clin Microbiol Rev* (1993) 6:89–117. doi:10.1128/CMR.6.2.89
2. Franco MF. Host parasite relationship in paracoccidioidomycosis. *J Med Vet Mycol* (1987) 25:5–18. doi:10.1080/02681218780000021
3. Benard G. An overview of the immunopathology of human paracoccidioidomycosis. *Mycopathologia* (2008) 165:209–21. doi:10.1007/s11046-007-9065-0
4. Felonato M, Pina A, Bernardino S, Loures FV, de Araujo EF, Calich VL. CD28 exerts protective and detrimental effects in a pulmonary model of paracoccidioidomycosis. *Infect Immun* (2010) 78:4922–35. doi:10.1128/IAI.00297-10
5. Felonato M, Pina A, de Araujo EF, Loures FV, Bazan SB, Feriotti C, et al. Anti-CD25 treatment depletes Treg cells and decreases disease severity in susceptible and resistant mice infected with *Paracoccidioides brasiliensis*. *PLoS One* (2012) 7:e51071. doi:10.1371/journal.pone.0051071
6. Loures FV, Pina A, Felonato M, Calich VL. TLR2 is a negative regulator of Th17 cells and tissue pathology in a pulmonary model of fungal infection. *J Immunol* (2009) 183:1279–90. doi:10.4049/jimmunol.0801599
7. Loures FV, Pina A, Felonato M, Araújo EF, Leite KRM, Calich VLG. TLR4 signaling leads to a more severe fungal infection associated with enhanced proinflammatory immunity and impaired expansion of regulatory T cells. *Infect Immun* (2010) 78:1078–88. doi:10.1128/IAI.01198-09
8. Loures FV, Araújo EF, Feriotti C, Bazan SB, Calich VLG. TLR-4 cooperates with dectin-1 and mannose receptor to expand Th17 and Tc17 cells induced by *Paracoccidioides brasiliensis* stimulated dendritic cells. *Front Microbiol* (2015) 6:261. doi:10.3389/fmicb.2015.00261
9. Bernardino S, Pina A, Felonato M, Costa TA, Frank de Araújo E, Feriotti C, et al. TNF-α and CD8+ T cells mediate the beneficial effects of nitric oxide synthase-2 deficiency in pulmonary paracoccidioidomycosis. *PLoS Negl Trop Dis* (2013) 7(8):e2325. doi:10.1371/journal.pntd.0002325
10. de Castro LF, Ferreira MC, da Silva RM, Blotta MH, Longhi LN, Mamoni RL. Characterization of the immune response in human paracoccidioidomycosis. *J Infect* (2013) 67:470–85. doi:10.1016/j.jinf.2013.07.019
11. Ferreira MC, de Oliveira RT, da Silva RM, Blotta MH, Mamoni RL. Involvement of regulatory T cells in the immunosuppression characteristic of patients with paracoccidioidomycosis. *Infect Immun* (2010) 78:4392–401. doi:10.1128/IAI.00487-10
12. Shoham S, Huang C, Chen JM, Golenbock DT, Levitz SM. Toll-like receptor 4 mediates intracellular signaling without TNF-alpha release in response to *Cryptococcus neoformans* polysaccharide capsule. *J Immunol* (2001) 166:4620–6. doi:10.4049/jimmunol.166.7.4620
13. Netea MG, Van Der Graaf CA, Vonk AG, Verschueren I, Van Der Meer JW, Kullberg BJ. The role of toll-like receptor (TLR) 2 and TLR4 in the host defense against disseminated candidiasis. *J Infect Dis* (2002) 185:1483–9. doi:10.1086/340511
14. Netea MG, Ferwerda G, van der Graaf CA, van der Meer JW, Kullberg BJ. Recognition of fungal pathogens by toll-like receptors. *Curr Pharm Des* (2006) 12:4195–201. doi:10.2174/138161206778743538
15. Calich VLG, Costa TA, Felonato M, Arruda C, Bernardino S, Loures FV, et al. Innate immunity to *Paracoccidioides brasiliensis* infection. *Mycopathologia* (2008) 165:223–36. doi:10.1007/s11046-007-9048-1
16. Chai LY, Vonk AG, Kullberg BJ, Verweij PE, Verschueren I, van der Meer JW, et al. *Aspergillus fumigatus* cell wall components differentially modulate host TLR2 and TLR4 responses. *Microbes Infect* (2011) 13:151–9. doi:10.1016/j.micinf.2010.10.005
17. Bonfim CV, Mamoni RL, Blotta MH. TLR-2, TLR-4 and dectin-1 expression in human monocytes and neutrophils stimulated by *Paracoccidioides brasiliensis*. *Med Mycol* (2009) 47:722–33. doi:10.3109/13693780802641425

18. Loures FV, Pina A, Felonato M, Feriotti C, de Araújo EF, Calich VL. MyD88 signaling is required for efficient innate and adaptative immune responses to *Paracoccidioides brasiliensis* infection. *Infect Immun* (2011) 79:2470–80. doi:10.1128/IAI.00375-10
19. Feriotti C, Loures FV, De Araujo EF, Costa TA, Calich VLG. Mannosyl-recognizing receptors induce an M1-like phenotype in macrophages of susceptible mice but an M2-like phenotype in mice resistant to a fungal infection. *PLoS One* (2013) 8:e54845. doi:10.1371/journal.pone.0054845
20. Loures FV, Araújo EF, Feriotti C, Bazan SB, Costa TA, Brown GD, et al. Dectin-1 induces M1 macrophages and prominent expansion of CD8+IL-17+ cells in pulmonary Paracoccidioidomycosis. *J Infect Dis* (2014) 210:762–73. doi:10.1093/infdis/jiu136
21. Feriotti C, Bazan SB, Loures FV, Araújo EF, Costa TA, Calich VLG. Expression of dectin-1 and enhanced activation of NALP3 inflammasome are associated with resistance to paracoccidioidomycosis. *Front Microbiol* (2015) 6:913. doi:10.3389/fmicb.2015.00913
22. Pina A, Bernardino S, Calich VLG. Alveolar macrophages from susceptible mice are more competent than those of resistant mice to control initial *Paracoccidioides brasiliensis* infection. *J Leukoc Biol* (2008) 83:1088–93. doi:10.1189/jlb.1107738
23. Matzinger P. The danger model: a renewed sense of self. *Science* (2002) 296(5566):301–5. doi:10.1126/science.1071059
24. Kumar H, Kawai T, Akira S. Pathogen recognition by the innate immune system. *Int Rev Immunol* (2011) 30:16–34. doi:10.3109/08830185.2010.529976
25. Schroder K, Tschopp J. The inflammasomes. *Cell* (2010) 140:821–32. doi:10.1016/j.cell.2010.01.040
26. Vanaja SK, Rathinam VA, Fitzgerald KA. Mechanisms of inflammasome activation: recent advances and novel insights. *Trends Cell Biol* (2015) 25:308–15. doi:10.1016/j.tcb.2014.12.009
27. Pétrilli V, Dostert C, Muruve DA, Tschopp J. The inflammasome: a danger sensing complex triggering innate immunity. *Curr Opin Immunol* (2007) 19:615–22. doi:10.1016/j.coi.2007.09.002
28. Fritz JH, Ferrero RL, Philpott DJ, Girardin SE. Nod-like proteins in immunity, inflammation and disease. *Nat Immunol* (2006) 7:1250–7. doi:10.1038/ni1412
29. Gabrielli E, Pericolini E, Luciano E, Sabbatini S, Roselletti E, Perito S, et al. Induction of caspase-11 by aspartyl proteinases of *Candida albicans* and implication in promoting inflammatory response. *Infect Immun* (2015) 83:1940–8. doi:10.1128/IAI.02895-14
30. He Y, Hara H, Núñez G. Mechanism and regulation of NLRP3 inflammasome activation. *Trends Biochem Sci* (2016) 41:1012–21. doi:10.1016/j.tibs.2016.09.002
31. Man SM, Kanneganti TD. Regulation of inflammasome activation. *Immunol Rev* (2015) 265:6–21. doi:10.1111/imr.12296
32. Said-Sadier N, Padilla E, Langsley G, Ojcius DM. *Aspergillus fumigatus* stimulates the NLRP3 inflammasome through a pathway requiring ROS production and the Syk tyrosine kinase. *PLoS One* (2010) 5:e10008. doi:10.1371/journal.pone.0010008
33. Wellington M, Koselny K, Sutterwala FS, Krysan DJ. *Candida albicans* triggers NLRP3-mediated pyroptosis in macrophages. *Eukaryot Cell* (2014) 13:329–40. doi:10.1128/EC.00336-13
34. Plato A, Hardison SE, Brown GD. Pattern recognition receptors in antifungal immunity. *Semin Immunopathol* (2015) 37:97–106. doi:10.1007/s00281-014-0462-4
35. Joly S, Sutterwala FS. Fungal pathogen recognition by the NLRP3 inflammasome. *Virulence* (2010) 1:276–80. doi:10.4161/viru.1.4.11482
36. Gross O, Poeck H, Bscheider M, Dostert C, Hannesschläger N, Endres SJ, et al. Syk kinase signalling couples to the Nlrp3 inflammasome for anti-fungal host defence. *Nature* (2009) 459:433–6. doi:10.1038/nature07965
37. Van De Veerdonk FL, Joosten LA, Shaw PJ, Smeekens SP, Malireddi RK, Van Der Meer JW, et al. The inflammasome drives protective Th1 and Th17 cellular responses in disseminated candidiasis. *Eur J Immunol* (2011) 41:2260–8. doi:10.1002/eji.201041226
38. Karki R, Man SM, Malireddi RK, Gurung P, Vogel P, Lamkanfi M, et al. Concerted activation of the AIM2 and NLRP3 inflammasomes orchestrates host protection against *Aspergillus* infection. *Cell Host Microbe* (2015) 17:357–68. doi:10.1016/j.chom.2015.01.006
39. Tavares AH, Magalhães KG, Almeida RD, Correa R, Burgel PH, Bocca AL. NLRP3 inflammasome activation by *Paracoccidioides brasiliensis*. *PLoS Negl Trop Dis* (2013) 7:e2595. doi:10.1371/journal.pntd.0002595
40. Ketelut-Carneiro N, Silva GK, Rocha FA, Milanezi CM, Cavalcanti-Neto FF, Zamboni DS, et al. IL-18 triggered by the Nlrp3 inflammasome induces host innate resistance in a pulmonary model of fungal infection. *J Immunol* (2015) 194:4507–17. doi:10.4049/jimmunol.1402321
41. Arruda C, Kashino SS, Fazioli RA, Calich VL. A primary subcutaneous infection with *Paracoccidioides brasiliensis* leads to immunoprotection or exacerbated disease depending on the route of challenge. *Microbes Infect* (2007) 9:308–16. doi:10.1016/j.micinf.2006.12.005
42. Kuida K, Lippke JA, Ku G, Harding MW, Livingston DJ, Su MS, et al. Altered cytokine export and apoptosis in mice deficient in interleukin-1 beta converting enzyme. *Science* (1995) 267:2000–3. doi:10.1126/science.7535475
43. Lara-Tejero M, Sutterwala FS, Ogura Y, Grant EP, Bertin J, Coyle AJ, et al. Role of the caspase-1 inflammasome in *Salmonella typhimurium* pathogenesis. *J Exp Med* (2006) 203:1407–12. doi:10.1084/jem.20060206
44. Sutterwala FS, Ogura Y, Szczepanik M, Lara-Tejero M, Lichtenberger GS, Grant EP, et al. Critical role for NALP3/CIAS1/cryopyrin in innate and adaptive immunity through its regulation of caspase-1. *Immunity* (2006) 24:317–27. doi:10.1016/j.immuni.2006.02.004
45. Solle M, Labasi J, Perregaux DG, Stam E, Petrushova N, Koller BH, et al. Altered cytokine production in mice lacking P2X(7) receptors. *J Biol Chem* (2001) 276:125–32. doi:10.1074/jbc.M006781200
46. Netto CF, Vegas VS, Sciannaméa IM, Guarnieri DB. The polysaccharidic antigen from *Paracoccidioides brasiliensis*. Study of the time of cultivation necessary for the preparation of the antigen. *Rev Inst Med Trop Sao Paulo* (1969) 11:177–81.
47. Cano LE, Singer-Vermes LM, Vaz CA, Russo M, Calich VLG. Pulmonary paracoccidioidomycosis in resistant and susceptible mice, relationship among progression of infection, bronchoalveolar cell activation, cellular immune response, and specific isotype patterns. *Infect Immun* (1995) 63:1777–83.
48. Singer-Vermes LM, Ciavaglia MC, Kashino S, Burger E, Calich VLG. The source of the growth-promoting factor(s) affects the plating efficiency of *Paracoccidioides brasiliensis*. *J Med Vet Mycol* (1992) 30:261–4. doi:10.1080/02681219280000331
49. Bazan SB, Costa TA, de Araújo EF, Feriotti C, Loures FV, Pretel FD, et al. Loss- and gain-of-function approaches indicate a dual role exerted by regulatory T cells in pulmonary paracoccidioidomycosis. *PLoS Negl Trop Dis* (2015) 9:e0004189. doi:10.1371/journal.pntd.0004189
50. Ribeiro LR, Loures FV, de Araújo EF, Feriotti C, Costa TA, Serezani CH, et al. Lipoxin inhibits fungal uptake by macrophages and reduces the severity of acute pulmonary infection caused by *Paracoccidioides brasiliensis*. *Mediators Inflamm* (2015) 2015:852574. doi:10.1155/2015/852574
51. Sollberger G, Strittmatter GE, Garstkiewicz M, Sand J, Beer HD. Caspase-1: the inflammasome and beyond. *Innate Immun* (2014) 20:115–25. doi:10.1177/1753425913484374
52. Lamkanfi M, Kalai M, Saelens X, Declercq W, Vandenabeele P. Caspase-1 activates nuclear factor of the kappa-enhancer in B cells independently of its enzymatic activity. *J Biol Chem* (2004) 279:24785–93. doi:10.1074/jbc.M400985200
53. Sarkar A, Duncan M, Hart J, Hertlein E, Guttridge DC, Wewers MD. Asc directs NF-kappaB activation by regulating receptor interacting protein-2 (Rip2) caspase-1 interactions. *J Immunol* (2006) 176:4979–86. doi:10.4049/jimmunol.176.8.4979
54. Miggin SM, Pålsson-McDermott E, Dunne A, Jefferies C, Pinteaux E, Banahan K, et al. NF- kappaB activation by the toll-IL-1 receptor domain protein MyD88 adapter-like is regulated by caspase-1. *Proc Natl Acad Sci U S A* (2007) 104:3372–7. doi:10.1073/pnas.0608100104
55. Kurokawa CS, Araujo JP Jr, Soares AM, Sugizaki MF, Peraçoli MT. Pro- and anti-inflammatory cytokines produced by human monocytes challenged in vitro with *Paracoccidioides brasiliensis*. *Microbiol Immunol* (2007) 51:421–8. doi:10.1111/j.1348-0421.2007.tb03929.x
56. Peraçoli M, Kurokawa CS, Calvi SA, Mendes RP, Pereira PC, Marques SA, et al. Production of pro- and anti-inflammatory cytokines by monocytes from patients with paracoccidioidomycosis. *Microbes Infect* (2003) 5:413–8. doi:10.1016/S1286-4579(03)00040-6

57. Amaral EP, Ribeiro SC, Lanes VR, Almeida FM, de Andrade MR, Bomfim CC, et al. Pulmonary infection with hypervirulent mycobacteria reveals a crucial role for the P2X7 receptor in aggressive forms of tuberculosis. *PLoS Pathog* (2014) 10(7):e1004188. doi:10.1371/journal.ppat.1004188
58. Darville T, Welter-Stahl L, Cruz C, Sater AA, Andrews CW Jr, Ojcius DM. Effect of the purinergic receptor P2X7 on *Chlamydia* infection in cervical epithelial cells and vaginally infected mice. *J Immunol* (2007) 179(3):707–14. doi:10.4049/jimmunol.179.6.3707
59. Figliuolo VR, Chaves SP, Savio LEB, Thorstenberg MLP, Salles EM, Takiya CM, et al. The role of the P2X7 receptor in murine cutaneous leishmaniasis: aspects of inflammation and parasite control. *Purinergic Signal* (2017) 13:143–52. doi:10.1007/s11302-016-9544-1
60. Lees MP, Fuller SJ, McLeod R, Boulter NR, Miller CM, Zakrzewski AM, et al. P2X7 receptor-mediated killing of an intracellular parasite, *Toxoplasma gondii*, by human and murine macrophages. *J Immunol* (2010) 184:7040–6. doi:10.4049/jimmunol.1000012
61. Mishra A, Guo Y, Zhang L, More S, Weng T, Chintagari NR, et al. A critical role for P2X7 receptor-induced VCAM-1 shedding and neutrophil infiltration during acute lung injury. *J Immunol* (2016) 197:2828–37. doi:10.4049/jimmunol.1501041
62. Dostert C, Ludigs K, Guarda G. Innate and adaptive effects of inflammasomes on T cell responses. *Curr Opin Immunol* (2013) 25:359–65. doi:10.1016/j.coi.2013.02.008
63. Bauernfeind F, Ablasser A, Bartok E, Kim S, Hornung V. Inflammasome: current understanding and open questions. *Cell Mol Life Sci* (2011) 68:765–83. doi:10.1007/s00018-010-0567-4
64. De Luca A, Zelante T, D'Angelo C, Zagarella S, Fallarino F, Spreca A, et al. IL-22 defines a novel immune pathway of antifungal resistance. *Mucosal Immunol* (2010) 3:361–73. doi:10.1038/mi.2010.22
65. Manel N, Unutmaz D, Littman DR. The differentiation of human T(H)-17 cells requires transforming growth factor-beta and induction of the nuclear receptor RORgammat. *Nat Immunol* (2008) 9:641–9. doi:10.1038/ni.1610
66. Acosta-Rodriguez EV, Rivino L, Geginat J, Jarrossay D, Gattorno M, Lanzavecchia A, et al. Surface phenotype and antigenic specificity of human interleukin 17-producing T helper memory cells. *Nat Immunol* (2007) 8:639–46. doi:10.1038/ni1467
67. Cano LE, Singer-Vermes LM, Mengel JA, Xidieh CF, Arruda C, André DC, et al. Depletion of CD8+ T cells in vivo impairs host defense of resistant and susceptible mice to pulmonary paracoccidioidomycosis. *Infect Immun* (2000) 68:352–9. doi:10.1128/IAI.68.1.352-359.2000
68. Chiarella AP, Arruda C, Pina A, Costa TA, Ferreira RC, Calich VL. The relative importance of CD4+ and CD8+ T cell in immunity to pulmonary paracoccidioidomycosis. *Microbes Infect* (2007) 9:1078–88. doi:10.1016/j.micinf.2007.04.016
69. Ben-Sasson SZ, Hu-Li J, Quiel J, Cauchetaux S, Ratner M, Shapira I, et al. IL-1 acts directly on CD4 T cells to enhance their antigen-driven expansion and differentiation. *Proc Natl Acad Sci U S A* (2009) 106:7119–24. doi:10.1073/pnas.0902745106
70. Nakanishi K, Yoshimoto T, Tsutsui H, Okamura H. Interleukin-18 is a unique cytokine that stimulates both Th1 and Th2 responses depending on its cytokine milieu. *Cytokine Growth Factor Rev* (2001) 12:53–72. doi:10.1016/S1359-6101(00)00015-0
71. Arruda C, Valente-Ferreira RC, Pina A, Kashino SS, Fazioli RA, Vaz CA. Dual role of interleukin-4 (IL-4) in pulmonary paracoccidioidomycosis: endogenous IL-4 can induce protection or exacerbation of disease depending on the host genetic pattern. *Infect Immun* (2004) 72:3932–40. doi:10.1128/IAI.72.7.3932-3940.2004
72. Hwang I, Yang J, Hong S, Ju Lee E, Lee SH, Fernandes-Alnemri T, et al. Non-transcriptional regulation of NLRP3 inflammasome signaling by IL-4. *Immunol Cell Biol* (2015) 93:591–9. doi:10.1038/icb.2014.125
73. Wang W, Wang X, Chun J, Vilaysane A, Clark S, French G, et al. Inflammasome-independent NLRP3 augments TGF-β signaling in kidney epithelium. *J Immunol* (2013) 190:1239–49. doi:10.4049/jimmunol.1201959

16

FIBCD1 Binds *Aspergillus fumigatus* and Regulates Lung Epithelial Response to Cell Wall Components

Christine Schoeler Jepsen[1†], *Lalit Kumar Dubey*[1,2†], *Kimmie B. Colmorten*[1], *Jesper B. Moeller*[1,3], *Mark A. Hammond*[1], *Ole Nielsen*[4], *Anders Schlosser*[1], *Steven P. Templeton*[5], *Grith L. Sorensen*[1] *and Uffe Holmskov*[1*]

[1] Cancer and Inflammation Research, Department of Molecular Medicine, University of Southern Denmark, Odense, Denmark, [2] Global Health Institute, School of Life Sciences, École Polytechnique Fédérale de Lausanne, Lausanne, Switzerland, [3] Jill Roberts Institute for Research in Inflammatory Bowel Disease, Weill Cornell Medicine, Cornell University, New York, NY, United States, [4] Department of Clinical Pathology, Odense University Hospital, Odense, Denmark, [5] Department of Microbiology and Immunology, Indiana University School of Medicine-Terre Haute, Terre Haute, IN, United States

***Correspondence:**
Uffe Holmskov
uholmskov@health.sdu.dk

† These authors have contributed equally to this work

Aspergillus fumigatus (*A. fumigatus*) is a ubiquitous fungus of clinical importance associated with development of various pulmonary diseases and allergic hypersensitivity reactions. It is protected against environmental stress by a cell wall that contains polysaccharides such as chitin. We previously demonstrated that fibrinogen C domain-containing protein 1 (FIBCD1) is a membrane-bound protein that binds chitin through a conserved S1 binding site and is expressed in intestinal epithelium and salivary glands. Here, we further localized FIBCD1 protein expression at the surface of bronchial and alveolar human lung epithelium, observed recognition of *A. fumigatus* cell wall with S1 site-independent recognition. We observed FIBCD1-mediated suppression of IL-8 secretion, mucin production, and transcription of genes associated with airway inflammation and homeostasis in FIBCD1-transfected lung epithelial cells. These modulations were generally enforced by stimulation with *A. fumigatus* cell wall polysaccharides. In parallel, we demonstrated a FIBCD1-mediated modulation of IL-8 secretion induced by TLR2,−4, and −5. Collectively, our findings support FIBCD1 as a human lung epithelial pattern recognition receptor that recognizes the complex *A. fumigatus* cell wall polysaccharides and modulates the lung epithelial inflammatory response by suppressing inflammatory mediators and mucins.

Keywords: FIBCD1, *Aspergillus fumigatus*, human, A549, lung, inflammation, IL-8, epithelium

INTRODUCTION

Aspergillus fumigatus (*A. fumigatus*) is a ubiquitous, filamentous fungus with the ability to cause invasive and allergic pulmonary diseases that is partly attributed to its ability to circumvent host immune defenses at airway mucosal sites (1–4). Humans inhale several hundred *A. fumigatus* conidia every day and their small size make them easily aerosolized and capable of reaching the lung alveoli. In healthy, immune-competent hosts, inhaled *A. fumigatus* conidia are cleared by innate defense mechanisms including mucociliary transport mechanisms and phagocytic activity of leukocytes, primarily residential macrophages and neutrophils recruited by epithelial secretion of chemotactic factors such as IL-8. Additionally, epithelial secretion of opsonizing mediators such as ficolins and complement components support the activity of these mechanisms (5, 6).

A cell wall, mainly composed of polysaccharides and secretory antigens, protects *A. fumigatus* conidia and hyphae against environmental stress (7). The structural skeleton of the cell wall is composed of chitin and galactomannan covalently bound to β-1,3-glucan (8), which are polysaccharide structures absent in mammals. Therefore, they serve as pathogen-associated molecular patterns (PAMPs) recognized by pattern recognition receptors (PRRs) on mammalian cells (9). The *A. fumigatus* cell wall is continuously remodeled during morphogenesis from inhaled, resting conidia to fully-grown hyphae (10). In resting conidia, the cell wall is protected by an additional layer of hydrophobic proteins and pigments, not produced in germ tubes and hyphae. This layer shields *A. fumigatus* cell wall PAMPs, which makes the resting conidia immunologically inert (9). During the first stages of germination, cell wall polysaccharides are hydrolyzed and *de novo* synthesis of cell wall components, e.g. chitin and β-1,3-glucan, is initiated (10). This causes the conidia to swell, disintegrating the outer layer and exposing cell wall PAMPs to host PRRs (9). Various PRRs are involved in the initiation, control, and resolution of the anti-*A. fumigatus* inflammatory response (11), including Toll-Like Receptors (TLRs) (5, 6) and the β-1,3-glucan receptor Dectin-1 (12). Several studies report a TLR-regulated anti-*A. fumigatus* response dependent on the fungus' morphotype (5, 6, 13). However, the underlying mechanisms remain unknown and may involve interplay between other PRRs that recognize *A. fumigatus*-associated PAMPs.

We have previously identified fibrinogen C domain-containing protein 1 (FIBCD1) as the first membrane-bound protein of the fibrinogen-related domain (FReD) superfamily (14). FIBCD1 is expressed as a tetramer on the apical surface of small and large intestinal epithelium and is composed of a cytoplasmic tail with three potential phosphorylation sites, a transmembrane region, and an ectodomain containing a coiled-coil region, a polycationic region, and a FReD (14). FIBCD1 exhibits calcium-dependent binding of acetylated structures including crab shell chitin through a conserved S1 binding site in FReD and facilitates endocytosis of bound ligands (14, 15). The crystal structure of FIBCD1-FReD (16) is homologous to FReD superfamily members involved in immune regulation, including ficolin-1 and −2 (17, 18). Both ficolin-1 and −2 recognize *A. fumigatus*-associated PAMPs (19, 20) and binds directly or indirectly to resting *A. fumigatus* conidia (21).

The aim of this study is to investigate the potential role of FIBCD1 in the immune response against *A. fumigatus*. We hypothesize that FIBCD1 is expressed in human lung epithelium and interacts with *A. fumigatus* by binding fungal cell wall chitin in the S1 binding site of FIBCD1-FReD. We hypothesize that interaction between FIBCD1 and ligand(s) modulates TLR- and lung epithelial cell-mediated inflammatory response to fungal cell wall components.

Abbreviations: acBSA, acetylated BSA; *A. fumigatus, Aspergillus fumigatus*; AIF, alkali-insoluble fraction; CNRQ, calibrated normalized relative quantity; DPBS, Dulbecco's PBS; FIBCD1, fibrinogen C domain-containing protein 1; FReD, fibrinogen-related domain; IAA, iodoacetamide; IHC, Immunohistochemical; MBL, mannan-binding lectin; MOPS, 3-(N-morpholino)propanesulfonic acid; MUC, mucin; PAMPs, pathogen-associated molecular patterns; PRR, pattern recognition receptor; qPCR, quantitative PCR; RT, room temperature; SD, sabouraud dextrose; WGA, wheat germ agglutinin.

METHODS AND MATERIALS

Buffers and Reagents

PBS: 140 mM NaCl, 3 mM KCl, 8 mM Na_2HPO_4, 1.5 mM KH_2PO_4. TBS: 10 mM Tris-base, 140 mM NaCl. SDS-PAGE sample buffer: 374 mM Tris-base, 40% (v/v) glycerol, 3 mM bromophenol blue, 8% (w/v) SDS. Acetylated BSA (acBSA), BSA, citric acid, EDTA, glycine, glycerol, silver nitrate ($AgNO_3$), SDS, sodium azide (NaN_3), Tris-base, Triton X-100, H_2SO_4, iodoacetamide (IAA), DTT, $CaCl_2$, sodium acetate, $NaHCO_3$, sterile PBS, curdlan (β-1,3-glucan, from *Alcaligenes faecalis*), RNase ZAP®, M-MLV reverse transcriptase, and oligo-dT primers were ordered from Sigma-Aldrich Co., St Louis, MO, United States. Alexa Fluor 488, Alexa Fluor 633-labeled wheat germ agglutinin (WGA), Gateway Technology® pDONR™-221 vector, 3-(N-morpholino)-propanesulfonic acid (MOPS) running buffer, RPMI media, FBS, L-glutamine, penicillin/streptomycin, hygromycin B, trypsin/EDTA, Dulbecco's PBS (DPBS), DMSO, TRIzol reagent, and RNaseOUT™ recombinant ribonuclease inhibitor were ordered from Invitrogen™, Thermo Fisher Scientific Inc., Waltham, MA, United states. Sabouraud dextrose (SD) agar, SD broth media, and 40-μm cell strainer were ordered from BD Biosciences, Franklin Lakes, NJ, United States. Acetic acid, bromophenol blue, formaldehyde, KCl, KH_2PO_4, NaCl, Na_2HPO_4, Na_2CO_3, NaOH, Tween 20, and mira cloth were ordered from Merck KGaA, Darmstadt, Germany. Four to twelve percent of polyacrylamide gradient gels, Precision Plus Protein™ KaleidoscopeTM Standards, and non-fat dry milk were ordered from Bio-Rad Laboratories, Inc., Hercules, CA, United States. Chitin beads were ordered from New England Biolabs Inc., Ipswich, Massachusetts, USA, and Dectin-1Fc was kindly provided by Prof Gordon Brown, Aberdeen University. HRP-conjugated rabbit anti-mouse Ig (#P0260), FITC-conjugated goat anti-mouse antibody (#F0479), and HRP-conjugated goat anti-rabbit Ig (#P0448) were ordered from Dako, Glostrup, Denmark. D-galacto-D-mannan (from Ceratonia Siliqua) and mouse monoclonal anti-GAPDH antibody (#sc32233) were ordered from Santa Cruz Biotechnologies, Inc., Dallas, TX, United States.

The anti-mucin (MUC) antibodies rabbit monoclonal anti-MUC-1 antibody (#ab45167), rabbit polyclonal anti-MUC-13 antibody (#ab65109), and mouse monoclonal anti-MUC-5AC antibody (#ab11335) were ordered from Abcam plc, Cambridge, United Kingdom. Protein G column, polyvinylidene difluoride membrane, filter paper, and ECL kit were ordered from GE Healthcare, Little Chalfont, United Kingdom. Ambion® nuclease-free water, custom TaqMan® array 96-well plates, and 2 X TaqMan® fast advanced master mix were ordered from Thermo Fisher Scientific Inc., Waltham, MA, United states.

The human TLR agonist kit was ordered from InvivoGen, San Diego, CA, United States. Alphazyme was ordered from PAA Laboratories GmbH, Pasching, Austria. O-phenylendiamid was ordered from Kem-En-Tec Diagnostics A/S, Taastrup, Denmark. Human CXCL8/IL-8 DuoSet kit was ordered from R&D Systems, Inc., Minneapolis, MN, United states. Limulus amebocyte lysate assay (QCL-1000™) was ordered from Lonza Group Ltd., Basel, Switzerland. Protease inhibitor cocktail tablets were ordered from Roche Diagnostics, Basel, Switzerland. Commercial cDNA library and FIBCD1 PerfectProbe™ assay were ordered from Primerdesign Ltd., United Kingdom. JetPEI transfection reagents were ordered from Polyplus transfection SA, Illkirch, France. Monoclonal anti-ovalbumin antibody was ordered from SSI, Copenhagen, Denmark. The murine Sp2/mIl-6 (CRL-2016) myeloma cells and human lung carcinoma type II epithelial-like A549 cell line were purchased from the American type culture collection (Rockville, MD, USA).

Real Time Analysis of FIBCD1 Expression in Human Tissues

The relative tissue distribution of human FIBCD1 mRNA was quantitated using a commercial cDNA library and a custom made FIBCD1 PerfectProbe™ assay with the primer sequences 5′-CACCGTGGCTGACTATTCC-3′ and 5′-TTCTCTGAATGGTCGCTGTC-3′. Analysis was performed in triplicates using the cycling conditions: 95°C for 10 min, followed by 50 cycles of 95°C for 15 s, 60°C for 30 s and 72°C for 15 s. The study was performed on a 7500 Real-time PCR system (Applied Biosystems®, Thermo Fisher Scientific Inc., Waltham, MA, USA) using 18S RNA for normalization.

Expression and Purification of Recombinant FIBCD1-FReD (rfibcd1-FReD)

rFIBCD1-FReD was expressed in insect cells and purified on N-acetylated immobilized resin as described previously (15).

Production of Monoclonal Anti-FIBCD1 Antibodies

Mouse monoclonal anti-FIBCD1 antibodies HG-HYB-12-2,−12-5, and −12-6 were produced as previously described (14). Mouse monoclonal anti-FIBCD1-FReD antibody HYB-11-14-25 was produced by immunization of *Fibcd1*$^{-/-}$ C57BL6/n mice. The mice were immunized twice with 20 µg of rFIBCD1-FReD using GERBU as adjuvant with more than 2 weeks between each immunization. The mice were boosted once by an intra-peritoneal injection with 20 µg rFIBCD1-FReD without adjuvant 3 days before isolation of B cells. Hybridoma cells were produced by fusion between isolated B cells and myeloma cells and adapted for serum-free media. Secreted antibodies were purified using a protein G column on a fast protein liquid chromatography apparatus (ÄKTA, GE Healthcare, Little Chalfont, United Kingdom). These experiments were performed under license from the National Animal Experiments Inspectorate (reference no. 2012-15-2934-00076).

Immunohistochemical Analysis of FIBCD1 in Human Lung Tissue

Human tissues were obtained from the tissue bank at the Department of Pathology, Odense University Hospital (Odense, Denmark). The tissues were fixed in 4% formalin in PBS for 24 h and then conventionally dehydrated and embedded in paraffin. A biotin-streptavidin immunoperoxidase technique was used on paraffin sections. Paraffin sections were pre-treated in TEG buffer (10 mmol/L Tris, 0.5 mmol/L EGTA, pH 9) in a microwave oven for three 5 min periods at 650 W. The sections were left in TEG buffer for 15 min, washed in TBS, pre-incubated with 2% (w/v) BSA in TBS for 10 min, and incubated for 30 min with the mouse anti-human FIBCD1 (HG-HYB-12-2, 0.5 mg/mL) in TBS containing 15% (w/v) BSA and otherwise processed as described by Madsen et al. (22). The specificity of the immuno-staining was verified by replacing the primary antibody with a non-specific antibody. The local ethical committee in Odense approved the use of human tissue samples (ref. no: VF20050070).

Fungal Strain and Growth Conditions

A. fumigatus conidia (101355, Centraalbureau von Schimmelcultures, Utrecht, Netherlands) were cultivated on SD agar plates at 37°C for 5 days and harvested using PBS/0.5% Tween, washed, and used immediately or stored at 4°C. *A. fumigatus* germination was obtained by inoculating SD broth media with freshly-harvested conidia (less than a week after harvest) and incubating at 37°C. For production of a 1-week-culture, 10^4 freshly-harvested conidia were added per mL media in an Erlenmeyer flask containing 1:4 volume media and incubating at 37°C, 100–140 rpm for 7 days.

Alexa Fluor 488-Labeling of rFIBCD1-FReD

Purified protein (2 mg/mL) was labeled with Alexa Fluor 488 in a 1:9 molar ratio at RT for 1–2 h according to manufacturer's recommendations followed by extensive dialysis against PBS to remove excess dye. Activity of labeled rFIBCD1-FReD was tested by binding to acBSA. Labeled protein was stored at 4°C until used.

Staining of *A. fumigatus*

Staining of *A. fumigatus* was performed by a modification of previously described methods (23) and imaged using an Olympus IX71 fluorescence microscope equipped with four laser optics and F-view fluorescence CCD camera (Olympus Corporation, Tokyo, Japan). All images were acquired and processed using Cell^F soft imaging software (Olympus Corporation, Tokyo, Japan).

Preparation of *A. fumigatus* Alkali-Insoluble Fraction (AIF)

A. fumigatus cell wall component suspension (i.e., alkali-insoluble fraction) was prepared as previously described with minor modifications (8). Briefly, mycelium was harvested from one-week-culture by filtration through mira cloth, washed with distilled PBS, and subjected to three hot alkali treatments (distilled 1 M NaOH, 65°C heat bath, 30 min), each followed by five washes with distilled water and one with distilled TBS at

10,000 × g for 10 min. The product was grinded with mortar and pestle, washed with sterile PBS, forced through a 40 μm cell strainer, pH adjusted to ~7, added 0.05% NaN_3, and the final product stored at 4°C. AIF was tested for endotoxin contamination using a limulus amebocyte lysate assay revealing an endotoxin level below 0.25 endotoxin units per mL. The absence of protein was confirmed by boiling AIF 1:2 in SDS-PAGE sample buffer on a 99°C heating block for 1 min and separating eluted protein on a 4–12% polyacrylamide gradient gel using MOPS running buffer and subsequently silver staining the gel as described in the following section. The concentration was determined by vacuum drying using a MAXI-dry vacuum centrifuge (Heto-Holten A/S, Alleroed, Denmark) at 55°C, 1,300 rpm.

Pull Down Assay

For protein staining, 2 mg of AIF was washed three times with TBS/0.05% Tween/5 mM $CaCl_2$ and incubated at 4°C overnight with 20 μg/mL Dectin-1Fc, recombinant mannan-binding lectin (rMBL), WGA, and rFIBCD1-FReD in a total volume of 1 mL. Pull down was performed by centrifugation at 4°C, 10,000 × g for 5 min. The insoluble pellets were washed three times with TBS/0.05% Tween/5 mM $CaCl_2$ and bound protein was eluted by boiling the pellets in SDS-PAGE sample buffer for 1 min. For Western blotting, 2 mg AIF and β-1,3-glucan and 200 μL chitin beads were washed three times with TBS/0.05% Tween and incubated at 4°C overnight with 5 μg/mL rFIBCD1-FReD in a total volume of 1 mL TBS/0.05% Tween supplemented with 5 mM $CaCl_2$, 10 mM EDTA, or 100 mM sodium acetate. Pull down was performed by centrifugation at 5,000 rpm (Minispin, Eppendorf AG, Hamburg, Germany) for 5 min. The insoluble pellets were washed three times with TBS/0.05% Tween supplemented with 5 mM $CaCl_2$, 10 mM EDTA, or 100 mM sodium acetate and bound protein was eluted by boiling the pellets in SDS-PAGE sample buffer on a 99°C heating block for 1 min. Pull down of mutant FIBCD1-FReD (A432V) by AIF and chitin beads was performed as previously described (15). Eluted protein was separated by SDS-PAGE on a 4–12% polyacrylamide gradient gel using MOPS running buffer and analyzed by silver staining or Western blotting as described in the following section.

Silver Staining

Silver staining of proteins separated by SDS-PAGE was performed as previously described (24) with some modifications (**Supplementary Datasheet 2**).

Generation of A549 Cells Expressing Full Length of FIBCD1

To generate A549 cells stably expressing full length FIBCD1, the cells were transfected with the expression vector pDEST-FIBCD1 using JetPEI transfection reagents according to manufacturer's instructions. The pDEST-FIBCD1 vector was constructed using Gateway Technology® and keeping to the recommendations of the manufacturer using cDNA containing the open reading frame of FIBCD1, donor vector pDONR™-221, and destination vector pDEST. A corresponding sham-transfected isogenic control cell type was constructed using a pDEST-sham vector. Cells were selected for stable integration of vectors using 500 μg/mL of hygromycin B. Successful expression of FIBCD1 protein was confirmed by Western blotting of cell lysates (**Supplementary Datasheet 2**) and surface expression of FIBCD1 was confirmed by flow cytometry. Unless otherwise stated, A549 cells were maintained in serial passages at 37°C, 5% CO_2 humidity in RPMI media supplemented with 10% FBS, 2 mM L-glutamine, 250 μg/mL hygromycin B, 50 U/mL penicillin, and 50 μg/mL streptomycin. When confluent, cells were subcultured by washing twice in sterile DPBS, detaching with 1 mL 0.5% trypsin/EDTA/sterile DPBS, and diluted using fresh complete media.

Flow Cytometry

A549 cells were harvested by incubation with alphazyme and centrifugation at 350 × g for 5 min. Cells were suspended in media, counted using a haemocytometer, portioned out in minisorp tubes (10^6 cells/tube), pelleted by centrifugation, and supernatant removed. The cells were incubated on ice for 2 h with 0.1 mg/mL monoclonal mouse anti-FIBCD1 antibody HG-HYB-12-5 in PBS/0.5% BSA diluted 1:2 in 100 μL cell suspension. Monoclonal anti-ovalbumin antibody was used as an isotype control. Then, the cells were washed three times and incubated in darkness on ice for 1 h with FITC-conjugated goat anti-mouse antibody diluted 1:10 in PBS/0.5% BSA and 1:2 in 100 μL cell suspension. Finally, the cells were washed three times, diluted in 1.5 mL PBS/0.5% BSA, and analyzed on a Benson Dickinson FACS Calibur (BD Biosciences, Franklin Lakes, NJ, United States) using CELL Quest™ (BD Biosciences, Franklin Lakes, NJ, United States) and FlowJo 8.8.6 software (FlowJo, LLC, Ashland, OR, United States).

Cell Culture Stimulation Conditions, Relative Gene Expression, and Protein Expression

For stimulations of transfected cells, A549 cells transfected with sham and FIBCD1, respectively, were harvested by incubation with 0.5% trypsin/EDTA in DPBS and centrifugation at 350 × g for 5 min. Cells were suspended in media, counted using a haemocytometer, and seeded at a density of 10^6 cells/well/2 mL media in 6-well culture plates or 250,000 cells/well/0.5 mL media in 24-well culture plates (80% confluence). After ~8 h, the adherent cells were washed with sterile DPBS, added 2 or 0.5 mL serum-free media, and incubated overnight. Then, cells were stimulated by removing the media and adding 2 mL of fresh serum-free media containing 100 μL conidia, AIF, β-1,3-glucan, chitin, galactomannan, or acBSA (ligand control) diluted in sterile DPBS or 0.5 mL of fresh serum-free media containing 22.2 μL human TLR agonist diluted in endotoxin-free water to each well and incubating 0, 4, and 8 h. All stimulations were performed as technical duplicates and biological triplicates.

At each time point, culture supernatant was removed from the cells and used for detection of secreted IL-8 by use of the human CXCL8/IL-8 DuoSet kit and keeping to the recommendations of the manufacturer. For RNA analysis, the cells were washed with DPBS, added TRIzol Reagent, and stored at −20°C. Total RNA was isolated from cells stimulated 8 h with 500 μg/mL AIF, β-1,3-glucan, or chitin, and cells incubated with DPBS for 8 h as a reference. TRIzol Reagent from technical duplicates of stimulated cells was pooled together, while five biological replicates from DPBS-incubated cells were pooled together to three independent samples. Total RNA was isolated from TRIzol Reagent according to the recommendations of the manufacturer in a fume cupboard treated with RNase ZAP®. cDNA synthesis by M-MLV reverse transcriptase and oligo-dT primers was subsequently performed in keep with manufacturer's instructions. The RNA concentration and purity (260/280) was determined by NanoDrop® ND-1000 spectrophotometry (Thermo Fisher Scientific Inc., Waltham, MA, United states). Then, quantitative PCR (qPCR) was performed targeting 21 different genes involved in immunological response and barrier function (CCL2, CCL5, CCL20, CXCL2, CSF2RA, TNF, TSLP, IL1B, IL6 IL8, IL10, IL12B, IL13, IL25, IL33, MUC1, MUC13, MUC5AC, TJP1, OCLN, ICAM1) and two housekeeping genes (GAPDH, TBP) for normalization. Custom TaqMan® Array 96-well Plates containing dried assay of these genes were added 10 μL cDNA diluted 1:2 in 2 X TaqMan® fast advanced master mix as single copies and qPCR was performed according to the recommendations of the manufacturer using a StepOnePlus™ Real-Time PCR System (Applied Biosystems®, Thermo Fisher Scientific Inc., Waltham, MA, USA) and StepOne™ v2.1 software (Applied Biosystems®, Thermo Fisher Scientific Inc., Waltham, MA, USA). A no-template control was included to exclude DNA contamination. Relative expression of the genes was calculated by qBase plus software (Biogazelle, Gent, Belgium), which uses threshold cycle values of target genes and reference genes to determine calibrated normalized relative quantities (CNRQs). For protein analysis, cells were washed twice with DPBS, added 11 μL/cm^2 RIPA buffer/protease inhibitors (1 tablet per 50 mL)/phosphatase inhibitors (1 tablet per 10 mL), and incubated on a shaker at 4°C for 60 min. Cellular debris were sedimented by centrifugation at 4°C, 10,000 rpm (Sigma 1-16 k refrigerated centrifuge, Sigma-Aldrich Co., St Louis, MO, United States) for 5 min and supernatants were stored at −20°C. Protein concentrations were determined by Bradford in accordance with the recommendations of the manufacturer and samples were prepared for SDS-PAGE by boiling three parts cell lysate with one part SDS-PAGE sample buffer on a 99°C heating block for 1 min. The samples were alkylated by adding one tenth 1.4 M IAA, separated on a 4–12% polyacrylamide gradient gel (19 μg protein per well) using MOPS running buffer, and analyzed by Western blotting as described in the following section.

Western Blotting

Proteins separated by SDS-PAGE were transferred onto a polyvinylidene difluoride membrane by semidry electroblotting (1.2 mA/cm^2 for 1 h or 0.2 mA/cm^2 overnight) using transfer buffer (75 mM Tris-base/39 mM glycine/0.037% (w/v) SDS/20% ethanol) and blocked with TBS/0.5 M NaCl/0.1% Tween/5% non-fat dry milk at 4°C for several hours. FIBCD1 was detected by probing the blot with 2 μg/mL mouse monoclonal anti-FIBCD1 antibody HG-HYB-12-2 or mouse monoclonal anti-FIBCD1-FReD antibody HYB-11-14-25 diluted in TBS/0.5 M NaCl/0.1 % Tween/2.5% non-fat dry milk at 4°C overnight. Mucins were detected by probing the blot with 0.22 μg/mL rabbit monoclonal anti-MUC-1 antibody, 2 μg/mL rabbit polyclonal anti-MUC-13 antibody, or 6.6 μg/mL mouse monoclonal anti-MUC-5AC antibody in 20 mL TBS/0.5 M NaCl/0.1% Tween/2.5% non-fat dry milk at 4°C overnight. Mouse monoclonal anti-GAPDH antibody (0.01 μg/mL) was used as control. Excess antibody was removed by extensive washing with TBS/0.5 M NaCl/0.1% Tween and the blot was incubated 1 h with either HRP-conjugated rabbit anti-mouse antibody diluted 1:10,000 or HRP-conjugated goat anti-rabbit antibody diluted 1:20,000 in TBS/0.5 M NaCl/0.1% Tween. The blot was washed, developed using ECL standard method, detected by Fusion Fx7 (Vilber Lourmat, Collégien, France), and depicted using FUSION-CAPT version 15.18 software (Vilber Lourmat, Collégien, France). Precision Plus Protein™ Kaleidoscope™ Standards were used as size markers. Between incubations with anti-mucin and -GAPDH antibodies, the membrane was stripped and blocked. Stripping was achieved by washing once with TBS/0.5 M NaCl/0.1% Tween, boiling in deionized water for 10 min, and washing twice with TBS/0.5 M NaCl/0.1% Tween.

Expression of Results and Statistics

Unless otherwise stated, data are expressed as mean ± SEM and differences were considered to be statistically significant when $p < 0.05$. Log2-transformed IL-8 secretion data was analyzed by one- or two-way ANOVA with Tukey's *post-hoc* tests depending on the number of independent variables using Prism software (version 6.0d, Graphpad, San Diego, CA, USA). Multilevel mixed-effects linear regression models were used to determine whether changed RNA expression of various genes was associated with stimulant, genotype, or a combined effect of these variables using the XTMIXED function of STATA13 (STATA Corp, College Station, TX, USA). Genes were analyzed separately using multilevel mixed-effects linear regression models to compensate for random effects. Log2 (CNRQ) was outcome, while stimulant, genotype, and interaction between these were fixed effects, and biological triplicate and culture plate variation were random effects (**Table S1**). Final models were evaluated for normality by prediction of residuals and assessment of their normal distribution by graphic (qq-plot, histogram, and box plot) and numeric methods (Skewness/Kurtosis and Shapiro-Wilk tests). *P*-values were extracted from the models using the LINCOM function.

RESULTS

FIBCD1 Is Expressed on the Apical Surface of Human Bronchial and Alveolar Epithelial Cells

We have previously shown that FIBCD1 is expressed apically by epithelial cells of mucous membranes, i.e. the small and large intestine and salivary glands (14), and therefore hypothesized that it is also expressed in the lung mucosal membrane. First, we determined FIBCD1 mRNA expression in a series of human tissues (**Figure 1A**). The highest expressional levels were found in the respiratory tract (lung and trachea), gastrointestinal tract (colon and small intestine), testis, placenta, and brain. Then, we performed an immunohistochemical (IHC) analysis of human, non-cancerous lung tissue (control) from patients with lung cancer (**Figures 1B–E**) and from patients with pulmonary *A. fumigatus* infection (**Figures 1F–I**). FIBCD1 immunostaining was detected in submucosal glands, alveoli, and bronchioles with more intense staining coincident with areas of inflammation (**Figures 1G,H**). Bronchiolar FIBCD1 was restricted to the apical surface of ciliated epithelial cells (**Figures 1E,I**) similar to the expression observed in the gastrointestinal tract (14). Similar results were observed by von Huth et al. (25) in non-malignant, non-inflammatory, and histologically normal, human tissues. Thus, FIBCD1 is expressed apically in the lung mucosal membrane and seemingly increased in areas of inflammation.

FIBCD1 Binds to *A. fumigatus* Dependent on Cell Wall PAMP Availability

We next examined if FIBCD1 is capable of recognizing *A. fumigatus* hyphae. Fluorescence microscopy revealed FIBCD1 recognition of fully-grown hyphae (**Figures 2A,B**), including chitin-rich septum regions (**Figures 2C,D**) and mycelial frame of budding hyphae (**Figures 2E,F**). We further examined co-localization between the chitin-binding fluorescent-labeled WGA and FIBCD1 in different morphological stages. Co-localization was observed in all stages characterized by exposed cell wall polysaccharides including swollen conidia, germ tubes, budding regions, and growing hyphae (**Figure 2G**), while no binding of FIBCD1 observed on resting conidia (**Figure S1**). Thus, FIBCD1 binds to *A. fumigatus* dependent on cell wall PAMP availability.

FIBCD1 Recognizes a Composite Structure in AIF Not Exclusively Through the S1 Binding Site

To evaluate if FIBCD1 binds fungal chitin, we isolated the chitin-containing structural skeleton of the *A. fumigatus* cell wall (AIF) and performed a pull-down assay (**Figure 3A**). We show that rFIBCD1-FReD binds AIF and pull-down using Dectin-1 fc, rMBL, and WGA demonstrated that cell wall components β-1,3-glucan, galactomannan, and chitin, respectively, were preserved after treatment (12, 26). We observed bands corresponding to FIBCD1-FReD monomeric, dimeric, trimeric, and tetrameric structures, at ~25, 50, 75, and 100 kDa, respectively, and large Dectin-1 fc structures of ~120 and 300 kDa. We observed bands corresponding to higher polymeric structures of rMBL, which assembles into trimers and hexamers of trimers. The smallest rMBL band is ~30 kDa, which is comparable to the rMBL monomer. Finally, we observed a band corresponding to the WGA monomer at ~18 kDa.

FIBCD1 exhibits calcium-dependent binding of chitin and other acetylated compounds through a conserved S1 hydrophobic pocket of the FReD (14, 15). Therefore, we hypothesized that FIBCD1 binds *A. fumigatus* AIF through a similar mechanism. To investigate this, we performed a pull-down assay using AIF in the presence or absence of calcium and

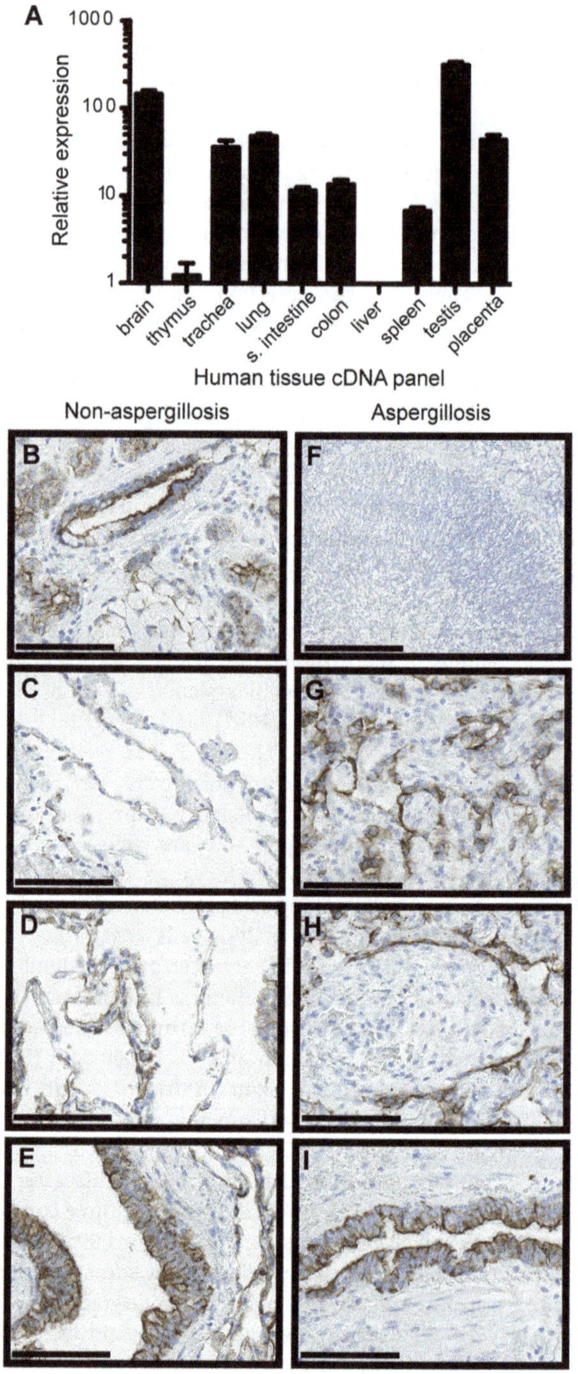

FIGURE 1 | FIBCD1 RNA is expressed in various human tissues and FIBCD1 protein is expressed on the apical site of lung epithelium and within submucosal glands. **(A)** Relative expression of FIBCD1 mRNA in various human tissues relative to expression in thymus. Technical triplicates. **(B–E)** IHC staining of FIBCD1 in non-cancerous lung tissue from a 68-year-old female patient with adenocarcinoma (scale bars: 100 μm, magnification: 40X). FIBCD1 was detected in submucosal glands **(B)**, non-inflamed alveoli **(C)**, inflamed alveoli **(D)**, and inflamed bronchioles **(E)**. **(G–I)** IHC staining of FIBCD1 in lung tissue from a 63-year-old male patient with *A. fumigatus* infiltration (scale bars: 100 μm, magnification: 40X). Formation of aspergilloma was observed (**F**, scale bar: 200 μm, magnification: 20X) and FIBCD1 was detected in alveoli with atelectasis **(G)** and pneumonia **(H)** and in bronchioles **(I)**.

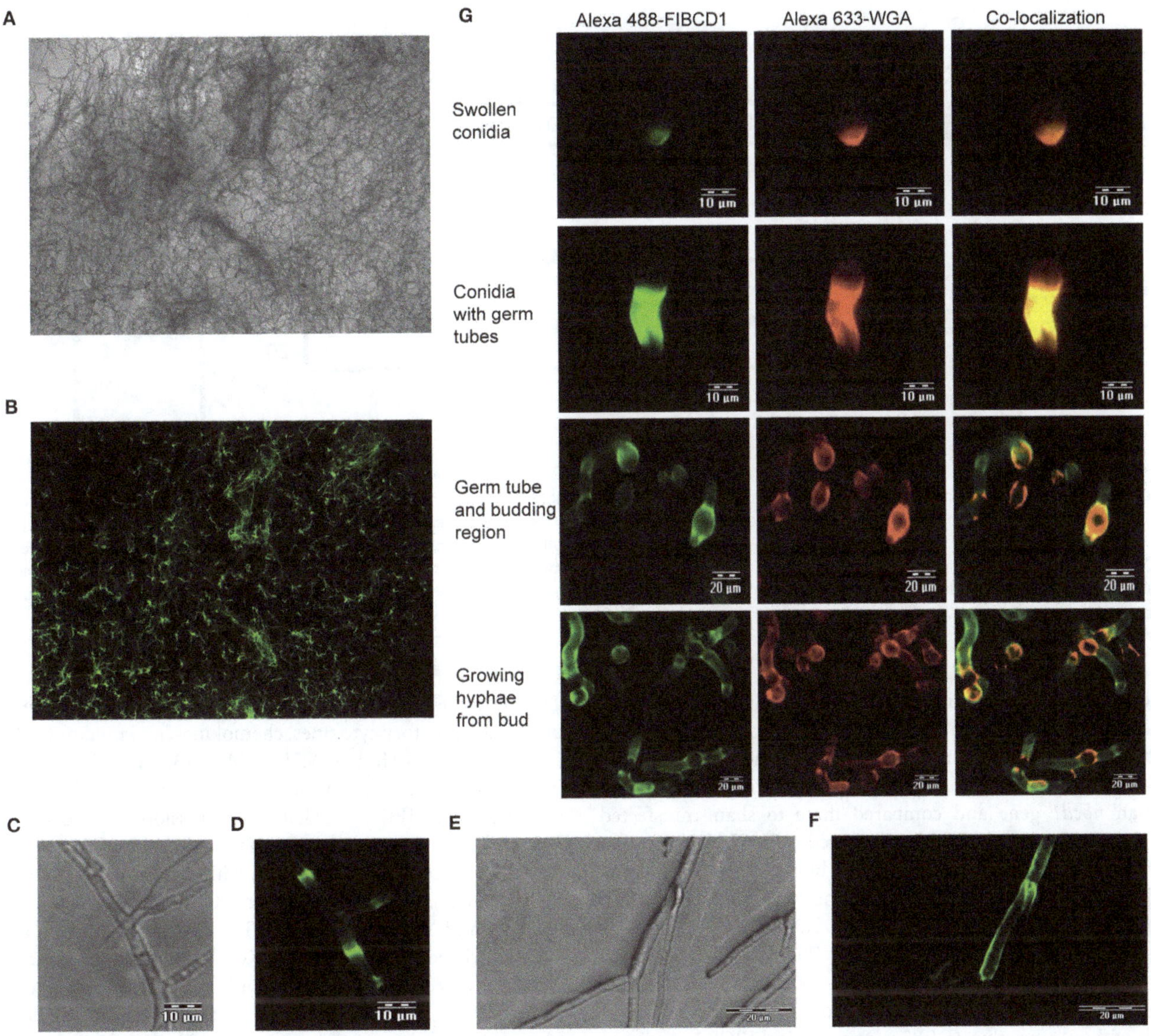

FIGURE 2 | FIBCD1 recognizes chitin-rich regions of *A. fumigatus* during different life stages. Bright field **(A,C,E)** and fluorescence **(B,D,F,G)** microscopy of *A. fumigatus*. **(A,B)** A total of 10^7 *A. fumigatus* conidia/mL was grown in SD medium to form fungal hyphae followed by staining with Alexa 488-labeled FIBCD1 as described in materials and methods. A clear recognition of fungal hyphae by FIBCD1 was observed. Image: 10X objective. **(C–F)** $5{\cdot}10^6$ *A. fumigatus* conidia/mL were grown in SD broth medium and stained with Alexa 488-labeled FIBCD1. rhFIBCD1 recognized the chitin-rich *A. fumigatus* septum of fully-grown hyphae. Image 40X and 20X objectives. **(G)** 10^4 *A. fumigatus* conidia/mL was grown in SD medium for various time points (6, 8, and 12 h) at 37°C and stained with Alexa 633-labeled WGA and Alexa 488-labeled FIBCD1. FIBCD1 failed to bind resting conidia (**Figure S1**). We observed co-localization of regions recognized by Alexa 488-labeled FIBCD1 and Alexa 633-labeled WGA.

acetate (**Figure 3B**). The insoluble, separate cell wall components β-1,3-glucan and chitin (beads) were used as negative and positive control, respectively (14). Surprisingly, our results show that FIBCD1 binding of AIF is calcium-independent and less sensitive to acetate than purified chitin, suggesting that FIBCD1 binds AIF through additional binding sites outside the S1 binding pocket, potentially involving other polysaccharide structures found in AIF. Therefore, we performed a pull-down assay of wild type FIBCD1-FReD and FIBCD1-FReD with a site-directed mutagenesis abolishing the binding properties of the S1 binding site, A432V (15), using AIF and chitin beads (positive control) (**Figure 3C**). Our results show that FIBCD1-FReD is capable of binding AIF when the binding activity of the S1 binding site is disrupted.

FIBCD1 Overexpression Suppresses IL-8 Secretion After Stimulation With *A. fumigatus* AIF and Galactomannan

A549 lung epithelial cells secrete IL-8 after exposure to *A. fumigatus* irradiated conidia and mycelium (27), and we confirmed a time- and dose-dependent induction of IL-8

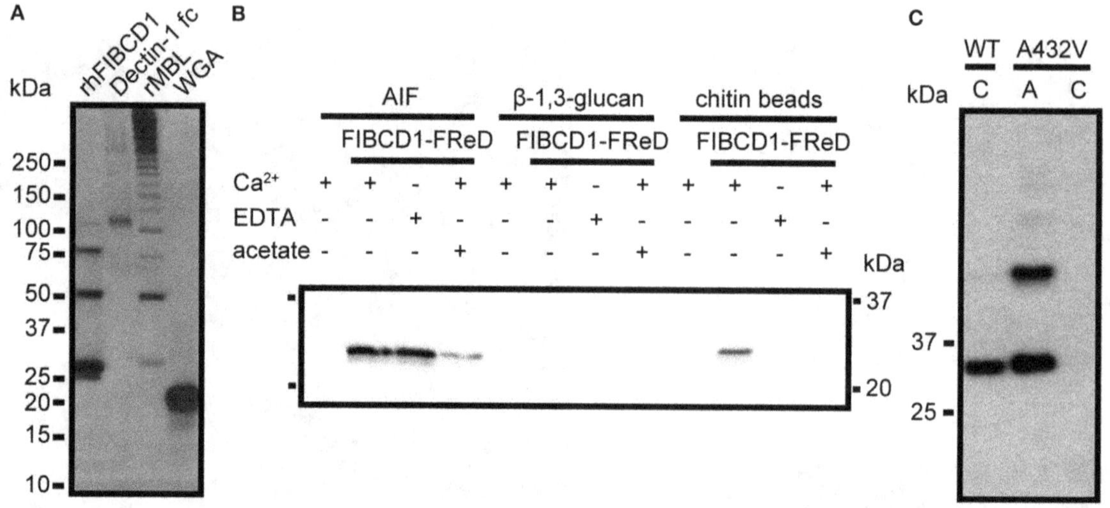

FIGURE 3 | rFIBCD1-FReD binds *A. fumigatus* AIF calcium- and acetate-independently. **(A)** The presence and binding activity of β-1,3-glucan, galactomannan, and chitin in AIF was validated by pull down of know ligands Dectin-1 fc, rMBL, and WGA. The samples were subjected to SDS-PAGE and analyzed by silver staining. Color is adjusted to gray scale. **(B)** Western blot showing FIBCD1-FReD pull down by AIF-associated polysaccharides in the presence of calcium (5 mM $CaCl_2$), EDTA (10 mM), and acetate (100 mM). 2 mg of AIF, β-1,3-glucan, and chitin beads were incubated with 5 μg/mL FIBCD1-FReD and pull down was performed as described. Data represent three independent experiments. **(C)** Western blot showing wild type and A432V mutant FIBCD1-FReD pull down by chitin beads and AIF. Color is adjusted to gray scale. Lane 1, 3: chitin beads, Lane 2: AIF.

following stimulation with live conidia and AIF (**Figure S2**). Since A549 cells constitutively expressed low or non-detectable levels of FIBCD1 protein (**Figure 4B**, top panel), we increased FIBCD1 expression by transfecting A549 cells with the full-length human *fibcd1* gene and compared these to sham-transfected A549 cells. In A549 FIBCD1-transfected cells, FIBCD1 protein expression was confirmed by Western blot analysis (**Figure 4A**) and surface expression by flow cytometry (**Figure 4B**, bottom panel). Stimulation of the transfected A549 cells with AIF, β-1,3-glucan, chitin, or galactomannan (**Figures 4C–L**) resulted in time- and dose-dependent IL-8 secretion. FIBCD1 over-expression mediated basal suppression of IL-8 secretion in cells without stimulus (DPBS alone). This FIBCD1-mediated IL-8 suppression was abolished during stimulation with β-1,3-glucan (**Figures 4E,F**) and chitin (**Figures 4G,H**). Chitin induced a very low IL-8 response, while β-1,3-glucan induced a high IL-8 response in both cell types. However, FIBCD1-mediated suppression of IL-8 secretion was increased by stimulation with AIF (**Figures 4C,D**) and galactomannan (**Figures 4I,J**). A similar response was observed against the positive control ligand acBSA (**Figures 4K,L**). Hence, FIBCD1 overexpression suppresses IL-8 secretion and maintains this suppression after stimulation with *A. fumigatus* AIF and galactomannan.

FIBCD1 Suppresses Mucin and Inflammatory Gene Expression and Increases Expression of Genes Involved in Mucosal Barrier Function

Next, we investigated the effect of FIBCD1 transfection on lung epithelial and immune response gene expression after incubation with AIF, β-1,3-glucan, and chitin (**Figure 5** and **Table S1**). Transfected FIBCD1 expression suppressed the RNA expression of proinflammatory cytokines, chemokines, and mucins (CCL20, CSF2RA, TNF, IL1B, IL8, MUC1, MUC13, and MUC5AC) and increased RNA expression of barrier function proteins (OCLN and ICAM1). FIBCD1-mediated suppression of CCL20, IL1B, IL8, and ICAM1 was reversed in the presence of β-1,3-glucan or chitin. In contrast, stimulation with AIF generally increased FIBCD1-mediated suppression of CCL2, CSF2RA, IL1B, IL8, MUC13, and MUC5AC and FIBCD1-mediated induction of the Th2-associated cytokine IL12B. CXCL2, IL6, IL10, IL25, and IL33 were not detected (data not shown). We further evaluated the protein expression of genes with threshold cycle values below 25 (data not shown) regulated at least 2-fold by FIBCD1 expression and not already examined (MUC-1, MUC-13, and MUC-5AC) (**Figure 6**). In keep with the qPCR data, we observed FIBCD1-mediated suppression of MUC-1,−13, and −5AC in the presence or absence of AIF. Increased FIBCD1-mediated suppression in the presence of AIF was only observed on MUC-13 and −5AC. Thus, FIBCD1 overexpression suppresses mucins and inflammatory gene expression and increases expression of genes involved in mucosal barrier function.

FIBCD1 Influences IL-8 Secretion From A549 Lung Epithelial Cells in Response to TLR2, TLR4, and TLR5 Agonists

Finally, we examined whether FIBCD1 expression modulated TLR-induced IL-8 secretion by stimulating A549 sham- and FIBCD1-transfected cells with 10 different TLR agonists and measuring IL-8 levels in culture supernatants (**Figure 7**). We found that FIBCD1 in particular suppressed TLR2 and −4 agonist-induced IL-8 secretion and that TLR5 agonist

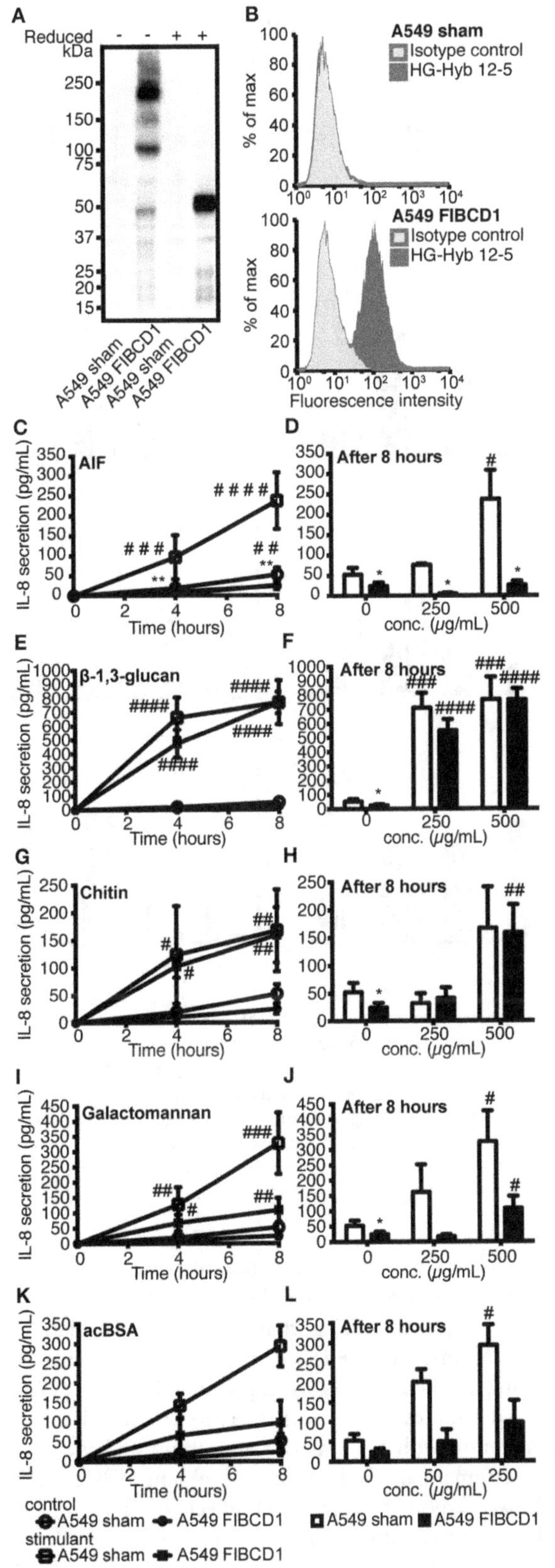

FIGURE 4 | Overexpression of FIBCD1 on the surface of A549 cells inhibits secretion of IL-8. The phenotype of sham- and FIBCD1-transfected A549 cells *(Continued)*

FIGURE 4 | was analyzed by Western blotting **(A)** and flow cytometry **(B)**. **(A)** Western blot of cell lysate from sham- and FIBCD1-transfected A549 cells under reducing and non-reducing conditions revealed the presence of four known oligomeric forms of FIBCD1 in the FIBCD1-transfected cells when probed with the anti-FIBCD1 mAb clone HG-HYB 12-2. **(B)** Flow cytometry of sham- and FIBCD1-transfected A549 cells showed surface expression of FIBCD1 on FIBCD1-transfected cells and none on sham-transfected cells when using anti-FIBCD1 antibody HG-HYB 12-5 for detection. **(C–L)** A549 sham- and FIBCD1-transfected cells were seeded at a density of one million cells in 2 mL of media per well of a 6-well tissue culture plate and serum-starved overnight prior to stimulation with two different concentrations of several components associated with *A. fumigatus* or FIBCD1 for 0, 4, and 8 h and the concentration of secreted IL-8 was determined by sandwich ELISA as described. Left column: Time-dependent IL-8 secretion to 1,000 μg AIF **(C)**, 1,000 μg β-1,3-glucan **(E)**, 1,000 μg chitin **(G)**, 1,000 μg galactomannan **(I)**, or 500μg acBSA **(K)** per 2 mL medium. Right column: Dose-dependent IL-8 secretion after 8 h of stimulation with AIF **(D)**, β-1,3-glucan **(F)**, chitin **(H)**, galactomannan **(J)**, or acBSA **(L)**. Data are presented as mean ± SEM from three independent experiments. Duplicate cell cultures were used for each of the three independent experiments and ELISA measurements were performed in duplicates on each of these. Data were analyzed by two-way ANOVA, following Tukey's test, $^{\#}p < 0.05$, $^{\#\#}p < 0.01$, $^{\#\#\#}p < 0.001$, and $^{\#\#\#\#}p < 0.0001$ relative to 0 h or DPBS-treated cells. $^{*}p < 0.05$ and $^{**}p < 0.01$, relative to A549 sham cells stimulated with the same stimulant for the same time period.

circumvented IL-8 suppression. These findings are supported by qPCR (**Figure S4**). Though TLR6/2,−7,−8, and −9 agonist-induced IL-8 secretion was suppressed by FIBCD1 expression, it differed little from the basal suppression. Contrary to this, TLR2,−4, and −5 agonist-induced IL-8 secretion was changed at least 2-fold from basal suppression. Similar results were observed after 4 h of stimulation (**Figure S3**). Hence, FIBCD1 expression influences TLR2,−4, and −5 agonist-induced IL-8 secretion.

DISCUSSION

We previously reported FIBCD1 protein expression at the brush border of human intestinal epithelium and identified binding of crab shell chitin in the S1 binding site of FIBCD1-FReD (14, 15). In the current study, we observed FIBCD1 protein expression at the apical site of human bronchial and alveolar epithelium and binding between FIBCD1 and *A. fumigatus* dependent on cell wall availability, as well as an S1 site-independent AIF recognition. We observed FIBCD1-mediated suppression of IL-8 secretion, mucin production, and transcription of genes involved in inflammatory signaling and FIBCD1-mediated induction of tight junction and cell adhesion molecule transcription. Additionally, we show that this regulation was modulated by stimulation with *A. fumigatus* cell wall and individual cell wall components, i.e., β-1,3-glucan and chitin, and FIBCD1 expression effected TLR agonist-induced IL-8 secretion.

Fluorescence microscopy of different *A. fumigatus* morphotypes (**Figure 2**) showed that soluble FIBCD1 binding was dependent on conidial germination and concomitant exposure of cell wall polysaccharides. Thus, FIBCD1's role in the immune response against *A. fumigatus* may be associated with the expanded immune response, i.e. opsonization

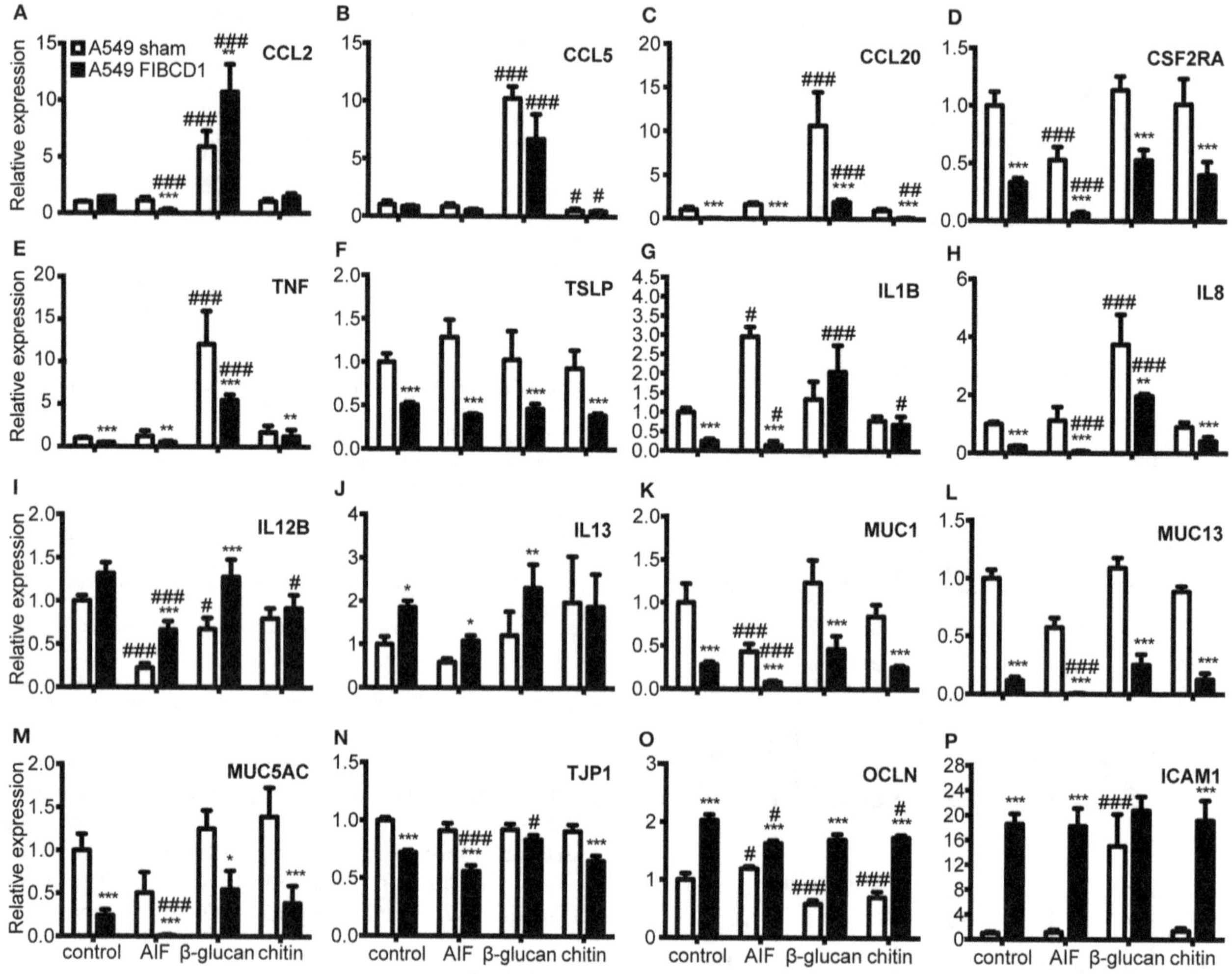

FIGURE 5 | Overexpression of FIBCD1 affects RNA expression of genes associated with immunological responses at mucosal sites. Relative RNA expression of cytokines **(A-J)**, mucins **(K-M)**, TJ proteins **(N-O)**, and adhesion protein **(P)** by A549 sham and A549 FIBCD1 cells in response to stimulation. One million A549 lung epithelial cells transfected with sham and hFIBCD1, respectively, were incubated with DPBS, 500 μg/mL AIF, β-1,3-glucan, and chitin in 2 mL serum-free complete medium for 8 h. The culture supernatants were removed, 1 mL TRIzol added to each well, RNA isolated, cDNA synthetized and tested, and qPCR performed. Data are presented as mean ± SEM from three independent experiments. *P*-values are extracted from the multilevel linear regression models. $^{\#}p < 0.05$, $^{\#\#}p < 0.01$, and $^{\#\#\#}p < 0.001$ relative to DPBS-treated cells. $^{*}p < 0.05$, $^{**}p < 0.01$, and $^{***}p < 0.001$ relative to A549 sham cells stimulated with the same stimulant.

and chemotactic attraction of neutrophils to the site of inflammation (1). Furthermore, we observed co-localization between chitin-rich zones and areas recognized by FIBCD1, which led us to investigate interaction between FIBCD1 and the chitin-containing structural skeleton of the *A. fumigatus* cell wall (AIF). Pull-down experiments (**Figure 3**) revealed that FIBCD1 recognizes AIF independently of calcium and the S1 binding site with less sensitivity to acetate compared to that of chitin.

Chitin is the only component of the cell wall known as a FIBCD1 ligand, which it binds through the S1 binding site (14). These findings support that FIBCD1 recognizes fungal chitin through the S1 binding site, but also recognizes other cell wall structures found in AIF, possibly through conjunctional binding sites or separately in other unknown binding sites.

Similar to a previous study using A549 lung epithelial cells (27), we observed a time- and dose-dependent secretion of IL-8, a proinflammatory chemokine that attracts neutrophils and thereby plays an important role in the inflammatory response against *A. fumigatus* hyphae (1). Stimulation of A549 lung epithelial cells overexpressing FIBCD1 (**Figure 4**) revealed a suppression of IL-8 secretion, which is abolished by stimulation with β-1,3-glucan and chitin and increased by AIF, galactomannan, and acBSA. As a non-FIBCD1 binding ligand, we expect the observed effect of β-1,3-glucan on FIBCD1-mediated suppression of IL-8 secretion to be caused by the activation of pathways that either deactivate FIBCD1, decrease its expression, or induce IL-8 production through circumventing pathways, possibly through the well-known β-1,3-glucan PRR Dectin-1 (12). Different effects of the FIBCD1

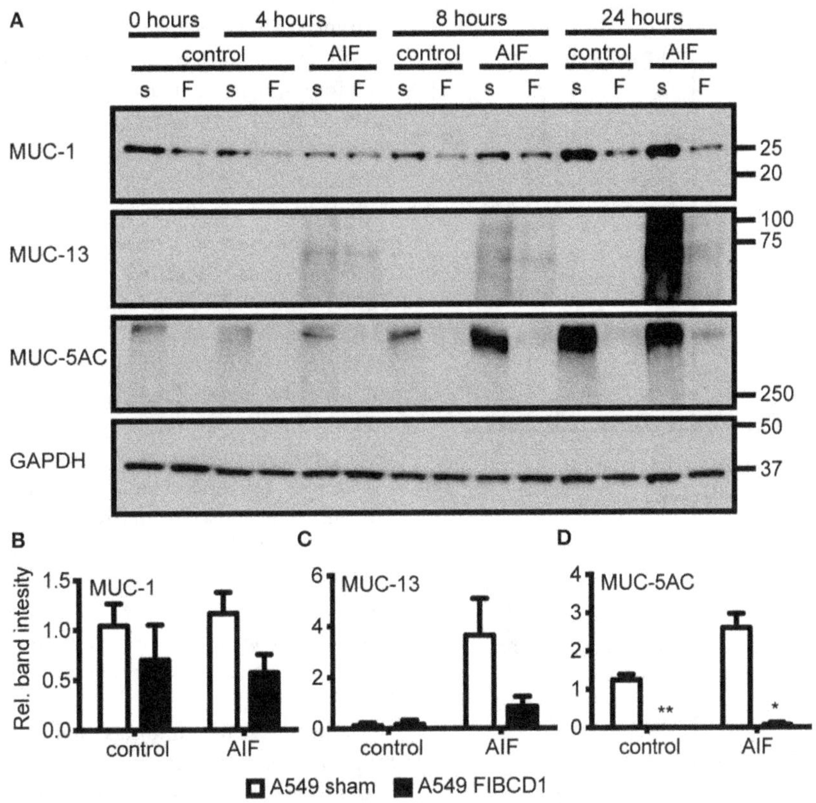

FIGURE 6 | Overexpression of FIBCD1 modulates mucin protein production. A549 sham- and FIBCD1-transfected cells were seeded at a density of one million cells in 2 mL of media per well of a 6-well tissue culture plate and serum-starved over night prior to incubation with DPBS or 500 μg/mL AIF in 2 mL serum-free media for 0, 4, 8, and 24 h. **(A)** Western blot analysis was performed as described using 19 μg of cell lysate per well. Lane 1, 3, 5, 7, 9, 11, 13: A549 sham-transfected cells, Lane 2, 4, 6, 8, 10, 12, 14: A549 FIBCD1-transfected cells. The Western blot shown is from one of three independent experiments yielding similar results. Color is adjusted to gray scale. **(B–D)** Western blots were quantified using ImageJ software. The values obtained after 8 h are expressed as mean ± SEM of the ratio of MUC-1 **(B)**, MUC-13 **(C)**, and MUC-5AC **(D)** to GAPDH from three independent experiments. Data were analyzed by two-way ANOVA, following Tukey's test, $^{\#}p < 0.05$, $^{\#\#}p < 0.01$, and $^{\#\#\#}p < 0.001$ relative to control cells. $^{*}p < 0.05$, $^{**}p < 0.01$, and $^{***}p < 0.001$ relative to A549 sham cells stimulated with the same stimulant.

ligands AIF, chitin, and acBSA were observed, which is likely caused by particle size and source differences known to impact epithelial responses against chitin (28, 29). Previous studies have shown that large particles fail to induce an inflammatory response, while intermediate and small particles protect against Th2-associated allergy (28, 29). In the current study, the exact size of the chitin particles is unknown, however, large, insoluble fragments were observed by bright field microscopy during the stimulation study, which may have effected the interaction between FIBCD1 and chitin. Contrary to this, AIF was administered in intermediate particle size (<40 μm) and acBSA and galactomannan are both soluble molecules. It is currently unclear if the FIBCD1-mediated suppression of IL-8 secretion in response to galactomannan is caused by mere particle size, intersections of signaling pathways or by direct or indirect interaction between FIBCD1 and galactomannan. It is, however, clear that galactomannan does not bind to the S1 binding site of FIBCD1-FReD (**Figure S5**).

We observed a FIBCD1-mediated transcriptional suppression of proinflammatory cytokines, chemokines, and mucins and an induction of barrier function gene expression (**Figure 5**). During the anti-fungal response, several proteins of the genes suppressed by FIBCD1 are released from epithelium to aid in the response. They cause increased inflammation, recruitment of neutrophils, monocytes, and mast cells to the site of inflammation, stimulation of naïve Th cell polarization to Th2 cells, and facilitate homing of these cells. Finally, they induce secretion of MUC-5AC and epithelial expression of MUC-1 and −13, and disrupt epithelial apical junctional complexes, which further enhances inflammation and antigen presentation by dendritic cells (30–40). Thus, FIBCD1 may serve as a general suppressor of airway inflammation. Similar to the IL-8 secretion observations, stimulation with β-1,3-glucan and chitin diminish and AIF increases FIBCD1-mediated suppression.

Mucociliary clearance is the primary defense mechanism against *A. fumigatus* in the bronchioles (6) and is highly dependent on the synthesis, glycosylation, and release of secreted and membrane-bound mucins (37, 41). FIBCD1-mediated suppression of MUC-1 and MUC-5AC and an AIF-increased

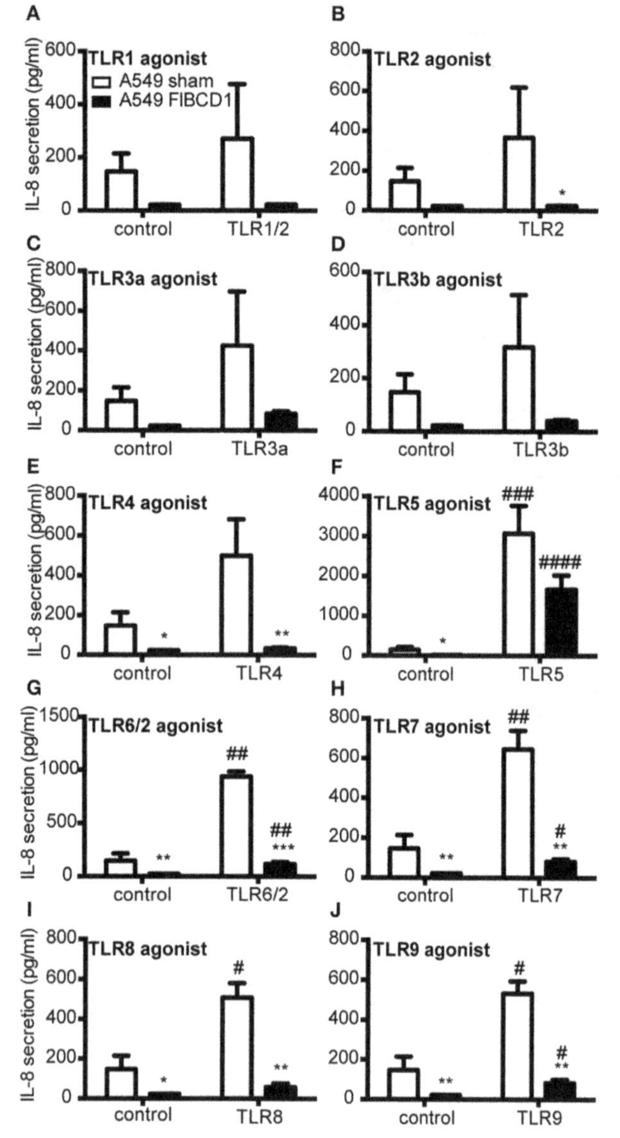

FIGURE 7 | Overexpression of FIBCD1 on the surface of A549 cells inhibits TLR agonist effects. A549 sham- and FIBCD1-transfected cells were seeded at a density of 250,000 cells in 0.5 mL of media per well of a 24-well tissue culture plate and serum-starved overnight prior to stimulation. The cells were stimulated with TLR1/2 **(A)**, 5 **(F)**, and 6/2 **(G)** agonists (0.67 μg/mL), TLR2 **(B)** agonist (6.7·107 cells/mL), TLR3a **(C)** and 3b **(D)** agonists (8.9 μg/mL), TLR4 **(E)** agonist (4.4 μg/mL), TLR7 **(H)** and 8 **(I)** agonists (1.8 μg/mL), and TLR9 **(J)** agonist (0.068 μg/mL) for 8 h and the concentration of secreted IL-8 was determined by sandwich ELISA as described in methods. Data are presented as mean ± SEM from three independent experiments. Duplicate cell cultures were used for each of the three independent experiments and ELISA measurements were performed in duplicates on each of these. Data were analyzed by two-way ANOVA, followed by Tukey's post-test, $^{\#}p < 0.05$, $^{\#\#}p < 0.01$, $^{\#\#\#}p < 0.001$, and $^{\#\#\#\#}p < 0.0001$ relative to DPBS-treated cells. $^{*}p < 0.05$, $^{**}p < 0.01$, and $^{***}p < 0.001$ relative to A549 sham cells stimulated with the same stimulant.

FIBCD1-mediated suppression of MUC-13 and MUC-5AC were observed by Western blotting of cell lysates from A549 lung epithelial cells (**Figure 6**). This indicates that FIBCD1 expression impacts mucus composition and thereby fungal clearance. However, whether these alterations are beneficial for fungi or host is unclear. Additionally, MUC-5AC is a secretory mucin (41) and the lack of vesicle storage in the A549 FIBCD1-transfected cells compared to the A549 sham-transfected cells may reflect increased release as well as decreased production.

Finally, we observed that FIBCD1 overexpression affects the inflammatory response mediated by TLRs in A549 lung epithelial cells (**Figure 7**). The overexpression decreases TLR2- and TLR4-induced IL-8 secretion and increases TLR5-induced IL-8 secretion. Intriguingly, these TLRs are associated with different outcomes of fungal infections. Several studies have investigated the role of TLR2 and TLR4 in the immunological response against *A. fumigatus* and found that their expression is required for optimal host defense (6, 42, 43). The investigation of TLR5's involvement in anti-*A. fumigatus* responses is fairly limited, and it has early been demonstrated that TLR5 have no influence on the anti-*A. fumigatus* response (42). However, Rodland et al. (44) observed an increased RNA expression of the receptor in human monocytes challenges with *A. fumigatus* and later found that TLR5 has an enhancing effect on the viability of conidia (45).

Collectively, our findings demonstrate FIBCD1 as human lung epithelial PRR that recognizes the cell wall of *A. fumigatus* and suppresses epithelial inflammatory signaling and mucin production. FIBCD1 activation may have a beneficial effect by decreasing inflammatory damage or an adverse effect by diminishing anti-fungal responses such as recruitment of neutrophils and mucin production.

AUTHOR CONTRIBUTIONS

The experiments were designed by CJ, LD, AS, GS, ST, and UH. CJ, LD, KC, JM, MH, and ON performed the experiments. CJ performed statistical analysis of the data. The reagents, materials, and analysis tools were provided by ON, AS, GS, and UH. CJ, ST, and UH wrote the paper.

FUNDING

This work was supported by The Danish Medical Research Council, The Independent Research Fund Denmark, The Novo Nordisk Foundation, The Lundbeck Foundation, Fonden til Lægevidenskabens Fremme, The Beckett foundation, and The Gangsted Foundation.

ACKNOWLEDGMENTS

We thank René Holst for help with the multilevel linear regression models, Theresa Thomsen for providing the FIBCD1 deletion mutants, and Jan Mollenhauer for providing the pDEST vector.

SUPPLEMENTARY MATERIAL

Figure S1 | FIBCD1 does not recognizes *A. fumigatus* resting conidia. Bright field **(A)** and fluorescence **(B)** microscopy of *A. fumigatus*. **(A,B)** *A. fumigatus* conidia/mL was grown in SD medium to form fungal hyphae followed by staining with Alexa 488-labeled FIBCD1 as described in materials and methods. A clear recognition of fungal hyphae by FIBCD1 was observed while no staining was seen of the resting conidia indicated by arrows was seen. Image: 20X objective.

Figure S2 | *A. fumigatus* conidia and AIF induce IL-8 secretion by A549 wild type cells time- and dose-dependently. Wild type A549 cells were seeded at a density of $3 \cdot 10^5$ cells in 2 mL of media per well of a 12-well tissue culture plate and serum-starved over night prior to stimulation and the concentration of secreted IL-8 was determined by sandwich ELISA as described in methods. Left panels: Time-dependent IL-8 secretion to $3 \cdot 10^5$ conidia **(A)** and 800µg AIF **(C)** per 2 mL medium. Right panels: Dose-dependent IL-8 secretion after 8 h of stimulation with conidia **(B)** and AIF **(D)**. Data are presented as mean ± SEM from three independent experiments. ELISA measurements were performed in triplicates **(A,C)** and duplicates **(B,D)** for each of the three independent experiments. Data were analyzed by two-way **(A,C)** and one-way **(B,D)** ANOVA, followed by Tukey's post-test. $^*p < 0.05$, $^{**}p < 0.01$, $^{***}p < 0.001$, and $^{****}p < 0.0001$ relative to previous time or dosage.

Figure S3 | Overexpression of FIBCD1 on the surface of A549 cells influences TLR agonist effects after 4 h. A549 sham- and FIBCD1-transfected cells were seeded at a density of 250,000 cells in 0.5 mL of media per well of a 24-well tissue culture plate and serum-starved overnight prior to stimulation. The cells were stimulated with TLR1/2 **(A)**, 5 **(F)**, and 6/2 **(G)** agonists (0.67 µg/mL), TLR2 **(B)** agonist (6.7·107 cells/mL), TLR3a **(C)** and 3b **(D)** agonists (8.9 µg/mL), TLR4 **(E)** agonist (4.4 µg/mL), TLR7 **(H)** and 8 **(I)** agonists (1.8 µg/mL), and TLR9 **(J)** agonist (0.068 µg/mL) for 4 h and the concentration of secreted IL-8 was determined by sandwich ELISA as described in methods. Data are presented as mean ± SEM from three independent experiments. Duplicate cell cultures were used for each of the three independent experiments and ELISA measurements were performed in duplicates on each of these. Data were analyzed by two-way ANOVA, following Tukey's test, $^{\#}p < 0.05$, $^{\#\#}p < 0.01$, $^{\#\#\#}p < 0.001$, and $^{\#\#\#\#}p < 0.001$ relative to DPBS-treated cells. $^*p < 0.05$, $^{**}p < 0.01$, and $^{***}p < 0.001$ relative to A549 sham cells stimulated with the same stimulant.

Figure S4 | Overexpression of FIBCD1 on the surface of A549 cells influences TLR agonist effects. A549 sham- and FIBCD1-transfected cells were seeded at a density of 250,000 cells in 0.5 mL of media per well of a 24-well tissue culture plate and serum-starved overnight prior to stimulation. The cells were stimulated with TLR1/2 and 5 agonists (0.67 µg/mL), TLR2 agonist ($6.7 \cdot 10^7$ cells/mL), and TLR4 agonist (4.4 µg/mL) for 4 h **(A)** and 8 h **(B)**. The culture supernatants were removed, 0.5 mL TRIzol added to each well, RNA isolated, cDNA synthetized, and qPCR performed. Data are presented as mean ± SEM from three independent experiments and qPCR measurements were performed in duplicates on each of these. Data were analyzed by two-way ANOVA, following Tukey's test, $^{\#}p < 0.05$, $^{\#\#}p < 0.01$ and $^{\#\#\#}p < 0.001$, relative to DPBS-treated cells. $^{**}p < 0.01$, and relative to A549 sham cells stimulated with the same stimulant.

Figure S5 | Competitive ELISA showing galactomannan's effect on binding between acBSA and FIBCD1-FReD. A maxisorp immuno plate was coated with 1 µg/mL acBSA in ELISA coating buffer overnight. PBS, acetate, mannan, and galactomannan were loaded in a 2-fold dilution series in TBS/0.05% tween/5 mM $CaCl_2$ starting at 100 mM, 2 mg/mL, and 2 mg/mL, respectively, along with 0.5 µg/mL FIBCD1-FReD. PBS was used as a control for decreased Ca^{2+} presence by the addition of polysaccharides suspended in PBS, calcium content started at 2.5 mM $CaCl_2$. FIBCD1-FReD was detected by 1 µg/mL HG-HYB-12-6 in TBS/0.05% tween/5 mM $CaCl_2$ and HRP-conjugated rabbit anti-mouse antibody. Data represent three independent experiments and is shown as mean ± SEM. ELISA measurements were performed in duplicates for each of the three independent experiments.

Table S1 | Multilevel linear regression models. Results of the multilevel linear regression models used to analyze relative mRNA expression of cytokines, mucins, adhesion proteins, and TJ proteins in A549 sham and A549 FIBCD1 cells in response to stimulation (**Figure 6**).

REFERENCES

1. Latge JP. *Aspergillus fumigatus* and aspergillosis. *Clin Microbiol Rev.* (1999) 12:310–50.
2. Zmeili OS, Soubani AO. Pulmonary aspergillosis: a clinical update. *QJM* (2007) 100:317–34. doi: 10.1093/qjmed/hcm035
3. Simon-Nobbe B, Denk U, Poll V, Rid R, Breitenbach M. The spectrum of fungal allergy. *Int Arch Allergy Immunol.* (2008) 145:58–86. doi: 10.1159/000107578
4. Chaudhary N, Marr KA. Impact of *Aspergillus fumigatus* in allergic airway diseases. *Clin Transl Allergy* (2011) 1:4. doi: 10.1186/2045-7022-1-4
5. Balloy V, Chignard M. The innate immune response to *Aspergillus fumigatus*. *Microbes Infect.* (2009)11:919–27. doi: 10.1016/j.micinf.2009.07.002
6. Park SJ, Mehrad B. Innate immunity to Aspergillus species. *Clin Microbiol Rev.* (2009) 22:535–51. doi: 10.1128/cmr.00014-09
7. Bernard M, Latge JP. *Aspergillus fumigatus* cell wall: composition and biosynthesis. *Med Mycol.* (2001) 39:9–17. doi: 10.1080/714030981
8. Fontaine T, Simenel C, Dubreucq G, Adam O, Delepierre M, Lemoine J, et al. Molecular organization of the alkali-insoluble fraction of *Aspergillus fumigatus* cell wall. *J Biol Chem.* (2000) 275:41528. doi: 10.1074/jbc.M909975199
9. Latge JP. Tasting the fungal cell wall. *Cell Microbiol.* (2010) 12:863–72. doi: 10.1111/j.1462-5822.2010.01474.x
10. Latge JP, Mouyna I, Tekaia F, Beauvais A, Debeaupuis JP, Nierman W. Specific molecular features in the organization and biosynthesis of the cell wall of *Aspergillus fumigatus*. *Med Mycol.* (2005) 43:S15–S22. doi: 10.1080/13693780400029155
11. Romani L. Immunity to fungal infections. *Nat Rev Immunol.* (2004) 4:1–23. doi: 10.1038/nri1255.
12. Steele C, Rapaka RR, Metz A, Pop SM, Williams DL, Gordon S, et al. The beta-glucan receptor dectin-1 recognizes specific morphologies of *Aspergillus fumigatus*. *PLoS Pathog.* (2005) 1:e42. doi: 10.1371/journal.ppat.0010042
13. Netea MG, Warris A, Van der Meer JWM, Fenton MJ, Verver-Janssen TJG, Jacobs LEH, et al. *Aspergillus fumigatus* evades immune recognition during germination through loss of toll-like receptor-4-mediated signal transduction. *J Infect Dis.* (2003) 188:320–6. doi: 10.1086/376456
14. Schlosser A, Thomsen T, Moeller JB, Nielsen O, Tornoe I, Mollenhauer J, et al. Characterization of FIBCD1 as an acetyl group-binding receptor that binds chitin. *J Immunol.* (2009) 183:3800–9. doi: 10.4049/jimmunol.0901526
15. Thomsen T, Moeller JB, Schlosser A, Sorensen GL, Moestrup SK, Palaniyar N, et al. The recognition unit of FIBCD1 organizes into a noncovalently linked tetrameric structure and uses a hydrophobic funnel (S1) for acetyl group recognition. *J Biol Chem.* (2010) 285:1229–38. doi: 10.1074/jbc.M109.061523
16. Shrive AK, Moeller JB, Burns I, Paterson JM, Shaw AJ, Schlosser A, et al. Crystal structure of the tetrameric fibrinogen-like recognition domain of fibrinogen c domain containing 1 (FIBCD1) protein. *J Biol Chem.* (2014) 289:2880–7. doi: 10.1074/jbc.M113.520577
17. Lynch NJ, Roscher S, Hartung T, Morath S, Matsushita M, Maennel DN, et al. L-ficolin specifically binds to lipoteichoic acid, a cell wall constituent of Gram-positive bacteria, and activates the lectin pathway of complement. *J Immunol.* (2004) 172:1198–202. doi: 10.4049/jimmunol.172.2.1198
18. Liu Y, Endo Y, Iwaki D, Nakata M, Matsushita M, Wada I, et al. Human M-ficolin is a secretory protein that activates the lectin complement pathway. *J Immunol.* (2005) 175:3150–6. doi: 10.4049/jimmunol.175.5.3150

19. Ma YG, Cho MY, Zhao MY, Park JW, Matsushita M, Fujita T, et al. Human mannose-binding lectin and L-ficolin function as specific pattern recognition proteins in the lectin activation pathway of complement. *J Biol Chem.* (2004) 279:25307–12. doi: 10.1074/jbc.M400701200
20. Jensen K, Lund KP, Christensen KB, Holm AT, Dubey LK, Moeller JB, et al. M-ficolin is present in *Aspergillus fumigatus* infected lung and modulates epithelial cell immune responses elicited by fungal cell wall polysaccharides. *Virulence* (2017) 8:1870–9. doi: 10.1080/21505594.2016.1278337
21. Ma YJ, Doni A, Hummelshoj T, Honore C, Bastone A, Mantovani A, et al. Synergy between ficolin-2 and pentraxin 3 boosts innate immune recognition and complement deposition. *J Biol Chem.* (2009) 284:28263–75. doi: 10.1074/jbc.M109.009225
22. Madsen J, Tornoe I, Nielsen O, Koch C, Steinhilber W, Holmskov U. Expression and localization of lung surfactant protein A in human tissues. *Am J Respir Cell Mol Biol.* (2003) 29:591–7. doi: 10.1165/rcmb.2002-0274OC
23. Fortwendel JR, Panepinto JC, Seitz AE, Askew DS, Rhodes JC. *Aspergillus fumigatus* rasA and rasB regulate the timing and morphology of asexual development. *Fung Genet Biol.* (2004) 41:129–39. doi: 10.1016/j.fgb.2003.10.004
24. Nesterenko MV, Tilley M, Upton SJ. A simple modification of blums silver stain method allows for 30 minute detection of proteins in polyacrylamide gels. *J Biochem Biophys Methods* (1994) 28:239–242. doi: 10.1016/0165-022x(94)90020-5
25. von Huth S, Moeller JB, Schlosser A, Marcussen N, Nielsen O, Nielsen V, et al. Immunohistochemical localization of fibrinogen c domain containing 1 on epithelial and mucosal surfaces in human tissues. *J Histochem Cytochem.* (2017) 66:85–97. doi: 10.1369/0022155417743694
26. Raikhel NV, Lee HI, Broekaert WF. Structure and function of chitin-binding proteins. *Ann Rev Plant Phys Plant Mol Biol.* (1993) 44:591–615. doi: 10.1146/annurev.pp.44.060193.003111
27. Zhang Z, Liu R, Noordhoek JA, Kauffman HF. Interaction of airway epithelial cells (A549) with spores and mycelium of *Aspergillus fumigatus. J Infect.* (2005) 51:375–82. doi: 10.1016/j.jinf.2004.12.012
28. Da Silva CA, Chalouni C, Williams A, Hartl D, Lee CG, Elias JA. Chitin is a size-dependent regulator of macrophage TNF and IL-10 production. *J Immunol.* (2009) 182:3573–82. doi: 10.4049/jimmunol.0802113
29. Alvarez FJ. The effect of chitin size, shape, source and purification method on immune recognition. *Molecules* (2014) 19:4433–51. doi: 10.3390/molecules19044433
30. Stadnyk AW. Cytokine production by epithelial cells. *FASEB J.* (1994) 8:1041–7. doi: 10.1096/fasebj.8.13.7926369
31. Duong M, Ouellet N, Simard M, Bergeron Y, Olivier M, Bergeron MG. Kinetic study of host defense and inflammatory response to *Aspergillus fumigatus* in steroid-induced immunosuppressed mice. *J Infect Dis.* (1998) 178:1472–82. doi: 10.1086/314425
32. Eisenbarth SC, Piggott DA, Huleatt JW, Visintin I, Herrick CA, Bottomly K. Lipopolysaccharide-enhanced, toll-like receptor 4-dependent T helper cell type 2 responses to inhaled antigen. *J Exp Med.* (2002) 196:1645–51. doi: 10.1084/jem.20021340.
33. Bruewer M, Luegering A, Kucharzik T, Parkos CA, Madara JL, Hopkins AM, et al. Proinflammatory cytokines disrupt epithelial barrier function by apoptosis-independent mechanisms. *J Immunol.* (2003) 171:6164–72. doi: 10.4049/jimmunol.171.11.6164
34. Li X, Wang L, Nunes DP, Troxler RF, Offner GD. Pro-inflammatory cytokines up-regulate MUC1 gene expression in oral epithelial cells. *J Dental Res.* (2003) 82:883–7. doi: 10.1177/154405910308201107
35. Song KS, Lee WJ, Chung KC, Koo JS, Yang EJ, Choi JY, et al. Interleukin-1 beta and tumor necrosis factor-alpha induce MUC5AC overexpression through a mechanism involving ERK/p38 mitogen-activated protein kinases-MSK1-CREB activation in human airway epithelial cells. *J Biol Chem.* (2003) 278:23243–50. doi: 10.1074/jbc.M300096200
36. Al-Sadi RM, Ma TY. IL-1beta causes an increase in intestinal epithelial tight junction permeability. *J Immunol.* (2007) 178:4641–9. doi: 10.4049/jimmunol.178.7.4641
37. Linden SK, Sutton P, Karlsson NG, Korolik V, McGuckin MA. Mucins in the mucosal barrier to infection. *Mucosal Immunol.* (2008) 1:183–97. doi: 10.1038/mi.2008.5
38. Bellanger AP, Millon L, Khoufache K, Rivollet D, Bieche I, Laurendeau I, et al. *Aspergillus fumigatus* germ tube growth and not conidia ingestion induces expression of inflammatory mediator genes in the human lung epithelial cell line A549. *J Med Microbiol.* (2009) 58(*Pt* 2):174–179. doi: 10.1099/jmm.0.005488-0
39. Capaldo CT, Nusrat A. Cytokine regulation of tight junctions. *Biochim Biophys Acta* (2009) 1788:864–71. doi: 10.1016/j.bbamem.2008.08.027
40. Ito T, Carson WF, Cavassani KA, Connett JM, Kunkel SL. CCR6 as a mediator of immunity in the lung and gut. *Exp Cell Res.* (2011) 317:613–9. doi: 10.1016/j.yexcr.2010.12.018
41. Fahy JV, Dickey BF. Airway mucus function and dysfunction. *N Engl J Med.* (2010) 363:2233–47. doi: 10.1056/NEJMra0910061
42. Meier A, Kirschning CJ, Nikolaus T, Wagner H, Heesemann J, Ebel F. Toll-like receptor (TLR) 2 and TLR4 are essential for Aspergillus-induced activation of murine macrophages. *Cell Microbiol.* (2003) 5:561–70. doi: 10.1046/j.1462-5822.2003.00301.x
43. Balloy V, Si-Tahar M, Takeuchi O, Philippe B, Nahori MA, Tanguy M, et al. Involvement of toll-like receptor 2 in experimental invasive pulmonary aspergillosis. *Infect Immunol.* (2005) 73:5420–5. doi: 10.1128/iai.73.9.5420-5425.2005
44. Rodland EK, Mattingsdal M, Olstad OK, Ovstebo R, Kierulf P, Muller F, et al. Expression of genes in normal human monocytes in response to *Aspergillus fumigatus. Med Mycol.* (2008) 46:327–36. doi: 10.1080/13693780701874507
45. Ernst KRO, Ager-Wick E, Halvorsen B, Muller F, Froland SS. Toll like receptor 5 (TLR5) may be involved in the immunological response to *Aspergillus fumigatus in vitro. Med Mycol.* (2011) 49:375–9. doi: 10.3109/13693786.2010.531772

17

Interaction of THP-1 Monocytes with Conidia and Hyphae of Different *Curvularia* Strains

Eszter Judit Tóth[1,2], Éva Boros[3], Alexandra Hoffmann[2], Csilla Szebenyi[1,2], Mónika Homa[1,2], Gábor Nagy[1], Csaba Vágvölgyi[2], István Nagy[3] and Tamás Papp[1,2]*

[1] MTA-SZTE Fungal Pathogenicity Mechanisms Research Group, Hungarian Academy of Sciences, University of Szeged, Szeged, Hungary, [2] Faculty of Science and Informatics, Department of Microbiology, University of Szeged, Szeged, Hungary, [3] Hungarian Academy of Sciences, Biological Research Centre, Szeged, Hungary

***Correspondence:**
Tamás Papp
pappt@bio.u-szeged.hu

Interaction of the human monocytic cell line, THP-1 with clinical isolates of three *Curvularia* species were examined. Members of this filamentous fungal genus can cause deep mycoses emerging in both immunocompromised and immunocompetent patients. It was found that monocytes reacted only to the hyphal form of *Curvularia lunata.* Cells attached to the germ tubes and hyphae and production of elevated levels of interleukin (IL)-8 and IL-10 and a low level of TNF-α were measured. At the same time, monocytes failed to produce IL-6. This monocytic response, especially with the induction of the anti-inflammatory IL-10, correlates well to the observation that *C. lunata* frequently cause chronic infections even in immunocompetent persons. Despite the attachment to the hyphae, monocytes could not reduce the viability of the fungus and the significant decrease in the relative transcript level of HLA-DRA assumes the lack of antigen presentation of the fungus by this cell type. *C. spicifera* and *C. hawaiiensis* failed to induce the gathering of the cells or the production of any analyzed cytokines. Monocytes did not recognize conidia of *Curvularia* species, even when melanin was lacking in their cell wall.

Keywords: *Curvularia*, monocyte, invasive mycosis, melanin, quantitative reverse transcription PCR, ELISA, interleukin-10

INTRODUCTION

Members of the ascomycete genus, *Curvularia* includes primarily saprotrophic and plant pathogenic filamentous fungi. Some of them, such as *Curvularia lunata*, *C. hawaiiensis*, and *C. spicifera*, however, are also considered as emerging agents of local and invasive human phaeohyphomycoses (1), i.e., infections caused by melanin producing molds. *Curvularia* species are frequently reported as agents of allergic fungal sinusitis and bronchopulmonary disease (2–4) but they can also be associated with mycotic keratitis (5, 6), cutaneous and subcutaneous mycoses (7, 8), and infections of the central nervous system (2, 9). Deep and disseminated *Curvularia* infections have been described in both immunocompromised and immunocompetent patients (4, 10–13). Increasing prevalence of these infections has been reported during recent years (4, 14, 15). Despite that *Curvularia* species are among the most common dematiaceous fungi isolated from clinical samples (16), experimental data concerning the background of their pathogenicity and interactions with the host are very limited (2).

Human monocytes are circulating cells of innate immunity that can further differentiate into macrophages or dendritic cells and capable of phagocytoses, cytokine production, and antigen presentation. They play a pivotal role in the host response to fungal infections and their activity against the conidia, germlings, and hyphae of *Aspergillus fumigatus* was proven and analyzed previously (17, 18).

THP-1 is a human monocytic cell line isolated from a patient with acute monocytic leukemia. This cell line can be differentiated into macrophages and are widely used to study monocyte and macrophage functions and in immune modulation studies (19). For example, THP-1 monocytes treated with LPS, showed altered expression of several inflammation related genes, such as *IL1B*, *IL6*, *IL8*, *IL10*, and *TNFA* (19, 20). Several studies have compared the responses of THP-1 monocytes and human peripheral blood mononuclear cell derived monocytes to a variety of stimuli and the two cell types showed relatively similar response patterns in most cases (19). THP-1 monocytes and macrophages has also been used successfully as *in vitro* models to examine host–pathogen interactions for various fungal agents, such as *A. fumigatus* (18, 21–23), *Candida albicans* (24), *Candida glabrata* (25), and *Cryptococcus neoformans* (26).

In this study, interactions of THP-1 monocytes with conidia and hyphae of three fungal strains representing *C. hawaiiensis*, *C. lunata*, and *C. spicifera* were analyzed to get a first insight into the host response to *Curvularia* species. For comparison, an *A. fumigatus* strain from a clinical origin was also involved in the study.

MATERIALS AND METHODS

Fungal Strains, Culture Conditions, and Inoculum Preparation

Curvularia lunata SZMC 23759 and *C. spicifera* SZMC 13064, *A. fumigatus* SZMC 23245 isolated from human eye infections and *C. hawaiiensis* CBS 103.97 isolated from human sinusitis with ophthalmic and cerebral involvement were used in the study. Strains were grown on potato dextrose agar (PDA; VWR International) at room temperature. To block melanin synthesis, PDA was supplemented with 20 μg/ml tricyclazole (Sigma-Aldrich) and 1% of agar (Merck). For the interaction studies, conidial suspensions (10^5 conidia/ml) were prepared in phosphate buffer saline (PBS; 137 mM NaCl, 2.7 mM KCl, 10 mM Na_2HPO_4, 2 mM KH_2PO_4, pH 7.4) by washing the conidia from 14 and 7 days old fungal cultures in case of the *Curvularia* strains and the *Aspergillus* strain, respectively. To get rid of hyphal debris, spore suspensions were filtered through a filter paper with a pore size of 45 μm (Millipore). Heat inactivation of the conidia was performed at 125°C for 25 min.

Culturing and Infection of the THP-1 Cells

THP-1 cells were maintained in RPMI 1640 medium (Gibco) supplemented with 10% (v/v) heat inactivated fetal bovine serum (FBS; Gibco) and 1% (v/v) antibiotic/antimycotic solution containing 10,000 U/ml of penicillin, 10,000 μg/ml of streptomycin and 25 μg/ml of Amphotericin B (Gibco) at 37°C in a humidified incubator with 5% CO_2. For interaction studies, THP-1 cells (10^5 cells/ml) were placed on 6-well or 12-well cell culture plates with flat bottoms (Sarstedt) in 3 or 1 ml RPMI 1640 medium supplemented with 10% heat inactivated FBS and without antibiotic the day before infection, respectively.

Number of the *Curvularia* conidia and cells were set to maintain an effector (THP-1) to target (conidia) (E:T) ratio of 20:1, while for *A. fumigatus* E:T ratio was 20:1 or 1:2. Because of the small size of the conidia of *A. fumigatus*, an E:T ratio of 1:2 proved to be optimal for this fungus in agreement with the literature data (18). For the *Curvularia* strains, we tested various E:T ratios and that of 20:1 proved to be applicable, mainly because of the large size and the relatively short germination time (approx. 1.5 h) of their conidia. Cells were incubated with or without the fungi at 37°C in a humidified incubator with 5% CO_2 for 3, 9, or 24 h. When monocytes were treated with lipopolysaccharide (LPS, *Escherichia coli* Q26:B6; Sigma-Aldrich), 1 μg/ml final concentration of LPS was used. Microscopic examination of the interactions was performed using a Leica DMI4000 B inverse microscope (Leica Microsystems). All experiments were performed in two technical and three biological replicates.

Phagocytosis Assay

THP-1 cells (10^5 cells/ml) were seated on a 12-well plate one day before the experiment. Four hours before the assay, cells were stained with CellMask Deep Red Plasma Membrane stain (Thermo Scientific) in a 0.5-fold concentration for 15 min and washed twice with PBS. Conidia were stained with AlexaFluor 488 carboxylic acid, succinimidyl ester (Thermo Scientific) for 15 min and washed twice with PBS at 4°C to prevent germination. The E:T ratio was 1:2 or 20:1. For analysis, collected samples were centrifuged with 1,000 rpm for 15 min and resuspended in 200 μl PBS supplemented with 0.05% Tween-20 (Reanal). Interaction and phagocytosis were measured after 1 or 3 h using a FlowSight Imaging Flow Cytometer (Amnis) and evaluated with the IDEAS Software (Amnis).

Real-time Quantitative Reverse Transcription PCR (qRT-PCR) Analysis

Total RNA was extracted from the THP-1 cells using the RNeasy Mini kit (Qiagen) according to the instructions of the manufacturer. The final elution volume was 20 μl. cDNA was synthesized using the SuperScript VILO Master Mix (Invitrogen) following the protocol of the manufacturer. qRT-PCR was carried out using StepOne Plus Real-Time PCR System (Applied Biosystems). Reactions were performed by either the TaqMan Gene expression Master Mix (Applied Biosystems) or the Sybr Select Master Mix (Applied Biosystems) using the probes and primers listed in **Tables 1** and **2**, respectively, according to the manufacturer's

TABLE 1 | TaqMan probe details (Applied Biosystems) used in the qRT-PCR analyses.

Target gene	TaqMan assay ID
18S rDNA	Hs99999901_s1
IL10	Hs00961522_m1
IL6	Hs00174131_m1
IL8	Hs00174103_m1
TNFA	Hs00174128_m1
NLRC3	Hs01054716_m1

TABLE 2 | Primer pairs used in the qRT-PCR analyses.

Target gene	Forward (5′–3′) primer	Reverse (5′–3′) primer	Product length (bp)
CCR1	TCTACGCCTTCGTTGGTGAG	TTTAACCAGGTGCACAGCCA	80
CCR2	TACCAACGAGAGCGGTGAAG	GCATGTTGCCCACAAAACCA	149
CCR5	TTACTGTCCCCTTCTGGGCT	AAGCAAACACAGCATGGACG	168
CXCR2	TTTCGCCATGGACTCCTCAA	GTAGTGGAAGTGTGCCCTGA	116
IL1B	AGCTGGAGAGTGTAGATCCCAA	GGGAACTGGGCAGACTCAAA	112
ITGAL	GCAAGGACATACCGCCCAT	TACTCAGGCTCAGCTCCACA	186
ITGAM	AGTCTGCCTCCATGTCCAGAA	CTGCGTGTGCTGTTCTTTGTC	144
ITGAX	AGTCTGCCTCCATGTCCAGAA	CTGCGTGTGCTGTTCTTTGTC	103
HLADRA	CCGATCACCAATGTACCTCCA	CGAAGCCACGTGACATTGAC	128

protocols. Relative transcript levels were calculated with the $\Delta\Delta C_T$ ($2^{-\Delta\Delta Ct}$) method (27) using a fragment of the 18S rRNA coding gene for normalization. All measurements were performed in two technical and three biological replicates.

Cytokine Assays

To confirm the cytokine concentrations in the culture supernatants, DuoSet ELISA Kits (R&D Systems) were used for tumor necrosis factor alpha (TNF-α), interleukin (IL)-6, and IL-8 according to the instructions of the manufacturer. To measure the IL-10 level, the Human IL-10 ELISA kit (Immunotools) was used. Cytokine titers were calculated by reference to standard curves generated by the four parameters logistic curve-fit method.

Viability Test

To measure the hyphal damage after the incubation with monocytes, a colorimetric assay using 3-(4,5-dimethylthiazol-2-yl)-2,5-diphenyltetrazolium bromide (MTT; Sigma-Aldrich) was performed (28) on 12-well culture plates. After incubation for 3, 6, or 24 h, monocytes were lysed with 0.5% sodium deoxycholate (Sigma-Aldrich) and the wells were washed three times with PBS. Then, 1 ml RPMI 1640 supplemented with 1% MTT was added to the wells and the plates were incubated at 37°C, under 5% CO_2 concentration for 3 h. After removing the supernatant, wells were washed two times with PBS and stored at −20°C overnight. Before detection, 1 ml acidic isopropanol (95% isopropanol and 5% 1 N HCl) was added into the wells and the plates were incubated until the blue color dissolved from hyphae. Absorbance of the supernatant was measured at the wavelength of 550 nm using a spectrophotometer (Spectrostar Nano, BMG Labtech). Viability of the hyphae was calculated using the following formula, where OD_{550} sample was the absorbance measured for the hyphae incubated with monocytes and OD_{550} control was the absorbance measured for the hyphae incubated without monocytes: $\text{Viability} = \left(\frac{OD550\ \text{sample}}{OD550\ \text{control}}\right) \times 100.$

Statistical Analysis

All measurements were performed in at least two technical and three biological replicates. Significance was calculated with paired *t*-test using Microsoft Excel of the Microsoft Office package. *P* values less than 0.05 were considered statistically significant.

RESULTS

THP-1 Cells Do Not Phagocytose *Curvularia* spp. Conidia and Hyphae

THP-1 cells were confronted with *C. lunata*, *C. hawaiiensis*, and *C. spicifera* by co-incubating heat inactivated or living conidia with the monocytes. Interactions were analyzed after 3 and 24 h of confrontation. In case of the living conidia, germination was already in progress and germ tubes were developed at 3 h postinoculation (**Figures 1A,B**) while branching hyphae were present at 24 h postinoculation (**Figures 1A,B**). Microscopic analysis revealed that the monocytes were not able to phagocytose the conidia of any tested strains; moreover, they did not attract to them at all (**Figures 1A,B**). The absence of the monocytic response did not depend on the melanin content as it also missed in case of those conidia of *C. lunata* where the melanin biosynthesis had been previously blocked. At the same time, THP-1 cells aggregated around and attached to the hyphae of *C. lunata* (**Figures 1C,D**). However, monocytes did not block the germination of the conidia and MTT assay did not detect hyphal damage in the tested *Curvularia* strains (**Figure 2**). For comparison, MTT assay was also performed with *A. fumigatus* under the same co-incubation conditions. In this case, viability of the hyphae decreased to 12.9% after 24 h of interaction with the THP-1 cells.

For quantification and a more detailed analysis, phagocytosis was also examined by imaging flow cytometry in case of *C. lunata* and *A. fumigatus* (**Figure 3**). THP-1 cells actively phagocytosed the living conidia of *A. fumigatus* already at 1 h after their confrontation; the mean ratio of the phagocyting cells counted from three biological replicates was found to be 2.4 (±0.4)% and 20.7 (±2.5)% at E:T ratios of 20:1 (**Figure 3C**) and 1:2 (**Figure 3B**), respectively. At the same time, the number of interacting cells and conidia proved to be insignificant in the case of *C. lunata*. Only 0.12 (±0.1)% of the monocytes were attached to or ingesting the conidia at 1 h after the start of the interaction (the E:T ratio was 20:1). Similar values were measured for heat inactivated and melanin blocked conidia, 0.35 (±0.2)% and 0.69 (±0.1)% after 1 h of interaction, respectively. Image analysis revealed that majority of these small numbers of interactions detected by flow cytometry was only attachment of the monocytes to the conidia instead of real phagocytosis (**Figure 3A**).

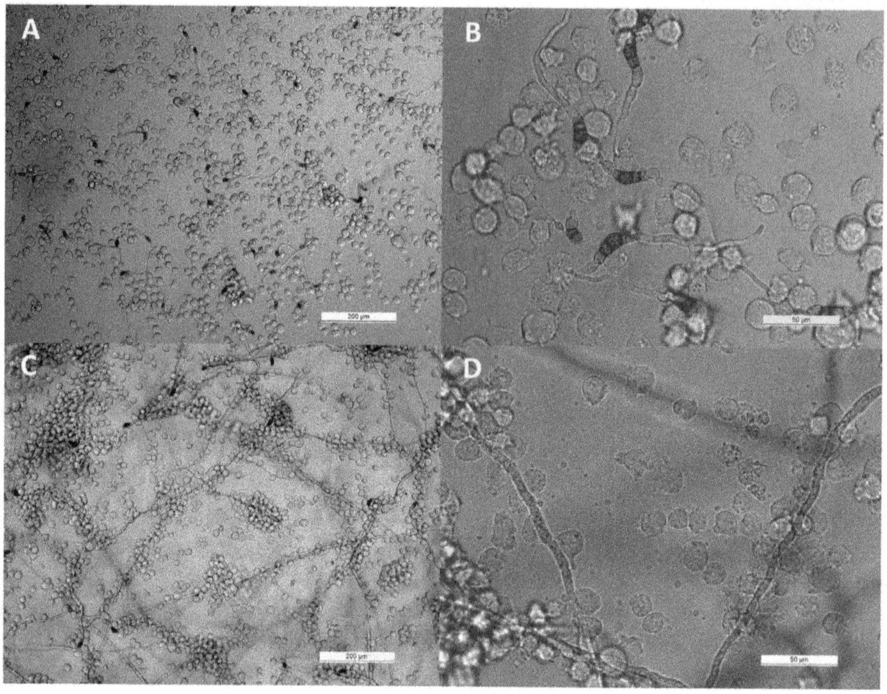

FIGURE 1 | Interaction of THP-1 monocytes with *Curvularia lunata*. Light micrographs were taken at 3 [panels **(A,B)**] and 24 h [panels **(C,D)**] postinoculation; the E:T ratio was 20:1.

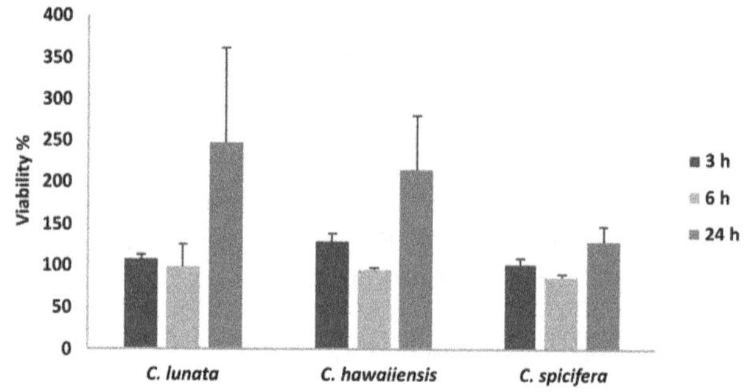

FIGURE 2 | Cell viability (MTT) assay of the three *Curvularia* strains incubated together with THP-1 monocytes for 3 and 24 h. Results are presented as averages of three independent experiments; error bars represent SDs.

qRT-PCR Analysis of Immune-Relevant Genes Induced by Germinating Conidia and Hyphae of *Curvularia* Species

Three and 24 h after the infection of THP-1 monocytes with conidia, cells were harvested and the relative transcript level of certain activation related and cytokine or chemokine coding genes were measured. Significant changes were not detected in the transcription of the genes encoding the chemokine receptors CCR5 (C-C chemokine receptor type 5), CXCR2 (IL-8 receptor, beta) and the cytokine IL-6 at both tested times in any interactions. Decreased relative transcript levels were detected for the genes of the chemokine receptors CCR1 (C-C chemokine receptor type 1) and CCR2 (C-C chemokine receptor type 2) after 24-h interaction with the tested *Curvularia* strains (**Figure 4**). Similarly, slightly decreased transcript levels were measured for the genes encoding the adhesion molecules ITGAL (integrin subunit alpha L), ITGAM (integrin subunit alpha M) and ITGAX (integrin subunit alpha X) after 24 h of co-incubation. In case of the gene encoding IL-1β, NLRC3 (NLR family CARD domain containing 3) either no significant changes in the transcription or decreased transcript levels were detected after 24 h of interaction (**Figure 4**). Transcription of gene of HLA-DRA (HLA class II histocompatibility antigen, DR alpha chain) showed significant reduction in case of *C. lunata*. Increased transcription of the gene encoding TNF-α was observed in response to all tested strains after both 3 and 24 h (**Figure 4**). A trend for increased transcript levels was detected for the genes of IL-8 and IL-10 but significant changes were detected only in interactions with certain strains (i.e., with *C. spicifera* for IL-8 and with *C. hawaiiensis* and *C. spicifera* for IL-10) (**Figure 4**).

In case of *A. fumigatus*, transcript levels were measured after 3, 9, and 24 h of interaction, because this fungus starts to germinate at about 7 h after inoculation. In accordance with the literature data (18), conidia did not induce the transcription of *IL6*, *IL8*, *IL10*, and *TNFA* while significantly increased relative transcript levels were measured for *TNFA* after 9 h of interaction (67.66 ± 10.9) and *IL8* at 9 (8.86 ± 0.73) and 24 h (24.03 ± 2.93) (see Figure S1 in Supplementary Material).

As control, THP-1 cells were also stimulated with LPS and the relative transcript levels of *IL1b*, *IL6*, *IL8*, *IL10*, *TNFA*, *CCR1*, and *CCR2* were measured as above. As expected, all tested genes showed significantly altered expression after LPS treatment. Expression of *IL1b*, *IL6*, *IL8*, *IL10*, and *TNFA* was induced showing

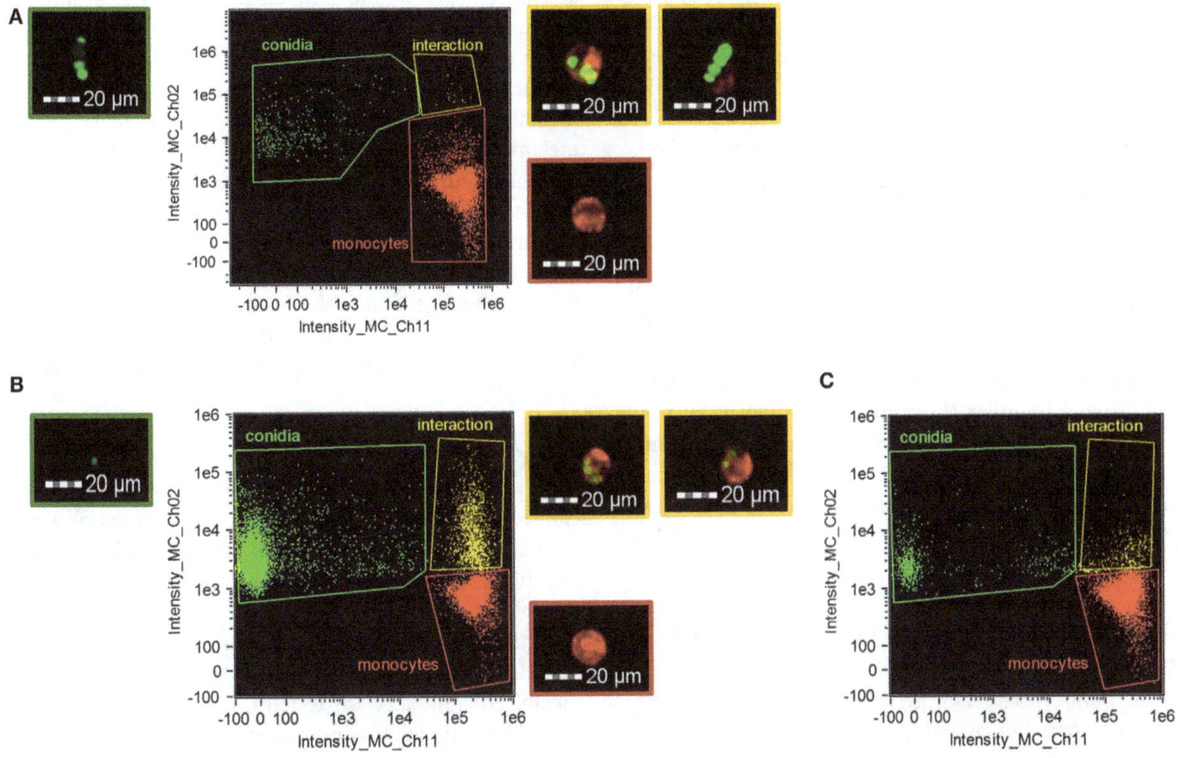

FIGURE 3 | Phagocytosis of *Curvularia lunata* **(A)** and *Aspergillus fumigatus* **(B,C)** conidia by THP-1 monocytes. THP-1 cells and conidia were stained with CellMask Deep Red Plasma Membrane Stain and Alexa Fluor 488 carboxylic acid, succinimidyl ester, respectively. Number of the *Curvularia* conidia and cells were set to maintain an E:T ratio of 20:1 **(A)**, while for *A. fumigatus* E:T ratio was 1:2 **(B)** or 20:1 **(C)**. Monocytes were identified by detecting fluorescence intensity on channel 11 (Intensity_MC_CH_11) while channel 2 (Intensity_MC_CH_2) was used to detect the conidia. Cells and conidia were co-incubated for 1 h. Fluorescent micrographs showing conidia (green border) and THP-1 cells alone (red border) and in interaction (i.e., phagocytosis or attachment) (yellow border) were recorded during the imaging flow cytometry.

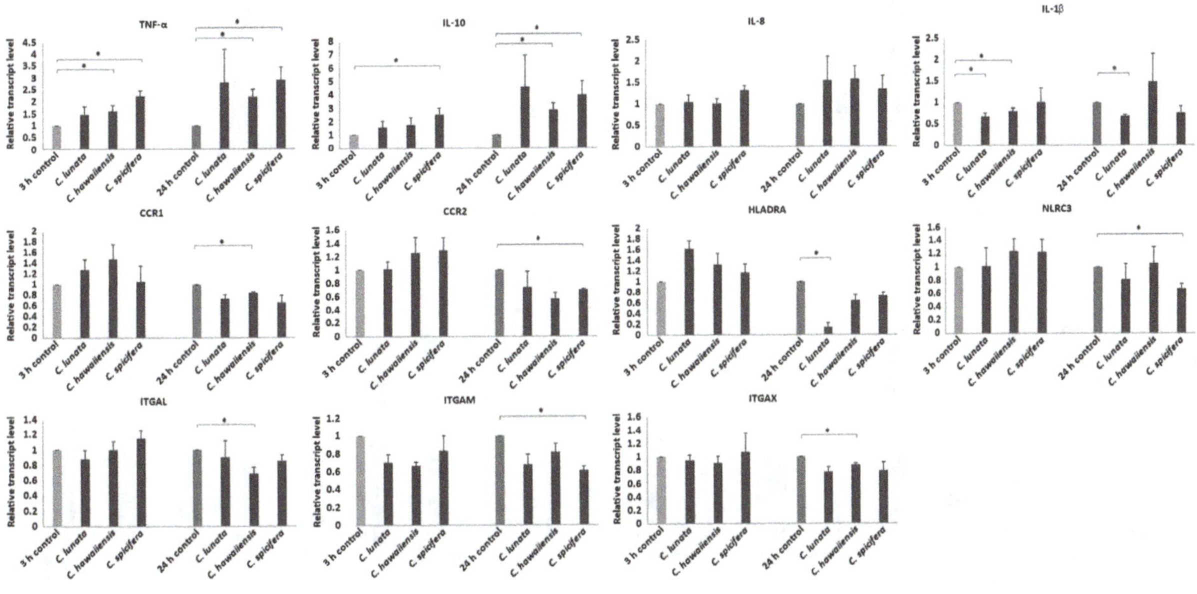

FIGURE 4 | Relative transcript levels of pro- and anti-inflammatory cytokines, activation and antigen presentation related genes. THP-1 monocytes were confronted with *Curvularia* strains for 3 and 24 h. After total RNA extraction from the monocytes, cDNA synthesis, and quantitative reverse transcription PCR were carried out. Relative transcript levels were calculated by the $2^{-\Delta\Delta Ct}$ method. Presented values are averages of the results of three independent experiments; error bars represent SDs. Relative transcript values followed by * significantly differed from the control (taken as 1), according to the paired *t*-test ($p < 0.05$).

significantly increased relative transcript levels compared to the untreated control, in contrast, relative transcript levels of *CCR1* and *CCR2* were found to be significantly decreased (see Figure S2 in Supplementary Material).

IL-6, IL-8, IL-10, and TNF-α Production in Response to Germinating Conidia and Hyphae of *Curvularia* Species

In agreement with the results of the transcription analysis, no significant IL-6 production was observed in all interactions (**Figure 5**). In response to *C. lunata*, THP-1 cells showed significant IL-8 (340 pg/ml) and IL-10 (318 pg/ml) production after 24 h of interaction (**Figure 5**). Confronting with *A. fumigatus*, monocytes displayed similar IL-8 production (376 pg/ml) but only a low amount of IL-10 (43 pg/ml) could be detected. Infection with the other two *Curvularia* strains did not cause significant change in the IL-8 and IL-10 level. In case of *C. lunata*, a moderate increase in the TNF-α level (45 pg/ml) was also measured at 24 h postinoculation (**Figure 5**).

Response of THP-1 Cells to the Conidia of *C. lunata*

Response of monocytes to non-germinating and germinating conidia were compared in case of *C. lunata*. In this experiment, activation of cytokine and chemotactic genes and cytokine production was analyzed by qRT-PCR and ELISA assays, respectively, after interactions of THP-1 cells with heat inactivated conidia (see Figures S3 and S4 in Supplementary Material). As melanin content may hamper the monocyte response, non-melanized and heat inactivated conidia, which were harvested after blocking the melanin biosynthesis during cultivation, were also tested. Compared to the germinating conidia and hyphae (**Figures 4** and **5**), presence of heat inactivated conidia, either melanized or non-melanized, did not affect the transcription of the examined genes and the production of any tested cytokines suggesting that only the germ tubes and the hyphae are able to activate the monocytes (Figures S3 and S4 in Supplementary Material).

DISCUSSION

Considering that activation of the innate immune system has a crucial role in recognition and control of filamentous fungal infections (18), present study was carried out to obtain information about the response of monocytic cell line THP-1 to the dematiaceous fungus *C. lunata* and related species.

THP-1 monocytes were not able to phagocytose the large and melanized conidia of any tested *Curvularia* species. Despite the lack of attraction to the conidia, monocytes recognized *C. lunata*,

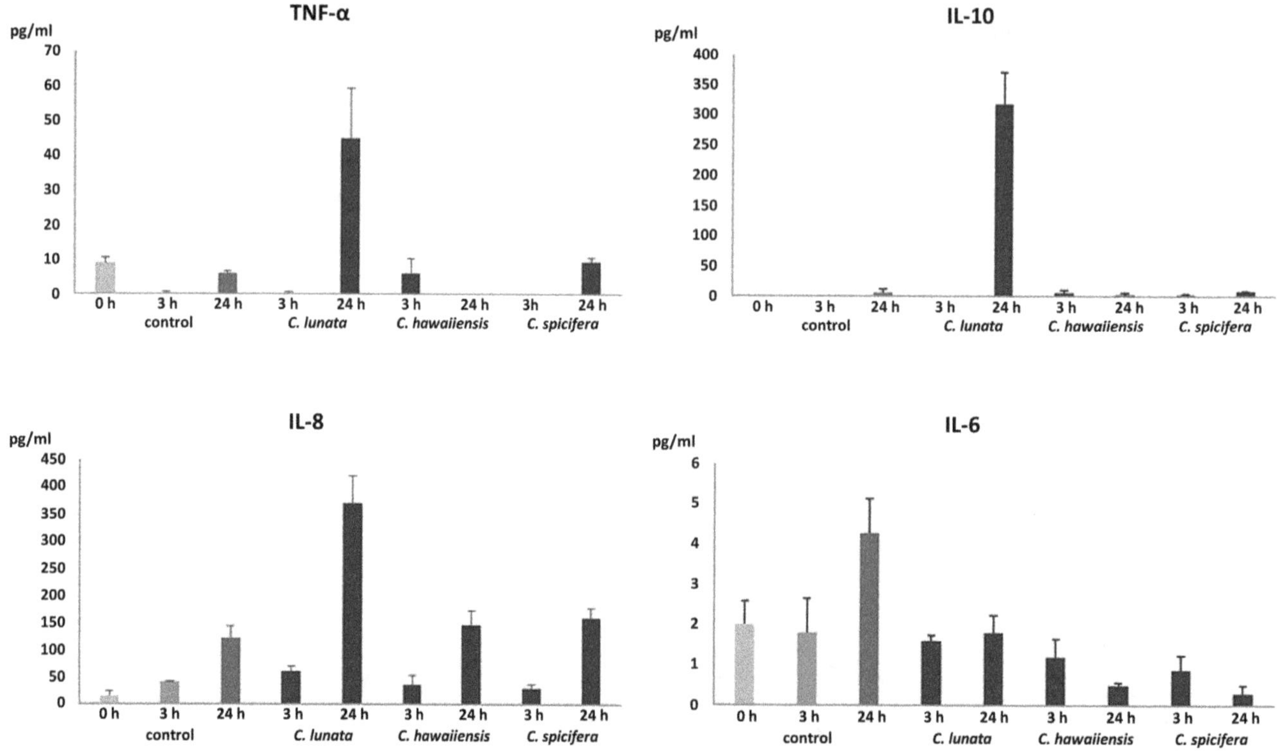

FIGURE 5 | Quantity of produced pro- and anti-inflammatory cytokines (pg/ml) after interaction with *Curvularia* strains for 3 and 24 h. THP-1 cells were interacted with the fungal conidia in an E:T ratio of 20:1. In case of the control, monocytes were incubated without the fungi. Concentrations of IL-6, IL-8, IL-10, and TNF-α in the culture supernatant were measured by ELISA. Cytokine titers were calculated by reference to standard curves generated by the four parameters logistic curve-fit method. Results are presented as averages from three independent experiments; error bars represent SDs.

but not *C. hawaiiensis* and *C. spicifera*, and preferably attached to the hyphae. In contrast to the *Curvularia* conidia, those of *A. fumigatus* were actively phagocytosed by the THP-1 cells in agreement with the results of previous studies (18). Different cell wall composition and highly distinct size of their conidia can explain this different affinity of the monocytes to the *Curvularia* and *Aspergillus* conidia. Although there are no available data about the response of monocytes to any similar dematiaceous mold, there are a few studies discussing the interaction of these fungi with other cell types. Recently, Reedy et al. (29) found that macrophages could not phagocytose the conidia of *Exserohilum rostratum*, another dematiaceous mold related to *Curvularia*. At the same time, macrophages also showed an attraction and attachment to the hyphae of *Exserohilum*. The different affinity of macrophages to the conidia and the hyphae was explained by the possibly different polysaccharide composition of the cell walls (29). Besides phagocytosis, only touching and dragging of the fungal cells, conidia and hyphal elements by macrophages to prevent the spread of the fungus into the different tissues was proven in cases of *A. fumigatus* and *C. albicans* (30).

Melanin is present in the cell wall of a wide range of fungal pathogens. Like Aspergilli, *Curvularia* species produce dihydroxynaphthalene-type melanin (DHN-melanin) (16). Melanin is generally considered as a virulence factor having role in the prevention of the immune recognition by masking the pathogen-associated molecular patterns on the surface of the conidia, as it was found in *A. fumigatus* (31–33). However, in our experiments, there was no difference in the response of monocytes to melanized and non-melanized conidia of *C. lunata* indicating that melanin content of the conidia has no significant effect on the recognition of this fungus by the THP-1 cells. Previously, comparison of killing rates of numerous dematiaceous yeasts by human neutrophils suggested that only melanization is not sufficient to assure the virulence (34).

MTT assay indicated that THP-1 cells did not damage significantly the *Curvularia* strains. Similarly, macrophages could not inhibit conidial germination and hyphal growth of *E. rostratum* (29). At the same time, THP-1 cells effectively decreased the viability of *A. fumigatus* during their interaction, as expected based on previous studies (20).

Transcription of immune-relevant genes of the monocytes during interaction with *C. lunata*, *C. hawaiiensis* and *C. spicifera* was examined by qRT-PCR analysis. A decrease in the transcription of the gene encoding CCR2, which is downregulated during monocytic differentiation (35), suggests the activation of THP-1 cells in response to *C. spicifera*. However, the unaltered or decreased expression of most tested genes, such as those encoding IL-6, IL-1β, CCR1, ITGAL, ITGAM, and ITGAX, suggests that *Curvularia* hyphae induce a moderate response in this cell type. After confrontation with *C. lunata*, transcription of HLA-DRA was significantly downregulated, assuming the lack of antigen presentation by monocytes despite of the attachment to the hyphae. In case of *A. fumigatus*, it was previously found that phagocytosis of the conidia did not induce the immediate expression of cytokine and chemokine genes in THP-1, which were activated only in the presence of the hyphae (18, 36). Similarly, we detected the induction of certain immune-relevant genes at 9 h postinoculation when the hyphae formation had already started.

In addition to the transcription analysis, production of certain cytokine proteins was measured after confrontation with the examined *Curvularia* strains. To the hyphae of *C. lunata*, THP-1 cells responded with intense IL-8 and IL-10 and moderate TNF-α production while they failed to produce IL-6. The chemokine IL-8 or CXCL8 is known to be involved in the immune response to fungal pathogens and it has a primary role in recruiting neutrophils to the site of infection (37, 38). IL-8 production and release by monocytes (including THP-1 cells) in response to confrontation with *A. fumigatus* is well documented by several studies (17, 18, 22). The low levels of the pro-inflammatory cytokines after interaction with *Curvularia* strains is somewhat surprising. These cytokines are involved in the effective immunity to fungal infections and their role has been studied and proven among others in response to *C. albicans*, *A. fumigatus*, and *C. neoformans* (37). In case of *C. lunata*, this situation can be partly explained by the high expression of the anti-inflammatory cytokine IL-10, which can repress pro-inflammatory responses and can inhibit the production of TNF-α, IL-6, and even IL-8 (39–41). In case of the THP-1 cells confronted with the *A. fumigatus* strain involved for comparison, this relatively high IL-10 production was not detected. Induction of IL-10 production in monocytes correlates well to that *Curvularia* strains and especially *C. lunata* can cause chronic infections even in immunocompetent persons (4) and are among the most frequent agents of allergic sinusitis and allergic bronchopulmonary disease (2, 4). It is known that certain pathogenic organisms possess mechanisms to modulate the immune response by enhancing IL-10 production and/or exploit the anti-inflammatory properties of IL-10 for their survival (42, 43). In the cases of *Histoplasma capsulatum* and *C. albicans*, the absence of IL-10 expression led to enhanced clearance of the fungi (44–46). Similarly, increased levels of serum IL-10 due to single nucleotide polymorphism in the *IL10* gene is associated with an increased susceptibility to *A. fumigatus* colonization and allergic bronchopulmonary aspergillosis (47). Despite the high IL-10 production, increased IL-8 level was measured after co-incubation with *C. lunata* that may suggest that neutrophils may have an important role in the immune response to this fungus as it was found in case of several other fungal species (33, 38). Interestingly, significantly increased relative transcript levels were measured for the genes encoding TNF-α and IL-10 in response to *C. spicifera* and *C. hawaiiensis* while secretion of these proteins by the monocytes could not be detected. Although the relative transcript level of *IL8* showed similar values as in case of *C. lunata*, there was no significant increase in protein release either. Considering that secretion of IL-10 and IL-8 is regulated primarily at a transcriptional level (48, 49), this is a surprising phenomenon. TNF-α production is regulated at a transcriptional and translational level as well (50, 51). Immune cells can display different attraction even to closely related fungal species. For example, different recognition of *C. albicans* and *C. glabrata* was observed by Netea et al. (52) and a distinct IL-1β release and ROS production of macrophages induced by *C. albicans* and *C. parapsilosis* (53). *Aspergillus* species (i.e., *A. fumigatus*, *A. flavus*, *A. niger*, and *A. terreus*) also induced significantly different release of IL-6 and TNF-α by human monocytes (54).

As a conclusion, our results show that THP-1 monocytes cannot effectively phagocytose the conidia of *Curvularia* species and there is a clear difference in response of these cells to the three investigated strains. They attach to the hyphae and respond to those of *C. lunata* by IL-10 and IL-8 production. Further studies to clarify the mechanisms in the background of the enhanced IL-10 production and the possible association of this phenomenon with the chronic mycoses caused by this fungus are needed. Considering the upregulation of IL-8, the role of neutrophils in the clearance of *Curvularia* infections is also worth to examine.

AUTHOR CONTRIBUTIONS

ET carried out most of the experimental work, performed the statistical analysis, and participated in the evaluation of the results and drafting the manuscript. ÉB, AH, CS, and MH performed experiments, analyzed data, and participated in the writing of the manuscript. GN performed experiments and participated in the evaluation of the results. IN, CV, and TP designed and coordinated the study and participated in the writing and the edition of the manuscript.

ACKNOWLEDGMENTS

The authors would like to thank Erik Zajta and Katalin Csonka for her help in the cell culturing and ELISA tests.

FUNDING

The study was supported by the "Lendület" Grant of the Hungarian Academy of Sciences (LP2016-8/2016) and the project GINOP-2.3.2-15-2016-00035. ÉB was funded by the European Union and the State of Hungary, co-financed by the European Social Fund in the framework of "National Excellence Program" (grant number A2-ELMH-12-0082); IN was supported by the János Bolyai Research Scholarship of the Hungarian Academy of Sciences. EJT is supported by the UNKP-17-3 New National Excellence Program of the Ministry of Human Capacities.

REFERENCES

1. Manamgoda DS, Cai L, Bahkali AH, Chukeatirote E, Hyde KD. Cochliobolus: an overview and current status of species. *Fungal Divers* (2011) 51(1):3–42. doi:10.1007/s13225-011-0139-4
2. Paredes K, Capilla J, Sutton DA, Mayayo E, Fothergill AW, Guarro J. Virulence of *Curvularia* in a murine model. *Mycoses* (2013) 56(5):512–5. doi:10.1111/myc.12064
3. Cavanna C, Seminari E, Pusateri A, Mangione F, Lallitto F, Esposto MC, et al. Allergic fungal rhinosinusitis due to *Curvularia lunata*. *New Microbiol* (2014) 37(2):241–5.
4. Krizsán KPT, Manikandan P, Shobana S, Chandrasekaran M, Vágvölgyi C, Kredics L. Clinical importance of the genus *Curvularia*. In: Razzaghi-Abyaneh M, Shams-Ghahfarokhi M, Rai M, editors. *Medical Mycology: Current Trends and Future Prospects*. Boca Raton, FL: CRC Press (2015). p. 147–204.
5. Bashir G, Hussain W, Rizvi A. *Bipolaris hawaiiensis* keratomycosis and endophthalmitis. *Mycopathologia* (2009) 167(1):51–3. doi:10.1007/s11046-008-9144-x
6. Mythili A, Babu Singh YR, Priya R, Shafeeq Hassan A, Manikandan P, Panneerselvam K, et al. In vitro and comparative study on the extracellular enzyme activity of molds isolated from keratomycosis and soil. *Int J Ophthalmol* (2014) 7(5):778–84. doi:10.3980/j.issn.2222-3959.2014.05.07
7. Moody MN, Tschen J, Mesko M. Cutaneous *Curvularia* infection of the forearm. *Cutis* (2012) 89(2):65–8.
8. Gunathilake R, Perera P, Sirimanna G. *Curvularia lunata*: a rare cause of black-grain eumycetoma. *J Mycol Med* (2014) 24(2):158–60. doi:10.1016/j.mycmed.2013.09.005
9. Skovrlj B, Haghighi M, Smethurst ME, Caridi J, Bederson JB. *Curvularia* abscess of the brainstem. *World Neurosurg* (2014) 82(1–2):e9–13. doi:10.1016/j.wneu.2013.07.014
10. Revankar SG, Patterson JE, Sutton DA, Pullen R, Rinaldi MG. Disseminated phaeohyphomycosis: review of an emerging mycosis. *Clin Infect Dis* (2002) 34(4):467–76. doi:10.1086/338636
11. Kobayashi H, Sano A, Aragane N, Fukuoka M, Tanaka M, Kawaura F, et al. Disseminated infection by *Bipolaris spicifera* in an immunocompetent subject. *Med Mycol* (2008) 46(4):361–5. doi:10.1080/13693780701883490
12. Balla A, Pierson J, Hugh J, Wojewoda C, Gibson P, Greene L. Disseminated cutaneous *Curvularia* infection in an immunocompromised host; diagnostic challenges and experience with voriconazole. *J Cutan Pathol* (2016) 43(4):383–7. doi:10.1111/cup.12648
13. Peghin M, Monforte V, Martin-Gomez MT, Ruiz-Camps I, Berastegui C, Saez B, et al. Epidemiology of invasive respiratory disease caused by emerging non-*Aspergillus* molds in lung transplant recipients. *Transpl Infect Dis* (2016) 18(1):70–8. doi:10.1111/tid.12492
14. El Khizzi NBS, Parvez S. *Bipolaris*: a plant pathogen causing human infections: an emerging problem in Saudi Arabia. *Res J Microbiol* (2010) 5(3):212–7. doi:10.3923/jm.2010.212.217
15. da Cunha KC, Sutton DA, Fothergill AW, Cano J, Gene J, Madrid H, et al. Diversity of *Bipolaris* species in clinical samples in the United States and their antifungal susceptibility profiles. *J Clin Microbiol* (2012) 50(12):4061–6. doi:10.1128/JCM.01965-12
16. Perfect JR, Alexander BD, Schell WA. Phaeohyphomycoses (brown–black moulds). 2nd ed. In: Kauffman C, Pappas P, Sobel JD, Dismukes WE, editors. *Essentials of Clinical Mycology*. New York, NY: Springer Science & Business Media (2011). p. 305–17.
17. Cortez KJ, Lyman CA, Kottilil S, Kim HS, Roilides E, Yang J, et al. Functional genomics of innate host defense molecules in normal human monocytes in response to *Aspergillus fumigatus*. *Infect Immun* (2006) 74(4):2353–65. doi:10.1128/IAI.74.4.2353-2365.2006
18. Loeffler J, Haddad Z, Bonin M, Romeike N, Mezger M, Schumacher U, et al. Interaction analyses of human monocytes co-cultured with different forms of *Aspergillus fumigatus*. *J Med Microbiol* (2009) 58(Pt 1):49–58. doi:10.1099/jmm.0.003293-0
19. Chanput W, Mes JJ, Wichers HJ. THP-1 cell line: an in vitro cell model for immune modulation approach. *Int Immunopharmacol* (2014) 23(1):37–45. doi:10.1016/j.intimp.2014.08.002
20. Sharif O, Bolshakov VN, Raines S, Newham P, Perkins ND. Transcriptional profiling of the LPS induced NF-kappaB response in macrophages. *BMC Immunol* (2007) 8:1. doi:10.1186/1471-2172-8-1
21. Marr KA, Koudadoust M, Black M, Balajee SA. Early events in macrophage killing of *Aspergillus fumigatus* conidia: new flow cytometric viability assay. *Clin Diagn Lab Immunol* (2001) 8(6):1240–7. doi:10.1128/CDLI.8.6.1240-1247.2001
22. Shalit I, Halperin D, Haite D, Levitov A, Romano J, Osherov N, et al. Anti-inflammatory effects of moxifloxacin on IL-8, IL-1beta and TNF-alpha secretion and NFkappaB and MAP-kinase activation in human monocytes stimulated with *Aspergillus fumigatus*. *J Antimicrob Chemother* (2006) 57(2):230–5. doi:10.1093/jac/dki441
23. Simitsopoulou M, Roilides E, Paliogianni F, Likartsis C, Ioannidis J, Kanellou K, et al. Immunomodulatory effects of voriconazole on monocytes challenged

with *Aspergillus fumigatus*: differential role of toll-like receptors. *Antimicrob Agents Chemother* (2008) 52(9):3301–6. doi:10.1128/AAC.01018-07
24. Barker KS, Liu T, Rogers PD. Coculture of THP-1 human mononuclear cells with *Candida albicans* results in pronounced changes in host gene expression. *J Infect Dis* (2005) 192(5):901–12. doi:10.1086/432487
25. Rai MN, Borah S, Bairwa G, Balusu S, Gorityala N, Kaur R. Establishment of an in vitro system to study intracellular behavior of *Candida glabrata* in human THP-1 macrophages. *J Vis Exp* (2013) 82:e50625. doi:10.3791/50625
26. Srikanta D, Yang M, Williams M, Doering TL. A sensitive high-throughput assay for evaluating host-pathogen interactions in *Cryptococcus neoformans* infection. *PLoS One* (2011) 6(7):e22773. doi:10.1371/journal.pone.0022773
27. Livak KJ, Schmittgen TD. Analysis of relative gene expression data using real-time quantitative PCR and the 2(-Delta Delta C(T)) method. *Methods* (2001) 25(4):402–8. doi:10.1006/meth.2001.1262
28. Levitz SM, Diamond RD. A rapid colorimetric assay of fungal viability with the tetrazolium salt MTT. *J Infect Dis* (1985) 152(5):938–45. doi:10.1093/infdis/152.5.938
29. Reedy JL, Negoro PE, Feliu M, Lord AK, Khan NS, Lukason DP, et al. The carbohydrate lectin receptor dectin-1 mediates the immune response to *Exserohilum rostratum*. *Infect Immun* (2017) 85(3):e903–16. doi:10.1128/IAI.00903-16
30. Behnsen J, Narang P, Hasenberg M, Gunzer F, Bilitewski U, Klippel N, et al. Environmental dimensionality controls the interaction of phagocytes with the pathogenic fungi *Aspergillus fumigatus* and *Candida albicans*. *PLoS Pathog* (2007) 3(2):e13. doi:10.1371/journal.ppat.0030013
31. Pihet M, Vandeputte P, Tronchin G, Renier G, Saulnier P, Georgeault S, et al. Melanin is an essential component for the integrity of the cell wall of *Aspergillus fumigatus* conidia. *BMC Microbiol* (2009) 9:177. doi:10.1186/1471-2180-9-1771471-2180-9-177
32. Chai LY, Netea MG, Sugui J, Vonk AG, van de Sande WW, Warris A, et al. *Aspergillus fumigatus* conidial melanin modulates host cytokine response. *Immunobiology* (2010) 215(11):915–20. doi:10.1016/j.imbio.2009.10.002
33. Erwig LP, Gow NA. Interactions of fungal pathogens with phagocytes. *Nat Rev Microbiol* (2016) 14(3):163–76. doi:10.1038/nrmicro.2015.21
34. Peltroche-Llacsahuanga H, Schnitzler N, Jentsch S, Platz A, De Hoog S, Schweizer KG, et al. Analyses of phagocytosis, evoked oxidative burst, and killing of black yeasts by human neutrophils: a tool for estimating their pathogenicity? *Med Mycol* (2003) 41(1):7–14. doi:10.1080/mmy.41.1.7.14
35. Fantuzzi L, Borghi P, Ciolli V, Pavlakis G, Belardelli F, Gessani S. Loss of CCR2 expression and functional response to monocyte chemotactic protein (MCP-1) during the differentiation of human monocytes: role of secreted MCP-1 in the regulation of the chemotactic response. *Blood* (1999) 94(3):875–83.
36. Said-Sadier N, Padilla E, Langsley G, Ojcius DM. *Aspergillus fumigatus* stimulates the NLRP3 inflammasome through a pathway requiring ROS production and the Syk tyrosine kinase. *PLoS One* (2010) 5(4):e10008. doi:10.1371/journal.pone.0010008
37. Antachopoulos C, Roilides E. Cytokines and fungal infections. *Br J Haematol* (2005) 129(5):583–96. doi:10.1111/j.1365-2141.2005.05498.x
38. Morton CO, Bouzani M, Loeffler J, Rogers TR. Direct interaction studies between *Aspergillus fumigatus* and human immune cells; what have we learned about pathogenicity and host immunity? *Front Microbiol* (2012) 3:413. doi:10.3389/fmicb.2012.00413
39. de Waal Malefyt R, Abrams J, Bennett B, Figdor CG, de Vries JE. Interleukin 10(IL-10) inhibits cytokine synthesis by human monocytes: an autoregulatory role of IL-10 produced by monocytes. *J Exp Med* (1991) 174(5):1209–20. doi:10.1084/jem.174.5.1209
40. Couper KN, Blount DG, Riley EM. IL-10: the master regulator of immunity to infection. *J Immunol* (2008) 180(9):5771–7. doi:10.4049/jimmunol.180.9.5771
41. Ouyang W, Rutz S, Crellin NK, Valdez PA, Hymowitz SG. Regulation and functions of the IL-10 family of cytokines in inflammation and disease. *Annu Rev Immunol* (2011) 29:71–109. doi:10.1146/annurev-immunol-031210-101312
42. Cyktor JC, Turner J. Interleukin-10 and immunity against prokaryotic and eukaryotic intracellular pathogens. *Infect Immun* (2011) 79(8):2964–73. doi:10.1128/IAI.00047-11
43. Iyer SS, Cheng G. Role of interleukin 10 transcriptional regulation in inflammation and autoimmune disease. *Crit Rev Immunol* (2012) 32(1):23–63. doi:10.1615/CritRevImmunol.v32.i1.30
44. Romani L, Puccetti P, Mencacci A, Cenci E, Spaccapelo R, Tonnetti L, et al. Neutralization of IL-10 up-regulates nitric oxide production and protects susceptible mice from challenge with *Candida albicans*. *J Immunol* (1994) 152(7):3514–21.
45. Deepe GS Jr, Gibbons RS. Protective and memory immunity to *Histoplasma capsulatum* in the absence of IL-10. *J Immunol* (2003) 171(10):5353–62. doi:10.4049/jimmunol.171.10.5353
46. Netea MG, Sutmuller R, Hermann C, Van der Graaf CA, Van der Meer JW, van Krieken JH, et al. Toll-like receptor 2 suppresses immunity against *Candida albicans* through induction of IL-10 and regulatory T cells. *J Immunol* (2004) 172(6):3712–8. doi:10.4049/jimmunol.172.6.3712
47. Romani L. Immunity to fungal infections. *Nat Rev Immunol* (2004) 4(1):1–23. doi:10.1038/nri1255
48. Le T, Leung L, Carroll WL, Schibler KR. Regulation of interleukin-10 gene expression: possible mechanisms accounting for its upregulation and for maturational differences in its expression by blood mononuclear cells. *Blood* (1997) 89(11):4112–9.
49. Roebuck KA. Regulation of interleukin-8 gene expression. *J Interferon Cytokine Res* (1999) 19(5):429–38. doi:10.1089/107999099313866
50. Spriggs DR, Deutsch S, Kufe DW. Genomic structure, induction, and production of TNF-alpha. *Immunol Ser* (1992) 56:3–34.
51. Parameswaran N, Patial S. Tumor necrosis factor-alpha signaling in macrophages. *Crit Rev Eukaryot Gene Expr* (2010) 20(2):87–103. doi:10.1615/CritRevEukarGeneExpr.v20.i2.10
52. Netea MG, Joosten LA, van der Meer JW, Kullberg BJ, van de Veerdonk FL. Immune defence against *Candida* fungal infections. *Nat Rev Immunol* (2015) 15(10):630–42. doi:10.1038/nri3897nri3897
53. Toth A, Zajta E, Csonka K, Vagvolgyi C, Netea MG, Gacser A. Specific pathways mediating inflammasome activation by *Candida parapsilosis*. *Sci Rep* (2017) 7:43129. doi:10.1038/srep43129
54. Warris A, Netea MG, Verweij PE, Gaustad P, Kullberg BJ, Weemaes CM, et al. Cytokine responses and regulation of interferon-gamma release by human mononuclear cells to *Aspergillus fumigatus* and other filamentous fungi. *Med Mycol* (2005) 43(7):613–21. doi:10.1080/13693780500088333

18

Fluorescent Tracking of Yeast Division Clarifies the Essential Role of Spleen Tyrosine Kinase in the Intracellular Control of *Candida glabrata* in Macrophages

*Zeina Dagher[1], Shuying Xu[1], Paige E. Negoro[1], Nida S. Khan[1,2], Michael B. Feldman[3], Jennifer L. Reedy[1], Jenny M. Tam[1], David B. Sykes[4] and Michael K. Mansour[1]**

[1] Division of Infectious Disease, Massachusetts General Hospital, Harvard Medical School, Boston, MA, United States, [2] Biomedical Engineering and Biotechnology, University of Massachusetts Medical School, Worcester, MA, United States, [3] Division of Pulmonary and Critical Care, Massachusetts General Hospital, Boston, MA, United States, [4] Center for Regenerative Medicine, Massachusetts General Hospital, Boston, MA, United States

***Correspondence:**
Michael K. Mansour
mkmansour@mgh.harvard.edu

Macrophages play a critical role in the elimination of fungal pathogens. They are sensed *via* cell surface pattern-recognition receptors and are phagocytosed into newly formed organelles called phagosomes. Phagosomes mature through the recruitment of proteins and lysosomes, resulting in addition of proteolytic enzymes and acidification of the microenvironment. Our earlier studies demonstrated an essential role of Dectin-1-dependent activation of spleen tyrosine kinase (Syk) in the maturation of fungal containing phagosomes. The absence of Syk activity interrupted phago-lysosomal fusion resulting in arrest at an early phagosome stage. In this study, we sought to define the contribution of Syk to the control of phagocytosed live *Candida glabrata* in primary macrophages. To accurately measure intracellular yeast division, we designed a carboxyfluorescein succinimidyl ester (CFSE) yeast division assay in which bright fluorescent parent cells give rise to dim daughter cells. The CFSE-labeling of *C. glabrata* did not affect the growth rate of the yeast. Following incubation with macrophages, internalized CFSE-labeled *C. glabrata* were retrieved by cellular lysis, tagged using ConA-647, and the amount of residual CFSE fluorescence was assessed by flow cytometry. *C. glabrata* remained undivided (CFSE bright) for up to 18 h in co-culture with primary macrophages. Treatment of macrophages with R406, a specific Syk inhibitor, resulted in loss of intracellular control of *C. glabrata* with initiation of division within 4 h. Delayed Syk inhibition after 8 h was less effective indicating that Syk is critically required at early stages of macrophage–fungal interaction. In conclusion, we demonstrate a new method of tracking division of *C. glabrata* using CFSE labeling. Our results suggest that early Syk activation is essential for macrophage control of phagocytosed *C. glabrata*.

Keywords: *Candida*, *Candida glabrata*, macrophages, spleen tyrosine kinase, phagosome, carboxyfluorescein succinimidyl ester

INTRODUCTION

The fungal pathogen *Candida glabrata* is a common cause of invasive bloodstream infections in immunocompromised patients (1). With the rise of organ transplantation, immunosuppressive chemotherapy, implanted medical devices, and antibacterial use, *C. glabrata* has emerged as a frequently isolated species, accounting for 20% of systemic bloodstream *Candida*-related infections in North America (2, 3).

In vitro, following interaction with human or murine macrophages, *C. glabrata* undergoes phagocytosis. Despite being internalized, *C. glabrata* survives and replicates inside host immune cells (4, 5). Intracellular killing of *C. glabrata* by macrophages is only about 10% effective (6). The capacity of this *Candida* species to evade the innate immune system complicates evaluation of intracellular pathogen control by simple phagocytosis assays. A more sensitive and accurate approach to quantifying *C. glabrata* intracellular proliferation is required to understand and identify the relevant pathogen–host interactions.

The carboxyfluorescein diacetate succinimidyl ester (CFSE) assay is a well-established method to fluorescently track lymphocyte cellular division (7, 8). The succinimidyl moiety of the dye covalently attaches to cellular aliphatic amine groups, forming stable amide bonds (9). This covalent-coupling dye allows for tracking of lymphocyte proliferation; each progressive cell division results in a twofold dilution of the fluorescent signal between daughter cells (10, 11). Unlike labeling techniques that rely on microscopic evaluation, CFSE can be visualized by both fluorescence microscopy and can be formally quantitated by flow cytometry (12). CFSE is highly fluorescent, has an excitation/emission profile at 491/518 nm, is stable in long-term tracking, and can be used *in vitro* and *in vivo* (10).

Although most published reports have used CFSE to monitor lymphocyte proliferation, recent studies have also used the dye to follow proliferation of other mammalian and non-mammalian cell types, such as bacterial cells and parasites (13, 14). CFSE also successfully labeled *Paracoccidioides* yeast in a flow cytometry based phagocytosis study, although the tracking of proliferation was not evaluated (15).

Here, we have applied the CFSE proliferation-tracking properties to *C. glabrata*, though several factors require special consideration. Unlike animal cells, fungi possess a cell wall composed of extracellular carbohydrate-rich polymers. CFSE brightly labels the cell wall, though does not permeate the yeast to label intracellular structures. Additionally, unlike mammalian cells where the cell membrane is shared symmetrically (in equal amounts) between daughter cells (16), the yeast cell wall is shared asymmetrically, with the budding yeast generating an almost-entirely new cell wall (17). This new (and CFSE-unlabeled) cell wall is synthesized at growing cell tips through the localization and activation of cell wall carbohydrate synthases (18, 19). Thus, unlike CFSE assays in lymphocytes, the CFSE labeling of yeast such as *C. glabrata* does not allow one to track beyond a single division.

Following infection, tissue macrophages sense fungi through the expression of pattern-recognition receptors (PRRs), such as Dectin-1 and Dectin-2, which recognize fungal cell wall carbohydrates (5, 20). Recognition through PRRs triggers phagocytosis, engulfing microorganisms within phagosomes, eventually fusing with additional subcellular compartments including lysosomes for acidification and killing (21). The process of acidification is termed phagosomal maturation, which in response to fungal cell wall ligands, is spleen tyrosine kinase (Syk)-dependent (22). Syk activation and signal transduction is central for immune activation in several immune cells (23). PRRs share the ability to associate with immunoreceptor tyrosine-based activation motifs (ITAM) in their cytoplasmic domains, leading to Syk recruitment and phosphorylation, resulting in downstream events including phagocytosis, and the production of reactive oxygen species (ROS) and proinflammatory cytokines (24–26). The central role of Syk in activation of several innate and adaptive immune cells has made this kinase a promising target for the development of anti-inflammatory therapeutics (27, 28).

Although the role of Syk in intracellular signaling has been studied extensively, its involvement in the response to intracellular pathogens in innate immune cells, such as macrophages, is not delineated (23, 26). In this study, we introduce a CFSE-labeling assay that allows for intracellular tracking of yeast proliferation in macrophage phagosomes. We demonstrate that CFSE is a reliable method of evaluating *C. glabrata* division by fluorescence microscopy and quantitatively by flow cytometry. Employing the CFSE assay, we show that Syk inhibition in macrophages results in the loss of the ability to control *C. glabrata* proliferation. This loss of *C. glabrata* division control is independent of phagocytosis and is not a result of failure to activate the Dectin-1 and Dectin-2 pathways. These observations highlight CFSE live labeling as a useful and convenient tool for measuring yeast proliferation accurately and support further investigation into the role of Syk in antifungal immunity.

MATERIALS AND METHODS

Reagents

R406 was purchased from Santa Cruz Biotechnology (Dallas, TX, USA), Nonidet P40 (NP40) and peptone from American Bioanalytical (Natick, MA, USA), CFSE dye, and all other chemicals from Sigma (St. Louis, MO, USA) unless otherwise stated. Wild type *C. glabrata* (ATCC2001) was purchased from the American Type Culture Collection (ATCC, Manassas, VA, USA). Cell lysis buffer consisted of 4× NP40 containing 40 mM Tris-hydrochloric acid, 600 mM sodium chloride, 20 mM magnesium chloride, and 4% NP40 titrated to pH 7.5. Yeast culture media liquid YPD contained 1% yeast extract (BD Biosciences, San Jose, CA, USA), 2% peptone, and 2% dextrose. Cell culture media (RPMI-complete) was composed of RPMI 1640 (Corning, Tewksbury, MA, USA) with 2 mM L-glutamine, 10% heat-inactivated fetal bovine serum, and 1% penicillin–streptomycin (ThermoFisher Scientific, Waltham MA, USA).

Yeast Culture and CFSE Staining

Candida glabrata were grown overnight shaking in liquid YPD at 30°C, washed three times in phosphate buffered saline (PBS), counted using a Luna automated cell counter (Logos Biosystems, Annandale, VA, USA), and resuspended in PBS at the desired inoculum.

To stain yeast with CFSE, wild type *C. glabrata* were grown to log phase in liquid YPD, washed twice in 1 mL PBS, and 160 million yeast were stained with 25 µg/mL CFSE for 30 min in 4 mL PBS at 30°C on a vertical rotator. Yeasts were washed twice in 10 mL PBS containing 2% bovine serum albumin (BSA) to remove excess CFSE. Stained yeast cells were resuspended in 1 mL PBS and passed through a 25G 7/8-inch needle 10 times to dissociate clumps into single cell suspension.

Calcofluor White Staining

To stain all intracellular yeast cells, macrophages were fixed and permeabilized with 4% paraformaldehyde (Electron Microscopy Sciences, Hatfield, PA, USA) for 20 min at room temperature in the dark. Cells were washed three times with PBS and incubated in 10% calcofluor white solution in PBS for 15 min and imaged using confocal microscopy with 405 nm laser excitation.

Collection of Murine Peritoneal Macrophages

Eight-week-old inbred C57BL/6 mice (Jackson Laboratory, ME, USA), Dectin-1$^{-/-}$ (B6 background, a gift from Dr. Gordon Brown, University of Aberdeen, UK) (29), or Dectin-2$^{-/-}$ (B6 background, a gift from Dr. Marcel Wuethrich, University of Wisconsin) (30) were housed in a specific pathogen-free facility at the Massachusetts General Hospital (MGH, Boston, MA, USA). All animal experiments were approved by the MGH Institutional Animal Care and Use Committee. Peritoneal macrophages were isolated from mice following intraperitoneally instillation of 2 mL thioglycollate (Northeast Laboratory, Waterville, ME, USA). After 3 days, the mice were euthanized and the peritoneum lavaged with 10 mL RPMI-complete to retrieve cells. Intraperitoneal cells were washed and plated at a density of 300,000 cells per well in 500 µL RPMI-complete in 24-well dishes and allowed to adhere overnight. Non-adherent contaminating cells were washed away after 24 h resulting in a >95% pure, viable macrophage population as determine by anti-Mac 1 staining using flow cytometry (data not shown).

Co-Culture of Peritoneal Macrophages and CFSE-*C. glabrata*

The media in each 24-well was reduced to 250 µL and wells were treated with R406 dissolved in DMSO or DMSO only either 10 min prior to *C. glabrata* inoculation or 2, 4, or 8 h after *C. glabrata* inoculation. A total of 200,000 CFSE-labeled *C. glabrata* were added for a final MOI of 0.6. Plates were centrifuged for 1 min at 700 × *g* to facilitate cell-ligand contacts and incubated at 37°C with 5% CO_2. After the time indicated, the macrophages were lysed with 100 µL of 4× NP40 on ice for 5 min. Well contents were centrifuged for 7.5 min at 10,000 rpm. The pellets were then fixed with 4% formaldehyde for 10 min in the dark and washed with PBS/2% BSA. Concanavalin A conjugated to Alexa Fluor 647 (ThermoFisher, Waltham, MA, USA) at a final concentration 3 µg/mL was added for 20 min in the dark to stain *C. glabrata*. Yeast were washed and resuspended in PBS/2% BSA for flow cytometry.

Macrophage Phagocytosis of *C. glabrata*

To assess macrophage phagocytosis, CFSE-*C. glabrata* were co-incubated with macrophages in the presence or absence of inhibitor for the time indicated. Plates were transferred onto ice, wells washed with PBS, then macrophages mechanically lifted, and strained through a 40-µm filter and immediately subjected to flow cytometry gating on the macrophage population. The phagocytosis percent was measured as the number of CFSE positive macrophages over the total macrophage cell number.

Reactive Oxygen Species

Reactive oxygen species was measured as described (31), briefly macrophages were plated at 5×10^4 cells/well in white wall 96-well plate (Costar, Cambridge, MA, USA). Cells were placed on ice and washed three times with PBS. Lucigenin solution (0.9 mM $CaCl_2$, 0.5 mM $MgCl_2$, 20 mM dextrose, and 20 µM lucigenin) was added, and cells were incubated on ice for 10 min. Heat-killed *C. glabrata* for 10 min were added at an effector to target ratio of 25, and then the plate was centrifuged at 750 × *g* for 1 min to facilitate cell-ligand contacts. An initial reading was then taken immediately after centrifugation for baseline. The plate was then incubated at 37°C and read with SpectraMax i3x reader (Molecular Devices, Sunnyvale, CA, USA) for total luminescence every 10 min for 2 h.

Confocal Microscopy

2×10^4 peritoneal macrophages were plated onto eight-chambered coverslip slides (LabTek, Thermo Scientific, Rochester, NY, USA) in RPMI-complete. CFSE-labeled *C. glabrata* were added at MOI 1:1, spun at 700 *g* × 1 min for immediate co-culture and slides mounted on a Nikon Ti-E inverted microscope equipped with an EM-CCD camera (Hamamatsu Photonics K.K., Hamamatsu, Japan). The excitation source was an 89 North MultiLine LaserBank (89 North, Burlington, VT, USA) A piezo stage (Prior Instruments, Rockland, MA, USA) capable of *X*, *Y*, and *Z* movement was used for acquisition. A polarizer (Nikon, MEN 51941) and Wollaston prisms (Nikon, MBH76190) were used to acquire differential interference contrast (DIC) images. Emission light from the samples was collected after passage through the appropriate emission filters (Semrock, Rochester, NY, USA) (32). Images were acquired using MetaMorph software (Molecular Devices, Downingtown, PA, USA), and processed using Adobe Photoshop CS5 and assembled in Adobe Illustrator, version CS5 (Adobe Systems, San Jose, CA, USA).

Flow Cytometric Analysis of CFSE

Carboxyfluorescein succinimidyl ester-labeled *C. glabrata* that were fixed and stained with concanavalin A-Alexa Fluor 647 were flowed using FACS Calibur flow cytometer (Becton-Dickinson, San Jose, CA, USA) and CellQuest software (Becton-Dickinson). ConA-647 (FL4) was plotted on the *y*-axis and CFSE (FL1) on the *x*-axis and the percentage of CFSE bright undivided population was determined with FlowJo 10 (FlowJo, Ashland, OR, USA).

Statistics

Statistical calculations were performed using GraphPad Prism 7 software. Data were analyzed by two-tailed, unpaired *t* test and were considered significantly different when $p \leq 0.05$.

RESULTS

CFSE Labeling Tracks Division of *C. glabrata*

We evaluated CFSE staining of *C. glabrata* using fluorescence microscopy. *C. glabrata* were homogenously fluorescent throughout the cell wall, likely due to the high content of fungal cell wall esterases that permit CFSE activation and labeling. The CFSE-labeled *C. glabrata* retained normal cell shape and morphology (**Figure 1**). Following 6 h in culture, CFSE-labeled *C. glabrata* were counter-stained with calcofluor white for chitin to delineate all yeast cells and visualized using confocal microscopy. All yeast cells were evenly stained with calcofluor white. Parent yeast cells were brightly CFSE-fluorescent, while daughter cells exhibited diluted CFSE leading to reduced fluorescence intensity as identified by flow cytometry (**Figure 2A**).

The consistent and predictable decrease in fluorescence permits quantitation of *C. glabrata* intracellular division as a marker of control by macrophages. While calcofluor allows visualization of all yeast cells using 405 nm laser excitation under confocal microscopy, our FACSCalibur is fitted with a blue and red laser incapable of exciting calcofluor. For these reasons, the total number of yeast were identified by labeling with concanavalin A conjugated to AF647 for flow cytometry. Therefore, a *C. glabrata* parent cell population is double-positive for CFSE and ConA-647, while divided daughter cells are CFSE-dim, but remain ConA-647 (**Figure 2B**).

With each cell division, the percent of the parent cells decrease, as daughter cell numbers rise and are easily distinguished *via* CFSE intensity. In fact, the diminished CFSE-bright parent cells was inversely proportional to the increase in the optical density of the growing yeast, confirming that the percentage of CFSE-bright cells accurately reflects yeast proliferation (**Figure 2C**). Moreover, CFSE-labeled and unlabeled *C. glabrata* proliferated at the same rate (as measured by OD_{600}) indicating that the CFSE-labeling process does not affect yeast proliferation.

Macrophages Control Intracellular *C. glabrata* Proliferation Using Syk

To evaluate the role of Syk in macrophages following exposure to *C. glabrata*, we used an *in vitro* co-culture system. Peritoneal macrophages were co-cultured with CFSE-labeled *C. glabrata* parent cells and monitored for evidence of intracellular proliferation. In wild type murine macrophages, yeast cells were phagocytosed by macrophages with high efficiency. There were rare numbers of extracellular yeast remaining as measured by microscopy (**Figure 3A**) and flow cytometry analysis of co-culture supernatant (data not shown). Following co-culture incubation, analysis of CFSE intensity of *C. glabrata* from lysed macrophages revealed that yeast did not divide for up to 16 h as measured by retained parent CFSE-bright (**Figure 3B**, top panel). However, in the presence of the reversible Syk inhibitor, R406, macrophages were unable to control *C. glabrata* division (**Figure 3B** bottom panel). Compared to untreated controls, R406-treated macrophages resulted in a diminished number of parent yeast and in a growing numbers of divided daughter population. While these yeast remained intracellular, they had escaped control and undergone division as noted by loss of CFSE (**Figure 3C**). To ensure that R406 does not alter growth kinetics of *C. glabrata*, division rates of *C. glabrata* in the presence of R406 and was not different from yeast control conditions (data not shown). These data suggest that loss of Syk activity significantly impaired the ability of macrophages to control *C. glabrata* intracellular division.

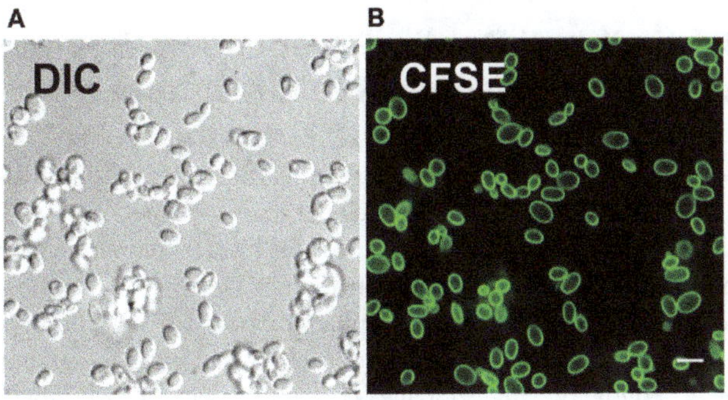

FIGURE 1 | Carboxyfluorescein succinimidyl ester (CFSE) labels cell wall of *Candida glabrata*. **(A)** Differential interference contrast and **(B)** fluorescence confocal microscopy image of live *C. glabrata* stained with CFSE showing labeling of all yeast cells prior to cell division. Scale bar represents 5 μm.

Early Syk Activity Is Required for Intracellular *C. glabrata* Control

Given that Syk is essential for control of *C. glabrata* division, we next sought to define the temporal relationship between Syk activity and yeast control. Macrophages that had engulfed *C. glabrata* were exposed to R406 continuously or following a 2, 4, or 8-h delay from time of coincubation. Syk inhibition at the start, or 2- or 4-h resulted in a loss of macrophage control as evidenced by the significant decrease in the percent of undivided yeast (**Figure 4**). The delayed addition of R406 to 8 h, and beyond, did not have an influence *C. glabrata* division. These data suggest that it is the early Syk activity following macrophage phagocytosis of yeast that is required for intracellular *C. glabrata* control.

Syk Inhibition Does Not Affect Macrophage Phagocytosis

In certain cell types, Syk has been shown to play a role in cytoskeletal rearrangement and endocytosis (33). If the process of macrophage phagocytosis was impaired by Syk inhibition (R406), this might leave extracellular *C. glabrata* in an actively dividing state. To determine if Syk inhibition impacts the process of phagocytosis of *C. glabrata* by peritoneal macrophages, we measured phagocytosis by flow cytometry in the presence and absence of R406. Cytochalasin D, an actin polymerization inhibitor, was used as a positive control inhibitor of phagocytosis.

We first determined the percent of macrophages that were associated with CFSE-bright *C. glabrata*. There was no difference in the ability of macrophages to phagocytose *C. glabrata* in the presence of R406 after 5 min (**Figure 5**). Macrophages that were treated with cytochalasin D showed dramatically reduced phagocytosis. The small percentage of yeast associated with cytochalasin D-treated macrophages as detected by flow possibly represents CFSE-bright *C. glabrata* attached extracellularly to the macrophage membrane or incomplete inhibition of

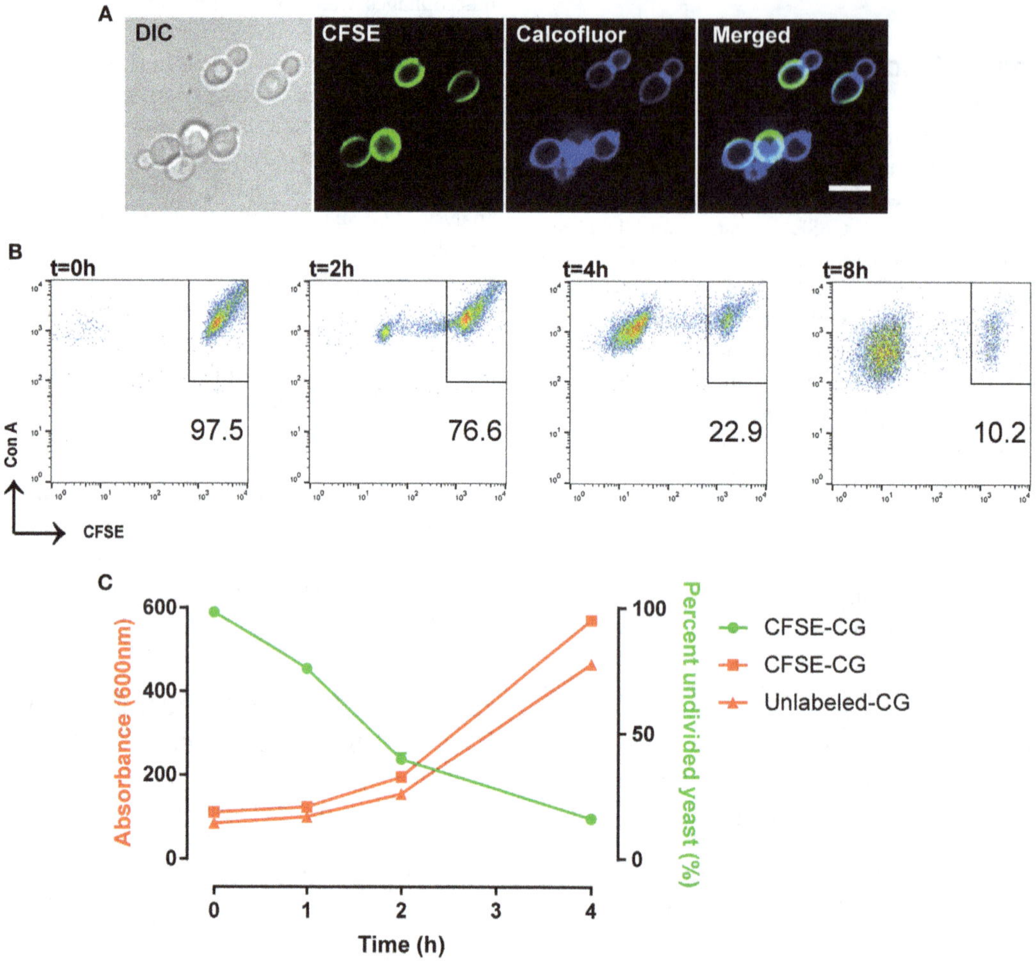

FIGURE 2 | Carboxyfluorescein succinimidyl ester (CFSE)-labeling marks *Candida glabrata* yeast division. **(A)** Differential interference contrast and fluorescence microscopy image of CFSE-labeled *C. glabrata* that have undergone division and stained with calcofluor white. Parental cells exhibit full CFSE labeling, while daughter cells have diluted CFSE labeling leading to dimmer fluorescence signal. Scale bar represents 5 μm. **(B)** Scatter plot of Con A-AF647 and CFSE fluorescence. CFSE-bright parental yeast population in upper right quadrant gate. Percent (scatter plot inset) of undivided CFSE-bright population was determined over time indicated. **(C)** Correlation of percent CFSE-bright population to OD_{600} nm of proliferating yeast. Data represent a minimum of three independent triplicate experiments.

phagocytosis by cytochalasin D. These findings indicate that Syk plays a minor role in the process of macrophage phagocytosis of *C. glabrata*.

R406 Inhibition of Syk Does Not Result in Permanent Macrophage Impairment

Given that Syk-mediated pathways are involved in multiple macrophage functions, we sought to determine if chemical Syk inhibition might result in a persistent hyporesponsive state. Given that ROS is a key mechanism in the response of macrophage to fungi, we evaluated ROS production in primary macrophages treated with R406 as compared to macrophages pulsed with R406 and then washed free of the inhibitor.

With constant R406, ROS production was completely suppressed (**Figure 6**). However, removal of R406 (following 2 h of exposure) restored ROS production to baseline levels. The observation that R406-pulsed macrophages were capable of generating robust ROS mirroring those of untreated control cells suggests that inhibition of Syk does not permanently alter the viability or biological activity of macrophages.

Dectin-1 and Dectin-2-Dependent Syk Activity Are Dispensable for Control of Intracellular *C. glabrata* Growth

Dectin-1 and Dectin-2 are upstream carbohydrate lectin PRRs that rely on Syk to regulate intracellular macrophage responses. To determine if the Syk activity required for intracellular *C. glabrata* control was derived through activation of Dectin-1 or Dectin-2, we compared peritoneal macrophages derived from wild type, to those derived from Dectin-1-deficient and Dectin-2-deficient mice. Following macrophage co-culture with CFSE-labeled *C. glabrata*, there was no difference in the control of intracellular *C. glabrata* growth between the macrophage genotypes signifying that the critical Syk activity required for yeast control is not related to individual Dectin-1 or Dectin-2 function (**Figure 7**).

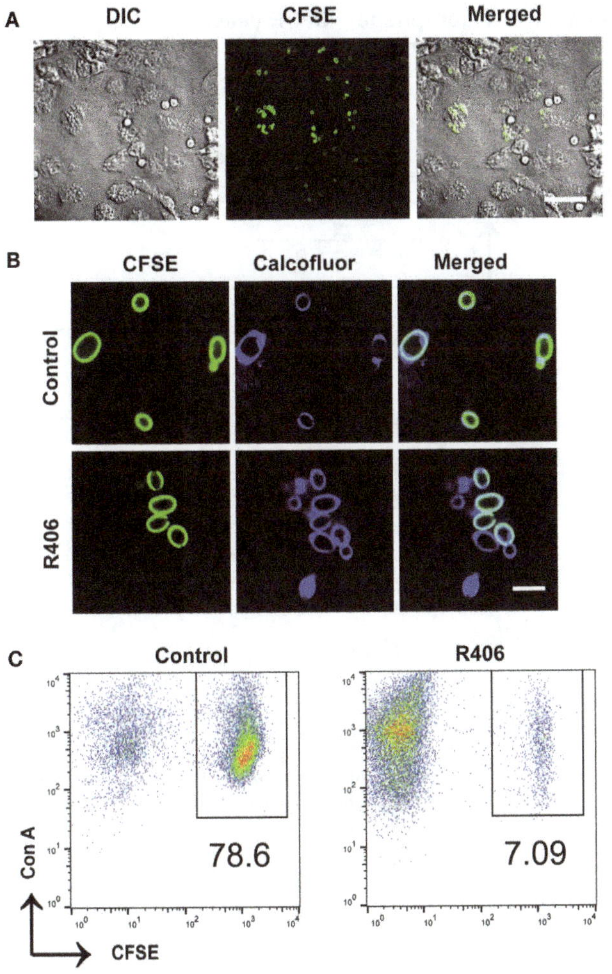

FIGURE 3 | Spleen tyrosine kinase is required for peritoneal macrophage control of *Candida glabrata*. **(A)** Differential interference contrast (DIC) and fluorescence microscopy image of carboxyfluorescein succinimidyl ester (CFSE)-*C. glabrata* and macrophage after 1 h of coculture indicating complete uptake of the yeast by the macrophages. Scale bar represents 50 µm. **(B)** DIC and fluorescence microscopy image of CFSE *C. glabrata* infected macrophages 16 h post inoculation. Macrophages control *C. glabrata* division in CFSE-bright undivided state, while treatment with R406 impaired the macrophages' ability in controlling *C. glabrata*. Scale bar represents 5 µm. **(C)** Flow cytometry scatter plots of Con A and CFSE showing macrophage controlling *C. glabrata* division and loss of control in R406-treated cells. Data represent three independent experiments.

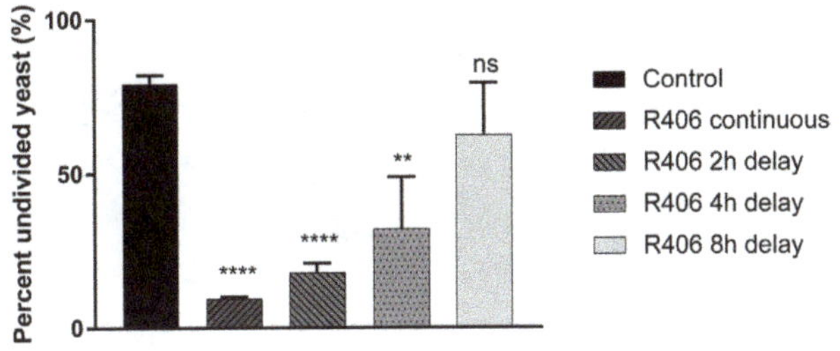

FIGURE 4 | Spleen tyrosine kinase (Syk) is required at an early stage for macrophage control of *Candida glabrata*. Macrophages were treated with chemical Syk inhibitor, R406, prior to addition of *C. glabrata* for 2, 4, and 8 h after infection. All wells were lysed after 16 h of co-culture and the yeast retrieved and stained with ConA-AF647. Percent of parental CFSE-bright population was assessed *via* flow cytometry, with R406 treatments initiated at indicated time. $^{**}p \leq 0.01$, $^{***}p \leq 0.001$, $^{****}p \leq 0.0001$. Data represent a minimum of three independent experiments.

DISCUSSION

Though the importance of the innate immune system in protecting against fungal pathogens has been articulated, defining the mechanisms responsible for the intracellular control of *C. glabrata* have yet to be defined. In this study, we define the role of Syk in the intracellular control of *C. glabrata* division in macrophages. Our approach outlines the CFSE-labeling technique as a new tool to track yeast division. We demonstrate that in macrophages, early Syk activity is essential for controlling *C. glabrata* division, and that this role is not solely dependent on the contribution of Dectin-1 or Dectin-2, both of which rely principally on Syk for intracellular signaling following ligand engagement.

We delineated a method of CFSE labeling that allows tracking of yeast multiplication. This process involved conjugating the cell wall of *C. glabrata* cells with CFSE, a fluorescent dye that links to amine groups through covalent bonds, and that can be visualized using confocal microscopy and flow cytometry. Microscopy demonstrated that CFSE does not change the morphology of *C. glabrata* cells. CFSE stained only the cell walls of parent yeasts, which permitted us to distinguish CFSE-bright parent populations and CFSE-dim daughter populations. The increase of CFSE-dim yeast cells, indicative of cell division and a growing daughter population, could be accurately measured by flow cytometry.

While CFSE assays have historically been used to follow the division of lymphocytes, our adaptation to track yeast division does face limitations. CFSE stains only the fungal cell wall rather than the contents of the cytoplasm, which allows us to track only a single generation of daughter cells. This observation is likely due to the presence of the esterase-rich fungal cell wall. Esterases are necessary for the activation of CFSE for covalent conjugation to amino groups on proteins. In mammalian cells, esterases are abundant within the cytoplasm, whereas in yeast, high levels of esterases are found within the fungal cell wall (34). This esterase distribution clarifies the reason for concentrated CFSE conjugation to the cell wall ultrastructure as opposed to homogenous cytoplasmic staining as seen in lymphocytes. Given the high concentration of CFSE in the cell wall, we confirmed that labeling did not alter the fungal cell wall or yeast division. By monitoring growth *via* optical density at 600 nm, we show that CFSE-labeled *C. glabrata* are capable of proliferating with normal kinetics as compared to unlabeled controls. While this method allows tracking of intracellular yeast division, it does not confirm killing of the yeast by macrophages.

Using CFSE-labeled yeast, we defined the role of Syk in the intracellular control of *C. glabrata* by macrophages. We hypothesized that Syk is indeed necessary for macrophages to maintain growth control of *C. glabrata* given its described contribution to phagolysosomal maturation (22) and autophagy (31). The downstream Syk-dependent molecular mechanisms critical for control of *C. glabrata* will require additional investigation and may involve sequestration of essential nutrients or disrupted

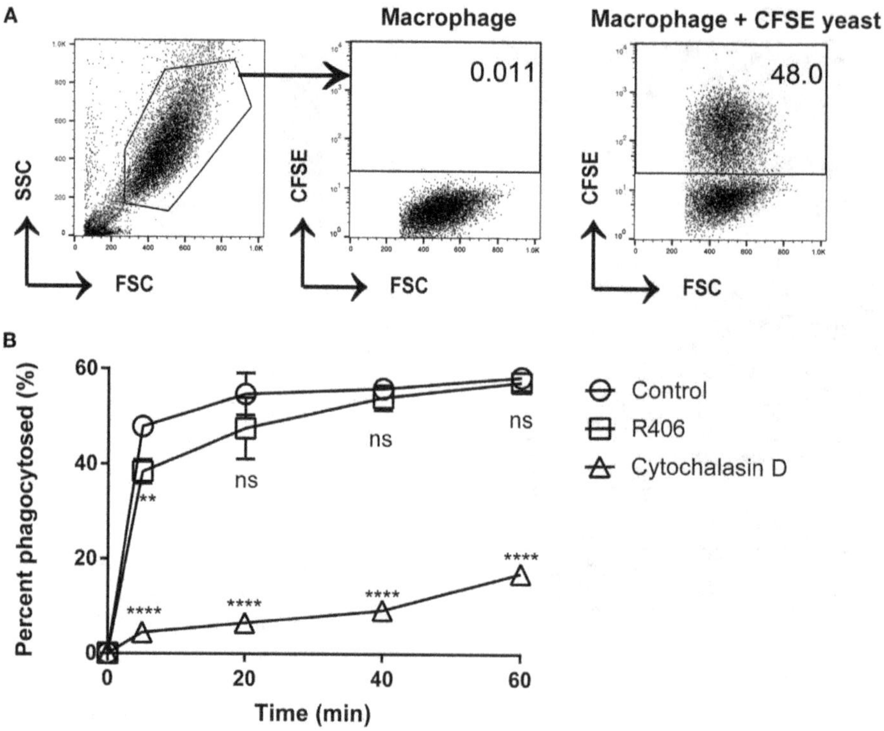

FIGURE 5 | R406-induced spleen tyrosine kinase inhibition does not affect macrophage phagocytosis of *C. glabrata*. **(A)** Gating scheme for calculated percentage of macrophages that have phagocytosed CFSE-labeled *C. glabrata* by flow cytometry. **(B)** Percent phagocytosis of *C. glabrata* by macrophages over time incubated with control, R406, or cytochalasin D by flow cytometry. $^{**}p \leq 0.01$, $^{****}p < 0.0001$. Data represent three independent experiments.

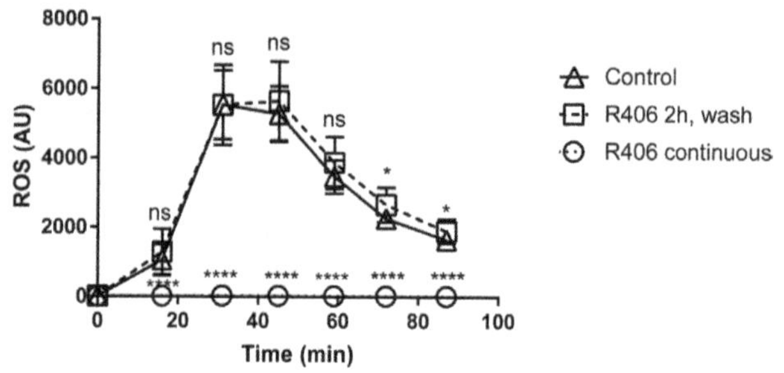

FIGURE 6 | R406 does not result in permanent macrophage response defects to fungal stimuli as measured by reactive oxygen species (ROS) production. Plated macrophages were treated with R406 for 2 h, and then washed to remove the inhibitor. ROS production measured by lucigenin after addition of heat-killed *Candida*. Arbitrary light unites (AU) represents total luminescence corresponding with ROS production. $^{*}p \leq 0.05$, $^{****}p \leq 0.0001$. Data represent a minimum of three independent experiments.

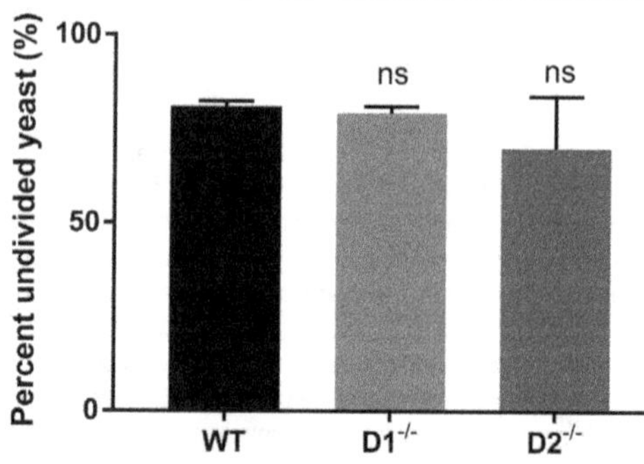

FIGURE 7 | Spleen tyrosine kinase-mediated control of *Candida glabrata* is independent of Dectin-1 and Dectin-2. Percent undivided carboxyfluorescein succinimidyl ester-bright *C. glabrata* population from peritoneal macrophages-yeast co-cultures. Macrophages were obtained from wild type, Dectin-1$^{-/-}$, and Dectin-2$^{-/-}$ mice. Comparisons between all groups are non-significant. Data represent a minimum of three independent experiments.

fusion of lysosomal content. The C-type lectin receptors, Dectin-1 and Dectin-2, recognize fungi and are linked through Syk for intracellular signaling (35). We determined the contribution of each receptor to Syk activity in macrophages following *Candida* exposure. Data reveal that loss of either receptor does not impact the control of intracellular *C. glabrata* suggesting that Syk activity is stimulated through redundant pathways.

In addition to Syk being important for *C. glabrata* control, we also demonstrates the importance of timing of Syk activity. Early Syk activation, within the first 4 h after macrophage phagocytosis *C. glabrata*, is the essential window for effective control of *C. glabrata* division. Macrophages in which Syk was inhibited 2 or 4 h after addition of *C. glabrata* enabled the yeast to divide unchecked. Syk may have less relevance when inhibited 8 h after co-infection because the macrophages retain their ability to control yeast division in similar fashion to untreated macrophages. These observations may be due to time-dependent phagosomal mechanisms, which have no further consequence on *C. glabrata* division at later stages following phagocytosis. In addition, *C. glabrata*-specific immune evasion pathways may be upregulated at later time points, and these may bypass Syk-related control mechanisms. In this study, we have only evaluated chemical Syk inhibition, and have yet to test Syk knockout models.

Spleen tyrosine kinase has an established role in cytoskeletal changes, which could potentially impact phagocytosis. To control for this possibility, we measured uptake of *C. glabrata* by macrophages and found no difference in phagocytosis between control and R406-treated macrophages. This observation is in line with our previous observation using tyrosine mutations in the hemi-ITAM of Dectin-1, which result in complete loss of Syk phosphorylation, yet maintains near normal rates of phagocytosis (22). In addition, to address the likelihood of a lasting effect triggered through Syk inhibition, we utilized ROS activity as a surrogate marker of macrophage activity. After washout of R406, ROS activity is fully restored, indicating that transient Syk inhibition does not result in a long-lasting inhibition of macrophages, and does not account for loss of intracellular *C. glabrata* activity.

In conclusion, our results demonstrate that macrophages control the division of *C. glabrata* in a Syk-dependent manner. A limitation of this observation is the use of a single ATCC strain and further investigation is required to determine if Syk-dependent control is generalizable to other *Candida* species. These observations were verified by a CFSE-labeling technique that accurately distinguished CFSE-bright parent and CFSE-dim daughter cell populations through flow cytometric analysis or microscopy. We show that Syk in macrophages is essential in the early stages of *C. glabrata* infection and that Dectin-1 or Dectin-2 are not individual contributors to Syk activity. Further investigations are required to define the precise downstream mechanisms of Syk activity in the intracellular control of fungal pathogens.

AUTHOR CONTRIBUTIONS

ZD, SX, PN, MM, and DS contributed to experimental design. ZD, SX, PN, JT, and MM executed the experiments. ZD, SX, PN, NK, MF, JR, JT, DS, and MM performed analysis and interpretation of experiments. ZD, SX, PN, and MM contributed in writing the manuscript.

FUNDING

This work was supported, in whole or in part, by NIH NIAID T32 AI007061 (to JR), NIH NIAID K08 AI110655 (to MM), and K08 CA201640 (to DS).

REFERENCES

1. Sardi JC, Scorzoni L, Bernardi T, Fusco-Almeida AM, Mendes Giannini MJ. *Candida* species: current epidemiology, pathogenicity, biofilm formation, natural antifungal products and new therapeutic options. *J Med Microbiol* (2013) 62(Pt 1):10–24. doi:10.1099/jmm.0.045054-0
2. Rodrigues CF, Silva S, Henriques M. *Candida glabrata*: a review of its features and resistance. *Eur J Clin Microbiol Infect Dis* (2014) 33(5):673–88. doi:10.1007/s10096-013-2009-3
3. Silva S, Henriques M, Hayes A, Oliveira R, Azeredo J, Williams DW. *Candida glabrata* and *Candida albicans* co-infection of an in vitro oral epithelium. *J Oral Pathol Med* (2011) 40(5):421–7. doi:10.1111/j.1600-0714.2010.00981.x
4. Kaur R, Ma B, Cormack BP. A family of glycosylphosphatidylinositol-linked aspartyl proteases is required for virulence of *Candida glabrata*. *Proc Natl Acad Sci U S A* (2007) 104(18):7628–33. doi:10.1073/pnas.0611195104
5. Kasper L, Seider K, Hube B. Intracellular survival of *Candida glabrata* in macrophages: immune evasion and persistence. *FEMS Yeast Res* (2015) 15(5):fov042. doi:10.1093/femsyr/fov042
6. Ifrim DC, Bain JM, Reid DM, Oosting M, Verschueren I, Gow NA, et al. Role of Dectin-2 for host defense against systemic infection with *Candida glabrata*. *Infect Immun* (2014) 82(3):1064–73. doi:10.1128/IAI.01189-13
7. Filby A, Begum J, Jalal M, Day W. Appraising the suitability of succinimidyl and lipophilic fluorescent dyes to track proliferation in non-quiescent cells by dye dilution. *Methods* (2015) 82:29–37. doi:10.1016/j.ymeth.2015.02.016
8. Tario JD Jr, Humphrey K, Bantly AD, Muirhead KA, Moore JS, Wallace PK. Optimized staining and proliferation modeling methods for cell division monitoring using cell tracking dyes. *J Vis Exp* (2012) (70):e4287. doi:10.3791/4287
9. Weston SA, Parish CR. New fluorescent dyes for lymphocyte migration studies. Analysis by flow cytometry and fluorescence microscopy. *J Immunol Methods* (1990) 133(1):87–97. doi:10.1016/0022-1759(90)90322-M
10. Hawkins ED, Hommel M, Turner ML, Battye FL, Markham JF, Hodgkin PD. Measuring lymphocyte proliferation, survival and differentiation using CFSE time-series data. *Nat Protoc* (2007) 2(9):2057–67. doi:10.1038/nprot.2007.297
11. Lastovicka J, Rataj M, Bartunkova J. Assessment of lymphocyte proliferation for diagnostic purpose: comparison of CFSE staining, Ki-67 expression and (3)H-thymidine incorporation. *Hum Immunol* (2016) 77(12):1215–22. doi:10.1016/j.humimm.2016.08.012
12. Parish CR. Fluorescent dyes for lymphocyte migration and proliferation studies. *Immunol Cell Biol* (1999) 77(6):499–508. doi:10.1046/j.1440-1711.1999.00877.x
13. Ludington JG, Ward HD. The *Cryptosporidium parvum* C-type lectin CpClec mediates infection of intestinal epithelial cells via interactions with sulfated proteoglycans. *Infect Immun* (2016) 84(5):1593–602. doi:10.1128/IAI.01410-15
14. Ueckert JE, Nebe von-Caron G, Bos AP, ter Steeg PF. Flow cytometric analysis of *Lactobacillus plantarum* to monitor lag times, cell division and injury. *Lett Appl Microbiol* (1997) 25(4):295–9. doi:10.1046/j.1472-765X.1997.00225.x
15. Batista VG, Toledo MS, Straus AH, Mendes-Giannini MJ, Duarte AJ, Takahashi HK, et al. Glycolipid sensing and innate immunity in paracoccidioidomycosis. *Mycopathologia* (2014) 178(3–4):153–62. doi:10.1007/s11046-014-9783-z
16. Bocharov G, Luzyanina T, Cupovic J, Ludewig B. Asymmetry of cell division in CFSE-based lymphocyte proliferation analysis. *Front Immunol* (2013) 4:264. doi:10.3389/fimmu.2013.00264
17. Seider K, Brunke S, Schild L, Jablonowski N, Wilson D, Majer O, et al. The facultative intracellular pathogen *Candida glabrata* subverts macrophage cytokine production and phagolysosome maturation. *J Immunol* (2011) 187(6):3072–86. doi:10.4049/jimmunol.1003730
18. Davi V, Minc N. Mechanics and morphogenesis of fission yeast cells. *Curr Opin Microbiol* (2015) 28:36–45. doi:10.1016/j.mib.2015.07.010
19. Piel M, Tran PT. Cell shape and cell division in fission yeast. *Curr Biol* (2009) 19(17):R823–7. doi:10.1016/j.cub.2009.08.012
20. Hohl TM, Rivera A, Pamer EG. Immunity to fungi. *Curr Opin Immunol* (2006) 18(4):465–72. doi:10.1016/j.coi.2006.05.003
21. Collette JR, Lorenz MC. Mechanisms of immune evasion in fungal pathogens. *Curr Opin Microbiol* (2011) 14(6):668–75. doi:10.1016/j.mib.2011.09.007
22. Mansour MK, Tam JM, Khan NS, Seward M, Davids PJ, Puranam S, et al. Dectin-1 activation controls maturation of beta-1,3-glucan-containing phagosomes. *J Biol Chem* (2013) 288(22):16043–54. doi:10.1074/jbc.M113.473223
23. Turner M, Schweighoffer E, Colucci F, Di Santo JP, Tybulewicz VL. Tyrosine kinase SYK: essential functions for immunoreceptor signalling. *Immunol Today* (2000) 21(3):148–54. doi:10.1016/S0167-5699(99)01574-1
24. Miller YI, Choi SH, Wiesner P, Bae YS. The SYK side of TLR4: signalling mechanisms in response to LPS and minimally oxidized LDL. *Br J Pharmacol* (2012) 167(5):990–9. doi:10.1111/j.1476-5381.2012.02097.x
25. Underhill DM, Rossnagle E, Lowell CA, Simmons RM. Dectin-1 activates Syk tyrosine kinase in a dynamic subset of macrophages for reactive oxygen production. *Blood* (2005) 106(7):2543–50. doi:10.1182/blood-2005-03-1239

26. Yi YS, Son YJ, Ryou C, Sung GH, Kim JH, Cho JY. Functional roles of Syk in macrophage-mediated inflammatory responses. *Mediators Inflamm* (2014) 2014:270302. doi:10.1155/2014/270302
27. Geahlen RL. Getting Syk: spleen tyrosine kinase as a therapeutic target. *Trends Pharmacol Sci* (2014) 35(8):414–22. doi:10.1016/j.tips.2014.05.007
28. Ruzza P, Biondi B, Calderan A. Therapeutic prospect of Syk inhibitors. *Expert Opin Ther Pat* (2009) 19(10):1361–76. doi:10.1517/13543770903207039
29. Taylor PR, Tsoni SV, Willment JA, Dennehy KM, Rosas M, Findon H, et al. Dectin-1 is required for beta-glucan recognition and control of fungal infection. *Nat Immunol* (2007) 8(1):31–8. doi:10.1038/ni1408
30. Saijo S, Ikeda S, Yamabe K, Kakuta S, Ishigame H, Akitsu A, et al. Dectin-2 recognition of alpha-mannans and induction of Th17 cell differentiation is essential for host defense against *Candida albicans*. *Immunity* (2010) 32(5):681–91. doi:10.1016/j.immuni.2010.05.001
31. Tam JM, Mansour MK, Khan NS, Seward M, Puranam S, Tanne A, et al. Dectin-1-dependent LC3 recruitment to phagosomes enhances fungicidal activity in macrophages. *J Infect Dis* (2014) 210(11):1844–54. doi:10.1093/infdis/jiu290
32. Reedy JL, Negoro PE, Feliu M, Lord AK, Khan NS, Lukason DP, et al. The carbohydrate lectin receptor dectin-1 mediates the immune response to *Exserohilum rostratum*. *Infect Immun* (2017) 85(3):e903–16. doi:10.1128/IAI.00903-16
33. Le Roux D, Lankar D, Yuseff MI, Vascotto F, Yokozeki T, Faure-Andre G, et al. Syk-dependent actin dynamics regulate endocytic trafficking and processing of antigens internalized through the B-cell receptor. *Mol Biol Cell* (2007) 18(9):3451–62. doi:10.1091/mbc.E06-12-1114
34. Peter J, Armstrong D, Lyman CA, Walsh TJ. Use of fluorescent probes to determine MICs of amphotericin B and caspofungin against *Candida* spp. and *Aspergillus* spp. *J Clin Microbiol* (2005) 43(8):3788–92. doi:10.1128/JCM.43.8.3788-3792.2005
35. Netea MG, Brown GD, Kullberg BJ, Gow NA. An integrated model of the recognition of *Candida albicans* by the innate immune system. *Nat Rev Microbiol* (2008) 6(1):67–78. doi:10.1038/nrmicro1815

19

The Absence of NOD1 Enhances Killing of *Aspergillus fumigatus* Through Modulation of Dectin-1 Expression

Mark S. Gresnigt[1,2], Martin Jaeger[2], R. K. Subbarao Malireddi[3], Orhan Rasid[1], Grégory Jouvion[4], Catherine Fitting[1], Willem J. G. Melchers[5], Thirumala-Devi Kanneganti[3], Agostinho Carvalho[6,7], Oumaima Ibrahim-Granet[1†] and Frank L. van de Veerdonk[2†]*

[1] Unité de recherche Cytokines and Inflammation, Institut Pasteur, Paris, France, [2] Laboratory for Experimental Internal Medicine, Department of Internal Medicine, Radboud University Medical Center, Nijmegen, Netherlands, [3] Department of Immunology, St. Jude Children's Research Hospital, Memphis, TN, United States, [4] Unité Histopathologie Humaine et Modèles Animaux, Département Infection et Epidémiologie, Institut Pasteur, Paris, France, [5] Department of Medical Microbiology, Radboud University Medical Centre, Nijmegen, Netherlands, [6] Life and Health Sciences Research Institute (ICVS), School of Medicine, University of Minho, Braga, Portugal, [7] ICVS/3B's – PT Government Associate Laboratory, Braga/Guimarães, Portugal

***Correspondence:**
Frank L. van de Veerdonk
frank.vandeveerdonk@radboudumc.nl

†These authors have contributed equally to this work.

One of the major life-threatening infections for which severely immunocompromised patients are at risk is invasive aspergillosis (IA). Despite the current treatment options, the increasing antifungal resistance and poor outcome highlight the need for novel therapeutic strategies to improve outcome of patients with IA. In the current study, we investigated whether and how the intracellular pattern recognition receptor NOD1 is involved in host defense against *Aspergillus fumigatus*. When exploring the role of NOD1 in an experimental mouse model, we found that *Nod1*$^{-/-}$ mice were protected against IA and demonstrated reduced fungal outgrowth in the lungs. We found that macrophages derived from bone marrow of *Nod1*$^{-/-}$ mice were more efficiently inducing reactive oxygen species and cytokines in response to *Aspergillus*. Most strikingly, these cells were highly potent in killing *A. fumigatus* compared with wild-type cells. In line, human macrophages in which NOD1 was silenced demonstrated augmented *Aspergillus* killing and NOD1 stimulation decreased fungal killing. The differentially altered killing capacity of NOD1 silencing versus NOD1 activation was associated with alterations in dectin-1 expression, with activation of NOD1 reducing dectin-1 expression. Furthermore, we were able to demonstrate that *Nod1*$^{-/-}$ mice have elevated dectin-1 expression in the lung and bone marrow, and silencing of *NOD1* gene expression in human macrophages increases dectin-1 expression. The enhanced dectin-1 expression may be the mechanism of enhanced fungal killing of *Nod1*$^{-/-}$ cells and human cells in which NOD1 was silenced, since blockade of dectin-1 reversed the augmented killing in these cells. Collectively, our data demonstrate that NOD1 receptor plays an inhibitory role in the host defense against *Aspergillus*. This provides a rationale to develop novel immunotherapeutic strategies for treatment of aspergillosis that target the NOD1 receptor, to enhance the efficiency of host immune cells to clear the infection by increasing fungal killing and cytokine responses.

Keywords: NOD1, *Aspergillus fumigatus*, nucleotide-binding oligomerization domain, dectin-1, fungal killing

INTRODUCTION

Invasive aspergillosis (IA) is an opportunistic fungal infection that globally affects hundreds of thousands severely immunocompromised patients on an annual basis (1). IA is associated with an unacceptable high mortality (2), yet modern antifungal drugs, patient isolation care, and prophylactic treatment strategies have not been able to reduce mortality over the past years. An increased knowledge of the antifungal host response is crucial for understanding the pathogenesis of the disease on one hand and on the other hand in the development of new immunomodulatory therapies, which are considered to be one of the few possibilities to decrease mortality associated with IA (3).

A fine-tuned interplay between recognition and signaling leads to the clearance of the fungus by the immune system, while defects in parts of these components or their absence have been associated with severe infections with the fungus. Although most types of PRRs, including toll-like receptors and C-type lectin receptors, have well-characterized roles in antifungal host defense (4, 5). Some PRRs have, however, not yet been evaluated for their role in antifungal host defense. Insights in these not yet explored PRRs might yield new insights in the pathogenesis of IA and provide potential candidate targets for novel treatment strategies.

The nucleotide-oligomerization domain (NOD) receptors play a crucial role in host defense against bacteria; however, only limited evidence is available regarding the role of these receptors in host defense against aspergillosis. One of the NOD receptors, NOD1, has been described to be able to activate NFκB in corneal epithelial cells in response to *Aspergillus fumigatus* (6). However, it is not yet investigated whether NOD1 plays a role in host defense against pulmonary aspergillosis. Overall, it is evident that NOD1 plays an important role in pulmonary host defense. NOD1 is highly expressed in the lung (7) and in lung epithelial cells (8). Human alveolar macrophages utilize NOD1 to induce proinflammatory cytokine responses and induce autophagy for an efficient host defense against *Mycobacterium tuberculosis* (9). Moreover, in host defense against *Legionella pneumophila*, NOD1 regulates neutrophil recruitment to the alveoli (10, 11). These studies of pulmonary host defense against bacteria reveal various mechanisms, induced by NOD1, that are known to play significant roles in host defense against *A. fumigatus*; e.g., autophagy machinery (12–15), neutrophil recruitment (16–18), and proinflammatory cytokines (19–21).

Therefore, the current study investigates the role of NOD1 in host defense against aspergillosis. Specifically, in a murine model representing immunocompromised hosts, we assess how NOD1 deficiency influences the host defense during aspergillosis. Using murine *Nod1*-deficient cells as well as silencing of *NOD1* gene expression in primary human cells, we systematically evaluated the importance of this receptor in the antifungal response. Novel insight into the exact biology of this receptor during aspergillosis can increase our understanding of the infection, which subsequently may lead to the development of immunotherapeutic strategies.

MATERIALS AND METHODS

Aspergillus fumigatus

A clinical isolate of *A. fumigatus* V05-27, which has been characterized previously (22), was used for all *ex vivo* and *in vitro* stimulations. Conidia and hyphae were prepared and heat-inactivated (HI) as previously described (23). A concentration of 1×10^7/mL was used in the experiments unless otherwise indicated. For *in vivo* experiments, the luciferase-expressing *A. fumigatus* 2/7/1 strain was used, which has been described previously (24); this strain has been reported to have a similar antifungal susceptibility and demonstrates no growth defects under various *in vitro* cultivation conditions such as different temperatures and carbon sources (24). In corticosteroid immunosuppressed mouse models of aspergillosis (25), the 2/7/1 strain demonstrated a similar virulence as observed for its parental strain CBS144.85 (26, 27).

In Vivo Experiments

Mice for *in vivo* experiments were supplied by the breeding center R. Janvier (Le Genest Saint-Isle, France). For the survival experiment in an immunosuppressed background C57/BL6 wild type (WT), and *Nod1*$^{-/-}$ mice (28 to 31 g, 10 weeks old) were used. Mice were immunosuppressed at day 4 and day 1 before infection by intraperitoneal injection of 200-μL cyclophosphamide (Sigma Aldrich) at 4 mg/mL. At the day of infection, mice were anesthetized by intramuscular injection (150 μL) of ketamine (10 mg/mL) and xylasine (10 mg/mL) hair was shaved from the ventral lung area and subsequently mice were inoculated intranasally with 5×10^4 luciferase-expressing *A. fumigatus* 2/7/1 conidia (24) in 25-μL PBS.

In all experiments, survival and weight was monitored during the course of infection. Bioluminescence imaging was acquired at day 1 post-infection (pi) and was continued on days 2, 3, 6, and 8 pi. Images were acquired using an IVIS 100 system (PerkinElmer, Waltham, MA, USA) as previously described (25).

For immunological and histological assessment female C57/BL6 and *Nod1*$^{-/-}$ mice (19–22 g, 8 weeks old) were used. They received similar immunosuppression regimen and were similarly infected as the mice for survival. Weight and bioluminescence were monitored daily during the course of infection. At day 3, the mice were euthanized. Serum and BAL were collected and lung homogenates were obtained following disruption in saline using the Retsch Mixer Mill 301 homogenizer. Cytokine concentrations in BAL and plasma were determined by ELISA as specified by the manufacturer (DuoSet; R&D Systems).

The fungal burden was determined by amplification of *Aspergillus* ITS2 regions. Briefly, homogenized tissue samples were used for DNA isolation by using the automated MagNA Pure system and the MagNA Pure LC Total Nucleic Acid Isolation Kit according to manufacturer's protocol (Roche Applied Science). PhHV was added to all samples as an internal isolation control C.

The concentration of total isolated DNA was measured by using the Quantus Fluorometer (Promega). *Aspergillus* loads were determined by real-time PCR using the LC480 instrument and the probes master kit (Roche applied Science). Thermocycling conditions were as follows: 37°C for 10 min,

95°C for 10 min, and 50 cycles: 95°C for 15 s, and 60°C for 45 s. The rDNA ITS2 region of *A. fumigatus* was detected by using primers 5′-GCGTCATTGCTGCCCTCAAGC-3′, 5′-ATATGC TTAAGTTCAGCGGGT-3′ and probe Cy5-TCCTCGAGCGTA TGGGGCTT-BBQ. The PhHV isolation control was detected by using primers 5′-GGGCGAATCACAGATTGAATC-3′, 5′-GCG GTTCCAAACGTACCAA-3′ and probe LC610-TTTTTATGT GTCCGCCACCATCTGGATC- BBQ. For the ITS2 detection, a twofold dilution series of the cloned PCR product was included to calculate the number of copies per reaction.

PBMC Isolation and Stimulation

Venous blood samples from healthy controls and patients were obtained after written informed consent. PBMCs were isolated as previously described (23). Briefly, blood was diluted in PBS (1:1) and fractions were separated by Ficoll (Ficoll-Paque Plus, GE Healthcare) density gradient centrifugation. Cells were washed twice with PBS and resuspended in RPMI-1640$^+$ (RPMI1640 Dutch modification supplemented with 10-μg/mL gentamycin, 2mM glutamax and 1mM pyruvate; Thermofisher).

PBMCs were plated in 96-well round-bottom plates (Corning) at a final concentration of 2.5×10^6 cells/mL and in a total volume of 200 μL and stimulated with medium (negative control) or live *Aspergillus* at a final concentration of 1×10^7/mL for 24 h. PBMCs in costimulation experiments were exposed to 10-μg/mL TriDAP (Invivogen) and subsequently stimulated with medium or live resting conidia (1×10^7/mL). After stimulation, culture supernatants were collected and stored at −20°C until cytokine measurement. Cells were either analyzed for surface receptor expression by flow cytometry or assessed for the fungal killing capacity.

Flow Cytometry

Surface pattern recognition receptor expression on human monocytes was assessed following stimulation of PBMCs with TriDAP as described above. Monocytes were stained with anti-human CD14 conjugated with FITC (BD) and anti-human CD45 conjugated with PE-Cy7 in combination with, anti-human CD282 (TLR2) Alexa647 (BD) and anti-human CD284 (TLR4) PE (Biolegend), or anti-human CD206 (Mannose Receptor) PE (Biolegend) and anti-human dectin-1 APC (R&D). CD14$^+$ monocytes were gated within the population of CD45$^+$ cells and subsequently, the mean fluorescence intensity (MFI) of TLR2, TLR4, Mannose receptor, and dectin-1 were assessed on the CD14$^+$/CD45$^+$ cells. For dectin-1 also a negative population was observed and the percentage of dectin-1$^+$ cells was assessed in addition to the MFI. The cells were measured on an FC500 flow cytometer (Beckman Coulter) and the data were analyzed using CXP analysis software v2.2 (Beckman Coulter).

Ex Vivo Stimulation of WT and *Nod1*$^{-/-}$ Murine Splenocytes and Bone Marrow-Derived Macrophages (BMDMs)

Wild-type and *Nod1*$^{-/-}$ C57Bl/6 mice were bred and maintained in the St. Jude Children's Research Hospital, Memphis, TN, USA. Spleens were homogenized in 0.4-μM cell strainer (BD) and the cell number was adjusted to 1×10^7/mL. The cell suspensions (500 μL/well) were placed in 24-well plates (corning) and incubated with culture medium or *Aspergillus* conidia for 1 or 5 days at 37°C and 5% CO_2.

Bone marrow from mice (age between 8 and 20 weeks old) was flushed out after dissecting mouse legs. Differentiation into macrophages (BMDMs) occurred in 5 days at 37°C (5% CO_2) in Dulbecco's modified eagles medium (DMEM) supplemented with 30% of L929 supernatant containing 10% fetal bovine serum (HI, Invitrogen), 100-U/mL penicillin and 100-mg/mL streptomycin. The BMDMs (1×10^5 /well) were placed in 96-well plates (corning) and incubated with culture medium or live *Aspergillus* conidia for 1 day at 37°C and 5% CO_2. After stimulation, culture supernatants were collected and stored at −20°C until cytokine measurement.

Silencing NOD1

Freshly isolated PBMCs were differentiated to macrophages using 6-day differentiation in 10% human serum (serum differentiated macrophages) or 10% human serum supplemented with 5-ng/mL GM-CSF (R&D Systems). After differentiation (1×10^5) macrophages were seeded in 96-well plates and left for 2 h at 37°C to subsequently transfect them with 25-nM NOD1 siRNA (on target) or scrambled (non-targeted siRNA) control siRNA (smartpool, Thermo Scientific) for 48 h at 37°C (Dharmafect, Thermo Scientific). Subsequently, the culture medium was refreshed and cells were used for killing, ROS assays, and PCR analysis.

Killing of *Aspergillus* by BMDMs, Human Macrophages, or PBMCs

Following differentiation, the mouse BMDMs (1×10^5), human MDMs (1×10^5), or freshly isolated PBMCs (5×10^5) were exposed to *Aspergillus* conidia (2×10^6) in 96-well plates a final volume of 200 μL. In several experiments dectin-1 was blocked using laminarin (100 μg/mL; Sigma Aldrich) or with a mouse dectin-1 blocking antibody (GE2; Thermo Fisher) or its isotype control. After 24 hat 37°C and 5% CO_2, the cells were washed in water and plated in serial dilution on Sabouraud agar plates. CFUs were counted after 24 h incubation at 37°C.

Quantitative Reverse Transcriptase PCR

RNA was isolated according to the protocol supplied with the TRIzol reagent. Isolated mRNA (1 μg) was reverse transcribed into cDNA using the iScript cDNA synthesis kit (BIORAD). Quantitative real-time PCR (qPCR) was performed using power SYBR Green PCR master mix (Applied Biosystems) and following primers for human samples hNOD1 Fwd 5′-AGAGGCTCTGCGGAACCA-3′ and Rev 5′-TGTGGAGATGCCGTTGGA-3′, hGAPDH Fwd 5′-AGGGGAGATTCAGTGTGGTG-3′ and Rev 5′-CGACC ACTTTGTCAAGCTCA-3′ hCLEC7A Fwd 5′-ACAATGCTG GCAACTGGGCT-3′ and Rev 5′-GCCGAGAAAGGCCTATC CAAAA-3′ hTLR2 Fwd 5′-GAATCCTCCAATCAGGCTTC TCT-3′ and Rev 5′-GCCCTGAGGGAATGGAGTTTA-3′ and the following primer sets form mouse samples mClec7a Fwd 5′-AGGTTTTTCTCAGCCTTGCCTTC-3′ and Rev 5′-GGG AGCAGTGTCTCTTACTTCC-3′, mGapdh Fwd 5′-AGGTC

GGTGTGAACGGATTTG-3′ and Rev 5′-TGTAGACCATGT AGTTGAGGTCA-3′. PCR was performed using an Applied Biosystems 7300 real-time PCR system using PCR conditions 2 min 50°C, 10 min 95°C followed by 40 cycles at 95°C for 15 s and 60°C for 1 min. The RNA genes of interest were corrected for differences in loading concentration using the signal of the housekeeping protein GAPDH.

IκBa Phosphorylation

For analysis of NFκB signaling pathways, the BMDMs were subcultured in 12-well cell culture plates for 16 h, and stimulated with live *Aspergillus* spores at 25 MOI of infection for indicated times. Protein lysates were prepared using the lysis buffer (10-mM Tris–HCl, 150-mM NaCl, 1% Nonidet P-40, supplemented with protease and phosphatase inhibitor cocktails; Roche). Protein samples were denatured by boiling in sample loading buffer-containing SDS and 100-mM DTT for 5 min and separated in denaturing SDS-PAGE. Separated proteins were transferred to PVDF membranes and immunoblotted with rabbit antibodies against total IκBa, Phospho-IκBa. All antibodies were purchased from Cell Signaling followed by secondary anti-rabbit HRP antibodies (JacksonImmunoResearch Laboratories).

Cytokine Measurements

The cytokine levels were measured using commercially available ELISA assays according to the protocol supplied by the manufacturer. IL-1β, TNFα, IL-17, and IL-22 assays were from R&D Systems and IFNγ was from Sanquin. Mouse IL-1β, TNFα, IL-6, KC, IL-17, IL-22, and IFNγ in splenocyte stimulations were measured using the Luminex multiplex platform (Millipore). In the *in vivo* experiments mouse IL-1β, TNFα, IL-6, KC, and G-CSF were measured using commercially available ELISA assays from R&D Systems according to the protocol supplied by the manufacturer.

NOD1 Immunofluorescence Staining

$CD14^+$ cells were isolated from PBMCs using magnetic bead isolation (MACS Miltenyi) according to the protocol supplied by the manufacturer. $CD14^+$ cells (1×10^5) were allowed to adhere for 1 h to 12-mm Ø glass coverslips. After adherence, the $CD14^+$ monocytes were exposed for 30 min to FITC labeled *Aspergillus* conidia in a ratio of (5:1/conidia/CD14 cells), after which the cells were fixed in Methanol. NOD1 was stained using rabbit anti-NOD1 and secondary stained with Goat anti-rabbit IgG H/L Alexa594 (Invitrogen). The coverslips were mounted in Vectashield with DAPI (Vector Laboratories) and immunofluorescence was observed at 1,000× magnification using a Zeiss LSM510 confocal microscope (Carl Zeiss).

Statistical Analysis

Data are presented as the mean ± SEM, or as scatterplots representing individual data points and a line indicating the median value of all the data obtained in experiments. Experiments were conducted at least twice and the number of biological replicates (mice/human donors) is indicated in the figure legends for each graph. Unless otherwise indicated the Mann–Whitney *U* test was used to determine statistical significant differences between experimental groups with $p < 0.05$ = *, $p < 0.01$ = **, $p < 0.001$ = ***, and $p < 0.0001$ = ****. All data were analyzed using Graphpad Prism v6.0.

RESULTS

NOD1 Localizes to *Aspergillus*-Containing Phagosomes

Since NOD1 is an intracellular pattern recognition receptor for bacterial ligands, we wanted to investigate at which cellular level NOD1 interacts with *Aspergillus*. To assess the location of NOD1 during the interaction of monocytes with *Aspergillus*, the monocytes of healthy human volunteers were allowed to engulf *Aspergillus*, both resting and swollen conidia, for 1 h. Subsequently, NOD1 was stained by immunofluorescence staining. We observed that engulfed *A. fumigatus* resting or swollen conidia demonstrate a halo of NOD1 surrounding the conidia, suggestion colocalization to the phagosomes containing *Aspergillus* (**Figure 1**). In addition to the halo surrounding the conidia, a diffuse cytoplasmic staining of NOD1 could be observed.

NOD1-Deficient Mice Do Not Develop IA

To investigate whether NOD1 plays a role in the susceptibility to aspergillosis, we subjected WT C57Bl6 and *Nod1*$^{-/-}$ mice to lethal *Aspergillus* infection. Survival experiments were performed in mice immunosuppressed with cyclophosphamide and subsequently infected with the bioluminescent *Aspergillus* strain 2/7/1 (24). In contrast to WT mice, *Nod1*$^{-/-}$ mice showed a significant improvement in 14-day survival (**Figure 2A**). Nine out of 12 *Nod1*$^{-/-}$ mice survived, whereas 12 out of 13 WT mice did not survive the infection. Bioluminescence imaging of the luciferase-expressing *Aspergillus* within the mice suggests that *Nod1*$^{-/-}$ mice more efficiently clear the fungi from the lung, whereas WT mice developed a progressing infection as indicated by the increasing luminescence signal (**Figure 2B**). When comparing the weight loss of mice post-infection we observed that *Nod1*$^{-/-}$ mice and a single-surviving WT mouse started to recover their weight from day 4 post-infection (pi), whereas all other WT mice sharply declined in weight and succumbed to the infection and the three non-surviving *Nod1*$^{-/-}$ mice demonstrated a similar weight loss as WT mice (**Figure 2C**).

Reduced Inflammation and Improved Fungal Clearance in Nod1-Deficient Mice

To investigate differences in fungal burden, histological damage and inflammation in a standardized fashion, an experiment was performed where cyclophosphamide immunosuppressed mice were infected with the bioluminescent *Aspergillus* strain 2/7/1, but were sacrificed at day 3 pi. The luminescence signal from the lung reveals that *Nod1*$^{-/-}$ mice have a significantly reduced fungal burden compared with WT mice (**Figure 3A**). This observation could be confirmed by a quantitative *Aspergillus* PCR, which revealed the absence of *Aspergillus* DNA in the lung homogenates of *Nod1*$^{-/-}$ mice. However, in the lung homogenates of WT mice *Aspergillus* could be detected (**Figure 3B**). To assess how fungal burden correlates with pathological

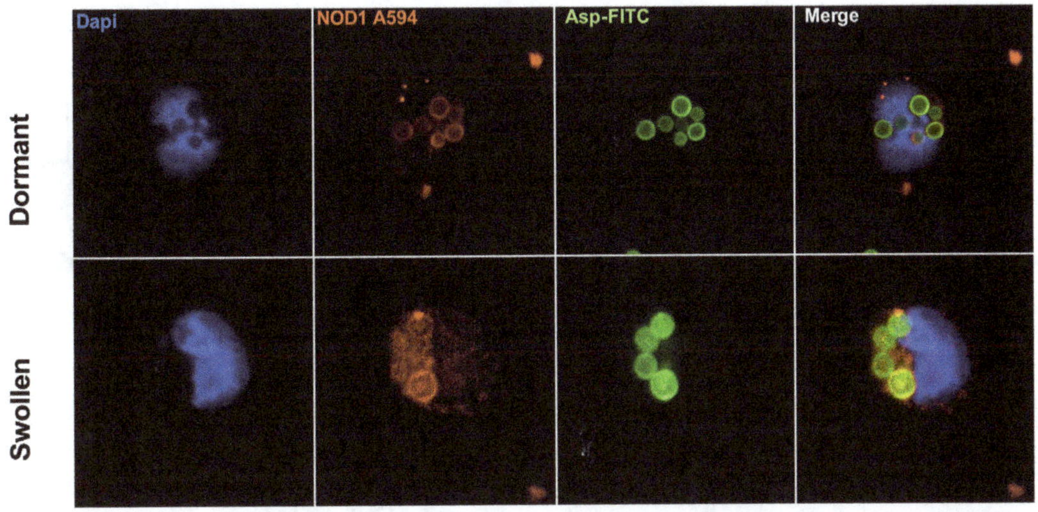

FIGURE 1 | NOD1 localizing to *Aspergillus*-containing phagosomes. Representative confocal immunofluorescence images at 100x magnification demonstrating co-localization of NOD1 (stained with rabbit-anti-humanNOD1, conjugated with Goat-anti-RabbitIgG-Alexa594) with engulfed FITC-labeled dormant or swollen *Aspergillus fumigatus* spores in human monocytes (nuclear stain: DAPI).

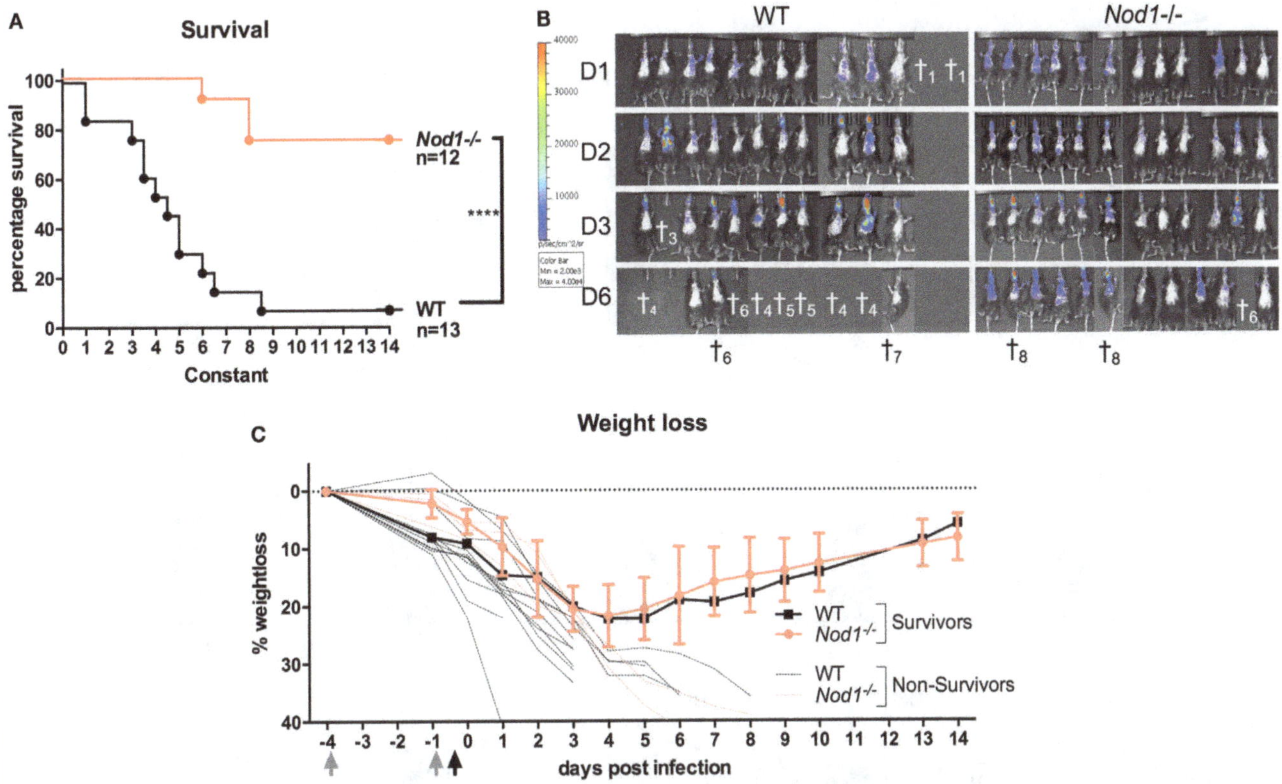

FIGURE 2 | Immunocompromised *Nod1*$^{-/-}$ mice protected against invasive aspergillosis. Assessment of survival, fungal burden and weight in cyclophosphamide immunosuppressed wild-type (WT) (n = 13) and *Nod1*$^{-/-}$ (n = 12) mice infected intranasally with 5 x 10^4 conidia in three separate experiments (WT:*Nod1*$^{-/-}$ 5:6; 3:3; 5:3). **(A)** Kaplan–Meier survival curve of WT (n = 13) and *Nod1*$^{-/-}$ (n = 12) mice. *P*-values of the Kaplan–Meier curve were determined using the log-rank test. Data represent the cumulative data of three separate experiments. **(B)** Bioluminescence imaging representing the fungal burden in the lungs of the mice during the course of the infection. **(C)** Representative graph of percentage weight loss of surviving mice in one of the experiments where survival of WT (n = 5; 4 died; n = 1 shown) and *Nod1*$^{-/-}$ (n = 6; 1 died; n = 5 shown) mice was compared.

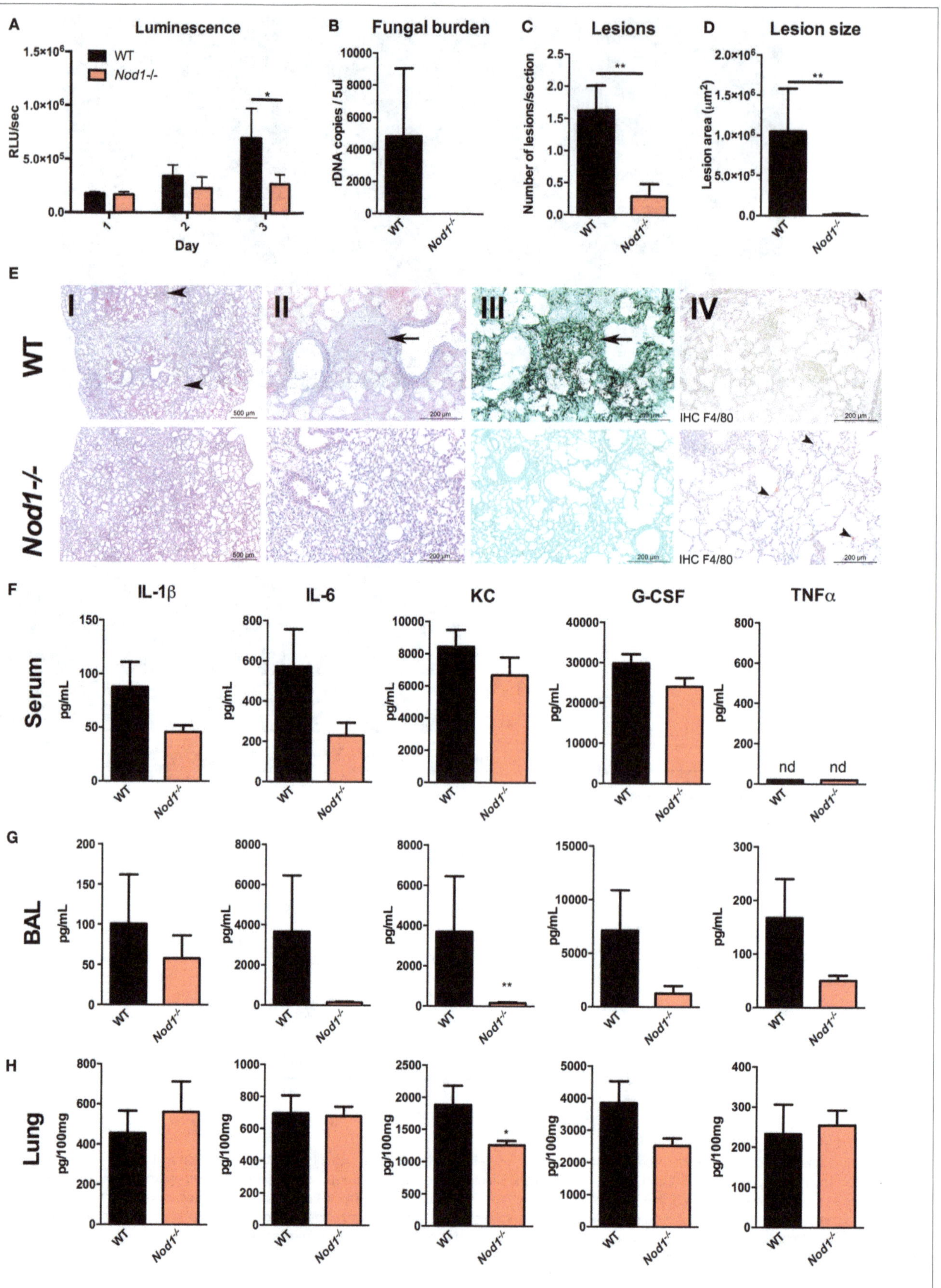

FIGURE 3 | Continued

FIGURE 3 | *Nod1*$^{-/-}$ mice reducing fungal burden, histological damage, and inflammation. Assessment of fungal burden, histopathological damage, and inflammation in *A. fumigatus*-infected wild-type (WT; $n = 8$) and *Nod1*$^{-/-}$ ($n = 7$) mice in two separate experiments (WT:*Nod1*$^{-/-}$ = 4:4 and 4:3). **(A)** Luminescence signal at day 1 to 3 post-infection revealing the fungal burden represented by the luminescence signal from live *Aspergillus* within infected WT and *Nod1*$^{-/-}$ mice. **(B)** Fungal burden as determined by amplification of *Aspergillus* ITS2 regions from lung homogenates. **(C–E)** Histology of lung sections of WT and *Nod1*$^{-/-}$ mice at day 3 pi, and morphometric analysis of the lesions in the whole lung sections using Image J software to quantify the lesions in **(C)** number and **(D)** size. Slides were stained by HE staining at [**(E)**; I] 2x and [**(E)**; II] 10x magnification, [**(E)**; III] Grocott's Methenamine Silver staining at 10x magnification or [**(E)**; IV] immunohistochemistry with anti-F4/80 antibody counterstained with HE staining. **(F–H)** IL-1β, IL-6, KC, G-CSF, and TNFα levels in **(F)** serum, **(G)** broncheoalveolar lavage (BAL), and **(H)** lung homogenates measured at day 3 pi. Data are represented as mean ± SEM and means were compared using the Mann–Whitney *U* test. *P*-values of statistical tests are shown within the graphs.

damage to the lungs, a histopathological analysis was performed. Morphometric analysis of the histology revealed significantly fewer lesions in the lung sections of *Nod1*$^{-/-}$ mice compared with WT mice (**Figure 3C**). Moreover, the size of the lesions affected a significantly smaller part of the lungs (**Figure 3D**). The morphometric analysis of pulmonary lesions corresponds with the finding that practically no fungi could be detected with Grocott methamine silver staining (**Figure 3E**, III). Based on immunohistochemistry for F4/80^{+} no differences in the presence of macrophages could be determined between WT and *Nod1*$^{-/-}$ mice (**Figure 3E**, IV). Systemic inflammation in the WT and *Nod1*$^{-/-}$ mice was assessed by measuring serum cytokine levels, and pulmonary inflammation was assessed by measuring cytokines in the BAL and in lung homogenates. Although *Nod1*$^{-/-}$ mice have a slight reduction in the levels of circulating proinflammatory cytokines, this was not significant compared with the WT mice (**Figure 3F**). In the BAL and lung homogenates, only a significant reduction in KC (CXCL1) levels were found when comparing *Nod1*$^{-/-}$ to the control group (**Figures 3G,H**, respectively). However, it must be noted that levels of other cytokines also tend to be lower in *Nod1*$^{-/-}$, but due to a large variation in the control group the differences are not significant.

Improved Cytokine Responses, Oxidative Burst, and Fungal Killing in Nod1 Deficient cells

Ex vivo cytokine responses to *Aspergillus* were investigated in *Nod1*-deficient cells to identify the underlying mechanisms of the phenotypes observed in *Nod1*$^{-/-}$ mice. Cytokine responses by WT and *Nod1*$^{-/-}$ BMDMs were investigated. *Nod1*$^{-/-}$ BMDMs demonstrated significantly higher cytokine responses, compared with WT BMDMs (**Figure 4A**). Moreover, splenocytes were isolated from naive *Nod1*$^{-/-}$ and WT C57Bl/6 mice and stimulated with *Aspergillus*. Although the cytokine responses produced by splenocytes in response to *Aspergillus* were generally low, *Nod1*$^{-/-}$ splenocytes produced significantly more TNFα and KC in response to *Aspergillus* (**Figure 4B**). The *Aspergillus*-induced, T-helper cell cytokines IL-17, and IFNγ were undetectable (ud) and IL-22 was very poorly induced by WT splenocytes, while these cytokines were significantly elevated in culture supernatants of *Nod1*$^{-/-}$ splenocytes (**Figure 4C**). In addition to cytokine release, zymosan- and *Aspergillus*-induced ROS by BMDMs was significantly higher in *Nod1*$^{-/-}$ BMDMs (**Figure 4D**). The area under the curve was calculated to illustrate the quantitative difference in ROS release, with zymosan or *Aspergillus*. We also investigated whether this increased responsiveness of *Nod1*$^{-/-}$ BMDMs correlated with an altered capacity to kill *A. fumigatus* conidia. *Nod1*$^{-/-}$ BMDMs were significantly more efficient in killing *Aspergillus* conidia than WT BMDMs (**Figure 4E**). Subsequently, we investigated whether the differential cytokine induction and activation of *Nod1*$^{-/-}$ cells was due to differences in the capacity of these cells to activate NFκB signaling. BMDMs were exposed to live *Aspergillus* spores and subsequently lysed to assess IκBa phosphorylation as a marker for NFκB activation by Western Blot. WT macrophages show a steady increase in IκBa phosphorylation after stimulation, whereas the level of IκBa phosphorylation varies over time in *Nod1*$^{-/-}$ BMDMs with a significant increase after 1 and 2 h (**Figure 4F**).

NOD1 Silencing Augments Oxidative Burst and Fungal Killing

Since *Nod1* deficiency impacts the killing capacity and ROS production in murine BMDMs, we validated these findings within a human background by silencing *NOD1* gene expression in human monocyte-derived macrophages (MDMs). *NOD1* silencing by siRNA targeting NOD1 (siNOD1) was confirmed by qPCR and a significant reduction of *NOD1* mRNA expression could be detected in both serum- and GM-CSF-differentiated MDMs (**Figure 5A**). Treatment with siNOD1 increased the killing capacity of MDMs when compared with cells that were transfected with scrambled siRNA (**Figure 5B**). ROS release was undetectable in the serum-differentiated MDMs; however, in GM-CSF-differentiated MDMs treated with siNOD1 the capacity to induce an oxidative burst was also slightly, yet significantly increased (**Figures 5C,D**).

NOD1 Signaling Suppresses Fungal Killing Capacity

Since we observed that NOD1 deficiency or silencing resulted in an increased capacity to eliminate *A. fumigatus* conidia, we investigated whether activation of NOD1 could thus have an inhibitory effect on the host response to *Aspergillus*. To assess the effect of NOD stimulation on oxidative burst, PBMCs were stimulated with TriDAP and subsequently exposed to zymosan. Oxidative burst induced by zymosan was also reduced by pre-stimulation with the NOD1 ligand (**Figure 6A**). NOD ligands could potentially induce an oxidative burst thereby exhausting the cells; however, we found no detectable oxidative burst induced by NOD ligands (**Figure 6B**). Monocytes were differentiated with GM-CSF into MDMs and exposed to the NOD1 ligand

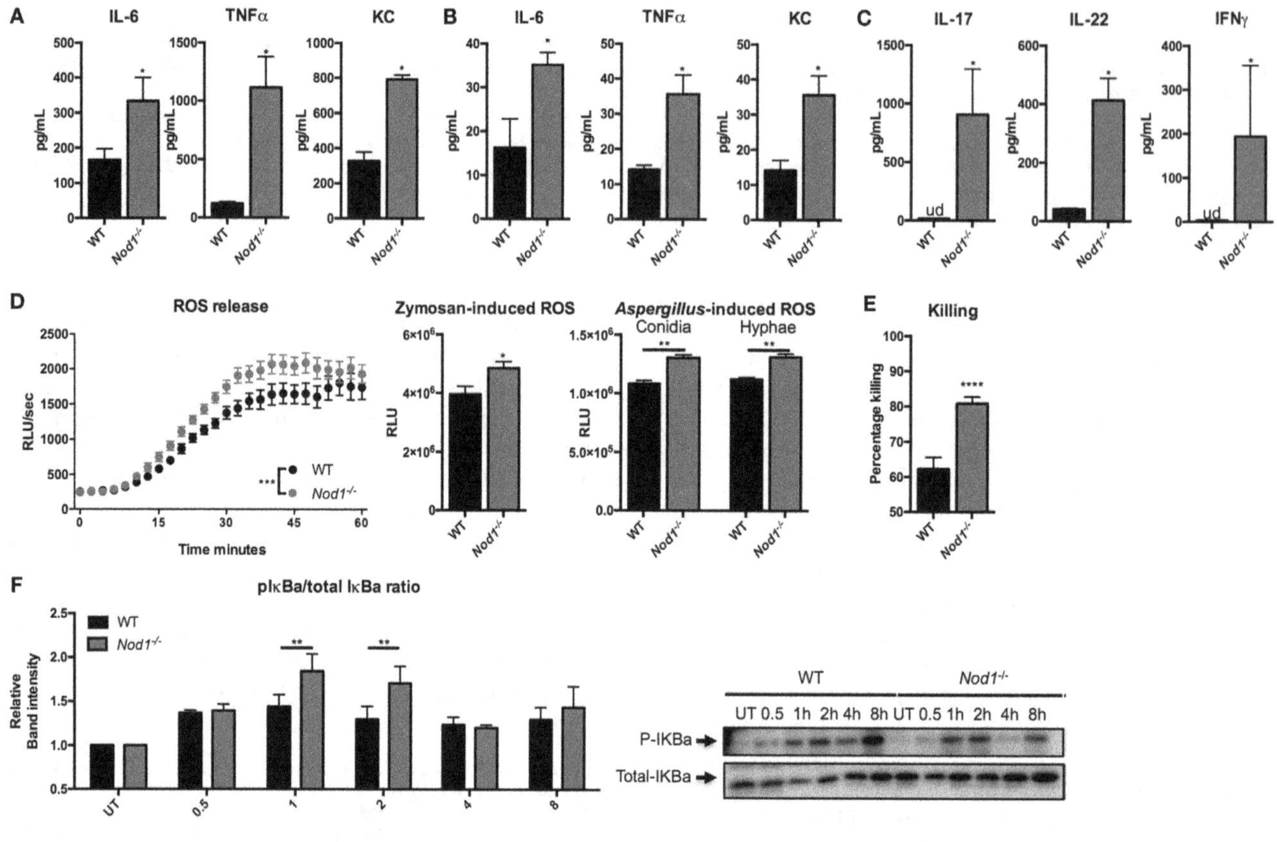

FIGURE 4 | *Nod1*-deficient cells showing an augmented antifungal host response. **(A)** IL-6, TNFα, KC, in culture supernatants of bone marrow-derived macrophages (BMDMs) (1×10^5) from wild-type (WT) and *Nod1*$^{-/-}$ mice ($n = 6$) that were stimulated for 24 h with heat inactivated *Aspergillus* conidia (2×10^6). **(B)** IL-6, TNFα, KC, and **(C)** IL-17, IL-22, and IFNγ levels in culture supernatants of splenocytes (1×10^6) from WT and *Nod1*$^{-/-}$ mice ($n = 5$ mice per group) that were stimulated for 5 days with heat inactivated *Aspergillus* conidia (2×10^7). **(D)** ROS release by WT and *Nod1*$^{-/-}$ BMDMs following exposure to zymosan ($n = 6$). Time points were compared for significance by two-way ANOVA. Area under the curve of the ROS luminescence data of *Aspergillus* spores ($n = 6$) and swollen conidia ($n = 6$) (1×10^7/mL) opsonized in 10% human serum and zymosan stimulated BMDMs. **(E)** CFU remaining of *A. fumigatus* plotted as percentage of input (2×10^6) following exposure for 24 h to WT ($n = 30$) and *Nod1*$^{-/-}$ ($n = 24$) BMDMs (1×10^5). **(F)** Representative Western Blot for phosphorylated and total IκBa in WT and *Nod1*$^{-/-}$ BMDMs following 0.5, 1, 2, 4, and 8 h of exposure to live *A. fumigatus spores*. IκBa phosphorylation measured as mean band intensity and corrected for total IκBa ($n = 3$). Data in bar plots are represented as mean ± SEM, data in scatter plots are represented as individual data points and median, and means were compared using the Mann–Whitney *U* test. ud = undetectable.

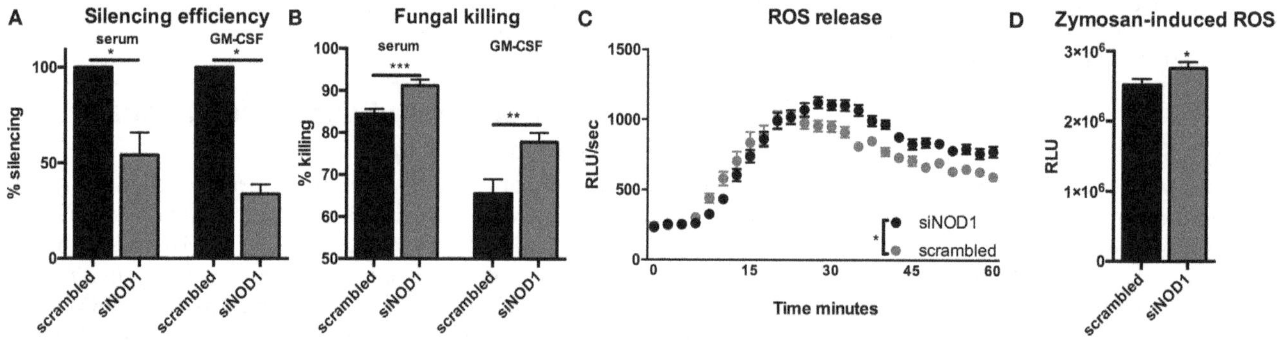

FIGURE 5 | Silencing of NOD1 gene expression in human monocyte-derived macrophages improves fungal killing and oxidative burst. **(A)** Silencing efficiency of siRNA targeting NOD1(siNOD1) compared with scrambled siRNA in human macrophages (1×10^5) differentiated in 10% serum ($n = 6$) or 10% serum with 5 ng/mL GM-CSF ($n = 7$). **(B)** CFU remaining of *A. fumigatus* plotted as percentage of input (2×10^6) following exposure for 24 h to human macrophages (1×10^5) differentiated in 10% serum or 10% serum with 5 ng/mL GM-CSF that were treated with scrambled siRNA or siNOD1. **(C,D)** ROS release by GM-CSF differentiated macrophages treated with scrambled siRNA or siNOD1following exposure to zymosan ($n = 5$). Time points were compared for significance by two-way ANOVA. Data in scatter plots are represented as individual data points and median. Means were compared using the Wilcoxon signed rank test. ud = undetectable.

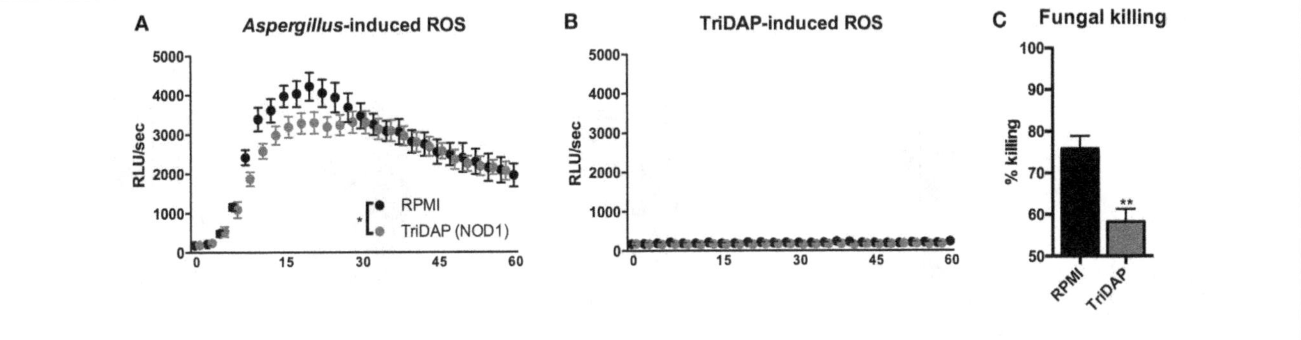

FIGURE 6 | NOD1 activation dampening protective antifungal effector functions in human cells. **(A,B)** ROS release by human PBMCs following exposure to **(A)** Zymosan, when cells were pre-stimulated for 24 h in presence or absence of (10 μg/mL) TriDAP (n = 5), or **(B)** culture medium or (10 μg/mL) TriDAP alone (n = 3). **(C)** Fungal killing capacity of human GM-CSF differentiated monocytes-derived macrophages assessed as CFU remaining of *A. fumigatus* plotted as percentage of input (2 × 10⁶) following exposure for 24 h to (1 × 10⁵), after 24-h pre-stimulation in the presence or absence of (10 μg/mL) TriDAP (n = 9). All plots represent mean ± SEM. Means were compared using the Wilcoxon signed rank test, except for ROS curves, which were compared for significance using two-way ANOVA.

TriDAP. MDMs that were exposed to TriDAP demonstrated a significantly reduced killing capacity compared with control cells (**Figure 6C**).

NOD1 Activation or Deficiency Modulates Expression of Dectin-1

Nucleotide-oligomerization domain receptors are known to interplay with TLRs *via* their downstream kinase RICK, and in particular with TLR2 (28–31). NOD1 deficiency or stimulation of NOD1 could very well impact killing, cytokine release, and ROS *via* modulation of PRRs. Therefore, surface expression of several PRRs, known to be involved in host defense against *Aspergillus*, were assessed by flow cytometry on PBMCs. Stimulation with TriDAP did not significantly affect TLR4 and MR expression on monocytes. dectin-1, however, was differentially regulated by NOD1 stimulation with a decrease of its expression (**Figure 7A**). This observation was also reflected by the number of dectin-1 positive monocytes (**Figure 7B**). To validate whether the reduced dectin-1 surface expression was regulated on a transcriptional level, RNA expression of *CLEC7A* (the gene encoding dectin-1) was assessed. Similarly, a decreased dectin-1 (*CLEC7A*) expression was observed (**Figure 7C**). In addition, siRNA treatment with siNOD1 of MDMs resulted in an increased dectin-1 (*CLEC7A*) expression (**Figure 7D**). To assess whether *Nod1*-deficient mice have altered dectin-1 expression, RNA was isolated from the lung, spleen, and bone marrow and dectin-1 (*Clec7A*) expression was measured. Compared with wild-type mice, *Nod1*-deficient mice had significantly elevated *Clec7A* expression in the lung and bone marrow, while only a trend toward increased *Clec7A* expression was observed in the spleen (**Figure 7E**). To determine whether the augmented killing capacity of human MDMs in which NOD1 is silenced is due to a functional enhancement of dectin-1 we systematically blocked dectin-1 using laminarin and dectin-1-blocking antibodies. The augmented killing capacity of human macrophages treated with *NOD1* targeting siRNA was abolished by dectin-1 blockade using laminarin or anti-human dectin-1 (**Figure 7F**). Similarly, laminarin mediated blockade of dectin-1 reversed the augmented fungal killing of *Nod1*$^{-/-}$ BMDMs (**Figure 7G**).

DISCUSSION

PRRs regulate the induction of an effective host defense against *A. fumigatus* through recognition of molecules present on the fungal cell wall and induction of potent antifungal effector mechanisms (4, 32). However, little is known about receptors that have a direct inhibitory effects on the induction of antifungal effector mechanisms. Here we demonstrate that the intracellular pattern recognition receptor NOD1 plays an inhibitory role in host response against *A. fumigatus*. We observed that NOD1 activation reduces fungal killing and the induction of oxidative burst. Conversely, murine *Nod1*-deficient cells or human cells in which *NOD1* gene expression was silenced show augmented fungal killing, oxidative burst, and cytokine responses. Most striking, despite being immunocompromised, *Nod1*$^{-/-}$ mice were observed to be less susceptible to *Aspergillus* infection, with reduced fungal burden, and pathological damage to the lungs. Finally, we demonstrate that the activity of NOD1 is inversely correlated with dectin-1 expression, where NOD1 stimulation reduces the expression of dectin-1, while *NOD1* silencing in human macrophages or murine *Nod1* deficiency was associated with increased *CLEC7A* (dectin-1) mRNA expression.

It is rarely observed that deficiency of a receptor is associated with decreased antifungal effector mechanisms. *Tlr9*$^{-/-}$ mice were found to be less susceptible to *Aspergillus* infection with reduced fungal burden (33). However, why TLR9 deficiency is protective is difficult to understand since TLR9 stimulation by CpG enhances the capacity of DCs to induce protective Th1 responses (34). Modulation of TLR5 in THP-1 cells is shown to negatively impact killing of *Aspergillus* conidia, with silencing of *TLR5* gene expression associated with increased fungal killing and activation of TLR5 with reduced fungal killing (35), reduced fungal killing was also observed in neutrophils (36). This modulation of fungal killing is similar to our data with NOD1 activation or siNOD1 in MDMs. However, a mutation in *TLR5* leading to a stop codon was identified as a risk factor for aspergillosis (37). Other than these PRRs, we are not aware of other receptors that negatively impact host defense against *Aspergillus*.

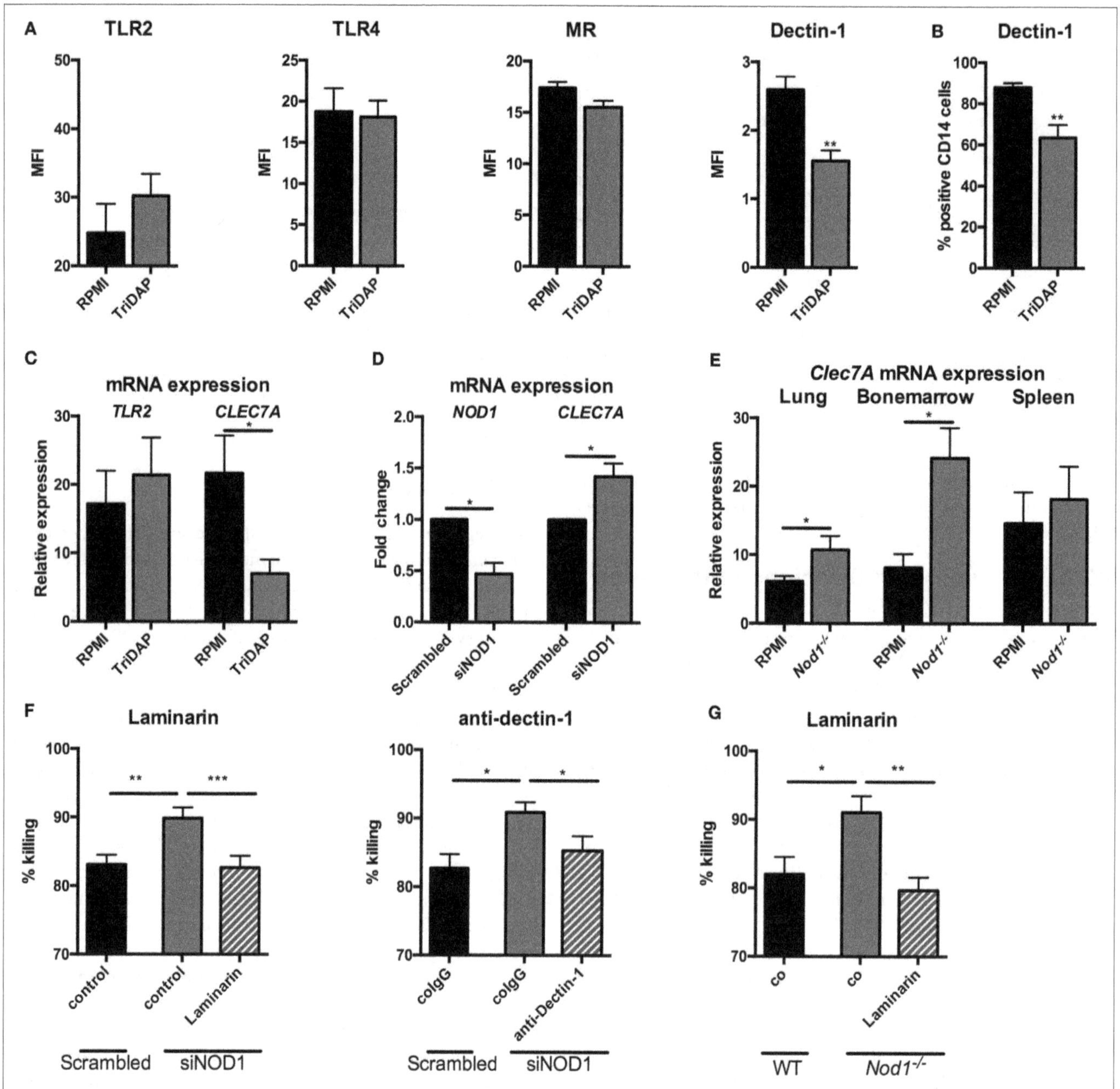

FIGURE 7 | NOD1 suppresses dectin-1 expression and NOD1 deficiency augmenting fungal killing through dectin-1. **(A)** Surface expression of TLR2 (n = 6), TLR4 (n = 6), MR (n = 9) and dectin-1 (n = 9) on human CD14$^+$ monocytes measured by flowcytometry following 24-h stimulation in the presence or absence of (10 μg/mL) TriDAP. **(B)** Percentage of dectin-1$^+$ CD14$^+$ monocytes following 24-h stimulation in the presence or absence of (10 μg/mL) TriDAP (n = 9). **(C)** mRNA expression of *TLR2* (n = 8) and *CLEC7A* (dectin-1) (n = 6) in human PBMCs following 24-h stimulation in the presence or absence of (10 μg/mL) TriDAP. **(D)** *NOD1* and *CLEC7A* (dectin-1) mRNA expression following siRNA treatment with scrambled siRNA or siRNA targeting NOD1(siNOD1) (n = 6). **(E)** *Clec7A* (dectin-1) expression in the lung, bone marrow and spleen of wild type (WT) (n = 8) and *Nod1*$^{-/-}$ (n = 6) at day 3 following *Aspergillus*-infection. Means were compared using the Mann–Whitney *U* test. **(F,G)** Fungal killing capacity assessed as CFU remaining of *A. fumigatus* plotted as percentage of input (2 × 10^6). **(F)** Fungi killed by human GM-CSF differentiated monocytes-derived macrophages treated with scrambled siRNA or NOD1 targeting siRNA, the latter in the presence or absence of Laminarin (100 μg/mL) or a dectin-1 blocking antibody. Means were compared using the Wilcoxon signed rank test. **(G)** Fungi were killed by murine BMDMs of WT and *Nod1*$^{-/-}$ mice, the latter in the presence or absence of laminarin. Means were compared using the Mann–Whitney *U* test. All plots represent mean ± SEM.

Following an otherwise lethal *Aspergillus* infection, *Nod1*-deficient mice demonstrated rapid fungal clearance, which was associated with an almost complete absence of pathological damage and fungal outgrowth in the lungs. In contrast, WT mice succumbed to the infection with severe fungal outgrowth in the lungs and significant pathological damage detected by histopathology. In contrast to our aspergillosis model, the NOD1 receptor is non-redundant in numerous bacterial infection models, such as *Mycobacterium tuberculosis* (9), *Pseudomonas aeruginosa* (38), *Shigella flexineri* (39), and *Helicobacter pylori* (40). In these models, NOD1 was required for an efficient cytokine response (38, 39) and killing of the pathogen (9, 38, 40). In contrast to these latter studies with bacteria, our data suggest that NOD1 has an inhibitory role on the antifungal host defense against *Aspergillus*. *Nod1* deficiency results in an increased capacity of BMDMs to kill live *Aspergillus* and an enhanced oxidative burst upon stimulation with zymosan. Strikingly, we also observe increased cytokine responses and enhanced NFκB translocation in murine *Nod1*-deficient cells. This is in contrast to a previous study that shows NOD1 to be required for NFκB translocation in the response of corneal epithelial cells to *A. fumigatus* (6). The fact that we observe similar results when we silence *NOD1* gene expression in human MDMs validates that the observed effects are due to the absence of NOD1. In contrast, we observed that NOD1 activation has the opposite effect of *NOD1* deficiency and silencing. Taken together, these data suggest that NOD1 inhibits crucial pathways in recognition of *Aspergillus* that limits the induction of protective antifungal effector mechanisms.

Mechanistically, we were able to demonstrate that activation of the NOD1 receptor by its ligand TriDAP reduces surface expression of the C-type lectin receptor dectin-1 on human monocytes, one of the most crucial receptors in host defense against *Aspergillus* (41–51). We found that the reduced surface expression was the result of a downregulation of *CLEC7A* mRNA expression when human monocytes were stimulated with the NOD1 ligand. Contrariwise, NOD1 silencing increased *CLEC7A* mRNA expression. Therefore, the activity of NOD1 seems to show a reverse correlation with *CLEC7A* transcription. Extending this to the *in vivo* model we observed increased *Clec7A* mRNA levels in the lungs and bone marrow of $Nod1^{-/-}$ mice, compared with WT controls. Dectin-1 is crucial for the induction of ROS by *Aspergillus*, which is in line with our data showing increased ROS by *Nod1*-deficient murine BMDMs or in human MDM where *NOD1* gene expression was silenced, which express more dectin-1 (52). We were able to pinpoint that the increased *dectin-1* expression, in the absence of NOD1, was responsible for augmented fungal killing by $Nod1^{-/-}$ BMDMs and human MDM in which NOD1 was silenced, as blockade of dectin-1 reversed the augmented killing.

ROS is essential for the host defense against *Aspergillus* and its importance is illustrated by patients with chronic granulomatous disease who are highly susceptible to infections with *Aspergillus* due to a defect in NADPH-dependent ROS production (53, 54). *Aspergillus* and Zymosan, which are used in our study to study the oxidative burst by murine and human macrophages, are both recognized by dectin-1 (55). We suggest that the modulation of dectin-1 expression by NOD1 could be the responsible mechanism for alterations in the capacity to induce an oxidative burst. Similarly we found that $Nod1^{-/-}$ BMDMs and human MDMs wherein *NOD1* gene expression was silenced have an increased capacity to kill conidia and a decreased conidial killing was observed in human MDMs when NOD1 was stimulated. These changes in conidial killing can also be explained by the differences in dectin-1 expression, as dectin-1 expression is required for efficient phagocytosis (45, 50, 51) and killing of *A. fumigatus* (48, 49) [reviewed in Ref. (42)].

In our *in vitro* studies, we observed that the absence of NOD1 improved fungal killing through enhancement of dectin-1 expression in BMDMs or human MDMs. Although it is evident that in host defense against *A. fumigatus* these cells employ dectin-1 to induce their antifungal effector functions, it is becoming increasingly evident that other cells also use dectin-1 to recognize *Aspergillus*. For example, the role of the pulmonary epithelium is an important tissue that must be taken into account, since these cells can also play an important role in anti-Aspergillus host defense. Dectin-1 on bronchial epithelial cells plays a role in the induction of innate immune responses to *Aspergillus* including the release of antimicrobial peptides such as defensins (51). Moreover, it has been demonstrated that enhancing dectin-1 on only the pulmonary epithelium promotes the resistance to IA (52). The role of dectin-1 in non-myeloid derived tissues is also highlighted by the observation that dectin-1 polymorphisms in the genotype of the recipients of hematopoietic stem cell transplants, which represent the non-myeloid tissues in the patient, predisposes to the development of aspergillosis (56). It cannot be concluded that the protection against aspergillosis that we observe in $Nod1^{-/-}$ mice is solely due to the increased dectin-1 expression on macrophages. We observed that dectin-1 expression in these mice is increased in both the bone marrow as well as the lung. Although resident macrophages in the lung could account for the changed dectin-1 expression, from our data it cannot be excluded that enhanced dectin-1 expression on the pulmonary epithelium does not play an additional role in the protection against *Aspergillus* infection.

Most interestingly, we were able to demonstrate that, in addition to its cytoplasmic expression, the NOD1 receptor localizes to *Aspergillus*-containing phagosome. Due to this localization to the phagosome, we suggest that NOD1 may also recognize fungal PAMPs that are exposed in the phagosome. Nevertheless, further studies are warranted to explore whether cytoplasmic sensing of fungal PAMPs or sensing of fungal PAMPs in the phagosome triggers the effects mediated by NOD1. Although NOD1 is crucial for recognition of bacterial cell wall products (57, 58) and activation of downstream protective immune mechanisms, we suggest that upon engagement of NOD1 with fungi, deleterious mechanisms are induced. Therefore, the potent protective effect of *Nod1* deficiency and beneficial effects of NOD1 silencing makes it tempting to suggest the blockade of NOD1 as a novel treatment strategy for IA. Currently, no pharmacological inhibitors are available to block NOD1 *in vivo*, but small molecule inhibitors that could potentially be used for therapy have been identified (59).

Collectively, we conclude that NOD1 induces a detrimental effect on protective antifungal mechanisms in host defense against *A. fumigatus*. The absence of NOD1 enhances the protective effector mechanisms such as cytokine production, oxidative burst, fungal killing, and dectin-1 expression. This observation paves the way for the development of new treatment strategies for IA that target NOD1.

ETHICS STATEMENT

The human study was carried out in accordance with the recommendations of the guidelines for human research from the Arnhem-Nijmegen Medical Ethical Committee, with written informed consent from all subjects. All subjects gave written informed consent in accordance with the Declaration of Helsinki. The protocol was approved by the Arnhem-Nijmegen Medical Ethical Committee. The animal study was carried out in accordance with the recommendations of Institut Pasteur guidelines, in compliance with European animal welfare regulation and under regulations of the St. Jude Children's Research Hospital Committee on Use and Care of Animals. The protocols were approved by the by the ethical committee for animal experimentation CETEA (Comité d'éthique en experimentation animale, Project license number 2013-0020) and by St. Jude Children's Research Hospital Committee on Use and Care of Animals (protocol no 482-100265-1-/13), respectively.

AUTHOR CONTRIBUTIONS

MG, OI-G, and FV conceived and designed the experiments. MG, MJ, RM, OR, GJ, CF, WM, and OI-G performed the experiments. MG, MJ, RM, OR, GJ, WM, TK, and OI-G analyzed the data. TK provided valuable reagents. MG, AC, OI-G, and FV wrote the manuscript. MG, MJ, WM, TK, AC, OI-G, and FV amended the manuscript.

ACKNOWLEDGMENTS

Part of this work was the doctoral thesis of M.S. Gresnigt, Recognition and Cytokine Signaling Pathways in Host Defense Against *Aspergillus fumigatus* (60). The authors thank C. Wertz and M. Fanton D'Andon for providing *Nod1*-deficient mice K. Schraa for her assistance with culturing BMDMs, B. Briard for help with western blot analysis.

FUNDING

MG was supported by the Erasmus lifelong learning program. FV was supported by the E-rare project EURO-CMC. TK was supported by the National Institutes of Health [grant numbers AI101935, AI124346, AR056296, and CA163507]. AC was supported by the Northern Portugal Regional Operational Programme (NORTE 2020), under the Portugal 2020 Partnership Agreement, through the European Regional Development Fund (FEDER) (NORTE-01-0145-FEDER-000013), and the Fundação para a Ciência e Tecnologia (FCT) (IF/00735/2014).

REFERENCES

1. Brown GD, Denning DW, Gow NA, Levitz SM, Netea MG, White TC. Hidden killers: human fungal infections. *Sci Transl Med* (2012) 4(165): 165rv13. doi:10.1126/scitranslmed.3004404
2. Ben-Ami R, Lewis RE, Kontoyiannis DP. Enemy of the (immunosuppressed) state: an update on the pathogenesis of *Aspergillus fumigatus* infection. *Br J Haematol* (2010) 150(4):406–17. doi:10.1111/j.1365-2141.2010.08283.x
3. Armstrong-James D, Brown GD, Netea MG, Zelante T, Gresnigt MS, van de Veerdonk FL, et al. Immunotherapeutic approaches to treatment of fungal diseases. *Lancet Infect Dis* (2017) 17(12):e393–402. doi:10.1016/S1473-3099(17)30442-5
4. Gresnigt MS, Netea MG, van de Veerdonk FL. Pattern recognition receptors and their role in invasive aspergillosis. *Ann N Y Acad Sci* (2012) 1273:60–7. doi:10.1111/j.1749-6632.2012.06759.x
5. Lamoth F, Rubino I, Bochud PY. Immunogenetics of invasive aspergillosis. *Med Mycol* (2011) 49(Suppl 1):S125–36. doi:10.3109/13693786.2010.516408
6. Zhang Y, Wu J, Xin Z, Wu X. *Aspergillus fumigatus* triggers innate immune response via NOD1 signaling in human corneal epithelial cells. *Exp Eye Res* (2014) 127:170–8. doi:10.1016/j.exer.2014.07.025
7. Su AI, Wiltshire T, Batalov S, Lapp H, Ching KA, Block D, et al. A gene atlas of the mouse and human protein-encoding transcriptomes. *Proc Natl Acad Sci U S A* (2004) 101(16):6062–7. doi:10.1073/pnas.0400782101
8. Opitz B, Puschel A, Schmeck B, Hocke AC, Rosseau S, Hammerschmidt S, et al. Nucleotide-binding oligomerization domain proteins are innate immune receptors for internalized *Streptococcus pneumoniae*. *J Biol Chem* (2004) 279(35):36426–32. doi:10.1074/jbc.M403861200
9. Juarez E, Carranza C, Hernandez-Sanchez F, Loyola E, Escobedo D, Leon-Contreras JC, et al. Nucleotide-oligomerizing domain-1 (NOD1) receptor activation induces pro-inflammatory responses and autophagy in human alveolar macrophages. *BMC Pulm Med* (2014) 14:152. doi:10.1186/1471-2466-14-152
10. Berrington WR, Iyer R, Wells RD, Smith KD, Skerrett SJ, Hawn TR. NOD1 and NOD2 regulation of pulmonary innate immunity to *Legionella pneumophila*. *Eur J Immunol* (2010) 40(12):3519–27. doi:10.1002/eji.201040518
11. Frutuoso MS, Hori JI, Pereira MS, Junior DS, Sonego F, Kobayashi KS, et al. The pattern recognition receptors Nod1 and Nod2 account for neutrophil recruitment to the lungs of mice infected with *Legionella pneumophila*. *Microbes Infect* (2010) 12(11):819–27. doi:10.1016/j.micinf.2010.05.006
12. Sprenkeler EG, Gresnigt MS, van de Veerdonk FL. LC3-associated phagocytosis: a crucial mechanism for antifungal host defence against *Aspergillus fumigatus*. *Cell Microbiol* (2016) 18(9):1208–16. doi:10.1111/cmi.12616
13. Chamilos G, Akoumianaki T, Kyrmizi I, Brakhage A, Beauvais A, Latge JP. Melanin targets LC3-associated phagocytosis (LAP): a novel pathogenetic mechanism in fungal disease. *Autophagy* (2016) 12(5):888–9. doi:10.1080/15548627.2016.1157242
14. Kanayama M, Shinohara ML. Roles of autophagy and autophagy-related proteins in antifungal immunity. *Front Immunol* (2016) 7:47. doi:10.3389/fimmu.2016.00047
15. Tam JM, Mansour MK, Acharya M, Sokolovska A, Timmons AK, Lacy-Hulbert A, et al. The role of autophagy-related proteins in *Candida albicans* infections. *Pathogens* (2016) 5(2):E34. doi:10.3390/pathogens5020034
16. Bonnett CR, Cornish EJ, Harmsen AG, Burritt JB. Early neutrophil recruitment and aggregation in the murine lung inhibit germination of *Aspergillus fumigatus* conidia. *Infect Immun* (2006) 74(12):6528–39. doi:10.1128/iai.00909-06
17. Mehrad B, Strieter RM, Moore TA, Tsai WC, Lira SA, Standiford TJ. CXC chemokine receptor-2 ligands are necessary components of neutrophil-mediated host defense in invasive pulmonary aspergillosis. *J Immunol* (1999) 163(11):6086–94.
18. Cunha C, Kurzai O, Loffler J, Aversa F, Romani L, Carvalho A. Neutrophil responses to aspergillosis: new roles for old players. *Mycopathologia* (2014) 178(5–6):387–93. doi:10.1007/s11046-014-9796-7
19. Phadke AP, Mehrad B. Cytokines in host defense against *Aspergillus*: recent advances. *Med Mycol* (2005) 43(Suppl 1):S173–6. doi:10.1080/13693780500052099
20. Gresnigt MS, van de Veerdonk FL. The role of interleukin-1 family members in the host defence against *Aspergillus fumigatus*. *Mycopathologia* (2014) 178(5–6):395–401. doi:10.1007/s11046-014-9776-y

21. Mencacci A, Cenci E, Bacci A, Montagnoli C, Bistoni F, Romani L. Cytokines in candidiasis and aspergillosis. *Curr Pharm Biotechnol* (2000) 1(3):235–51. doi:10.2174/1389201003378924
22. Netea MG, Warris A, Van der Meer JW, Fenton MJ, Verver-Janssen TJ, Jacobs LE, et al. *Aspergillus fumigatus* evades immune recognition during germination through loss of toll-like receptor-4-mediated signal transduction. *J Infect Dis* (2003) 188(2):320–6. doi:10.1086/376456
23. Chai LY, Kullberg BJ, Vonk AG, Warris A, Cambi A, Latge JP, et al. Modulation of toll-like receptor 2 (TLR2) and TLR4 responses by *Aspergillus fumigatus*. *Infect Immun* (2009) 77(5):2184–92. doi:10.1128/IAI.01455-08
24. Galiger C, Brock M, Jouvion G, Savers A, Parlato M, Ibrahim-Granet O. Assessment of efficacy of antifungals against *Aspergillus fumigatus*: value of real-time bioluminescence imaging. *Antimicrob Agents Chemother* (2013) 57(7):3046–59. doi:10.1128/AAC.01660-12
25. Brock M, Jouvion G, Droin-Bergere S, Dussurget O, Nicola MA, Ibrahim-Granet O. Bioluminescent *Aspergillus fumigatus*, a new tool for drug efficiency testing and in vivo monitoring of invasive aspergillosis. *Appl Environ Microbiol* (2008) 74(22):7023–35. doi:10.1128/AEM.01288-08
26. Dubourdeau M, Athman R, Balloy V, Huerre M, Chignard M, Philpott DJ, et al. *Aspergillus fumigatus* induces innate immune responses in alveolar macrophages through the MAPK pathway independently of TLR2 and TLR4. *J Immunol* (2006) 177(6):3994–4001. doi:10.4049/jimmunol.177.6.3994
27. Philippe B, Ibrahim-Granet O, Prevost MC, Gougerot-Pocidalo MA, Sanchez Perez M, Van der Meeren A, et al. Killing of *Aspergillus fumigatus* by alveolar macrophages is mediated by reactive oxidant intermediates. *Infect Immun* (2003) 71(6):3034–42. doi:10.1128/IAI.71.6.3034-3042.2003
28. Joosten LA, Heinhuis B, Abdollahi-Roodsaz S, Ferwerda G, Lebourhis L, Philpott DJ, et al. Differential function of the NACHT-LRR (NLR) members Nod1 and Nod2 in arthritis. *Proc Natl Acad Sci U S A* (2008) 105(26):9017–22. doi:10.1073/pnas.0710445105
29. Netea MG, Ferwerda G, de Jong DJ, Jansen T, Jacobs L, Kramer M, et al. Nucleotide-binding oligomerization domain-2 modulates specific TLR pathways for the induction of cytokine release. *J Immunol* (2005) 174(10):6518–23. doi:10.4049/jimmunol.174.10.6518
30. Watanabe T, Kitani A, Murray PJ, Strober W. NOD2 is a negative regulator of toll-like receptor 2-mediated T helper type 1 responses. *Nat Immunol* (2004) 5(8):800–8. doi:10.1038/ni1092
31. Oosting M, Berende A, Sturm P, Ter Hofstede HJ, de Jong DJ, Kanneganti TD, et al. Recognition of *Borrelia burgdorferi* by NOD2 is central for the induction of an inflammatory reaction. *J Infect Dis* (2010) 201(12):1849–58. doi:10.1086/652871
32. Becker KL, Ifrim DC, Quintin J, Netea MG, van de Veerdonk FL. Antifungal innate immunity: recognition and inflammatory networks. *Semin Immunopathol* (2015) 37(2):107–16. doi:10.1007/s00281-014-0467-z
33. Bellocchio S, Montagnoli C, Bozza S, Gaziano R, Rossi G, Mambula SS, et al. The contribution of the toll-like/IL-1 receptor superfamily to innate and adaptive immunity to fungal pathogens in vivo. *J Immunol* (2004) 172(5):3059–69. doi:10.4049/jimmunol.172.5.3059
34. Bozza S, Gaziano R, Lipford GB, Montagnoli C, Bacci A, Di Francesco P, et al. Vaccination of mice against invasive aspergillosis with recombinant *Aspergillus* proteins and CpG oligodeoxynucleotides as adjuvants. *Microbes Infect* (2002) 4(13):1281–90. doi:10.1016/S1286-4579(02)00007-2
35. Rodland EK, Ager-Wick E, Halvorsen B, Muller F, Froland SS. Toll-like receptor 5 (TLR5) may be involved in the immunological response to *Aspergillus fumigatus* in vitro. *Med Mycol* (2011) 49(4):375–9. doi:10.3109/13693786.2010.531772
36. Bellocchio S, Moretti S, Perruccio K, Fallarino F, Bozza S, Montagnoli C, et al. TLRs govern neutrophil activity in aspergillosis. *J Immunol* (2004) 173(12):7406–15. doi:10.4049/jimmunol.173.12.7406
37. Grube M, Loeffler J, Mezger M, Kruger B, Echtenacher B, Hoffmann P, et al. TLR5 stop codon polymorphism is associated with invasive aspergillosis after allogeneic stem cell transplantation. *Med Mycol* (2013) 51(8):818–25. doi:10.3109/13693786.2013.809630
38. Chung D, Barker BM, Carey CC, Merriman B, Werner ER, Lechner BE, et al. ChIP-seq and in vivo transcriptome analyses of the *Aspergillus fumigatus* SREBP SrbA reveals a new regulator of the fungal hypoxia response and virulence. *PLoS Pathog* (2014) 10(11):e1004487. doi:10.1371/journal.ppat.1004487
39. Kroll K, Pahtz V, Hillmann F, Vaknin Y, Schmidt-Heck W, Roth M, et al. Identification of hypoxia-inducible target genes of *Aspergillus fumigatus* by transcriptome analysis reveals cellular respiration as an important contributor to hypoxic survival. *Eukaryot Cell* (2014) 13(9):1241–53. doi:10.1128/ec.00084-14
40. Ben-Ami R. Angiogenesis at the mold-host interface: a potential key to understanding and treating invasive aspergillosis. *Future Microbiol* (2013) 8(11):1453–62. doi:10.2217/fmb.13.114
41. Chamilos G, Ganguly D, Lande R, Gregorio J, Meller S, Goldman WE, et al. Generation of IL-23 producing dendritic cells (DCs) by airborne fungi regulates fungal pathogenicity via the induction of T(H)-17 responses. *PLoS One* (2010) 5(9):e12955. doi:10.1371/journal.pone.0012955
42. Drummond RA, Brown GD. The role of dectin-1 in the host defence against fungal infections. *Curr Opin Microbiol* (2011) 14(4):392–9. doi:10.1016/j.mib.2011.07.001
43. Gessner MA, Werner JL, Lilly LM, Nelson MP, Metz AE, Dunaway CW, et al. Dectin-1-dependent interleukin-22 contributes to early innate lung defense against *Aspergillus fumigatus*. *Infect Immun* (2012) 80(1):410–7. doi:10.1128/IAI.05939-11
44. Hohl TM, Van Epps HL, Rivera A, Morgan LA, Chen PL, Feldmesser M, et al. *Aspergillus fumigatus* triggers inflammatory responses by stage-specific beta-glucan display. *PLoS Pathog* (2005) 1(3):e30. doi:10.1371/journal.ppat.0010030
45. Kyrmizi I, Gresnigt MS, Akoumianaki T, Samonis G, Sidiropoulos P, Boumpas D, et al. Corticosteroids block autophagy protein recruitment in *Aspergillus fumigatus* phagosomes via targeting dectin-1/Syk kinase signaling. *J Immunol* (2013) 191(3):1287–99. doi:10.4049/jimmunol.1300132
46. Said-Sadier N, Padilla E, Langsley G, Ojcius DM. *Aspergillus fumigatus* stimulates the NLRP3 inflammasome through a pathway requiring ROS production and the Syk tyrosine kinase. *PLoS One* (2010) 5(4):e10008. doi:10.1371/journal.pone.0010008
47. Sainz J, Lupianez CB, Segura-Catena J, Vazquez L, Rios R, Oyonarte S, et al. Dectin-1 and DC-SIGN polymorphisms associated with invasive pulmonary aspergillosis infection. *PLoS One* (2012) 7(2):e32273. doi:10.1371/journal.pone.0032273
48. Steele C, Rapaka RR, Metz A, Pop SM, Williams DL, Gordon S, et al. The beta-glucan receptor dectin-1 recognizes specific morphologies of *Aspergillus fumigatus*. *PLoS Pathog* (2005) 1(4):e42. doi:10.1371/journal.ppat.0010042
49. Werner JL, Metz AE, Horn D, Schoeb TR, Hewitt MM, Schwiebert LM, et al. Requisite role for the dectin-1 beta-glucan receptor in pulmonary defense against *Aspergillus fumigatus*. *J Immunol* (2009) 182(8):4938–46. doi:10.4049/jimmunol.0804250
50. Luther K, Torosantucci A, Brakhage AA, Heesemann J, Ebel F. Phagocytosis of *Aspergillus fumigatus* conidia by murine macrophages involves recognition by the dectin-1 beta-glucan receptor and toll-like receptor 2. *Cell Microbiol* (2007) 9(2):368–81. doi:10.1111/j.1462-5822.2006.00796.x
51. Gersuk GM, Underhill DM, Zhu L, Marr KA. Dectin-1 and TLRs permit macrophages to distinguish between different *Aspergillus fumigatus* cellular states. *J Immunol* (2006) 176(6):3717–24. doi:10.4049/jimmunol.176.6.3717
52. Underhill DM, Rossnagle E, Lowell CA, Simmons RM. Dectin-1 activates Syk tyrosine kinase in a dynamic subset of macrophages for reactive oxygen production. *Blood* (2005) 106(7):2543–50. doi:10.1182/blood-2005-03-1239
53. Antachopoulos C. Invasive fungal infections in congenital immunodeficiencies. *Clin Microbiol Infect* (2010) 16(9):1335–42. doi:10.1111/j.1469-0691.2010.03289.x
54. Segal BH, DeCarlo ES, Kwon-Chung KJ, Malech HL, Gallin JI, Holland SM. *Aspergillus nidulans* infection in chronic granulomatous disease. *Medicine (Baltimore)* (1998) 77(5):345–54. doi:10.1097/00005792-199809000-00004
55. Gantner BN, Simmons RM, Canavera SJ, Akira S, Underhill DM. Collaborative induction of inflammatory responses by dectin-1 and toll-like receptor 2. *J Exp Med* (2003) 197(9):1107–17. doi:10.1084/jem.20021787
56. Cunha C, Di Ianni M, Bozza S, Giovannini G, Zagarella S, Zelante T, et al. Dectin-1 Y238X polymorphism associates with susceptibility to invasive aspergillosis in hematopoietic transplantation through impairment of both recipient- and donor-dependent mechanisms of antifungal immunity. *Blood* (2010) 116(24):5394–402. doi:10.1182/blood-2010-04-279307
57. Chamaillard M, Hashimoto M, Horie Y, Masumoto J, Qiu S, Saab L, et al. An essential role for NOD1 in host recognition of bacterial

peptidoglycan containing diaminopimelic acid. *Nat Immunol* (2003) 4(7):702–7. doi:10.1038/ni945

58. Girardin SE, Boneca IG, Carneiro LA, Antignac A, Jehanno M, Viala J, et al. Nod1 detects a unique muropeptide from gram-negative bacterial peptidoglycan. *Science* (2003) 300(5625):1584–7. doi:10.1126/science.1084677
59. Shepardson KM, Ngo LY, Aimanianda V, Latge JP, Barker BM, Blosser SJ, et al. Hypoxia enhances innate immune activation to *Aspergillus fumigatus* through cell wall modulation. *Microbes Infect* (2013) 15(4):259–69. doi:10.1016/j.micinf.2012.11.010
60. Gresnigt MS. *Recognition and Cytokine Signalling Pathways in Host Defence against Aspergillus fumigatus [Doctoral Dissertation]*. Radboud University Nijmegen (2015). Available from: http://repository.ubn.ru.nl

20

Antifungal Activity of Plasmacytoid Dendritic Cells and the Impact of Chronic HIV Infection

Samuel Maldonado[1,2] *and Patricia Fitzgerald-Bocarsly*[1,2]*

[1] *Rutgers School of Graduate Studies, Newark, NJ, United States,* [2] *Department of Pathology and Laboratory Medicine, New Jersey Medical School, Newark, NJ, United States*

Correspondence:
Patricia Fitzgerald-Bocarsly
Bocarsly@njms.rutgers.edu

Due to the effectiveness of combined antiretroviral therapy, people living with HIV can control viral replication and live longer lifespans than ever. However, HIV-positive individuals still face challenges to their health and well-being, including dysregulation of the immune system resulting from years of chronic immune activation, as well as opportunistic infections from pathogenic fungi. This review focuses on one of the key players in HIV immunology, the plasmacytoid dendritic cell (pDC), which links the innate and adaptive immune response and is notable for being the body's most potent producer of type-I interferons (IFNs). During chronic HIV infection, the pDC compartment is greatly dysregulated, experiencing a substantial depletion in number and compromise in function. This immune dysregulation may leave patients further susceptible to opportunistic infections. This is especially important when considering a new role for pDCs currently emerging in the literature: in addition to their role in antiviral immunity, recent studies suggest that pDCs also play an important role in antifungal immunity. Supporting this new role, pDCs express C-type lectin receptors including dectin-1, dectin-2, dectin-3, and mannose receptor, and toll-like receptors-4 and -9 that are involved in recognition, signaling, and response to a wide variety of fungal pathogens, including *Aspergillus fumigatus*, *Cryptococcus neoformans, Candida albicans,* and *Pneumocystis jirovecii*. Accordingly, pDCs have been demonstrated to recognize and respond to certain pathogenic fungi, measured *via* activation, cytokine production, and fungistatic activity *in vitro*, while *in vivo* mouse models indicated a strikingly vital role for pDCs in survival against pulmonary *Aspergillus* challenge. Here, we discuss the role of the pDC compartment and the dysregulation it undergoes during chronic HIV infection, as well as what is known so far about the role and mechanisms of pDC antifungal activity.

Keywords: plasmacytoid dendritic cells, C-type lectin receptors, toll-like receptors, innate antifungal immunity, HIV

INTRODUCTION

An estimated 33 million people were living with HIV/AIDS worldwide in 2015 (1). Although the development of combined antiretroviral therapy has allowed HIV patients to suppress viral replication and live longer lifespans (2, 3), HIV evades the immune system and persists, causing chronic immune activation and inflammation (4). The persistence of infection and immune activation leads to significant detrimental changes that occur in the body, and pose major threats to patients' well-being; in fact, in 2010, HIV/AIDS was still the fifth leading cause of disease burden worldwide (5).

Arguably the most significant pathological process faced by treated and untreated patients alike is the erosion of the immune system. HIV infection famously depletes $CD4^+$ T-helper (T_H) cells, first quickly in the acute phase of infection, followed by a near-total recovery in numbers, and finally a steady decline over a number of years (4) leaving the adaptive immune system at a tremendous disadvantage. T-cell depletion occurs *via* mechanisms such as direct infection, bystander effects due to chronic inflammation, and senescence (4, 6). The dysfunction of the immune system is also much broader; almost every known immune cell type has been associated with a dysfunction due to chronic HIV infection. Because HIV gains access to a cell *via* its interaction with CD4 and co-receptors CXCR4 and CCR5, it also has the capacity to infect other cells that express those receptors, including monocytes, macrophages, and plasmacytoid dendritic cells (pDCs) (4). In addition, the immune system may be further dysregulated due to chronic innate immune activation and the continued production of normally beneficial cytokines (7).

This erosion of the immune system leaves patients hypersusceptible to a variety of opportunistic infections, including fungal infections not commonly seen in the general population. For example, *Candida albicans* infection is the most common fungal infection in HIV patients. While it usually presents as oropharyngeal thrush, it can span a broad spectrum of severity from asymptomatic to invasive candidiasis (8). The most common systemic fungal infection in the HIV population is cryptococcal meningitis, caused by *Cryptococcus neoformans*. Cryptococcal meningitis causes 181,000 deaths a year in HIV-positive patients, accounting for 15% of global AIDS-related deaths (9, 10). *Aspergillus fumigatus* is the causative agent of invasive Aspergillosis, which is less common in the context of HIV infection but is particularly aggressive and difficult to treat, resulting in a median survival of only 3 months after diagnosis (11, 12). These and other pathogenic fungi take advantage of an HIV patient's impaired immune system. Studies early in the HIV epidemic suggested that HIV patients are much more likely to develop opportunistic infections when two events occur: absolute $CD4^+$ cell counts drop below 250 cells/mm^3, and interferon (IFN)-α production by virus-stimulated peripheral blood mononuclear cells (PBMCs) drops below 300 IU/ml (13). It is the latter that makes pDCs a cell type of great interest when studying HIV infection, as they are the body's most potent producers of type-I IFNs. pDCs produce up to 100-fold more IFN-α than any other cell type in response to viral stimulation and serve as an important link between the innate and the adaptive branches of the immune system (14–16). pDC IFN production and influence over the rest of the immune response has made these cells the subject of extensive investigation in human and mouse models. Importantly, murine systems do not perfectly represent human ones, and studies on mouse pDC function must also be investigated in humans. For example, toll-like receptor (TLR) 9 is broadly expressed by murine myeloid cells, but is more limited to pDCs and B-cells in humans (17). Similarly, murine pDCs commonly produce IL-12 while human pDCs rarely, if ever, produce IL-12 (18).

Plasmacytoid dendritic cell dysregulation during chronic HIV infection has garnered attention due to the potentially far-reaching effects on patient outcome and well-being. However, an interesting development in the field of pDC research is the investigation into their role in fungal infection. Studies have demonstrated that pDCs have the machinery needed to recognize and respond to fungal stimulation, that they in fact do respond with certain cellular functions, and that they are necessary *in vivo* for a successful antifungal immune response. In this review, we outline the current paradigm concerning pDCs' role in viral immunity and describe the dysregulation of the pDC compartment during chronic HIV infection. We then switch gears to the role of pDCs in antifungal immunity, where we highlight the components of fungal immunity that pDCs possess, and summarize what has been discovered to date concerning the mechanisms of pDC antifungal activity.

pDCs IN ANTIVIRAL IMMUNITY

Both the innate and the adaptive immune responses play active roles in combating viral infections such as HIV. The adaptive immune response includes a strong $CD4^+$ and $CD8^+$ T-cell response, as well as the production of neutralizing antibodies that begins during the acute phase of infection (19, 20). Mobilization of the adaptive immune response depends in part on pDCs, a lineage-negative subtype of dendritic cells that derives its name from a plasma-cell-like morphology. Although pDCs comprise only 0.2–0.8% of PBMC (14, 15, 21), their powerful immunomodulating capabilities make pDCs highly influential to the development of the immune response to HIV infection, and a lack of sufficient pDC numbers or function corresponds with high viral loads and opportunistic infections (22).

Human pDCs are generally found in peripheral blood and lymphoid tissue, so if an infection occurs in a different tissue (e.g., the lung or mucosa), they must migrate to sites of infection or inflammation by responding to chemokines. This occurs primarily *via* the chemokine receptors CMKLR1, CCR7, CXCR3, and CXCR4 (22–24) as well as through homing molecules, such as CD62L, which binds L-selectin and allows pDCs to track to high endothelial venules and the gut homing receptor $\alpha4\beta7$ (25). Once at the site of infection, pDCs directly recognize and respond to viral stimulation. The initial interaction between pDCs and HIV virions is possible because pDCs express the surface molecules that are targeted by HIV: CD4, CCR4, and CXCR5, as reviewed in Ref. (16). The interaction between the virus and CD4 allows the pDC to endocytose the virus, which induces activation in a TLR-dependent or -independent manner.

In the TLR-dependent pathway, the endocytosed virus is delivered to endosomes in pDC that contain TLR-7 and 9. Acidification of the endosomes allows TLR-7 and 9 to access viral RNA or unmethylated CpG motifs, including that in viral DNA, respectively (26, 27). These TLRs have the capacity to recognize a host of viral, bacterial, and fungal nucleic acids, as well as small molecule artificial ligands such as imiquimod and resiquimod (28, 29). Ligation of TLR-7 or 9 induces a MyD88-dependent activation pathway that ultimately leads to pDC activation and cytokine production (30). Although less well-characterized than the TLR-dependent pathway, evidence exists for a TLR-independent activation pathway in pDCs. For example, one study found that IFN-α production by murine pDCs in response to Sendai virus was not abrogated in MyD88$^{-/-}$ mice and was not dependent on endosomal acidification, both of which are required for TLR9 signaling (31). Another study found that murine pDC IFN-α production in response to HSV-1 was not completely dependent on TLR9 (32). However, specific mechanisms of TLR-independent pDC activation and cytokine production are still under investigation.

Both the TLR-dependent and -independent signaling pathways converge on interferon regulatory factor (IRF) 7, the master regulator of IFN production which is constitutively expressed by pDCs at uniquely high levels (30, 33, 34). Phosphorylation of IRF7 causes it to translocate into the nucleus and induce the transcription of IFN genes, producing high concentrations of type-I IFN (35). TLR-7 and -9 ligation also lead to the activation of transcription factor NF-κB, which induces the production of inflammatory cytokines/chemokines and the upregulation of co-stimulatory molecules (21, 36). Activated pDCs can then produce type-I IFNs, type-III IFNs, and a network of other cytokines and chemokines. They also have the ability to become antigen-presenting cells, at which point they develop a morphology resembling conventional DCs (cDCs) (36–38).

Perhaps the most significant contribution of pDCs to antiviral immunity is the production of massive amounts of type-I IFNs (mainly α and β) in response to viral stimulation. Most notably, pDCs can produce 100–1,000 times more type-I IFN than any other cell type (39–41). It has even been reported that as much as 60% of genes expressed in an activated pDC are dedicated to the production of type-I and type-III IFNs (42). Type-I IFNs all bind the same receptor, the IFN-α/β receptor, which is widely expressed by most nucleated cells in the body. The IFN-α/β receptor is composed of two subunits, IFNAR1 and IFNAR2, that form a heterodimer upon ligation of type-I IFN (43). IFNAR-associated Janus kinases then phosphorylate STAT1 and STAT2, which form a complex with IRF9 called the ISGF3 complex. The resulting signaling cascade activates gene transcription for factors that produce an antiviral state in surrounding tissues and mobilizes virtually all types of immune cells to combat viral infection (44, 45). For example, IFN-α acts as a survival, maturation, and cytokine/chemokine production factor for pDCs (46, 47) and cDCs (48), activates natural killer cells (26), biases the immune system toward a T_H1 response (49, 50), primes CD8$^+$ T-cells and induces memory CD8$^+$ T-cells (51–53), promotes the development of regulatory T (Treg) cells (54), and enhances antibody production against soluble antigen (55). These effects, among others, are critical for the inhibition of viral replication and are why type-I IFNs are arguably the most important cytokines in antiviral immunity.

In addition to type-I IFNs, pDCs also produce type-III IFNs (IFN-λ1–3) after viral stimulation (38). The IFN-λ receptor is expressed on a much more limited scale than the IFN-α/β receptor—primarily epithelial cells and pDCs (38, 56)—suggesting that the biological activity of IFN-λ is more narrow than that of type-I IFN. However, type-I and type-III IFN share many common features: their signaling pathways include many of the same factors, including STAT1, STAT2, and the formation of the ISGF3 complex; they also activate several common genes (57, 58). Functionally, IFN-λ also has antiviral effects, especially for the protection of epithelial cells (59), the enhancement of TLR-mediated signaling in pDCs (56), development of Treg cells (60), and biasing toward a T_H1 response by reducing IL-13 expression (61). However, it has also been reported that IFN-λ can be antagonistic to type-I IFN antiviral activity (62).

Other than IFNs, pDCs are able to produce several other cytokines and chemokines. NF-κB activation after viral stimulation induces pDCs to produce inflammatory cytokines and chemokines such as IL-12 (in murine but not human pDC), TNF-α, RANTES, IL-10, IP-10, IL-6, MIP-1α, and MIP-1β (36, 63). One study identified 12 chemokines that are produced in three distinct waves by pDCs in the hours following influenza virus infection (64). Furthermore, pDCs are also capable of other innate immune functions. Although resting pDCs are less efficient than myeloid DCs at capturing, processing, and presenting antigen (65, 66), activation of pDCs in response to influenza virus induces a change into a dendritic morphology and the upregulation of MHC-II, enhancing their ability to present antigen to naïve and memory T-cells (67, 68). In 2012, Tel et al. reported that pDCs could not only present tumor antigens but could also directly kill tumor cells. They termed these cells "killer pDCs" (69). Another interesting feature of the pDC is the expression of several surface receptors usually restricted to myeloid cells. On pDCs, these receptors include the C-type lectin receptors (CLRs) dectin-1, dectin-2, dectin-3, and mannose receptor (MR) (70–72), which will be discussed later. These receptors are of particular interest because they are involved in antifungal immunity.

pDC DYSREGULATION DURING CHRONIC HIV INFECTION

Despite the impressive antiviral functions of pDCs, HIV still manages to evade the immune system and persist in the body. The observation that HIV patient blood cells produced less IFN after stimulation led to the discovery of what were termed natural IFN-producing cells, which would later be known as pDCs (73–76). After the discovery of pDCs as the major IFN-α-producing cell, observations surfaced that showed chronic HIV infection leads to a decline in pDC number and function (77). The decline in absolute pDC numbers correlated directly with a decline in CD4$^+$ T-cell count and increased viral load (22, 78), while pDC functional decline (percent of IFN-α-producing pDC after viral stimulation) correlated with an increase in patient viral load, but not CD4$^+$ T-cell count (76). Although ART treatment results in a partial recovery of pDC numbers, they do not make a full recovery (79). The specific cause of this decline in pDC number is still under investigation. Studies on macaque models indicate that pDCs are recruited to lymph nodes where they die rapidly (80, 81); this was supported by a study that found higher numbers and accelerated pDC death in human lymph nodes (82). Other studies show that pDCs are susceptible to HIV infection, which can cause syncytia formation and cell death (83, 84). Other possible mechanisms include recruitment to mucosal tissues, bystander apoptosis similar to T-cells, and bone marrow suppression (85).

Along with lower numbers, HIV also causes functional differences in pDCs. One of the earliest observations in HIV patients was the high levels of circulating IFN-α seen in some untreated patients, which was associated with disease progression (13, 86). The pDCs that accumulate in HIV patient lymph nodes were also described as producing significantly higher levels of IFN-α than non-infected healthy controls (82). This suggests that at certain points during infection, pDCs are chronically activated and are continuously producing IFN-α. This chronic immune activation may be driving pathology, including the immune exhaustion of T-cell compartments (7, 87). Supporting this hypothesis, one study found that humanized pDC-depleted mice infected with HIV-1 show dramatically reduced cell death and immune cell depletion, a phenomenon they suggested stems from the lack of persistent pDC activation and IFN production (88). In addition, other pDC functions are found to be dysregulated in HIV patients: pDCs become less able to stimulate T-cell proliferation in mixed lymphocyte reactions (89), show a partial activation phenotype (90), and have a reduced ability to respond to TLR7 and -9 agonists (91).

Another area of research concerns the possibility that pDCs may be inducing the differentiation of human Treg cells that lead to tolerogenicity and suppression of T-cell proliferation during chronic HIV infection. Human pDCs have been shown to induce both $CD8^+$ and $CD4^+$ Treg cell development in certain circumstances. For example, pDCs stimulated with type B CpG oligodeoxynucleotides (CpGb) induced $CD4^+CD25^-$ naïve T-cells to differentiate into $CD4^+CD25^+$ Treg cells, which suppressed T-cell proliferation and promoted tolerance (92). Another study found that pDCs activated with CD40L induced naïve $CD8^+$ T-cells to proliferate, but the resulting $CD8^+$ T-cells were poorly cytotoxic, had poor responses to secondary re-stimulation, and produced IL-10 (93). To that end, a study by Boasso et al. (94) found that T-cell proliferation in HIV-infected patients was being inhibited by pDCs through the expression of indoleamine-2,3-dioxygenase (IDO) (94). IDO is the first and rate-limiting enzyme in the catabolism of tryptophan, and its expression can be used by APCs as an immune modulator to limit T-cell proliferation (95). In the study, IDO mRNA expression in the blood of HIV-infected patients was directly correlated with viral load, and was responsible for impaired $CD4^+$ T-cell proliferation. Using flow cytometric analysis, they found that pDCs were the main producers of IDO, and that pDC IDO expression was a direct response to HIV that did not require the presence of other leukocytes. This phenomenon may represent yet another way that pDCs contribute to the dysfunction of the immune system during chronic HIV infection. In addition, another study found that IDO expression by pDCs blocks T-cell differentiation into T_H17 cells, which could further negatively impact adaptive immunity to fungal infection (96). This dysfunction, along with the dysregulation of virtually every immune cell type, leaves patients at higher risk of opportunistic infections and other comorbidities, including fungal infections with *C. albicans* and *C. neoformans*.

SELECT COMPONENTS OF THE IMMUNE RESPONSE TO FUNGAL INFECTION

A discussion of HIV patient susceptibility to fungal infections requires an understanding of normal antifungal immunity. Although some fungi are commensal with the human host, this review focuses on pathogenic fungal infections. Fungal pathogens, such as *A. fumigatus* and *C. neoformans*, tend to be ubiquitous to the environment and are introduced into the human host through inhalation of spores or small yeast cells (97, 98). In the case of *A. fumigatus* and other sporulating fungi, spores (termed "resting conidia," RC) that reach a suitable host begin to swell (termed "swollen conidia," SC), and germinate (termed "germinating conidia," GC), finally growing into filamentous hyphae (99). Fortunately, fungal pathogens express pathogen-associated molecular patterns (PAMPs), which are not found on mammalian cells and alert the immune system to the presence of non-self organisms (100). PAMPs can vary depending on the species, growth stage, and environment of the fungus (101, 102). Three significant PAMPs on fungal cell walls include β-glucans (polymers of glucose, typically with 1,3 linkages and occasional 1,6 branches), chitin (a polymer of *N*-acetylglucosamine), and mannans (polymers of mannose linked to fungal proteins) (97, 103). Fungi that make it into a human host can be recognized by innate immune cells through pattern recognition receptors (PRRs), such as TLRs and CLRs (100).

Once the PAMPs on fungi are recognized by cellular PRRs, a complex immune response begins that, incorporates both the innate and adaptive branches of the immune system (104). Phagocytes, such as monocytes, neutrophils, and macrophages, phagocytose and kill fungal pathogens directly (105), spread out over hyphae and kill them *via* oxidative and non-oxidative means, and in the case of neutrophils produce extracellular traps (106, 107). In addition to uptake and direct killing, cDCs also transport and present fungal antigen to T-cells and induce their differentiation into T_H1, T_H17, or Treg cells, depending on the environment and the fungus (108–110). While T_H1 cells are thought to be the most protective, patients with defects in the T_H1 compartment are not overly susceptible to certain fungal infections (97). This is because the T_H17 compartment is also protective and sometimes essential to fungal clearance, depending on the species and route of infection (111). Conversely, inborn errors in IL-17 immunity can result in chronic mucocutaneous candidiasis in humans (112), and more broad susceptibility to *C. albicans* infection in mice, including cutaneous and oropharyngeal infection (113). Finally, the development of protective antibodies after vaccination of mice with *C. albicans* adhesins suggests that humoral immunity may also get involved during fungal infection, although in those studies the main effector cells responsible for vaccine efficacy were CD4+ T-cells, and neither B-cell transfer nor passive immunization with serum of vaccinated mice were protective to unvaccinated mice (114).

The TLRs involved in fungal recognition that are expressed on pDCs are TLR4 and TLR9 (17, 35). TLR4 (CD284) is mainly known for recognizing bacterial lipopolysaccharide, but it also appears to recognize mannan structures of fungal cell walls, leading to cytokine/chemokine production and recruitment of neutrophils.

TLR4 is composed of a 608 residue extracellular domain, which contains 21 leucine-rich repeats and can be subdivided into N-, central, and C-terminal domains, and a 187-residue intracellular domain that signals *via* the TLR-associated adaptor MyD88 (115). Interruption of TLR4 signaling has been shown to increase susceptibility to *C. albicans* (116), *A. fumigatus* (117, 118), and *Pneumocystis jirovecii* (119) in mice. However, it is worth noting that TLR4 signaling did not induce cytokine production after recognizing mannans on *C. neoformans* cell walls (120), indicating fungal species-specific responses.

TLR9 (CD289) recognizes unmethylated CpG DNA sequences, which may allow it to recognize fungal DNA. As mentioned earlier, TLR9 is located in endosomes of pDCs, where it is known for responding to viral DNA in a MyD88-dependent manner. TLR9 has 25 intra-endosomal leucine-rich repeats, but a detailed structure for TLR9 has not yet been discovered (121). Studies show TLR9 induces IL-10 production by macrophages in response to *C. albicans* (120), pro-inflammatory cytokine secretion by mouse bone marrow-derived dendritic cells in response to *A. fumigatus* DNA (122), and IL-12p40 production and CD40 upregulation in DCs in response to *C. neoformans* (123). It is interesting to note that while MyD88 serves as a signaling adaptor for all of the TLRs except TLR3, patients with MyD88 deficiencies or mutations do not suffer from severe or recurrent fungal infections, suggesting that TLR signaling enhances but is not indispensable for antifungal immune responses (124).

C-type lectin receptors are a large family of receptors that contain C-type lectin-like domains (CTLDs), which, depending on the receptor, recognize a wide array of carbohydrates, proteins, or lipids (125). CLRs are a diverse family of receptors with a multitude of functions, but this review will focus on the four CLRs that have a role in fungal recognition and have been identified on human pDCs: dectin-1, dectin-2, dectin-3, and MR.

Dectin-1 (CLEC7A) recognizes β(1,3)- and β(1,6)-linked glucans, which are present on bacterial and fungal cell walls. B-glucans can comprise up to 50% of the cell walls of common pathogenic fungi, including *A. fumigatus*, *C. neoformans*, *P. jirovecii*, and *C. albicans* (126–130). Dectin-1 is composed of an extracellular CTLD, a single transmembrane domain, and an intracellular immunoreceptor tyrosine-based activation motif (ITAM) (126). The dimerization of dectin-1 and the phosphorylation of its intracellular ITAM recruits spleen tyrosine kinase (Syk), and induces a signaling cascade that includes the signaling adaptor caspase recruitment domain-containing protein 9 (CARD9). CARD9 is a major point of regulation within the signaling cascade of several CLRs, including dectin-1 and dectin-2, and is indispensable for the cell activation and cytokine production caused by dectin-1 and -2 ligation (131, 132). CARD9 deficiency has been linked to chronic and recurring fungal infections, especially by *C. albicans* (133, 134). In addition, pDCs from CARD9 knockout mice produced significantly less IL-6 and TNF-α than wild-type mice in response to influenza virus, while type-I IFN production was unaffected (135). Dectin-1/Syk/CARD9 signaling ultimately leads to the canonical activation and nuclear translocation of NF-κB subunits Rel-A (p65) and c-Rel. Dectin-1 also activates the NF-κB unit Rel-B through a non-canonical pathway, *via* Raf-1 instead of Syk (136). Dectin-1 has been shown to have an array of immune functions, including the recognition, uptake, and killing of fungi (137, 138), as well as cellular signaling leading to maturation, production of a respiratory burst, cytokine and chemokine production, enhanced survival and differentiation of T_H cells that helps control fungal infection in the GI tract, and cytotoxic T-lymphocyte priming (128, 139–143).

Dectin-2 (CLEC6A) recognizes α-mannose structures present on the surface of many viruses, bacteria, and fungal pathogens. Dectin-2 has been shown to have a role in immunity to fungi, including *C. albicans*, *A. fumigatus*, and non-encapsulated *C. neoformans*, with a preference for hyphal as opposed to yeast or conidial forms of fungal cell walls (144–146). It is composed of an extracellular CTLD and a short cytoplasmic tail, which couples with FcRγ to initiate downstream signaling. The phosphorylation of FcRγ again recruits Syk and CARD9 (147, 148). Dectin-2 signaling also induces the activation of NF-κB, but in contrast to dectin-1, dectin-2 selectively activates the c-Rel subunit of NF-κB *via* MALT1. This selectivity suggests that dectin-2 is more specific for the production of cytokines that induce T_H17 polarization (149). Dectin-2 signaling induces internalization of the fungus and the production of an array of cytokines, including TNF-α and IL-1β, 2, 6, 10, 12, and 23 (145, 147). Furthermore, blocking dectin-2 in mice abrogated the development of T_H1 and T_H17 cells, which left mice significantly more susceptible to *C. albicans* infection (150).

Similar to dectin-2, dectin-3 (CLEC4D, CLECSF8) also has a single extracellular CRD with a short cytoplasmic tail. The CRD of dectin-3 is highly homologous with that of dectin-2, and similarly recognizes α-mannans (151). In fact, dectin-3 was found to dimerize with dectin-2, and the resulting heterodimer was more adept at recognizing fungal PAMPs than the respective homodimers (152). Although the cytoplasmic tail of dectin-3 lacks a signaling motif and does not associate with any known signaling adaptor, including FcRγ, it does induce signaling *via* Syk and the CARD9/Bcl10/Malt1 complex and activates NF-κB (153). The cellular processes that are induced include phagocytosis, cytokine production, and a respiratory burst in macrophages (154). To illustrate its physiological relevance, murine bone marrow-derived macrophages pretreated with dectin-3-blocking monoclonal antibodies were inhibited from NF-κB nuclear translocation and cytokine production after *C. albicans* stimulation, and mice treated with dectin-3-blocking antibody succumbed rapidly to sub-lethal *C. albicans* IV challenge (152). Similarly, mice deficient in dectin-3 were more susceptible to DSS-induced colitis, and murine bone marrow-derived macrophages were impaired in phagocytic and fungicidal ability, NF-κB nuclear translocation, and cytokine production (155). Conversely, no role was found for dectin-3 in defense against *C. neoformans*, as dectin-3-deficient mice did not differ in pulmonary leukocyte recruitment, pulmonary cytokine profiles, or overall survival after pulmonary *C. neoformans* challenge. In addition, macrophages and DCs isolated from dectin-3 knockout mice did not differ in their phagocytic or fungicidal ability against *C. neoformans* (156).

Mannose receptor (CD206) is a highly endocytic receptor with three categories of extracellular binding domains, a single transmembrane domain, and a short cytoplasmic tail (157). The extracellular binding domains include an N-terminal cysteine-rich (CR) domain, which binds sulfated carbohydrates; a fibronectin type II (FNII) domain, which binds collagen; and eight CTLDs, which bind carbohydrates that terminate in D-mannose, L-fucose, or *N*-acetyl glucosamine, as reviewed in Ref. (158, 159). While the CR and FNII extracellular domains are involved in glycoprotein homeostasis (160, 161), it is the CTLDs that are responsible for recognizing carbohydrate entities on pathogens (159). For one particularly interesting example, MR binds the gp120 glycoprotein on HIV and mediates binding of the virus by dendritic cells (70) and macrophages (162). In the context of fungal infection, the MR has been shown to enhance uptake and clearance of pathogenic fungi, including *A. fumigatus* (163) *C. albicans* (164, 165), *C. neoformans* (166), and *Pneumocystis carinii* (167). However, MR seems to not be phagocytic in its own right; MR was unable to induce phagocytosis of its ligands when transfected onto Chinese hamster ovary cells (168). MR instead influences the signaling of other receptors. For example, Tachado et al. (169) discovered that human embryonic kidney 293 cells required transfection of both TLR2 and the MR in order to produce IL-8 in response to *Pneumocystis*. Similarly, in alveolar macrophages, *Pneumocystis* challenge led to direct interaction of TLR2 and MR, while blocking MR and TLR2 simultaneously abrogated IL-8 production (169). The downstream results of MR signaling are varied and dependent on many factors, including signaling from other receptors and the route of ligand delivery (158). A summary of the TLRs and CLRs discussed here can be found in **Table 1**.

pDCs IN ANTIFUNGAL IMMUNITY

The involvement of pDCs in antifungal immunity is a topic of study currently emerging in the literature. An early indication came in 2004, when Romani et al. described how thymosin alpha 1, a peptide produced by the thymus, served to activate human cDCs and pDCs by enhancing their phagocytic capacity and IL-10 production in response to *A. fumigatus* stimulation (171). Later, Dan et al. found that mannoproteins from *C. neoformans* and CpG-containing DNA synergistically induced pDCs to produce greater amounts of pro-inflammatory cytokines, although stimulation with mannoproteins alone did not induce any cytokine production (170). This implied that pDCs were able to sense mannoproteins, which are classically recognized by CLRs, and that recognition of mannoproteins acted as an adjuvant for TLR9-dependent pDC activation by CpG. That same year, Ramirez-Ortiz et al. found that *A. fumigatus* DNA contained unmethylated CpG motifs, which triggered TLR9 in mouse and human pDCs and induced cytokine production *in vitro* (122). Perruccio et al. then confirmed that *A. fumigatus* DNA stimulated TLR-9 in pDCs and induced the production of IL-12p70, IL-10, and IFN-α (172).

The response of pDCs to fungal recognition is still under investigation, but a few studies have shed some light on mechanisms of pDC antifungal activity (summarized in **Figure 1**). Direct pDC antifungal activity was first demonstrated in 2011, when Ramirez-Ortiz et al. found that human pDCs directly inhibited growth of *A. fumigatus* hyphae and produced IFN-α and TNF-α in response to *in vitro* hyphal stimulation (173). They found that pDCs spread out over the surface of hyphae and inhibited hyphal viability by up to 80%. However, this strong antifungal activity was observed with a pDC:fungal ratio of 50:1, which seems highly unlikely to occur in a live organism. At a pDC-fungal ratio of 1:10, a 40% decrease in hyphal viability was still observed. At the

TABLE 1 | A summary of the pattern recognition receptors (PRRs) on plasmacytoid dendritic cells (pDCs) that have a role in antifungal immunity.

Receptor	Structure	Fungal ligand	Cellular functions	Fungal pathogen	Reference
TLR4 (CD284)	Extracellular 608 residue domain, composed of an N-, central, and C-terminal domain. 21 leucine-rich repeats	Mannan structures	Cytokine/chemokine production, recruitment of neutrophils	*Candida albicans, Aspergillus fumigatus, Pneumocystis.* Not TLR4-dependent in *C. neoformans* models.	(17, 35, 115–120)
TLR9 (CD289)	25 leucine-rich repeats. Detailed structure not yet described	Unmethylated CpG DNA	IL-10, pro-inflammatory cytokine production including IL-12p40 production by murine DCs	*C. albicans, A. fumigatus, Cryptococcus neoformans*	(120–123)
Dectin-1 (CLEC7A)	Single extracellular C-type lectin-like domain (CTLD), intracellular immunoreceptor tyrosine-based activation motif	β(1,3)- and β(1,6)-linked glucans	Phagocytosis, cell maturation, respiratory burst, cytokine/chemokine production, direction of T_H cell differentiation, CTL priming	*A. fumigatus, C. neoformans, C. albicans, Pneumocystis*	(126, 127, 129, 130, 136–139, 141, 142)
Dectin-2 (CLEC6A)	Single extracellular CTLD, short cytoplasmic tail (couples with FcRγ)	a-mannose structures	Cytokine production, T_H1 and T_H17 differentiation	*A. fumigatus, C. albicans, C. neoformans*	(144–147, 150)
Dectin-3 (CLEC4D, CLECSF8)	Single extracellular CTLD, short cytoplasmic tail (does not couple with FcRγ)	a-mannose structures	Phagocytosis, cytokine production, respiratory burst (macrophages)	*C. albicans, C. neoformans* (conflicting studies)	(151, 152, 155, 156, 163)
Mannose receptor (MR, CD206)	Extracellular CR domain, fibronectin type II domain, and 8 CTLDs. Short cytoplasmic tail	Carbohydrates that terminate in D-mannose, L-fucose, or *N*-acetyl glucosamine	Phagocytosis (possibly requires TLR2), fungal clearance, IL-8 production	*A. fumigatus, C. albicans, C. neoformans, Pneumocystis*	(155, 157, 158, 163–166, 168, 170)

Listed are receptors that have been shown to have a role in fungal infection and are expressed on pDCs. Each receptor is then summarized with a brief description of their structures, their fungal ligands, the major downstream cellular functions, and a selection of sources from which this information was gathered. TLR9, Dectin-1, Dectin-2, Dectin-3, and MR have been implicated specifically in pDC–fungal interaction, while TLR4 has been investigated on other cell types but not yet on pDCs.

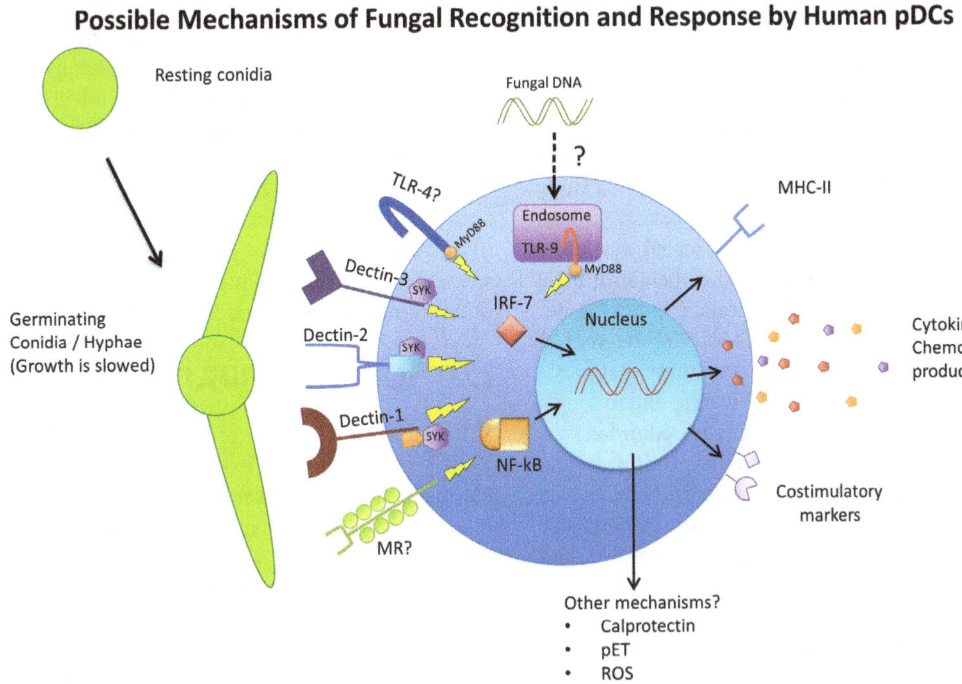

FIGURE 1 | Schematic representing the available receptors and cellular responses of plasmacytoid dendritic cells (pDCs) to fungal pathogens. Resting conidia (RC) or yeast cells are less immunogenic than germinating and hyphal forms of fungi due to the increased availability of ligands such as beta-glucans and alpha-mannan structures of the cell wall. The receptors TLR4, TLR9, Dectin-1, Dectin-2, Dectin-3, and MR have been implicated in antifungal immunity in various models and studies and have also been observed to be expressed by pDCs. The cellular responses of pDCs to fungal stimulation have only begun to be characterized, but include phagocytosis, activation/maturation, cytokine and chemokine production, and MHC-II upregulation. Other pDC antifungal mechanisms that have been proposed include the release of calprotectin by apoptotic pDCs, the production of pDC extracellular traps (pETs), and the production of reactive oxygen species (ROS).

same time, they found fungal stimulation lead to a large increase in pDC death, mediated partially by the production of gliotoxin by *A. fumigatus.* They also discovered that pDC lysates had the same antifungal activity as live cells, and implicated the release of calprotectin from dying pDCs as a contributor to the inhibition of fungal growth. Calprotectin has a documented role in antifungal immunity as a component of neutrophil extracellular traps (174). However, this was the first indication that pDCs may also use calprotectin. A later study by the same group indicated that pDC-*Aspergillus* interaction seemed to induce the production of pDC extracellular traps (pETs), similar to those extracellular traps laid by neutrophils (175). The production of extracellular traps by pDCs is a novel concept that has not been described elsewhere, and requires careful follow-up. Transcriptome analysis after *A. fumigatus* stimulation revealed the upregulation of several genes involved in activation, chemokine production, and antigen presentation, as well as genes associated with apoptosis. *In vivo*, mice depleted of pDCs were significantly more susceptible to *Aspergillus*-induced mortality, both after pulmonary and intravenous challenge (173). In addition, pulmonary challenge with *A. fumigatus* caused a six-fold increase in pDC number in the lungs. In a *C. neoformans* model, Hole et al. indicated that murine and human pDCs could phagocytose yeast cells and could directly inhibit *C. neoformans* growth through the use of reactive oxygen species (72).

As mentioned above, pDCs express receptors that are known to be involved in fungal recognition (summarized on **Figure 1**). As early as 2002, Taylor et al. mentioned that murine pDCs express dectin-1, although the data were not shown. Seeds et al. (71) later confirmed that finding, and added that murine pDCs also expressed the CLRs dectin-2 and MR (71). Because murine pDCs are not perfect representations of human pDCs, these receptors also needed to be investigated on human pDCs. Studies on human pDCs observed the expression of dectin-1 (176), dectin-2 (177), and MR (70, 178). However, attempts to identify which pDC receptor is responsible for fungal recognition have delivered mixed results. One study singled out dectin-2 as the main receptor responsible for recognition of *A. fumigatus* hyphae by human pDCs (175). They used laminarin and mannan to block dectin-1 and dectin-2, respectively, and found that while both blocking agents decreased the ability of pDCs to associate with fungal hyphae, only mannan's effect reached statistical significance. However, the definition and use of mannan as a dectin-2 blocker may be problematic, as it can be the ligand for other CLRs, including dectin-3 and MR. The study did follow-up by blocking with specific antibodies against dectin-1 and dectin-2, which recapitulated their results that dectin-2 was more responsible for pDC–hyphal association. Hole et al. observed the presence of dectin-3 on murine pDCs, and demonstrated that blocking dectin-3 on human pDCs resulted in a blunted reaction to *C. neoformans* stimulation (72). In their study, pDCs from dectin-3 knockout mice experienced the greatest reduction in fungal uptake and growth inhibition, greater than dectin-1, dectin-2, and MR knockout mice. Accordingly, pDCs from dectin-3 knockout mice were greatly deficient in their ability to phagocytose *C. neoformans* yeast cells. It is interesting to note that these findings stand in contrast to the aforementioned study where dectin-3 was not required for protection against *C. neoformans* (156). Nevertheless, the data again indicated that while dectin-3 knockout mice were the most affected in their antifungal activity and the only ones to achieve significance, knocking out dectin-1, dectin-2, and MR also resulted in varying degrees of reduced antifungal activity. This allows the possibility that pDCs use a combination of receptors to recognize and respond to fungal pathogens and that these PRRs have a measure of redundancy.

Considered together, this evidence strongly indicates that pDCs play an important role in antifungal immunity. However, there remains much to be discovered concerning the mechanisms of pDC–fungal interaction, cellular responses to recognition, and the role of pDCs in the broader landscape of antifungal immunity.

CONCLUDING REMARKS

One of the most insidious threats to the health and well-being of immunocompromised individuals, including those living with HIV, is the threat of opportunistic infections. Opportunistic fungal infections can be particularly fast, lethal, and difficult to treat. The main contributing factor for increased susceptibility to fungal infection in immunocompromised patients is the depletion and dysregulation of many components of the immune system; even when infection is well-controlled with antiretroviral medication, over time this dysregulation is measurable in individuals chronically infected with HIV. The pDC is no exception; HIV patients have a decline in number and functionality of their pDC compartment. This is especially problematic when considering the role of pDCs in fungal infection that is currently emerging in the literature. Studies have shown that pDCs have the machinery to recognize and respond to fungal infection, and do so in a manner that indicates pDCs are involved in a successful antifungal immune response. Therefore, dysregulation of the pDC compartment may be a contributing factor to the increased susceptibility of fungal infections that afflict HIV patients and other immunocompromised populations.

AUTHOR CONTRIBUTIONS

SM performed all literature searches and writing of this review. PF-B provided focused expertise and guidance on the field of plasmacytoid dendritic cell and HIV biology, extensive revision of this manuscript, and final approval of the version for publication.

ACKNOWLEDGMENTS

The authors would like to acknowledge the contributions of fellow lab members PD, HH, ZR, and HD as well as past members JD, VS, TS, MP, MN, and DD.

FUNDING

SM is supported by National Institutes of Health Integrated T32 Training Program in *Infection, Immunity and Inflammation* (Grant # 5T32AI125185) and the MD/PhD program at Rutgers New Jersey Medical School. PF-B is funded by NIH grants AI026806 and AI106125.

REFERENCES

1. WHO. *Global Health Sector Strategy on HIV 2016–2021*. Geneva, Switzerland: WHO Press (2016). 60 p.
2. Zaidi J, Grapsa E, Tanser F, Newell ML, Barnighausen T. Dramatic increase in HIV prevalence after scale-up of antiretroviral treatment. *AIDS* (2013) 27(14):2301–5. doi:10.1097/QAD.0b013e328362e832
3. May MT, Gompels M, Delpech V, Porter K, Orkin C, Kegg S, et al. Impact on life expectancy of HIV-1 positive individuals of CD4+ cell count and viral load response to antiretroviral therapy. *AIDS* (2014) 28(8):1193–202. doi:10.1097/QAD.0000000000000243
4. Maartens G, Celum C, Lewin SR. HIV infection: epidemiology, pathogenesis, treatment, and prevention. *Lancet* (2014) 384(9939):258–71. doi:10.1016/S0140-6736(14)60164-1
5. Ortblad KF, Lozano R, Murray CJ. The burden of HIV: insights from the Global Burden of Disease Study 2010. *AIDS* (2013) 27(13):2003–17. doi:10.1097/QAD.0b013e328362ba67
6. Cooper A, Garcia M, Petrovas C, Yamamoto T, Koup RA, Nabel GJ. HIV-1 causes CD4 cell death through DNA-dependent protein kinase during viral integration. *Nature* (2013) 498(7454):376–9. doi:10.1038/nature12274
7. Boasso A, Shearer GM. Chronic innate immune activation as a cause of HIV-1 immunopathogenesis. *Clin Immunol* (2008) 126(3):235–42. doi:10.1016/j.clim.2007.08.015
8. Anwar KP, Malik A, Subhan KH. Profile of candidiasis in HIV infected patients. *Iran J Microbiol* (2012) 4(4):204–9.
9. Park BJ, Wannemuehler KA, Marston BJ, Govender N, Pappas PG, Chiller TM. Estimation of the current global burden of cryptococcal meningitis among persons living with HIV/AIDS. *AIDS* (2009) 23(4):525–30. doi:10.1097/QAD.0b013e328322ffac
10. Rajasingham R, Smith RM, Park BJ, Jarvis JN, Govender NP, Chiller TM, et al. Global burden of disease of HIV-associated cryptococcal meningitis: an updated analysis. *Lancet Infect Dis* (2017) 17(8):873–81. doi:10.1016/S1473-3099(17)30243-8
11. Denning DW, Follansbee SE, Scolaro M, Norris S, Edelstein H, Stevens DA. Pulmonary aspergillosis in the acquired immunodeficiency syndrome. *N Engl J Med* (1991) 324(10):654–62. doi:10.1056/NEJM199103073241003
12. Holding KJ, Dworkin MS, Wan PC, Hanson DL, Klevens RM, Jones JL, et al. Aspergillosis among people infected with human immunodeficiency virus: incidence and survival. Adult and Adolescent Spectrum of HIV Disease Project. *Clin Infect Dis* (2000) 31(5):1253–7. doi:10.1086/317452
13. Lopez C, Fitzgerald PA, Siegal FP. Severe acquired immune deficiency syndrome in male homosexuals: diminished capacity to make interferon-alpha in vitro associated with severe opportunistic infections. *J Infect Dis* (1983) 148(6):962–6. doi:10.1093/infdis/148.6.962
14. McKenna K, Beignon AS, Bhardwaj N. Plasmacytoid dendritic cells: linking innate and adaptive immunity. *J Virol* (2005) 79(1):17–27. doi:10.1128/JVI.79.1.17-27.2005
15. Fitzgerald-Bocarsly P, Dai J, Singh S. Plasmacytoid dendritic cells and type I IFN: 50 years of convergent history. *Cytokine Growth Factor Rev* (2008) 19(1):3–19. doi:10.1016/j.cytogfr.2007.10.006
16. Fitzgerald-Bocarsly P, Jacobs ES. Plasmacytoid dendritic cells in HIV infection: striking a delicate balance. *J Leukoc Biol* (2010) 87(4):609–20. doi:10.1189/jlb.0909635

17. Kadowaki N, Ho S, Antonenko S, Malefyt RW, Kastelein RA, Bazan F, et al. Subsets of human dendritic cell precursors express different toll-like receptors and respond to different microbial antigens. *J Exp Med* (2001) 194(6):863–9. doi:10.1084/jem.194.6.863
18. Krug A, Towarowski A, Britsch S, Rothenfusser S, Hornung V, Bals R, et al. Toll-like receptor expression reveals CpG DNA as a unique microbial stimulus for plasmacytoid dendritic cells which synergizes with CD40 ligand to induce high amounts of IL-12. *Eur J Immunol* (2001) 31(10):3026–37. doi:10.1002/1521-4141(2001010)31:10<3026::AID-IMMU3026>3.0.CO;2-H
19. McMichael AJ, Rowland-Jones SL. Cellular immune responses to HIV. *Nature* (2001) 410(6831):980–7. doi:10.1038/35073658
20. Douek DC, Picker LJ, Koup RA. T cell dynamics in HIV-1 infection. *Annu Rev Immunol*(2003)21:265–304.doi:10.1146/annurev.immunol.21.120601.141053
21. O'Brien M, Manches O, Bhardwaj N. Plasmacytoid dendritic cells in HIV infection. *Adv Exp Med Biol* (2013) 762:71–107. doi:10.1007/978-1-4614-4433-6_3
22. Schmidt B, Fujimura SH, Martin JN, Levy JA. Variations in plasmacytoid dendritic cell (PDC) and myeloid dendritic cell (MDC) levels in HIV-infected subjects on and off antiretroviral therapy. *J Clin Immunol* (2006) 26(1):55–64. doi:10.1007/s10875-006-8401-3
23. Zabel BA, Silverio AM, Butcher EC. Chemokine-like receptor 1 expression and chemerin-directed chemotaxis distinguish plasmacytoid from myeloid dendritic cells in human blood. *J Immunol* (2005) 174(1):244–51. doi:10.4049/jimmunol.174.1.244
24. Lande R, Gilliet M. Plasmacytoid dendritic cells: key players in the initiation and regulation of immune responses. *Ann N Y Acad Sci* (2010) 1183:89–103. doi:10.1111/j.1749-6632.2009.05152.x
25. Bargatze RF, Jutila MA, Butcher EC. Distinct roles of L-selectin and integrins alpha 4 beta 7 and LFA-1 in lymphocyte homing to Peyer's patch-HEV in situ: the multistep model confirmed and refined. *Immunity* (1995) 3(1):99–108. doi:10.1016/1074-7613(95)90162-0
26. Krug A, French AR, Barchet W, Fischer JA, Dzionek A, Pingel JT, et al. TLR9-dependent recognition of MCMV by IPC and DC generates coordinated cytokine responses that activate antiviral NK cell function. *Immunity* (2004) 21(1):107–19. doi:10.1016/j.immuni.2004.06.007
27. Beignon AS, McKenna K, Skoberne M, Manches O, DaSilva I, Kavanagh DG, et al. Endocytosis of HIV-1 activates plasmacytoid dendritic cells via toll-like receptor-viral RNA interactions. *J Clin Invest* (2005) 115(11):3265–75. doi:10.1172/JCI26032
28. Gibson SJ, Lindh JM, Riter TR, Gleason RM, Rogers LM, Fuller AE, et al. Plasmacytoid dendritic cells produce cytokines and mature in response to the TLR7 agonists, imiquimod and resiquimod. *Cell Immunol* (2002) 218(1–2):74–86. doi:10.1016/S0008-8749(02)00517-8
29. Colak E, Leslie A, Zausmer K, Khatamzas E, Kubarenko AV, Pichulik T, et al. RNA and imidazoquinolines are sensed by distinct TLR7/8 ectodomain sites resulting in functionally disparate signaling events. *J Immunol* (2014) 192(12):5963–73. doi:10.4049/jimmunol.1303058
30. Honda K, Yanai H, Negishi H, Asagiri M, Sato M, Mizutani T, et al. IRF-7 is the master regulator of type-I interferon-dependent immune responses. *Nature* (2005) 434(7034):772–7. doi:10.1038/nature03464
31. Hornung V, Schlender J, Guenthner-Biller M, Rothenfusser S, Endres S, Conzelmann KK, et al. Replication-dependent potent IFN-alpha induction in human plasmacytoid dendritic cells by a single-stranded RNA virus. *J Immunol* (2004) 173(10):5935–43. doi:10.4049/jimmunol.173.10.5935
32. Hochrein H, Schlatter B, O'Keeffe M, Wagner C, Schmitz F, Schiemann M, et al. Herpes simplex virus type-1 induces IFN-alpha production via toll-like receptor 9-dependent and -independent pathways. *Proc Natl Acad Sci U S A* (2004) 101(31):11416–21. doi:10.1073/pnas.0403555101
33. Izaguirre A, Barnes BJ, Amrute S, Yeow WS, Megjugorac N, Dai J, et al. Comparative analysis of IRF and IFN-alpha expression in human plasmacytoid and monocyte-derived dendritic cells. *J Leukoc Biol* (2003) 74(6):1125–38. doi:10.1189/jlb.0603255
34. O'Brien M, Manches O, Sabado RL, Baranda SJ, Wang Y, Marie I, et al. Spatiotemporal trafficking of HIV in human plasmacytoid dendritic cells defines a persistently IFN-alpha-producing and partially matured phenotype. *J Clin Invest* (2011) 121(3):1088–101. doi:10.1172/JCI44960
35. Dai J, Megjugorac NJ, Amrute SB, Fitzgerald-Bocarsly P. Regulation of IFN regulatory factor-7 and IFN-alpha production by enveloped virus and lipopolysaccharide in human plasmacytoid dendritic cells. *J Immunol* (2004) 173(3):1535–48. doi:10.4049/jimmunol.173.3.1535
36. Fuchsberger M, Hochrein H, O'Keeffe M. Activation of plasmacytoid dendritic cells. *Immunol Cell Biol* (2005) 83(5):571–7. doi:10.1111/j.1440-1711.2005.01392.x
37. Decalf J, Fernandes S, Longman R, Ahloulay M, Audat F, Lefrerre F, et al. Plasmacytoid dendritic cells initiate a complex chemokine and cytokine network and are a viable drug target in chronic HCV patients. *J Exp Med* (2007) 204(10):2423–37. doi:10.1084/jem.20070814
38. Yin Z, Dai J, Deng J, Sheikh F, Natalia M, Shih T, et al. Type III IFNs are produced by and stimulate human plasmacytoid dendritic cells. *J Immunol* (2012) 189(6):2735–45. doi:10.4049/jimmunol.1102038
39. Feldman M, Fitzgerald-Bocarsly P. Sequential enrichment and immunocytochemical visualization of human interferon-alpha-producing cells. *J Interferon Res* (1990) 10(4):435–46. doi:10.1089/jir.1990.10.435
40. Siegal FP, Kadowaki N, Shodell M, Fitzgerald-Bocarsly PA, Shah K, Ho S, et al. The nature of the principal type 1 interferon-producing cells in human blood. *Science* (1999) 284(5421):1835–7. doi:10.1126/science.284.5421.1835
41. Liu Y-J. IPC: professional type 1 interferon-producing cells and plasmacytoid dendritic cell precursors. *Annu Rev Immunol* (2005) 23:275–306. doi:10.1146/annurev.immunol.23.021704.115633
42. Ito T, Kanzler H, Duramad O, Cao W, Liu YJ. Specialization, kinetics, and repertoire of type 1 interferon responses by human plasmacytoid predendritic cells. *Blood* (2006) 107(6):2423–31. doi:10.1182/blood-2005-07-2709
43. Novick D, Cohen B, Rubinstein M. The human interferon alpha/beta receptor: characterization and molecular cloning. *Cell* (1994) 77(3):391–400. doi:10.1016/0092-8674(94)90154-6
44. Biron CA. Role of early cytokines, including alpha and beta interferons (IFN-a/b), in innate and adaptive immune responses to viral infections. *Semin Immunol* (1998) 10:383–90. doi:10.1006/smim.1998.0138
45. Fitzgerald-Bocarsly P, Feng D. The role of type I interferon production by dendritic cells in host defense. *Biochimie* (2007) 89(6–7):843–55. doi:10.1016/j.biochi.2007.04.018
46. Ito T, Amakawa R, Inaba M, Ikehara S, Inaba K, Fukuhara S. Differential regulation of human blood dendritic cell subsets by IFNs. *J Immunol* (2001) 166(5):2961–9. doi:10.4049/jimmunol.166.5.2961
47. Schmidt B, Ashlock BM, Foster H, Fujimura SH, Levy JA. HIV-infected cells are major inducers of plasmacytoid dendritic cell interferon production, maturation, and migration. *Virology* (2005) 343(2):256–66. doi:10.1016/j.virol.2005.09.059
48. Honda K, Sakaguchi S, Nakajima C, Watanabe A, Yanai H, Matsumoto M, et al. Selective contribution of IFN-alpha/beta signaling to the maturation of dendritic cells induced by double-stranded RNA or viral infection. *Proc Natl Acad Sci U S A* (2003) 100(19):10872–7. doi:10.1073/pnas.1934678100
49. Brinkmann V, Geiger T, Alkan S, Heusser CH. Interferon alpha increases the frequency of interferon gamma-producing human CD4+ T cells. *J Exp Med* (1993) 178(5):1655–63. doi:10.1084/jem.178.5.1655
50. Cella M, Facchetti F, Lanzavecchia A, Colonna M. Plasmacytoid dendritic cells activated by influenza virus and CD40L drive a potent TH1 polarization. *Nat Immunol* (2000) 1(4):305–10. doi:10.1038/79747
51. Rothenfusser S, Hornung V, Ayyoub M, Britsch S, Towarowski A, Krug A, et al. CpG-A and CpG-B oligonucleotides differentially enhance human peptide-specific primary and memory CD8+ T-cell responses in vitro. *Blood* (2004) 103(6):2162–9. doi:10.1182/blood-2003-04-1091
52. Yoneyama H, Matsuno K, Toda E, Nishiwaki T, Matsuo N, Nakano A, et al. Plasmacytoid DCs help lymph node DCs to induce anti-HSV CTLs. *J Exp Med* (2005) 202(3):425–35. doi:10.1084/jem.20041961
53. Niessner A, Sato K, Chaikof EL, Colmegna I, Goronzy JJ, Weyand CM. Pathogen-sensing plasmacytoid dendritic cells stimulate cytotoxic T-cell function in the atherosclerotic plaque through interferon-alpha. *Circulation* (2006) 114(23):2482–9. doi:10.1161/CIRCULATIONAHA.106.642801
54. Dikopoulos N, Bertoletti A, Kroger A, Hauser H, Schirmbeck R, Reimann J. Type I IFN negatively regulates CD8+ T cell responses through IL-10-producing CD4+ T regulatory 1 cells. *J Immunol* (2005) 174(1):99–109. doi:10.4049/jimmunol.174.1.99
55. Le Bon A, Schiavoni G, D'Agostino G, Gresser I, Belardelli F, Tough DF. Type I interferons potently enhance humoral immunity and can promote isotype switching by stimulating dendritic cells in vivo. *Immunity* (2001) 14(4):461–70. doi:10.1016/S1074-7613(01)00126-1
56. Ank N, Iversen MB, Bartholdy C, Staeheli P, Hartmann R, Jensen UB, et al. An important role for type III interferon (IFN-lambda/IL-28)

in TLR-induced antiviral activity. *J Immunol* (2008) 180(4):2474–85. doi:10.4049/jimmunol.180.4.2474
57. Ank N, West H, Bartholdy C, Eriksson K, Thomsen AR, Paludan SR. Lambda interferon (IFN-lambda), a type III IFN, is induced by viruses and IFNs and displays potent antiviral activity against select virus infections in vivo. *J Virol* (2006) 80(9):4501–9. doi:10.1128/JVI.80.9.4501-4509.2006
58. Onoguchi K, Yoneyama M, Takemura A, Akira S, Taniguchi T, Namiki H, et al. Viral infections activate types I and III interferon genes through a common mechanism. *J Biol Chem* (2007) 282(10):7576–81. doi:10.1074/jbc.M608618200
59. Sommereyns C, Paul S, Staeheli P, Michiels T. IFN-lambda (IFN-lambda) is expressed in a tissue-dependent fashion and primarily acts on epithelial cells in vivo. *PLoS Pathog* (2008) 4(3):e1000017. doi:10.1371/journal.ppat.1000017
60. Mennechet FJ, Uze G. Interferon-lambda-treated dendritic cells specifically induce proliferation of FOXP3-expressing suppressor T cells. *Blood* (2006) 107(11):4417–23. doi:10.1182/blood-2005-10-4129
61. Jordan WJ, Eskdale J, Srinivas S, Pekarek V, Kelner D, Rodia M, et al. Human interferon lambda-1 (IFN-lambda1/IL-29) modulates the Th1/Th2 response. *Genes Immun* (2007) 8(3):254–61. doi:10.1038/sj.gene.6364382
62. Bordi L, Lalle E, Lapa D, Caglioti C, Quartu S, Capobianchi MR, et al. Type III interferon (IFN-lambda) antagonizes the antiviral activity of interferon-alpha in vitro. *J Biol Regul Homeost Agents* (2013) 27(4):1001–9.
63. Megjugorac NJ, Young HA, Amrute SB, Olshalsky SL, Fitzgerald-Bocarsly P. Virally stimulated plasmacytoid dendritic cells produce chemokines and induce migration of T and NK cells. *J Leukoc Biol* (2004) 75(3):504–14. doi:10.1189/jlb.0603291
64. Piqueras B, Connolly J, Freitas H, Palucka AK, Banchereau J. Upon viral exposure, myeloid and plasmacytoid dendritic cells produce 3 waves of distinct chemokines to recruit immune effectors. *Blood* (2006) 107(7):2613–8. doi:10.1182/blood-2005-07-2965
65. Colonna M, Trinchieri G, Liu YJ. Plasmacytoid dendritic cells in immunity. *Nat Immunol* (2004) 5(12):1219–26. doi:10.1038/ni1141
66. Fanning SL, George TC, Feng D, Feldman SB, Megjugorac NJ, Izaguirre AG, et al. Receptor cross-linking on human plasmacytoid dendritic cells leads to the regulation of IFN-alpha production. *J Immunol* (2006) 177(9):5829–39. doi:10.4049/jimmunol.177.9.5829
67. Villadangos JA, Young L. Antigen-presentation properties of plasmacytoid dendritic cells. *Immunity* (2008) 29(3):352–61. doi:10.1016/j.immuni.2008.09.002
68. Sadaka C, Marloie-Provost MA, Soumelis V, Benaroch P. Developmental regulation of MHC II expression and transport in human plasmacytoid-derived dendritic cells. *Blood* (2009) 113(10):2127–35. doi:10.1182/blood-2008-10-178152
69. Tel J, Smits EL, Anguille S, Joshi RN, Figdor CG, de Vries IJ. Human plasmacytoid dendritic cells are equipped with antigen-presenting and tumoricidal capacities. *Blood* (2012) 120(19):3936–44. doi:10.1182/blood-2012-06-435941
70. Milone MC, Fitzgerald-Bocarsly P. The mannose receptor mediates induction of IFN-alpha in peripheral blood dendritic cells by enveloped RNA and DNA viruses. *J Immunol* (1998) 161(5):2391–9.
71. Seeds RE, Gordon S, Miller JL. Characterisation of myeloid receptor expression and interferon alpha/beta production in murine plasmacytoid dendritic cells by flow cytomtery. *J Immunol Methods* (2009) 350(1–2):106–17. doi:10.1016/j.jim.2009.07.016
72. Hole CR, Leopold Wager CM, Mendiola AS, Wozniak KL, Campuzano A, Lin X, et al. Antifungal activity of plasmacytoid dendritic cells against *Cryptococcus neoformans* in vitro requires expression of dectin-3 (CLEC4D) and reactive oxygen species. *Infect Immun* (2016) 84(9):2493–504. doi:10.1128/IAI.00103-16
73. Siegal FP, Lopez C, Fitzgerald PA, Shah K, Baron P, Leiderman IZ, et al. Opportunistic infections in acquired immune deficiency syndrome result from synergistic defects of both the natural and adaptive components of cellular immunity. *J Clin Invest* (1986) 78(1):115–23. doi:10.1172/JCI112539
74. Howell DM, Feldman SB, Kloser P, Fitzgerald-Bocarsly P. Decreased frequency of functional natural interferon-producing cells in peripheral blood of patients with the acquired immune deficiency syndrome. *Clin Immunol Immunopathol* (1994) 71(2):223–30. doi:10.1006/clin.1994.1076
75. Feldman SB, Milone MC, Kloser P, Fitzgerald-Bocarsly P. Functional deficiencies in two distinct interferon alpha-producing cell populations in peripheral blood mononuclear cells from human immunodeficiency virus seropositive patients. *J Leukoc Biol* (1995) 57(2):214–20.
76. Feldman S, Stein D, Amrute S, Denny T, Garcia Z, Kloser P, et al. Decreased interferon-alpha production in HIV-infected patients correlates with numerical and functional deficiencies in circulating type 2 dendritic cell precursors. *Clin Immunol* (2001) 101(2):201–10. doi:10.1006/clim.2001.5111
77. Soumelis V, Scott I, Gheyas F, Bouhour D, Cozon G, Cotte L, et al. Depletion of circulating natural type 1 interferon-producing cells in HIV-infected AIDS patients. *Blood* (2001) 98(4):906–12. doi:10.1182/blood.V98.4.906
78. Donaghy H, Pozniak A, Gazzard B, Qazi N, Gilmour J, Gotch F, et al. Loss of blood CD11c(+) myeloid and CD11c(-) plasmacytoid dendritic cells in patients with HIV-1 infection correlates with HIV-1 RNA virus load. *Blood* (2001) 98(8):2574–6. doi:10.1182/blood.V98.8.2574
79. Chehimi J, Azzoni L, Farabaugh M, Creer SA, Tomescu C, Hancock A, et al. Baseline viral load and immune activation determine the extent of reconstitution of innate immune effectors in HIV-1-infected subjects undergoing antiretroviral treatment. *J Immunol* (2007) 179(4):2642–50. doi:10.4049/jimmunol.179.4.2642
80. Malleret B, Maneglier B, Karlsson I, Lebon P, Nascimbeni M, Perie L, et al. Primary infection with simian immunodeficiency virus: plasmacytoid dendritic cell homing to lymph nodes, type I interferon, and immune suppression. *Blood* (2008) 112(12):4598–608. doi:10.1182/blood-2008-06-162651
81. Brown KN, Wijewardana V, Liu X, Barratt-Boyes SM. Rapid influx and death of plasmacytoid dendritic cells in lymph nodes mediate depletion in acute simian immunodeficiency virus infection. *PLoS Pathog* (2009) 5(5):e1000413. doi:10.1371/journal.ppat.1000413
82. Lehmann C, Lafferty M, Garzino-Demo A, Jung N, Hartmann P, Fatkenheuer G, et al. Plasmacytoid dendritic cells accumulate and secrete interferon alpha in lymph nodes of HIV-1 patients. *PLoS One* (2010) 5(6):e11110. doi:10.1371/journal.pone.0011110
83. Patterson S, Rae A, Hockey N, Gilmour J, Gotch F. Plasmacytoid dendritic cells are highly susceptible to human immunodeficiency virus type 1 infection and release infectious virus. *J Virol* (2001) 75(14):6710–3. doi:10.1128/JVI.75.14.6710-6713.2001
84. Schmidt B, Scott I, Whitmore RG, Foster H, Fujimura S, Schmitz J, et al. Low-level HIV infection of plasmacytoid dendritic cells: onset of cytopathic effects and cell death after PDC maturation. *Virology* (2004) 329(2):280–8. doi:10.1016/j.virol.2004.08.016
85. Wijewardana V, Brown KN, Barratt-Boyes SM. Studies of plasmacytoid dendritic cell dynamics in simian immunodeficiency virus infection of nonhuman primates provide insights into HIV pathogenesis. *Curr HIV Res* (2009) 7(1):23–9. doi:10.2174/157016209787048483
86. Barron MA, Blyveis N, Palmer BE, MaWhinney S, Wilson CC. Influence of plasma viremia on defects in number and immunophenotype of blood dendritic cell subsets in human immunodeficiency virus 1-infected individuals. *J Infect Dis* (2003) 187(1):26–37. doi:10.1086/345957
87. Khaitan A, Unutmaz D. Revisiting immune exhaustion during HIV infection. *Curr HIV/AIDS Rep* (2011) 8(1):4–11. doi:10.1007/s11904-010-0066-0
88. Li G, Cheng M, Nunoya J, Cheng L, Guo H, Yu H, et al. Plasmacytoid dendritic cells suppress HIV-1 replication but contribute to HIV-1 induced immunopathogenesis in humanized mice. *PLoS Pathog* (2014) 10(7):e1004291. doi:10.1371/journal.ppat.1004291
89. Donaghy H, Gazzard B, Gotch F, Patterson S. Dysfunction and infection of freshly isolated blood myeloid and plasmacytoid dendritic cells in patients infected with HIV-1. *Blood* (2003) 101(11):4505–11. doi:10.1182/blood-2002-10-3189
90. Dillon SM, Robertson KB, Pan SC, Mawhinney S, Meditz AL, Folkvord JM, et al. Plasmacytoid and myeloid dendritic cells with a partial activation phenotype accumulate in lymphoid tissue during asymptomatic chronic HIV-1 infection. *J Acquir Immune Defic Syndr* (2008) 48(1):1–12. doi:10.1097/QAI.0b013e3181664b60
91. Martinson JA, Roman-Gonzalez A, Tenorio AR, Montoya CJ, Gichinga CN, Rugeles MT, et al. Dendritic cells from HIV-1 infected individuals are less responsive to toll-like receptor (TLR) ligands. *Cell Immunol* (2007) 250(1–2):75–84. doi:10.1016/j.cellimm.2008.01.007
92. Moseman EA, Liang X, Dawson AJ, Panoskaltsis-Mortari A, Krieg AM, Liu YJ, et al. Human plasmacytoid dendritic cells activated by CpG oligodeoxynucleotides induce the generation of CD4+CD25+ regulatory T cells. *J Immunol* (2004) 173(7):4433–42. doi:10.4049/jimmunol.173.7.4433

93. Gilliet M, Liu YJ. Generation of human CD8 T regulatory cells by CD40 ligand-activated plasmacytoid dendritic cells. *J Exp Med* (2002) 195(6): 695–704. doi:10.1084/jem.20011603
94. Boasso A, Herbeuval JP, Hardy AW, Anderson SA, Dolan MJ, Fuchs D, et al. HIV inhibits CD4+ T-cell proliferation by inducing indoleamine 2,3-dioxygenase in plasmacytoid dendritic cells. *Blood* (2007) 109(8): 3351–9. doi:10.1182/blood-2006-07-034785
95. Munn DH, Shafizadeh E, Attwood JT, Bondarev I, Pashine A, Mellor AL. Inhibition of T cell proliferation by macrophage tryptophan catabolism. *J Exp Med* (1999) 189(9):1363–72. doi:10.1084/jem.189.9.1363
96. Baban B, Chandler PR, Sharma MD, Pihkala J, Koni PA, Munn DH, et al. IDO activates regulatory T cells and blocks their conversion into Th17-like T cells. *J Immunol* (2009) 183(4):2475–83. doi:10.4049/jimmunol.0900986
97. Romani L. Immunity to fungal infections. *Nat Rev Immunol* (2011) 11:275–88. doi:10.1038/nri2939
98. Vallabhaneni S, Mody RK, Walker T, Chiller T. The global burden of fungal diseases. *Infect Dis Clin North Am* (2016) 30(1):1–11. doi:10.1016/j.idc.2015.10.004
99. Tronchin G, Bouchara JP, Ferron M, Larcher G, Chabasse D. Cell surface properties of *Aspergillus fumigatus* conidia: correlation between adherence, agglutination, and rearrangements of the cell wall. *Can J Microbiol* (1995) 41(8):714–21. doi:10.1139/m95-098
100. van de Veerdonk FL, Kullberg BJ, van der Meer JW, Gow NA, Netea MG. Host-microbe interactions: innate pattern recognition of fungal pathogens. *Curr Opin Microbiol* (2008) 11(4):305–12. doi:10.1016/j.mib.2008.06.002
101. Hohl TM, Van Epps HL, Rivera A, Morgan LA, Chen PL, Feldmesser M, et al. *Aspergillus fumigatus* triggers inflammatory responses by stage-specific beta-glucan display. *PLoS Pathog* (2005) 1(3):e30. doi:10.1371/journal.ppat.0010030
102. Latge JP. Tasting the fungal cell wall. *Cell Microbiol* (2010) 12(7):863–72. doi:10.1111/j.1462-5822.2010.01474.x
103. Levitz SM. Innate recognition of fungal cell walls. *PLoS Pathog* (2010) 6(4):e1000758. doi:10.1371/journal.ppat.1000758
104. Hamad M. Innate and adaptive antifungal immune responses: partners on an equal footing. *Mycoses* (2011) 55:205–17. doi:10.1111/j.1439-0507.2011.02078.x
105. Brown GD. Innate antifungal immunity: the key role of phagocytes. *Annu Rev Immunol* (2011) 29:1–21. doi:10.1146/annurev-immunol-030409-101229
106. Hohl TM, Feldmesser M. *Aspergillus fumigatus*: principles of pathogenesis and host defense. *Eukaryot Cell* (2007) 6(11):1953–63. doi:10.1128/EC.00274-07
107. Bruns S, Kniemeyer O, Hasenberg M, Aimanianda V, Nietzsche S, Thywissen A, et al. Production of extracellular traps against *Aspergillus fumigatus* in vitro and in infected lung tissue is dependent on invading neutrophils and influenced by hydrophobin RodA. *PLoS Pathog* (2010) 6(4):e1000873. doi:10.1371/journal.ppat.1000873
108. Bozza S, Gaziano R, Spreca A, Bacci A, Montagnoli C, di Francesco P, et al. Dendritic cells transport conidia and hyphae of *Aspergillus fumigatus* from the airways to the draining lymph nodes and initiate disparate Th responses to the fungus. *J Immunol* (2002) 168(3):1362–71. doi:10.4049/jimmunol.168.3.1362
109. Huang H, Ostroff GR, Lee CK, Wang JP, Specht CA, Levitz SM. Distinct patterns of dendritic cell cytokine release stimulated by fungal beta-glucans and toll-like receptor agonists. *Infect Immun* (2009) 77(5):1774–81. doi:10.1128/IAI.00086-09
110. Roy RM, Klein BS. Dendritic cells in antifungal immunity and vaccine design. *Cell Host Microbe* (2012) 11(5):436–46. doi:10.1016/j.chom.2012.04.005
111. Peck A, Mellins ED. Precarious balance: Th17 cells in host defense. *Infect Immun* (2010) 78(1):32–8. doi:10.1128/IAI.00929-09
112. Puel A, Cypowyj S, Marodi L, Abel L, Picard C, Casanova JL. Inborn errors of human IL-17 immunity underlie chronic mucocutaneous candidiasis. *Curr Opin Allergy Clin Immunol* (2012) 12(6):616–22. doi:10.1097/ACI.0b013e328358cc0b
113. Ling Y, Puel A. IL-17 and infections. *Actas Dermosifiliogr* (2014) 105(Suppl 1): 34–40. doi:10.1016/S0001-7310(14)70016-X
114. Spellberg B, Ibrahim AS, Lin L, Avanesian V, Fu Y, Lipke P, et al. Antibody titer threshold predicts anti-candidal vaccine efficacy even though the mechanism of protection is induction of cell-mediated immunity. *J Infect Dis* (2008) 197(7):967–71. doi:10.1086/529204
115. Medzhitov R, Preston-Hurlburt P, Janeway CA Jr. A human homologue of the *Drosophila* toll protein signals activation of adaptive immunity. *Nature* (1997) 388(6640):394–7. doi:10.1038/41131
116. Netea MG, Van Der Graaf CA, Vonk AG, Verschueren I, Van Der Meer JW, Kullberg BJ. The role of toll-like receptor (TLR) 2 and TLR4 in the host defense against disseminated candidiasis. *J Infect Dis* (2002) 185(10):1483–9. doi:10.1086/340511
117. Mambula SS, Sau K, Henneke P, Golenbock DT, Levitz SM. Toll-like receptor (TLR) signaling in response to *Aspergillus fumigatus*. *J Biol Chem* (2002) 277(42):39320–6. doi:10.1074/jbc.M201683200
118. Bellocchio S, Montagnoli C, Bozza S, Gaziano R, Rossi G, Mambula SS, et al. The contribution of the toll-like/IL-1 receptor superfamily to innate and adaptive immunity to fungal pathogens in vivo. *J Immunol* (2004) 172(5):3059–69. doi:10.4049/jimmunol.172.5.3059
119. Ding K, Shibui A, Wang Y, Takamoto M, Matsuguchi T, Sugane K. Impaired recognition by toll-like receptor 4 is responsible for exacerbated murine *Pneumocystis* pneumonia. *Microbes Infect* (2005) 7(2):195–203. doi:10.1016/j.micinf.2004.10.010
120. Nakamura K, Miyagi K, Koguchi Y, Kinjo Y, Uezu K, Kinjo T, et al. Limited contribution of toll-like receptor 2 and 4 to the host response to a fungal infectious pathogen, *Cryptococcus neoformans*. *FEMS Immunol Med Microbiol* (2006) 47(1):148–54. doi:10.1111/j.1574-695X.2006.00078.x
121. Botos I, Segal DM, Davies DR. The structural biology of toll-like receptors. *Structure* (2011) 19(4):447–59. doi:10.1016/j.str.2011.02.004
122. Ramirez-Ortiz ZG, Specht CA, Wang JP, Lee CK, Bartholomeu DC, Gazzinelli RT, et al. Toll-like receptor 9-dependent immune activation by unmethylated CpG motifs in *Aspergillus fumigatus* DNA. *Infect Immun* (2008) 76(5):2123–9. doi:10.1128/IAI.00047-08
123. Nakamura K, Miyazato A, Xiao G, Hatta M, Inden K, Aoyagi T, et al. Deoxynucleic acids from *Cryptococcus neoformans* activate myeloid dendritic cells via a TLR9-dependent pathway. *J Immunol* (2008) 180(6):4067–74. doi:10.4049/jimmunol.180.6.4067
124. Picard C, von Bernuth H, Ghandil P, Chrabieh M, Levy O, Arkwright PD, et al. Clinical features and outcome of patients with IRAK-4 and MyD88 deficiency. *Medicine (Baltimore)* (2010) 89(6):403–25. doi:10.1097/MD.0b013e3181fd8ec3
125. Vautier S, Sousa Mda G, Brown GD. C-type lectins, fungi and Th17 responses. *Cytokine Growth Factor Rev* (2010) 21(6):405–12. doi:10.1016/j.cytogfr.2010.10.001
126. Brown GD, Gordon S. Immune recognition. A new receptor for beta-glucans. *Nature* (2001) 413(6851):36–7. doi:10.1038/35092620
127. Odabasi Z, Paetznick VL, Rodriguez JR, Chen E, McGinnis MR, Ostrosky-Zeichner L. Differences in beta-glucan levels in culture supernatants of a variety of fungi. *Med Mycol* (2006) 44(3):267–72. doi:10.1080/13693780500474327
128. Dennehy KM, Brown GD. The role of the beta-glucan receptor Dectin-1 in control of fungal infection. *J Leukoc Biol* (2007) 82(2):253–8. doi:10.1189/jlb.1206753
129. Seeds RE, Mukhopadhyay S, Jones IM, Gordon S, Miller JL. The role of myeloid receptors on murine plasmacytoid dendritic cells in induction of type I interferon. *Int Immunopharmacol* (2011) 11(7):794–801. doi:10.1016/j.intimp.2011.01.013
130. Rhein J, Bahr NC, Morawski BM, Schutz C, Zhang Y, Finkelman M, et al. Detection of high cerebrospinal fluid levels of (1 - >3)-beta-d-Glucan in cryptococcal meningitis. *Open Forum Infect Dis* (2014) 1(3):ofu105. doi:10.1093/ofid/ofu052.1014
131. Gross O, Gewies A, Finger K, Schafer M, Sparwasser T, Peschel C, et al. Card9 controls a non-TLR signalling pathway for innate anti-fungal immunity. *Nature* (2006) 442(7103):651–6. doi:10.1038/nature04926
132. Drummond RA, Lionakis MS. Mechanistic insights into the role of C-type lectin receptor/CARD9 signaling in human antifungal immunity. *Front Cell Infect Microbiol* (2016) 6:39. doi:10.3389/fcimb.2016.00039
133. Drewniak A, Gazendam RP, Tool AT, van Houdt M, Jansen MH, van Hamme JL, et al. Invasive fungal infection and impaired neutrophil killing in human CARD9 deficiency. *Blood* (2013) 121(13):2385–92. doi:10.1182/blood-2012-08-450551
134. Alves de Medeiros AK, Lodewick E, Bogaert DJ, Haerynck F, Daele S. Van, Lambrecht B, et al. Chronic and invasive fungal infections in a family with CARD9 deficiency. *J Clin Immunol* (2016) 36(3):204–9. doi:10.1007/s10875-016-0255-8

135. Uematsu T, Iizasa E, Kobayashi N, Yoshida H, Hara H. Loss of CARD9-mediated innate activation attenuates severe influenza pneumonia without compromising host viral immunity. *Sci Rep* (2015) 5:17577. doi:10.1038/srep17577
136. Gringhuis SI, den Dunnen J, Litjens M, van der Vlist M, Wevers B, Bruijns SC, et al. Dectin-1 directs T helper cell differentiation by controlling noncanonical NF-kappaB activation through Raf-1 and Syk. *Nat Immunol* (2009) 10(2):203–13. doi:10.1038/ni.1692
137. Herre J, Marshall AS, Caron E, Edwards AD, Williams DL, Schweighoffer E, et al. Dectin-1 uses novel mechanisms for yeast phagocytosis in macrophages. *Blood* (2004) 104(13):4038–45. doi:10.1182/blood-2004-03-1140
138. Hefter M, Lother J, Weiss E, Schmitt AL, Fliesser M, Einsele H, et al. Human primary myeloid dendritic cells interact with the opportunistic fungal pathogen *Aspergillus fumigatus* via the C-type lectin receptor Dectin-1. *Med Mycol* (2017) 55(5):573–8. doi:10.1093/mmy/myw105
139. Gantner BN, Simmons RM, Underhill DM. Dectin-1 mediates macrophage recognition of *Candida albicans* yeast but not filaments. *EMBO J* (2005) 24(6):1277–86. doi:10.1038/sj.emboj.7600594
140. Brown GD. Dectin-1: a signalling non-TLR pattern-recognition receptor. *Nat Rev Immunol* (2006) 6:33–43. doi:10.1038/nri1745
141. Werner JL, Metz AE, Horn D, Schoeb TR, Hewitt MM, Schwiebert LM, et al. Requisite role for the dectin-1 beta-glucan receptor in pulmonary defense against *Aspergillus fumigatus*. *J Immunol* (2009) 182(8):4938–46. doi:10.4049/jimmunol.0804250
142. Rivera A, Hohl TM, Collins N, Leiner I, Gallegos A, Saijo S, et al. Dectin-1 diversifies *Aspergillus fumigatus*-specific T cell responses by inhibiting T helper type 1 CD4 T cell differentiation. *J Exp Med* (2011) 208(2):369–81. doi:10.1084/jem.20100906
143. Drummond RA, Dambuza IM, Vautier S, Taylor JA, Reid DM, Bain CC, et al. CD4(+) T-cell survival in the GI tract requires dectin-1 during fungal infection. *Mucosal Immunol* (2016) 9(2):492–502. doi:10.1038/mi.2015.79
144. McGreal EP, Rosas M, Brown GD, Zamze S, Wong SY, Gordon S, et al. The carbohydrate-recognition domain of Dectin-2 is a C-type lectin with specificity for high mannose. *Glycobiology* (2006) 16(5):422–30. doi:10.1093/glycob/cwj077
145. Sato K, Yang XL, Yudate T, Chung JS, Wu J, Luby-Phelps K, et al. Dectin-2 is a pattern recognition receptor for fungi that couples with the Fc receptor gamma chain to induce innate immune responses. *J Biol Chem* (2006) 281(50):38854–66. doi:10.1074/jbc.M606542200
146. Kerscher B, Willment JA, Brown GD. The Dectin-2 family of C-type lectin-like receptors: an update. *Int Immunol* (2013) 25(5):271–7. doi:10.1093/intimm/dxt006
147. Bi L, Gojestani S, Wu W, Hsu YM, Zhu J, Ariizumi K, et al. CARD9 mediates dectin-2-induced IkappaBalpha kinase ubiquitination leading to activation of NF-kappaB in response to stimulation by the hyphal form of *Candida albicans*. *J Biol Chem* (2010) 285(34):25969–77. doi:10.1074/jbc.M110.131300
148. Drummond RA, Saijo S, Iwakura Y, Brown GD. The role of Syk/CARD9 coupled C-type lectins in antifungal immunity. *Eur J Immunol* (2011) 41(2):276–81. doi:10.1002/eji.201041252
149. Gringhuis SI, Wevers BA, Kaptein TM, van Capel TM, Theelen B, Boekhout T, et al. Selective C-Rel activation via Malt1 controls anti-fungal T(H)-17 immunity by dectin-1 and dectin-2. *PLoS Pathog* (2011) 7(1):e1001259. doi:10.1371/journal.ppat.1001259
150. Robinson MJ, Osorio F, Rosas M, Freitas RP, Schweighoffer E, Gross O, et al. Dectin-2 is a Syk-coupled pattern recognition receptor crucial for Th17 responses to fungal infection. *J Exp Med* (2009) 206(9):2037–51. doi:10.1084/jem.20082818
151. Arce I, Martinez-Munoz L, Roda-Navarro P, Fernandez-Ruiz E. The human C-type lectin CLECSF8 is a novel monocyte/macrophage endocytic receptor. *Eur J Immunol* (2004) 34(1):210–20. doi:10.1002/eji.200324230
152. Zhu LL, Zhao XQ, Jiang C, You Y, Chen XP, Jiang YY, et al. C-type lectin receptors Dectin-3 and Dectin-2 form a heterodimeric pattern-recognition receptor for host defense against fungal infection. *Immunity* (2013) 39(2):324–34. doi:10.1016/j.immuni.2013.05.017
153. Zhao XQ, Zhu LL, Chang Q, Jiang C, You Y, Luo T, et al. C-type lectin receptor dectin-3 mediates trehalose 6,6'-dimycolate (TDM)-induced Mincle expression through CARD9/Bcl10/MALT1-dependent nuclear factor (NF)-kappaB activation. *J Biol Chem* (2014) 289(43):30052–62. doi:10.1074/jbc.M114.588574
154. Graham LM, Gupta V, Schafer G, Reid DM, Kimberg M, Dennehy KM, et al. The C-type lectin receptor CLECSF8 (CLEC4D) is expressed by myeloid cells and triggers cellular activation through Syk kinase. *J Biol Chem* (2012) 287(31):25964–74. doi:10.1074/jbc.M112.384164
155. Wang T, Pan D, Zhou Z, You Y, Jiang C, Zhao X, et al. Dectin-3 deficiency promotes colitis development due to impaired antifungal innate immune responses in the Gut. *PLoS Pathog* (2016) 12(6):e1005662. doi:10.1371/journal.ppat.1005662
156. Campuzano A, Castro-Lopez N, Wozniak KL, Leopold Wager CM, Wormley FL Jr. Dectin-3 is not required for protection against *Cryptococcus neoformans* infection. *PLoS One* (2017) 12(1):e0169347. doi:10.1371/journal.pone.0169347
157. Ezekowitz RA, Sastry K, Bailly P, Warner A. Molecular characterization of the human macrophage mannose receptor: demonstration of multiple carbohydrate recognition-like domains and phagocytosis of yeasts in Cos-1 cells. *J Exp Med* (1990) 172(6):1785–94. doi:10.1084/jem.172.6.1785
158. Gazi U, Martinez-Pomares L. Influence of the mannose receptor in host immune responses. *Immunobiology* (2009) 214(7):554–61. doi:10.1016/j.imbio.2008.11.004
159. Martinez-Pomares L. The mannose receptor. *J Leukoc Biol* (2012) 92(6):1177–86. doi:10.1189/jlb.0512231
160. Lee SJ, Evers S, Roeder D, Parlow AF, Risteli J, Risteli L, et al. Mannose receptor-mediated regulation of serum glycoprotein homeostasis. *Science* (2002) 295(5561):1898–901. doi:10.1126/science.1069540
161. Napper CE, Drickamer K, Taylor ME. Collagen binding by the mannose receptor mediated through the fibronectin type II domain. *Biochem J* (2006) 395(3):579–86. doi:10.1042/BJ20052027
162. Nguyen DG, Hildreth JE. Involvement of macrophage mannose receptor in the binding and transmission of HIV by macrophages. *Eur J Immunol* (2003) 33(2):483–93. doi:10.1002/immu.200310024
163. Wang Q, Zhao G, Lin J, Li C, Jiang N, Xu Q, et al. Role of the mannose receptor during *Aspergillus fumigatus* infection and interaction with dectin-1 in corneal epithelial cells. *Cornea* (2016) 35(2):267–73. doi:10.1097/ICO.0000000000000710
164. Marodi L, Korchak HM, Johnston RB Jr. Mechanisms of host defense against *Candida* species. I. Phagocytosis by monocytes and monocyte-derived macrophages. *J Immunol* (1991) 146(8):2783–9.
165. Porcaro I, Vidal M, Jouvert S, Stahl PD, Giaimis J. Mannose receptor contribution to *Candida albicans* phagocytosis by murine E-clone J774 macrophages. *J Leukoc Biol* (2003) 74(2):206–15. doi:10.1189/jlb.1202608
166. Dan JM, Kelly RM, Lee CK, Levitz SM. Role of the mannose receptor in a murine model of *Cryptococcus neoformans* infection. *Infect Immun* (2008) 76(6):2362–7. doi:10.1128/IAI.00095-08
167. Ezekowitz RA, Williams DJ, Koziel H, Armstrong MY, Warner A, Richards FF, et al. Uptake of *Pneumocystis carinii* mediated by the macrophage mannose receptor. *Nature* (1991) 351(6322):155–8. doi:10.1038/351155a0
168. Le Cabec V, Emorine LJ, Toesca I, Cougoule C, Maridonneau-Parini I. The human macrophage mannose receptor is not a professional phagocytic receptor. *J Leukoc Biol* (2005) 77(6):934–43. doi:10.1189/jlb.1204705
169. Tachado SD, Zhang J, Zhu J, Patel N, Cushion M, Koziel H. *Pneumocystis*-mediated IL-8 release by macrophages requires coexpression of mannose receptors and TLR2. *J Leukoc Biol* (2007) 81(1):205–11. doi:10.1189/jlb.1005580
170. Dan JM, Wang JP, Lee CK, Levitz SM. Cooperative stimulation of dendritic cells by *Cryptococcus neoformans* mannoproteins and CpG oligodeoxynucleotides. *PLoS One* (2008) 3(4):e2046. doi:10.1371/journal.pone.0002046
171. Romani L, Bistoni F, Gaziano R, Bozza S, Montagnoli C, Perruccio K, et al. Thymosin alpha 1 activates dendritic cells for antifungal Th1 resistance through toll-like receptor signaling. *Blood* (2004) 103(11):4232–9. doi:10.1182/blood-2003-11-4036
172. Perruccio K, Bozza S, Montagnoli C, Bellocchio S, Aversa F, Martelli M, et al. Prospects for dendritic cell vaccination against fungal infections in hematopoietic transplantation. *Blood Cells Mol Dis* (2004) 33(3):248–55. doi:10.1016/j.bcmd.2004.08.011
173. Ramirez-Ortiz ZG, Lee CK, Wang JP, Boon L, Specht CA, Levitz SM. A nonredundant role for plasmacytoid dendritic cells in host defense against

the human fungal pathogen *Aspergillus fumigatus*. *Cell Host Microbe* (2011) 9(5):415–24. doi:10.1016/j.chom.2011.04.007

174. Urban CF, Ermert D, Schmid M, Abu-Abed U, Goosmann C, Nacken W, et al. Neutrophil extracellular traps contain calprotectin, a cytosolic protein complex involved in host defense against *Candida albicans*. *PLoS Pathog* (2009) 5(10):e1000639. doi:10.1371/journal.ppat.1000639
175. Loures FV, Rohm M, Lee CK, Santos E, Wang JP, Specht CA, et al. Recognition of *Aspergillus fumigatus* hyphae by human plasmacytoid dendritic cells is mediated by dectin-2 and results in formation of extracellular traps. *PLoS Pathog* (2015) 11(2):e1004643. doi:10.1371/journal.ppat.1004643
176. Joo H, Upchurch K, Zhang W, Ni L, Li D, Xue Y, et al. Opposing roles of dectin-1 expressed on human plasmacytoid dendritic cells and myeloid dendritic cells in Th2 polarization. *J Immunol* (2015) 195(4):1723–31. doi:10.4049/jimmunol.1402276
177. Gavino AC, Chung JS, Sato K, Ariizumi K, Cruz PD Jr. Identification and expression profiling of a human C-type lectin, structurally homologous to mouse dectin-2. *Exp Dermatol* (2005) 14(4):281–8. doi:10.1111/j.0906-6705.2005.00312.x
178. Lundberg K, Rydnert F, Greiff L, Lindstedt M. Human blood dendritic cell subsets exhibit discriminative pattern recognition receptor profiles. *Immunology* (2014) 142(2):279–88. doi:10.1111/imm.12252

Permissions

All chapters in this book were first published by Frontiers; hereby published with permission under the Creative Commons Attribution License or equivalent. Every chapter published in this book has been scrutinized by our experts. Their significance has been extensively debated. The topics covered herein carry significant findings which will fuel the growth of the discipline. They may even be implemented as practical applications or may be referred to as a beginning point for another development.

The contributors of this book come from diverse backgrounds, making this book a truly international effort. This book will bring forth new frontiers with its revolutionizing research information and detailed analysis of the nascent developments around the world.

We would like to thank all the contributing authors for lending their expertise to make the book truly unique. They have played a crucial role in the development of this book. Without their invaluable contributions this book wouldn't have been possible. They have made vital efforts to compile up to date information on the varied aspects of this subject to make this book a valuable addition to the collection of many professionals and students.

This book was conceptualized with the vision of imparting up-to-date information and advanced data in this field. To ensure the same, a matchless editorial board was set up. Every individual on the board went through rigorous rounds of assessment to prove their worth. After which they invested a large part of their time researching and compiling the most relevant data for our readers.

The editorial board has been involved in producing this book since its inception. They have spent rigorous hours researching and exploring the diverse topics which have resulted in the successful publishing of this book. They have passed on their knowledge of decades through this book. To expedite this challenging task, the publisher supported the team at every step. A small team of assistant editors was also appointed to further simplify the editing procedure and attain best results for the readers.

Apart from the editorial board, the designing team has also invested a significant amount of their time in understanding the subject and creating the most relevant covers. They scrutinized every image to scout for the most suitable representation of the subject and create an appropriate cover for the book.

The publishing team has been an ardent support to the editorial, designing and production team. Their endless efforts to recruit the best for this project, has resulted in the accomplishment of this book. They are a veteran in the field of academics and their pool of knowledge is as vast as their experience in printing. Their expertise and guidance has proved useful at every step. Their uncompromising quality standards have made this book an exceptional effort. Their encouragement from time to time has been an inspiration for everyone.

The publisher and the editorial board hope that this book will prove to be a valuable piece of knowledge for researchers, students, practitioners and scholars across the globe.

List of Contributors

Raffael Júnio Araújo de Castro, Isaque Medeiros Siqueira, Márcio Sousa Jerônimo, Angelina Maria Moreschi Basso, Paulo Henrique de Holanda Veloso Junior, Luiza Chaves Leonhardt, Stephan Alberto Machado de Oliveira, Pedro Henrique Bürgel, Aldo Henrique Tavares and Anamélia Lorenzetti Bocca
Laboratory of Applied Immunology, Department of Cellular Biology, Institute of Biological Sciences, University of Brasília, Brasília, Brazil

Kelly Grace Magalhães
Laboratory of Immunology and Inflammation, Department of Cellular Biology, Institute of Biological Sciences, University of Brasília, Brasília, Brazil

Alicia Yoke Wei Wong
Singapore Immunology Network, Agency for Science, Technology and Research, Singapore, Singapore
National University of Singapore Graduate School for Integrative Sciences and Engineering, National University of Singapore, Singapore, Singapore

Vasilis Oikonomou, Giuseppe Paolicelli, Antonella De Luca and Marilena Pariano
Department of Experimental Medicine, University of Perugia, Perugia, Italy

Jan Fric
Singapore Immunology Network, Agency for Science, Technology and Research, Singapore, Singapore
Center for Translational Medicine (CTM), International Clinical Research Center (ICRC), St. Anne's University Hospital Brno, Brno, Czechia

Hock Soon Tay
Singapore Immunology Network, Agency for Science, Technology and Research, Singapore, Singapore

Paola Ricciardi-Castagnoli
Singapore Immunology Network, Agency for Science, Technology and Research, Singapore, Singapore
Toscana Life Sciences Foundation, Siena, Italy

Teresa Zelante
Singapore Immunology Network, Agency for Science, Technology and Research, Singapore, Singapore
Department of Experimental Medicine, University of Perugia, Perugia, Italy

Alayna K. Caffrey-Carr and Kelly M. Shepardson
Department of Microbiology and Immunology, Montana State University, Bozeman, MT, United States
Department of Microbiology and Immunology, Geisel School of Medicine at Dartmouth, Lebanon, NH, United States

Kimberly M. Hilmer
Department of Microbiology and Immunology, Montana State University, Bozeman, MT, United States

Caitlin H. Kowalski, Rachel M. Temple, Robert A. Cramer and Joshua J. Obar
Department of Microbiology and Immunology, Geisel School of Medicine at Dartmouth, Lebanon, NH, United States

Taise N. Landgraf and Wander C. Ribeiro
Department of Biochemistry and Immunology, Ribeirão Preto Medical School, University of São Paulo, Ribeirão Preto, Brazil

Marcelo V. Costa and Ademilson Panunto-Castelo
Department of Biology, Faculty of Philosophy, Sciences and Letters of Ribeirão Preto, University of São Paulo, Ribeirão Preto, Brazil

Aline F. Oliveira and Fabrício F. Fernandes
Department of Cell and Molecular Biology, Ribeirão Preto Medical School, University of São Paulo, Ribeirão Preto, Brazil

Anna-Maria Hellmann, Jasmin Lother, Sebastian Wurster, Anna Lena Schmitt, Kristin Czakai, Hermann Einsele and Juergen Loeffler
Medizinische Klinik & Poliklinik II, Universitätsklinikum Würzburg, Würzburg, Germany

Manfred B. Lutz
Institute of Virology and Immunobiology, University of Würzburg, Würzburg, Germany

Charles Oliver Morton
School of Science and Health, Western Sydney University, Campbelltown, NSW, Australia

Matthias Eyrich
Kinderklinik und Poliklinik, Universitätsklinikum Würzburg, Würzburg, Germany

Nycolas Willian Preite, Claudia Feriotti, Dhêmerson Souza de Lima, Bruno Borges da Silva, Antônio Condino-Neto, Alessandra Pontillo, Eliseu Frank de Araújo, Tania Alves da Costa, Vera Lúcia Garcia Calich, Nayane Alves de Lima Galdino and Flávio Vieira Loures
Departamento de Imunologia, Instituto de Ciências Biomédicas, Universidade de São Paulo, São Paulo, Brazil

Stanislaw Schmidt, Lars Tramsen and Thomas Lehrnbecher
Division for Pediatric Hematology and Oncology, Hospital for Children and Adolescents, Johann Wolfgang Goethe-University, Frankfurt, Germany

Liliane Mukaremera
Aberdeen Fungal Group, Institute of Medical Sciences, Foresterhill, University of Aberdeen, Aberdeen, United Kingdom
Department of Microbiology and Immunology, Medical School, University of Minnesota, Minneapolis, MN, United States

Keunsook K. Lee and Neil A. R. Gow
Aberdeen Fungal Group, Institute of Medical Sciences, Foresterhill, University of Aberdeen, Aberdeen, United Kingdom

Hector M. Mora-Montes
Departamento de Biología, Divisi0n de Ciencias Naturales y Exactas, Universidad de Guanajuato, Guanajuato, Mexico

Heather L. Clark
Department of Ophthalmology and Visual Sciences, Case Western Reserve University, Cleveland, OH, United States
Department of Ophthalmology, University of California Irvine, Irvine, CA, United States
Department of Physiology and Biophysics, University of California Irvine, Irvine, CA, United States

Serena Abbondante, Martin S. Minns, Elyse N. Greenberg and Eric Pearlman
Department of Ophthalmology, University of California Irvine, Irvine, CA, United States
Department of Physiology and Biophysics, University of California Irvine, Irvine, CA, United States

Yan Sun
Department of Ophthalmology and Visual Sciences, Case Western Reserve University, Cleveland, OH, United States

Tristan Hayes
Department of Biological Sciences, Virginia Tech, Blacksburg, VA, United States
Department of Pediatrics, School of Medicine, Indiana University Bloomington, Indianapolis, IN, United States

Amanda Rumore
Department of Biology, Randolph College, Lynchburg, VA, United States

Brad Howard, Xin He, Mengyao Luo, Liwu Li and Christopher B. Lawrence
Department of Biological Sciences, Virginia Tech, Blacksburg, VA, United States

Sabina Wuenschmann and Martin Chapman
Indoor Biotechnologies, Charlottesville, VA, United States

Shiv Kale
Biocomplexity Institute, Virginia Tech, Blacksburg, VA, United States

Hirohito Kita
Division of Allergic Diseases, Internal Medicine, Mayo Clinic, Rochester, MN, United States

Mohamed F. Ali, Harika Dasari, Virginia P. Van Keulen and Eva M. Carmona
The Thoracic Diseases Research Unit and the Division of Pulmonary and Critical Care, Department of Medicine Mayo Clinic and Foundation, Rochester, MN, United States

Jintao Xu, Lori M. Neal, Jeffrey L. Curtis, John J. Osterholzer and Michal A. Olszewski
Division of Pulmonary and Critical Care Medicine, Department of Internal Medicine, University of Michigan Health System, Ann Arbor, MI, United States
Department of Veterans Affairs Health System, VA Ann Arbor Healthcare System (VHA), Ann Arbor, MI, United States

Adam Flaczyk, Zhenzong Fa, Daphne Cheng and Mike Ivey
Department of Veterans Affairs Health System, VA Ann Arbor Healthcare System (VHA), Ann Arbor, MI, United States

Bethany B. Moore
Division of Pulmonary and Critical Care Medicine, Department of Internal Medicine, University of Michigan Health System, Ann Arbor, MI, United States
Department of Microbiology and Immunology, University of Michigan Medical School, Ann Arbor, MI, United States

Shengjie Xu
Department of Immunology, Duke University School of Medicine, Durham, NC, United States

Mari L. Shinohara
Department of Immunology, Duke University School of Medicine, Durham, NC, United States
Department of Molecular Genetics and Microbiology, Duke University School of Medicine, Durham, NC, United States

Juan Tang and Lijian Tao
Department of Nephrology, Xiangya Hospital, Central South University, Changsha, Hunan, China

Guoxin Lin
Department of Pathology, The University of Iowa, Iowa City, IA, United States
Department of Anesthesiology, The Third Xiangya Hospital, Central South University, Changsha, Hunan, China

Wallace Y. Langdon
School of Biological Sciences, University of Western Australia, Perth, WA, Australia

Jian Zhang
Department of Pathology, The University of Iowa, Iowa City, IA, United States

Dario Simões Zamboni
Department of Cell Biology, School of Medicine of Ribeirão Preto, University of São Paulo, São Paulo, Brazil

Christine Schoeler Jepsen, Kimmie B. Colmorten, Mark A. Hammond, Anders Schlosser, Grith L. Sorensen and Uffe Holmskov
Cancer and Inflammation Research, Department of Molecular Medicine, University of Southern Denmark, Odense, Denmark

Lalit Kumar Dubey
Cancer and Inflammation Research, Department of Molecular Medicine, University of Southern Denmark, Odense, Denmark
Global Health Institute, School of Life Sciences, École Polytechnique Fédérale de Lausanne, Lausanne, Switzerland

Steven P. Templeton
Department of Microbiology and Immunology, Indiana University School of Medicine-Terre Haute, Terre Haute, IN, United States

Jesper B. Moeller
Cancer and Inflammation Research, Department of Molecular Medicine, University of Southern Denmark, Odense, Denmark
Jill Roberts Institute for Research in Inflammatory Bowel Disease, Weill Cornell Medicine, Cornell University, New York, United States

Ole Nielsen
Department of Clinical Pathology, Odense University Hospital, Odense, Denmark

Eszter Judit Tóth, Csilla Szebenyi, Mónika Homa and Tamás Papp
MTA-SZTE Fungal Pathogenicity Mechanisms Research Group, Hungarian Academy of Sciences, University of Szeged, Szeged, Hungary
Faculty of Science and Informatics, Department of Microbiology, University of Szeged, Szeged, Hungary

Éva Boros and István Nagy
Hungarian Academy of Sciences, Biological Research Centre, Szeged, Hungary

Alexandra Hoffmann and Csaba Vágvölgyi
Faculty of Science and Informatics, Department of Microbiology, University of Szeged, Szeged, Hungary

Gábor Nagy
MTA-SZTE Fungal Pathogenicity Mechanisms Research Group, Hungarian Academy of Sciences, University of Szeged, Szeged, Hungary

Zeina Dagher, Shuying Xu, Paige E. Negoro, Jennifer L. Reedy, Jenny M. Tam and Michael K. Mansour
Division of Infectious Disease, Massachusetts General Hospital, Harvard Medical School, Boston, MA, United States

Nida S. Khan
Division of Infectious Disease, Massachusetts General Hospital, Harvard Medical School, Boston, MA, United States
Biomedical Engineering and Biotechnology, University of Massachusetts Medical School, Worcester, MA, United States

Michael B. Feldman
Division of Pulmonary and Critical Care, Massachusetts General Hospital, Boston, MA, United States

David B. Sykes
Center for Regenerative Medicine, Massachusetts General Hospital, Boston, MA, United States

Mark S. Gresnigt
Unité de recherche Cytokines and Inflammation, Institut Pasteur, Paris, France
Laboratory for Experimental Internal Medicine, Department of Internal Medicine, Radboud University Medical Center, Nijmegen, Netherlands

Willem J. G. Melchers
Department of Medical Microbiology, Radboud University Medical Centre, Nijmegen, Netherlands

Martin Jaeger and Frank L. van de Veerdonk
Laboratory for Experimental Internal Medicine, Department of Internal Medicine, Radboud University Medical Center, Nijmegen, Netherlands

R. K. Subbarao Malireddi and Thirumala-Devi Kanneganti
Department of Immunology, St. Jude Children's Research Hospital, Memphis, TN, United States

Orhan Rasid, Catherine Fitting and Oumaima Ibrahim-Granet
Unité de recherche Cytokines and Inflammation, Institut Pasteur, Paris, France

Grégory Jouvion
Unité Histopathologie Humaine et Modèles Animaux, Département Infection et Epidémiologie, Institut Pasteur, Paris, France

Agostinho Carvalho
Life and Health Sciences Research Institute (ICVS), School of Medicine, University of Minho, Braga, Portugal
ICVS/3B's - PT Government Associate Laboratory, Braga/Guimarães, Portugal

Samuel Maldonado and Patricia Fitzgerald-Bocarsly
Rutgers School of Graduate Studies, Newark, NJ, United States
Department of Pathology and Laboratory Medicine, New Jersey Medical School, Newark, NJ, United States

Index